Operative Techniques in Hepato-Pancreato-Biliary Surgery

Second Edition

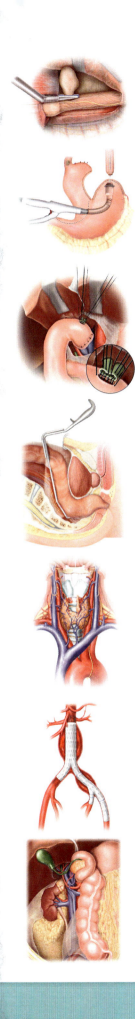

Operative Techniques in Hepato-Pancreato-Biliary Surgery

Second Edition

Mary T. Hawn, MD, MPH
EDITOR-IN-CHIEF

Emile Holman Professor and Chair
Department of Surgery
Stanford University School of Medicine
Stanford, California

EDITOR

Steven J. Hughes, MD

Professor of Surgery
Vice Chair, General Surgery
Chief, Division of Surgical Oncology
University of Florida
College of Medicine
Gainesville, Florida

Illustrations by: Body Scientific International, LLC

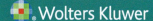

Philadelphia • Baltimore • New York • London
Buenos Aires • Hong Kong • Sydney • Tokyo

Senior Acquisitions Editor: Keith Donnellan
Senior Development Editor: Ashley Fischer
Development Editor: Barton Dudlick
Editorial Coordinator: Erin E. Hernandez
Marketing Manager: Kirsten Watrud
Production Project Manager: Bridgett Dougherty
Manager, Graphic Arts & Design: Stephen Druding
Manufacturing Coordinator: Beth Welsh
Prepress Vendor: TNQ Technologies

Copyright © 2024 Wolters Kluwer.

Copyright © 2015 Wolters Kluwer Health/Lippincott Williams & Wilkins. All rights reserved. This book is protected by copyright. No part of this book may be reproduced or transmitted in any form or by any means, including as photocopies or scanned-in or other electronic copies, or utilized by any information storage and retrieval system without written permission from the copyright owner, except for brief quotations embodied in critical articles and reviews. Materials appearing in this book prepared by individuals as part of their official duties as U.S. government employees are not covered by the above-mentioned copyright. To request permission, please contact Wolters Kluwer at Two Commerce Square, 2001 Market Street, Philadelphia, PA 19103, via email at permissions@lww.com, or via our website at shop.lww.com (products and services).

9 8 7 6 5 4 3 2 1

Printed in United States of America.

Library of Congress Cataloging-in-Publication Data

ISBN-13: 978-1-9751-7658-7

Cataloging in Publication data available on request from publisher.

This work is provided "as is," and the publisher disclaims any and all warranties, express or implied, including any warranties as to accuracy, comprehensiveness, or currency of the content of this work.

This work is no substitute for individual patient assessment based upon healthcare professionals' examination of each patient and consideration of, among other things, age, weight, gender, current or prior medical conditions, medication history, laboratory data and other factors unique to the patient. The publisher does not provide medical advice or guidance and this work is merely a reference tool. Healthcare professionals, and not the publisher, are solely responsible for the use of this work including all medical judgments and for any resulting diagnosis and treatments.

Given continuous, rapid advances in medical science and health information, independent professional verification of medical diagnoses, indications, appropriate pharmaceutical selections and dosages, and treatment options should be made and healthcare professionals should consult a variety of sources. When prescribing medication, healthcare professionals are advised to consult the product information sheet (the manufacturer's package insert) accompanying each drug to verify, among other things, conditions of use, warnings and side effects and identify any changes in dosage schedule or contraindications, particularly if the medication to be administered is new, infrequently used or has a narrow therapeutic range. To the maximum extent permitted under applicable law, no responsibility is assumed by the publisher for any injury and/or damage to persons or property, as a matter of products liability, negligence law or otherwise, or from any reference to or use by any person of this work.

shop.lww.com

Contributing Authors

David B. Adams, MD
Distinguished University Professor Emeritus
Department of Surgery
The Medical University of South Carolina
Charleston, South Carolina

Reid B. Adams, MD
S. Hurt Watts Professor and Chair
Department of Surgery
Chief Medical Officer
University of Virginia Health System
Charlottesville, Virginia

David L. Bartlett, MD
Professor
Department of Surgery
Drexel University College of Medicine
Philadelphia, Pennsylvania
System Chair, AHN Cancer Institute
AHN Surgery Institute
Allegheny Health Network
Pittsburgh, Pennsylvania

Kevin E. Behrns, MD
Professor of Surgery
Department of Surgery
University of Florida College of Medicine
Chief Medical Officer
Department of Surgery
UF Health
The Villages Hospital
The Villages, Florida

Walter L. Biffl, MD
Division Head, Trauma/Acute Care Surgery
Vice-Chair Department of Surgery
Scripps Clinic Medical Group
Trauma Medical Director
Department of Surgery
Scripps Memorial Hospital La Jolla
La Jolla, California

Mark Bloomston, MD, FACS, FSSO
Surgical Oncologist
South Florida Surgical Oncology
GenesisCare
Fort Myers, Florida

Richard J. Bold, MD, MBA
Physician-In-Chief
UC Davis Comprehensive Cancer Center
Professor and Chief
Division of Surgical Oncology
Department of Surgery
University of California Davis School of Medicine
Sacramento, California

Morgan M. Bonds, MD
Assistant Professor
Department of Surgery
University of Oklahoma Health Sciences Center
Oklahoma City, Oklahoma

Brian A. Boone, MD, FACS
Assistant Professor
Department of Surgery
Department of Microbiology, Immunology and Cell Biology
West Virginia University
Morgantown, West Virginia

Adam S. Brinkman, MD
Assistant Professor
Pediatric Trauma Director
Pediatric Surgical Critical Care Medical Director
Department of Surgery
American Family Children's Hospital
University of Wisconsin Health
Madison, Wisconsin

Zachary J. Brown, DO
Complex General Surgical Oncology Fellow
Department of Surgical Oncology
The Ohio State University Wexner Medical Center
Columbus, Ohio

Emily F. Cantrell, MD, FACS
Assistant Professor
Division of Acute Care Surgery
Department of Surgery
University of Nebraska Medical Center
Omaha, Nebraska

Hop S. Tran Cao, MD, FACS
Associate Professor
Department of Surgical Oncology
The University of Texas MD Anderson Cancer Center
Houston, Texas

Patrick R. Carney, PhD
Department of Surgery
University of Wisconsin School of Medicine and Public Health
Madison, Wisconsin

Jason A. Castellanos, MD, MS
Assistant Professor of Surgical Oncology
Department of Surgical Oncology
Fox Chase Cancer Center
Philadelphia, Pennsylvania

Eugene P. Ceppa, MD, FACS
Associate Professor
Department of Surgery
Indiana University School of Medicine
Indianapolis, Indiana

Shailendra S. Chauhan, MD
Clinical Associate Professor of Medicine
Department of Gastroenterology and Hepatology
Atrium Health
Charlotte, North Carolina

Jordan M. Cloyd, MD
Assistant Professor
Ward Family Professor of Surgical Oncology
Department of Surgery
The Ohio State Wexner Medical Center
Columbus, Ohio

Charles S. Cox, Jr., MD
George and Cynthia Mitchell Distinguished Chair
Professor of Pediatric Surgery
Department of Pediatric Surgery
McGovern Medical School at University of Texas
UT Health Science Center at Houston
Houston, Texas

v

CONTRIBUTING AUTHORS

Kaitlyn Crespo, BS
Digestive Health Institute
AdventHealth Tampa
University of Central Florida
Tampa, Florida

Kimberly A. Davis, MD, MBA
Professor of Surgery
Chief, Division of General Surgery,
  Trauma and Surgical Critical Care
Department of Surgery
Yale School of Medicine
New Haven, Connecticut

Christopher J. Dente, MD
Professor of Surgery
Department of Surgery
Emory University
Senior Surgeon
Department of Surgery
Grady Memorial Hospital
Atlanta, Georgia

Mary E. Dillhoff, MD, MS, FACS
Associate Professor
Division of Surgical Oncology
Department of Surgery
The Ohio State University School of
  Medicine
Columbus, Ohio

Matthew E. Dixon, MD, FACS
Assistant Professor of Surgery
Department of Surgery
Penn State College of Medicine
Hepatopancreatobiliary Surgery
Division of Surgical Oncology
Department of Surgery
Penn State Hershey Medical Center
Hershey, Pennsylvania

Epameinondas Dogeas, MD
Fellow
Division of Surgical Oncology
University of Pittsburgh Medical Center
Pittsburgh, Pennsylvania

Barish H. Edil, MD
John A. Schilling Chair and Professor of
  Surgery
Department of Surgery
University of Oklahoma Health Sciences
  Center
Oklahoma City, Oklahoma

Rony Eshkenazy, MD, PhD
Surgeon
Department of Hepato-Biliary and Pancreatic
  Surgery
Tel Aviv University
Department of Hepato-Biliary and Pancreatic
  Surgery
Sheba - Tel Hashomer Hospital Medical
  Center
Ramat-Gan, Israel

William Edward Fisher, MD
Professor and Vice Chair, Clinical Affairs
George L. Jordan, M.D. Chair of General
  Surgery
Michael E. DeBakey Department of Surgery
Baylor College of Medicine
Vice President
Baylor St. Luke's Medical Center
Texas Medical Center
Houston, Texas

Jared A. Forrester, MD
HPB Fellow
Hepatobiliary and Pancreatic Surgery Program
Providence Cancer Institute
Providence Portland Medical Center
Portland, Oregon

T. Clark Gamblin, MD, MS, MBA, FACS
Professor and Chief of Surgical Oncology
Department of Surgery
The Medical College of Wisconsin
Milwaukee, Wisconsin

Brian S. Geller, MD
Assistant Professor
Department of Radiology
University of Florida College of Medicine
UF Health
Gainesville, Florida

Jon M. Gerry, MD
Associate Program Director HPB Fellowship
Providence Cancer Institute
Providence Portland Medical Center
Portland, Oregon

Ryan T. Groeschl, MD
Hepatopancreatobiliary Surgeon
Department of Surgical Oncology
Essentia Health
Duluth, Minnesota

Julie Gail Grossman, MD
Surgical Oncology Fellow
Department of Surgery
Jackson Memorial Hospital
University of Miami
Miami, Florida

Niraj J. Gusani, MD, MS, FACS, FSSO
Chief, Section of Surgical Oncology
Department of Surgery
Baptist MD Anderson Cancer Center
Jacksonville, FL

Nathania M. Figueroa Guilliani, MD
HPB Fellow
Hepatobiliary and Pancreatic Surgery
  Program
Providence Cancer Institute
Providence Portland Medical Center
Portland, Oregon

Samuel Han, MD, MS
Assistant Professor
Section of Therapeutic Endoscopy
Division of Gastroenterology, Hepatology,
  and Nutrition
The Ohio State University Wexner Medical
  Center
Columbus, Ohio

Alan William Hemming, MD, MSc
Professor
Department of Surgery
University of Iowa
Director Liver Transplantation & HPB
  Surgery
Department of Surgery
University of Iowa Hospitals & Clinics
Iowa City, Iowa

O. Joe Hines, MD
Professor and Interim Chair
Department of Surgery
David Geffen School of Medicine at UCLA
Los Angeles, California

Steven J. Hughes, MD
Professor of Surgery
Vice Chair, General Surgery
Chief, Division of Surgical Oncology
University of Florida College of Medicine
Gainesville, Florida

Kamran Idrees, MD, MSCI, MMHC, FSSO
Chief, Division of Surgical Oncology and
  Endocrine Surgery
Ingram Associate Professor of Cancer
  Research, Department of Surgery
Vanderbilt University Medical Center
Nashville, Tennessee

Saleem Islam, MD, MPH
Professor and Division Chief, Pediatric
  Surgery
Department of Surgery
University of Florida College of Medicine
Gainesville, Florida

Crystal N. Johnson-Mann, MD
Assistant Professor
Department of Surgery
University of Florida College of Medicine
Gainesville, Florida

Rebecca Y. Kim, MD, MPH
Assistant Professor
Department of Surgery
Huntsman Cancer Institute
University of Utah
Salt Lake City, Utah

CONTRIBUTING AUTHORS

Song Cheol Kim, MD, PhD
Professor
Division of Hepatobiliary and Pancreatic Surgery
Department of Surgery
University of Ulsan College of Medicine
Asan Medical Center
Seoul, South Korea

Stephanie S. Kim, MD
Department of Surgery
David Geffen School of Medicine at UCLA
UCLA Medical Center
Los Angeles, California

KMarie King, MD, MS, MBA, FACS
Henry and Sally Schaffer Chair
Department of Surgery
Albany Medical College
Chief of Surgery
Department of Surgery
Albany Medical Center
Albany, New York

Kelly Lynn Koch, MD
Surgical Oncology Fellow
Division of Surgical Oncology
Department of Surgery
University of Miami Sylvester Cancer Center
Jackson Memorial Hospital
Miami, Florida

Shawn D. Larson, MB, ChB, FACS
Associate Professor
Division of Pediatric Surgery
Department of Surgery
University of Florida College of Medicine
Gainesville, Florida

Kenneth K. W. Lee, MD
Jane and Carl Citron Professor of Surgery
Department of Surgery
University of Pittsburgh School of Medicine
Pittsburgh, Pennsylvania

Aijun Li, MD, PhD
Professor
The 2nd Department of Special Therapy
Naval Medical University
Eastern Hepatobiliary Surgery Hospital
Shanghai, China

Tyler John Loftus, MD
Assistant Professor
Department of Surgery
University of Florida College of Medicine
Gainesville, Florida

Priyadarshini Manay, MBBS
Clinical Associate
Organ Transplant Center
Department of General Surgery
Carver College of Medicine
University of Iowa Hospitals and Clinics
Iowa City, Iowa

David McAneny, MD, FACS
Vice Chair and Professor of Surgery
Department of Surgery
Boston University School of Medicine
Chief Medical Officer
Department of Surgery
Boston Medical Center
Boston, Massachusetts

Sarah Meade, DO
Assistant Professor of Surgery
Department of Surgery
Boston University School of Medicine
Transplant Surgeon
Department of Surgery
Boston Medical Center
Boston, Massachusetts

Nipun B. Merchant, MD
Professor of Surgery
Department of Surgery
University of Miami
University of Miami Hospital
Miami, Florida

Rebecca M. Minter, MD, FACS
A.R. Curreri Professor and Chair
Department of Surgery
University of Wisconsin School of Medicine and Public Health
Madison, Wisconsin

Alicia M. Mohr, MD, FACS, FCCM
Division Chief, Acute Care Surgery
Department of Surgery
University of Florida College of Medicine
Gainesville, Florida

Katherine A. Morgan, MD, FACS
Professor
Director, Division of Gastrointestinal Surgery
Department of Surgery
Medical University of South Carolina
Charleston, South Carolina

Catalina Mosquera, MD
Surgical Oncologist
South Florida Surgical Oncology
GenesisCare
Fort Meyers, Florida

Ido Nachmany, MD
Senior lecturer
Sackler School of Medicine
Tel Aviv University
Chief, Department of Surgery B
Sheba - Tel Hashomer Hospital Medical Center
Ramat-Gan, Israel

Ibrahim Nassour, MD, MSCS
Assistant Professor
Division of Surgical Oncology
Department of Surgery
University of Florida College of Medicine
Gainesville, Florida

Timothy E. Newhook, MD
Assistant Professor
Department of Surgical Oncology
The University of Texas MD Anderson Cancer Center
Houston, Texas

Ankesh Nigam, MD
Associate Professor
Director of Surgical Oncology
Department of Surgery
Albany Medical College
Albany, New York

Alessandro Paniccia, MD
Assistant Professor of Surgery
Department of Surgery
University of Pittsburgh Medical Center
Pittsburgh, Pennsylvania

Georgios Papachristou, MD, PhD
Professor of Medicine
Section of Therapeutic Endoscopy
Division of Gastroenterology, Hepatology, and Nutrition
The Ohio State University Wexner Medical Center
Columbus, Ohio

Alexander A. Parikh, MD, MPH, FACS, FSSO
Professor of Surgery
Chief, Division of Surgical Oncology
Director of Hepatobiliary and Pancreas Surgery
East Carolina University The Brody School of Medicine
Greenville, North Carolina

Timothy M. Pawlik, MD, MPH, MTS, PhD, FACS, FRACS (Hon.)
Professor and Chair
Department of Surgery
The Urban Meyer III and Shelley Meyer Chair for Cancer Research
Professor of Surgery, Oncology, and Health Services Management and Policy
Surgeon in Chief
The Ohio State University Wexner Medical Center
Columbus, Ohio

CONTRIBUTING AUTHORS

Niv Pencovich, MD, PhD
Associate Professor
Faculty of Medicine
Attending Surgeon
Department of Surgery B
Sheba - Tel Hashomer Hospital Medical Center
Ramat-Gan, Israel

June S. Peng, MD
Assistant Professor
Division of Surgical Oncology
Department of Surgery
Penn State College of Medicine
Hershey, Pennsylvania

Darren W. Postoak, MD
Assistant Professor
Division of Vascular and Interventional Radiology
Department of Radiology
University of Florida College of Medicine
Gainesville, Florida

Martin D. Rosenthal, MD
Assistant Professor
Director, Abdominal Wall Reconstruction and Intestinal Rehab
Chair, UF Nutrition Committee
Department of Surgery
University of Florida College of Medicine
Gainesville, Florida

Lucy Ruangvoravat, MD, FACS
Assistant Professor
Division of General Surgery, Trauma, and Surgical Critical Care
Department of Surgery
Yale School of Medicine
New Haven, Connecticut

Jorge Sanchez-Garcia, MD
Research Fellow
Abdominal Transplant Services
Intermountain Medical Center
Salt Lake City, Utah

Courtney L. Scaife, MD
Professor
Department of Surgery
Huntsman Cancer Institute
University of Utah
Salt Lake City, Utah

Cameron Schlegel, MD
Clinical Instructor
Allegheny Health Network Surgery Institute
Allegheny Health Network
Pittsburgh, Pennsylvania

C. Max Schmidt, MD, PhD, MBA, FACS
Vice Chair and Professor of Surgery
Professor of Biochemistry and Molecular Biology
Indiana University School of Medicine
Chief of Surgery
IU Health University Hospital
Indianapolis, Indiana

Michael Collins Scott, MD, MPH
Department of Surgery
University of Texas Health Science Center
Children's Memorial Hermann Hospital
Houston, Texas

Randi N. Smith, MD, MPH
Assistant Professor
Department of Surgery
Emory University
Trauma Surgeon
Department of Acute Care Surgery
Grady Memorial Hospital
Atlanta, Georgia

Rebecca A. Snyder, MD, MPH, FACS, FSSO
Assistant Professor
Division of Surgical Oncology
East Carolina University The Brody School of Medicine
Greenville, North Carolina

Ki Byung Song, MD, PhD
Associate Professor
Division of Hepatobiliary and Pancreatic Surgery
Department of Surgery
University of Ulsan College of Medicine
Asan Medical Center
Seoul, South Korea

Iswanto Sucandy, MD, FACS
Associate Professor of Surgery
Department of Surgery
University of Central Florida
Director, Liver Surgery and Disorders Program
Digestive Health Institute
AdventHealth Tampa
Tampa, Florida

Jennifer F. Tseng, MD, MPH, FACS
James Utley Professor and Chair of Surgery
Department of Surgery
Boston University School of Medicine
Surgeon-in-Chief
Department of Surgery
Boston Medical Center
Boston, Massachusetts

Allan Tsung, MD
Professor of Surgery
Chief, Division of Surgical Oncology
Department of Surgery
The Ohio State University School of Medicine
The Ohio State University Wexner Medical Center
Columbus, Ohio

George Van Buren II, MD
Associate Professor
Department of Surgery
Baylor College of Medicine
Houston Texas

Erin L. Vanzant, MD
Assistant Professor
Department of Surgery
University of Florida College of Medicine
Gainesville, Florida

Roberto J. Vidri, MD, MPH, FACS
Division of Surgical Oncology
Department of Surgery
University of Wisconsin School of Medicine and Public Health
Madison, Wisconsin

Charles M. Vollmer, Jr., MD
Professor of Surgery
Department of Surgery
Perelman School of Medicine at the University of Pennsylvania
Director, Pancreatic Surgery
Department of Surgery
Hospital of the University of Pennsylvania
Philadelphia, Pennsylvania

Kojo Wallace, MD
Surgical Critical Care Fellow
Department of Surgery
Emory University School of Medicine
Grady Memorial Hospital
Atlanta, Georgia

Sharon M. Weber, MD
Professor
Chief, Division of Surgical Oncology
Medical Director of Surgical Oncology
Department of Surgery
University of Wisconsin Health
Madison, Wisconsin

Ujwal R. Yanala, MBBS
Advanced GI/MIS/Bariatric Surgery Fellow
Department of Surgery
University of Nebraska Medical Center
Omaha, Nebraska

Dennis Yang, MD
Associate Professor of Medicine
Division of Gastroenterology and
 Hepatology
Department of Internal Medicine
University of Florida College of
 Medicine
Interventional Endoscopist
University of Florida Health
Gainesville, Florida

Victor M. Zaydfudim, MD, MPH
Associate Professor of Surgery
Department of Surgery
University of Virginia Health System
Charlottesville, Virginia

Herbert J. Zeh III, MD
Professor and Chair of Surgery
Department of Surgery
UT Southwestern
Dallas, Texas

Ivan R. Zendejas, MD
Transplant and Hepatobiliary
 Surgeon
Abdominal Transplant Services
Intermountain Medical Center
Salt Lake City, Utah

Amer H. Zureikat, MD
Associate Professor of Surgery
University of Pittsburgh School of Medicine
Chief, Division of Surgical Oncology
Director, Surgical Oncology
UPMC Hillman Cancer Center
Vice Chair of Surgery for Surgical Oncology
Department of Surgery
University of Pittsburgh Medical Center
Pittsburgh, Pennsylvania

Nicholas J. Zyromski, MD
Professor of Surgery
Department of Surgery
Indiana University School of Medicine
Indianapolis, Indiana

Series Preface

Operative interventions are complex, technically demanding, and rapidly evolving. *Operative Techniques in Surgery* seeks to provide highly visual step-by-step instructions to perform these complex tasks. The series is organized anatomically with volumes covering foregut surgery, hepato-pancreato-biliary surgery, and colorectal surgery. Breast and endocrine surgery as well as other topics related to surgical oncology are included in a separate volume. Modern approaches to vascular surgery are covered in a standalone volume. We also have a first edition standalone volume dedicated to trauma surgery. Additionally, many chapters are augmented by video clips dynamically demonstrating the critical steps of the procedure throughout the series.

The series editors are renowned surgeons with expertise in their respective fields. Each is a leader in the discipline of surgery, each recognized for superb surgical judgment and outstanding operative skill. Breast surgery, endocrine procedures, and surgical oncology topics were edited by Dr. Michael S. Sabel of the University of Michigan. Thoracic and upper gastrointestinal surgery topics were edited by Dr. Aurora D. Pryor of Donald and Barbara Zucker School of Medicine at Hofstra/Northwell, with Dr. Steven J. Hughes of the University of Florida directing the section on hepato-pancreatico-biliary surgery. Dr. Daniel Albo of University of Texas Rio Grande directed the section dedicated to colorectal surgery. Dr. Kellie R. Brown of Medical College of Wisconsin edited topics related to vascular surgery, including both open and endovascular approaches. New this year, we have added a section on Trauma and Critical Surgery, led by Dr. Amy J. Goldberg of Temple University.

In turn, the series editors recruited contributors that are world-renowned; the resulting volumes have a distinctly international flavor. Surgery is a visual discipline. *Operative Techniques in Surgery* is lavishly illustrated with a compelling combination of line art and intraoperative photography. The illustrated material provides a uniform style emphasizing clarity and strong, clean lines. Intraoperative photographs are taken from the perspective of the operating surgeon so that operations might be visualized as they would be performed.

The accompanying text is intentionally sparse, with a focus on crucial operative details and important aspects of postoperative management and potential complications. The series is designed for surgeons at all levels of practice, from surgical residents to advanced practice fellows to surgeons of wide experience.

Operative Techniques in Surgery would be possible only at Wolters Kluwer, an organization of unique vision, organization, and talent of Brian Brown, executive editor, Keith Donnellan, senior acquisition editor, and Ashley Fischer, senior development editor.

I am deeply indebted to Dr. Michael W. Mulholland, a master surgeon and leader and the editor in chief of the first series for *Operative Techniques in Surgery*. Without his leadership, this project would not have been successful. I am grateful to our new and returning series editors for their vision on how to make the second edition even more impactful. Curating and editing a major surgical techniques textbook during a worldwide pandemic has not been seamless, yet the outcome is masterful.

Mary T. Hawn, MD, MPH

Preface

Operative Techniques in Hepato-Pancreato-Biliary Surgery is truly unique and thus essential to surgeons in training, fellowship, and practice. Particular attention is devoted to the rapid evolution of the field of hepato-pancreato-biliary surgery to minimally invasive and robotic approaches. To this end, this second edition proved necessary. As endoscopic and catheter-based therapies continue to evolve, complementing or replacing operative approaches, renowned authors from the fields of gastroenterology and radiology provide chapters specifically written for surgeons in the context of multidisciplinary care. Most learners now access the content electronically; hence streaming videos are embedded in the second edition, further emphasizing the uniqueness and value of the resource.

Hepato-pancreato-biliary system operative planning and execution require a thorough understanding of complex, often variable anatomy and is now routinely based on cross-sectional imaging of three-dimensional space. Addressing this challenge was the charge to each author—the result is a book replete with imaging and intraoperative photography supported by consistently exceptional artwork. When alternative approaches to those presented by the author are viable, they are included. The contemporary surgeon must focus on efficiency and needs a reliable resource that can effectively refresh or educate in this context. To meet this need, chapters are presented in outline form, organized to include key aspects of preoperative assessment and preparation. They then break down the operative procedures into logical steps, summarize essential postoperative care issues, and finally tabulate invaluable pearls and pitfalls. The need for versatility also means the content must be readily available; hence, the ability to install the book on various electronic media devices.

The sum product is an optimal resource for surgeons of all levels in preparation for virtually any surgical procedure of the liver, pancreas, bile ducts, and spleen. Editor-in-chief Dr. Mary T. Hawn and the editors at Wolters Kluwer deserve special recognition for their vision and execution in producing this valuable reference.

Steven J. Hughes, MD

Contents

Contributing Authors v
Series Preface xi
Operative Techniques in Hepato-Pancreato-Biliary Surgery Preface xiii
Video Contents List xvii

Section I Surgery of the Biliary System

1 Laparoscopic Cholecystectomy 1
Emily F. Cantrell and Ujwal R. Yanala

2 Open Cholecystectomy 12
Erin L. Vanzant, Martin D. Rosenthal, and Alicia M. Mohr

3 Radical Cholecystectomy 19
Richard J. Bold

4 Endoscopic Retrograde Cholangiopancreatography 29
Shailendra S. Chauhan and Dennis Yang

5 Laparoscopic Cholangiography, Common Bile Duct Exploration, and Endobiliary Stent Placement 39
Tyler John Loftus

6 Percutaneous Transhepatic Biliary Imaging and Intervention 44
Brian S. Geller and Steven J. Hughes

7 Surgically Assisted Endoscopic Retrograde Cholangiopancreatoscopy 51
Crystal N. Johnson-Mann and Steven J. Hughes

8 Roux-en-Y Choledochojejunostomy 55
Catalina Mosquera and Mark Bloomston

9 Minimally Invasive Choledochojejunostomy 61
Eugene P. Ceppa and C. Max Schmidt

10 Choledochoduodenostomy 67
Katherine A. Morgan and David B. Adams

11 Resection of Hilar Cholangiocarcinoma 73
Ryan T. Groeschl and T. Clark Gamblin

12 Intrahepatic Biliary-Enteric Anastomosis 81
Reid B. Adams and Victor M. Zaydfudim

13 Operative Management of Choledochal Cyst 92
Charles S. Cox Jr. and Michael Collins Scott

14 Operative Treatment of Biliary Atresia 103
Charles S. Cox Jr. and Michael Collins Scott

Section II Surgery of the Liver

15 Surgical Anatomy of the Liver 111
Jordan M. Cloyd and Timothy M. Pawlik

16 Intraoperative Ultrasound of the Liver 120
Ankesh Nigam and KMarie King

17 Hepatic Neoplasm Ablation and Related Technology 132
Ido Nachmany, Niv Pencovich, and Rony Eshkenazy

18 Catheter-Based Treatment of Hepatic Neoplasms 138
Darren W. Postoak

19 Segmental Hepatectomy 146
June S. Peng, Matthew E. Dixon, and Niraj J. Gusani

20 Minimally Invasive Segmental Hepatic Resection 153
Timothy E. Newhook and Hop S. Tran Cao

21 Right Hepatectomy 160
Rebecca A. Snyder and Alexander A. Parikh

22 Minimally Invasive Right Hepatectomy 170
Iswanto Sucandy, Kaitlyn Crespo, and Allan Tsung

23 Left Hepatectomy 179
Rebecca Y. Kim and Courtney L. Scaife

24 Minimally Invasive Left Hepatic Lobectomy 187
Epameinondas Dogeas and Amer H. Zureikat

25 Robotic Liver Resection 196
Cameron Schlegel and David L. Bartlett

26 **Vena Cava Resection During Hepatectomy** 205
Aijun Li and Steven J. Hughes

27 **Right Hepatic Trisegmentectomy** 214
Jorge Sanchez-Garcia and Ivan R. Zendejas

28 **Left Hepatic Trisectionectomy** 221
Jason A. Castellanos and Kamran Idrees

29 **Ex Vivo Hepatic Resection** 229
Priyadarshini Manay and Alan William Hemming

30 **Surgical Management of Hepatic Trauma** 236
Walter L. Biffl

Section III Surgery of the Pancreas

31 **Pancreaticoduodenectomy: Resection** 245
George Van Buren II and William Edward Fisher

32 **Pancreaticoduodenectomy: Minimally Invasive Resection** 257
Song Cheol Kim and Ki Byung Song

33 **Pancreaticoduodenectomy: Robotic-Assisted Resection** 266
Brian A. Boone and Herbert J. Zeh III

34 **Pancreaticoduodenectomy: Pancreaticojejunostomy** 273
Charles M. Vollmer Jr.

35 **Pancreaticoduodenectomy: Pancreaticogastrostomy** 284
Sarah Meade, Jennifer F. Tseng, and David McAneny

36 **Laparoscopic and Robotic Pancreaticojejunostomy** 289
Ibrahim Nassour and Steven J. Hughes

37 **Portal Vein Resection and Reconstruction** 298
Ibrahim Nassour, Alessandro Paniccia, and Steven J. Hughes

38 **Open Distal Pancreatectomy** 311
Roberto J. Vidri and Rebecca M. Minter

39 **Minimally Invasive Distal Pancreatectomy** 319
Jon M. Gerry, Jared A. Forrester, and Nathania M. Figueroa Guilliani

40 **Distal Pancreatectomy With Splenic Preservation** 332
Patrick R. Carney, Adam S. Brinkman, and Sharon M. Weber

41 **Enucleation of Pancreatic Neuroendocrine Tumor** 340
Morgan M. Bonds and Barish H. Edil

42 **Operative Treatment of Gastrinoma** 345
Kelly Lynn Koch, Julie Gail Grossman, and Nipun B. Merchant

43 **Lateral Pancreaticojejunostomy With (Frey) or Without (Puestow) Resection of the Pancreatic Head** 355
Kevin E. Behrns

44 **Enteric Drainage of Pancreatic Pseudocysts: Pancreatic Cyst Gastrostomy and Cyst Jejunostomy** 362
Kenneth K. W. Lee

45 **Pancreatic Necrosectomy** 372
Nicholas J. Zyromski

46 **Laparoscopic Pancreatic Necrosectomy** 381
O. Joe Hines and Stephanie S. Kim

47 **Endoscopic Pancreatic Debridement and Drainage** 386
Samuel Han and Georgios Papachristou

48 **Pancreas: Drainage, Distal Pancreatectomy/Splenectomy** 394
Kojo Wallace, Randi N. Smith, and Christopher J. Dente

Section IV Surgery of the Spleen

49 **Elective Splenectomy (Open and Minimally Invasive Techniques)** 398
Zachary J. Brown and Mary E. Dillhoff

50 **Splenorrhaphy** 407
Shawn D. Larson and Saleem Islam

51 **Splenic Injury: Splenectomy and Splenorrhaphy** 417
Lucy Ruangvoravat and Kimberly A. Davis

Index I-1

Video Contents List

Section I — Surgery of the Biliary System

Chapter 1 — Laparoscopic Cholecystectomy
- Video 1: Laparoscopic cholecystectomy
- Video 2: Using ICG to identify anatomy during cholecystectomy
- Video 3: Using ICG to identify aberrant biliary anatomy

Chapter 2 — Open Cholecystectomy
- Video 1: Open cholecystectomy technique

Chapter 4 — Endoscopic Retrograde Cholangiopancreatography
- Video 1: ERCP with stone removal
- Video 2: EHL for the management of large common bile duct stones
- Video 3: Biliary stent placement during ERCP
- Video 4: Endoscopic ampullectomy

Chapter 5 — Laparoscopic Cholangiography, Common Bile Duct Exploration, and Endobiliary Stent Placement
- Video 1: Balloon sphincterotomy

Chapter 7 — Surgically Assisted Endoscopic Retrograde Cholangiopancreatoscopy
- Video 1: Surgically assisted ERCP technique, part 1
- Video 2: Surgically assisted ERCP technique, part 2

Section II — Surgery of the Liver

Chapter 16 — Intraoperative Ultrasound of the Liver
- Video 1: Intraoperative ultrasound of the liver

Chapter 19 — Segmental Hepatectomy
- Video 1: Laparoscopic left lateral sectionectomy

Chapter 22 — Minimally Invasive Right Hepatectomy
- Video 1: Robotic right hepatectomy

Chapter 29 — Ex Vivo Hepatic Resection
- Video 1: Ex-vivo liver resection steps

Section III — Surgery of the Pancreas

Chapter 32 — Pancreaticoduodenectomy: Minimally Invasive Resection
- Video 1: LPD techniques
- Video 2: RPD techniques

Chapter 33 — Pancreaticoduodenectomy: Robotic-Assisted Resection
- Video 1: Robotic pancreaticoduodenectomy, resection

Chapter 36 — Laparoscopic and Robotic Pancreaticojejunostomy
- Video 1: Laparoscopic intussuscepting pancreatojejunostomy
- Video 2: Robotic modified Blumgart pancreatojejunostomy

Chapter 37 — Portal Vein Resection and Reconstruction
- Video 1: Robotic dissection of the uncinate and resection

Chapter 44 — Enteric Drainage of Pancreatic Pseudocysts: Pancreatic Cyst Gastrostomy and Cyst Jejunostomy
- Video 1: Transgastric cyst gastrostomy
- Video 2: Laparoendoscopic intragastric cyst gastrostomy
- Video 3: Roux-en-Y cyst jejunostomy

xviii VIDEO CONTENTS LIST

Chapter 45 Pancreatic Necrosectomy
Video 1 Goals of pancreatic debridement

Chapter 46 Laparoscopic Pancreatic Necrosectomy
Video 1 Retroperitoneal pancreatic necrosectomy

Chapter 47 Endoscopic Pancreatic Debridement and Drainage
Video 1 Lumen-apposing metal stent insertion
Video 2 Multiple-gateway technique
Video 3 Direct endoscopic necrosectomy
Video 4 Necrosectomy morcellator

SECTION I: Surgery of the Biliary System

Chapter 1: Laparoscopic Cholecystectomy

Emily F. Cantrell and Ujwal R. Yanala

DEFINITION
- Laparoscopic cholecystectomy describes a procedure involving the removal of the gallbladder using a laparoscope, a fiberoptic instrument inserted into the abdomen.[1]

Differential Diagnosis
- There are a number of indications for a laparoscopic cholecystectomy. The widespread use of ultrasonography has led to an increasing number of patients diagnosed with asymptomatic gallstones. The management of these patients is controversial as only approximately 2% to 3% of these patients become symptomatic per year.
- Indications in asymptomatic patients are the following:
  - Patients who are immunocompromised, awaiting organ allotransplantation, or have sickle cell disease
  - Presence of gallbladder polyps greater than 10 mm or those rapidly increasing in size
  - Porcelain gallbladder
  - Gallstones bigger than 3 cm in diameter in areas with high prevalence of gallbladder cancer
- Indications in symptomatic patients are the following:
  - Episodes of biliary colic in patients with identified gallstones
  - Acute cholecystitis
  - Patients with biliary dyskinesia diagnosed with cholecystokinin-HIDA cholescintigraphy
  - Patients with gallstone pancreatitis with no choledocholithiasis based on imaging and laboratory values
  - Patients with choledocholithiasis. In most situations, cholecystectomy follows ERCP for extraction of the common bile duct stones

PATIENT HISTORY AND PHYSICAL FINDINGS
- A good medical history is necessary to provide information about associated comorbidities that may affect the patient's tolerance to pneumoperitoneum or operative treatment in general.
- Patients with cardiorespiratory disease may not tolerate the impact of CO_2 pneumoperitoneum on cardiac output or CO_2 elimination.
- Coagulopathic disorders or anticoagulants should be identified and managed.
- Medical history can identify the patients who have a higher risk for choledocholithiasis (patients with jaundice, gallstone pancreatitis, or cholangitis).
- Physical examination of the abdomen reveals any surgical scars, hernias, or stomas that may alter port placement or approach to entering the abdomen. Previous abdominal surgery does not preclude attempt at laparoscopic cholecystectomy. Adhesive disease is a rare indication for conversion to an open procedure.

IMAGING AND OTHER DIAGNOSTIC STUDIES
- Ultrasonography is now the gold standard for the noninvasive diagnosis of cholelithiasis. This imaging test is highly accurate (>96%), can be performed at the patient's bedside, and does not require the use of ionizing radiation. Gallstones must fulfill three major sonographic criteria. They must (1) show an echogenic focus, (2) cast an acoustic shadow, and (3) seek gravitational dependence (**FIGURE 1**). Presence of a dilated common bile duct (>6-7 mm depending on age) during ultrasonography is suggestive of choledocholithiasis. In the case of acute cholecystitis, ultrasound can demonstrate pericholecystic fluid, gallbladder wall thickening, and even a sonographic Murphy sign, documenting tenderness specifically over the gallbladder.
- In atypical cases, a hepatobiliary iminodiacetic acid (HIDA) cholescintigraphy scan may be used to demonstrate obstruction of the cystic duct, which definitively diagnoses cholecystitis. Filling of the gallbladder during a HIDA scan essentially eliminates the diagnosis of cholecystitis (**FIGURE 2**).

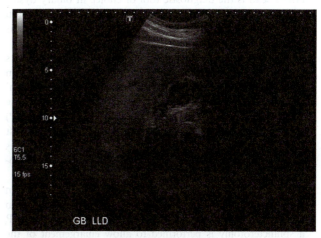

FIGURE 1 • Ultrasound of the abdomen showing multiple gallstones in the lumen of the gallbladder. There is no gallbladder thickening or pericholecystic fluid, thus acute cholecystitis is ruled out.

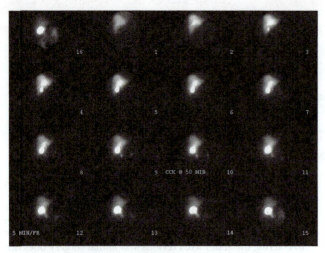

FIGURE 2 • HIDA cholescintigraphy scan. Filling of the gallbladder during a HIDA scan, as in this study, essentially eliminates the diagnosis of cholecystitis.

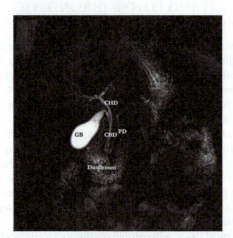

FIGURE 3 • Magnetic resonance cholangiopancreatography (MRCP). Note the filling defect in the distal common bile duct suggestive of choledocholithiasis. CBD, common bile duct; CHD, common hepatic duct; GB, gallbladder; PD, pancreatic duct.

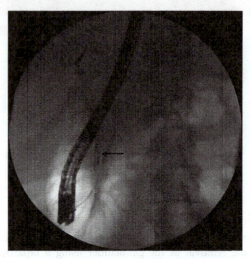

FIGURE 4 • Endoscopic retrograde cholangiopancreatography (ERCP). The *solid arrow* shows filling defect in the distal common bile duct, suggestive of choledocholithiasis.

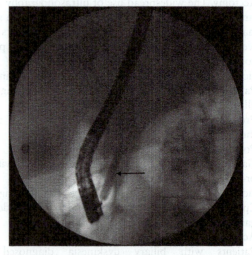

FIGURE 5 • ERCP on the same patient with sphincterotomy and balloon sweeping of all common bile duct stones. The *solid arrow* shows the endoscopic balloon.

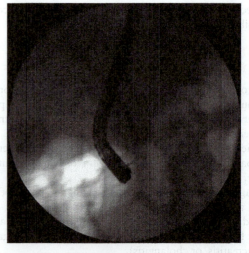

FIGURE 6 • Completed ERCP showing a patent common bile duct and absence of filling defects.

- HIDA scan is the diagnostic tool of choice in biliary dyskinesia and is performed with the concurrent administration of cholecystokinin. An ejection fraction of less than 20% is suggestive of the disease.
- If there is suspicion of choledocholithiasis, as in patients with jaundice, pancreatitis, cholangitis, or dilated common bile duct on ultrasonography, the biliary tree can be delineated and inspected for presence of gallstones with the use of magnetic resonance cholangiopancreatography (MRCP) (**FIGURE 3**). MRCP is highly sensitive (>90%) and almost has 100% specificity. As a noninvasive test, MRCP provides accurate imaging of the biliary tree, but in the setting of choledocholithiasis, it does not provide a therapeutic solution.
- Endoscopic retrograde cholangiopancreatography (ERCP) can be used as a diagnostic and therapeutic modality (**FIGURE 4**). In the presence of stones in the common bile duct during ERCP, a sphincterotomy is performed to allow enlargement of the papilla and subsequent extraction of stones with a balloon or basket (**FIGURES 5** and **6**). With this approach, over 80% of stones can be removed successfully. Larger stones may require additional removal techniques such as mechanical or

intraductal lithotripsy. ERCP has a complication rate of around 8%. Complications following ERCP include sedation-related issues, pancreatitis, bleeding, perforation, and infection.
- Preoperative laboratory studies should include amylase or lipase, liver function tests, renal function tests, electrolytes, and coagulation studies. Abnormal liver function studies may reflect choledocholithiasis or primary hepatic dysfunction.

SURGICAL MANAGEMENT

Preoperative Planning

- In the preoperative area, the patient should be assessed and asked if there have been any changes or updates to their medical history that were not present during the last clinic visit or assessment, particularly conditions that would factor into operative decision making (ie, a recent myocardial infarction, recent cerebrovascular event, current/active infections, worsening pulmonary status, initiation of antiplatelet or anticoagulant medications, etc).
- The patient is asked to void just prior to transfer to the operating room. If able to void, Foley catheter is usually not indicated for an elective laparoscopic cholecystectomy.
- The operative consent, imaging, and preoperative laboratory values are reviewed.

Positioning

- The patient is placed in a supine position with the right arm extended and the left arm is secured along the patient's torso (FIGURE 7), as this allows access for fluoroscopy should an intraoperative cholangiogram need to be performed.
- The patient should be secured to the operating room table with a strap at the level of the thighs. Additionally, a footboard can be placed at the patient's feet as well as additional straps around the lower legs to avoid sliding or a fall from the bed during steep reverse Trendelenburg position (FIGURE 8).
- Heel pads, sequential compression devices for deep venous thrombosis prophylaxis, and warming devices are also placed.
- An orogastric tube is inserted to decompress the stomach.
- The primary surgeon stands at the patient's left and the assistant surgeon at the patient's right (FIGURE 7).
- Two monitors are placed at the head of the bed, one on the right and one on the left, facing the surgeon and the assistant.
- The laparoscopic camera, light source, insufflation tubing, suction, and electrocautery are passed to a tower usually positioned at the foot or to the right of the operating room table.

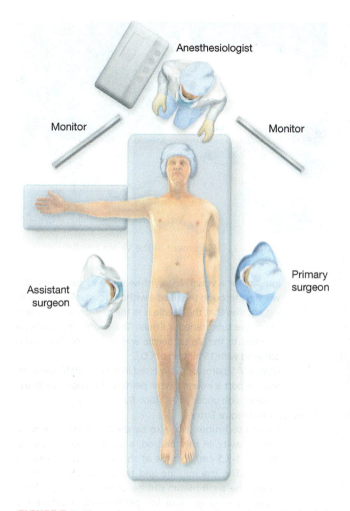

FIGURE 7 • The patient is placed in a supine position with the left arm tagged and the right arm extended. The primary surgeon stands to the left of the patient and the assistant to the right of the patient.

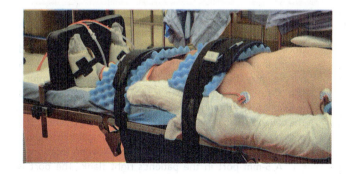

FIGURE 8 • The patient is strapped at the thighs and legs and a footboard is placed to support the patient during reverse Trendelenburg.

ENTRY INTO THE PERITONEAL CAVITY AND ACHIEVING PNEUMOPERITONEUM

- Veress Needle Entry
  - The base of the umbilicus is grasped with two penetrating towel clips and is elevated for easier access. A 5-mm incision is created in the superior aspect of the umbilicus with the use of a no. 11 blade. The base of the umbilicus is chosen because it gives a better cosmetic result.
- Alternatively, if the patient has a midline scar and a history of multiple intra-abdominal procedures or if it is the surgeon's preference, entry into the peritoneal cavity can also be achieved through an incision in the left subcostal area just inferior to the rib in the anterior axillary line (Palmer's point).
- Through this incision, a Veress needle is introduced into the peritoneal cavity (FIGURE 9). A syringe with saline is attached to the Veress needle. First, aspirate the syringe to rule out placement of the Veress needle in the lumen of

SECTION I SURGERY OF THE BILIARY SYSTEM

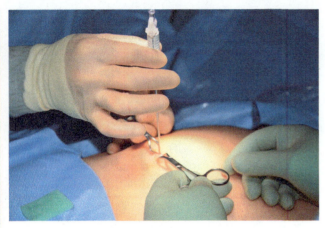

FIGURE 9 • Placement of the Veress needle.

intestine or a vessel. Then, infuse saline to determine if it will flow through the needle without resistance. This finding signifies that the needle is in the peritoneal cavity and not in the subcutaneous tissues. The insufflation tubing is attached to the Veress needle and pneumoperitoneum is achieved with 15 mm Hg of CO_2.
- Next, a 0° laparoscope is inserted in a 5-mm OptiView port, and the port is inserted in the peritoneal cavity through the same incision under direct vision (**FIGURE 10**).
- Hasson Technique Entry
    - Hasson technique can also be used to enter the peritoneal cavity. In this method, a small incision (approximately 1-1.5 cm) is made at the umbilicus. The fascia is incised in the midline and the peritoneum is identified. The peritoneum can be entered bluntly with a clamp or sharply. Once the peritoneum is entered, a finger is inserted to confirm position within the peritoneal cavity as well as sweep down any adhesions

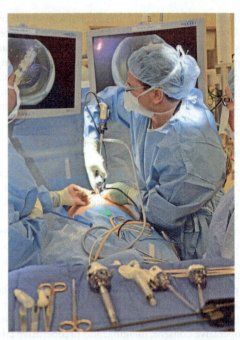

FIGURE 10 • With the laparoscope inserted in a 5-mm port, the surgeon places the first port under direct vision. Notice that the surgeon watches the monitor as he advances the port.

surrounding the port site. A Hasson trocar is inserted into the abdomen. Stay sutures can be placed on either side of the fascia to help secure the trocar into place. Insufflation of the abdomen is performed through the Hasson trocar.
- Hasson technique should be considered if the patient has a history of multiple prior intra-abdominal operations.

PLACEMENT OF THE OTHER PORTS

- Once the first port is in place, inspect the intestines and organs immediately beneath the incision (and site of Veress needle entry if different) to rule out any inadvertent injury. The 0° scope is replaced with a 30° scope that allows views through different angles.
- The patient is then placed in reverse Trendelenburg position. The gallbladder is typically easy to visualize following this maneuver.
- Additional ports are then placed in the following locations:
    - A 5-mm port in the patient's right flank. The port is placed in the anterior axillary line around two fingerbreadths below the costal margin. Through this port, the assistant surgeon grasps the fundus of the gallbladder and retracts the gallbladder and the liver in an anterior and cephalad direction toward the diaphragm. This facilitates visualization of the triangle of Calot.

If the gallbladder is very distended and inflamed, making it hard to be grasped, the gallbladder may be deflated with an endoscopic needle.
- A 12-mm port (or 5-mm port if Hasson technique was used to enter the abdomen) is placed in the epigastrium just below the xiphoid process and to the right of the falciform ligament. Ideally, the port is situated above the triangle of Calot just inferior to the liver edge.
- A 5-mm port in the midclavicular line, allowing for adequate spacing between the ports (**FIGURE 11**).
- If the anatomy of the liver precludes visualization of the triangle of Calot, an additional 5-mm port is placed in the left anterior axillary line at the level of the costal margin and a liver retractor is inserted.
- The assistant surgeon holds the camera and the right flank port retracting the gallbladder, whereas the primary surgeon works through the epigastric and midclavicular ports.

Chapter 1 LAPAROSCOPIC CHOLECYSTECTOMY 5

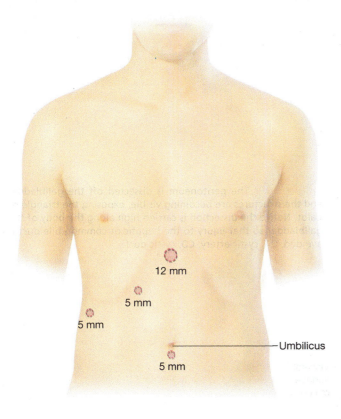

FIGURE 11 • Placement of the four ports.

EXPOSURE OF THE TRIANGLE OF CALOT

- With the use of a blunt dissector through the epigastric port, any adhesions between the gallbladder and the omentum or transverse mesocolon are divided, always taking such adhesions along the wall of the gallbladder to minimize bleeding (FIGURE 12).
- A grasping forceps, through the 5-mm midclavicular line port, is used to grasp the gallbladder at the Hartman's pouch and provide lateral traction (FIGURE 13). This maneuver retracts the gallbladder away from vital structures and,

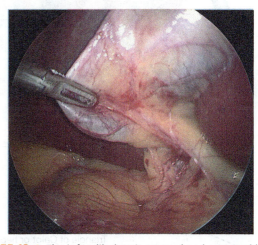

FIGURE 13 • The infundibulum is grasped and retracted lateral to the patient's right side. This is a very important maneuver as it places the cystic duct at a 90° angle to the common bile duct and minimizes confusion and potential injury to the common bile duct.

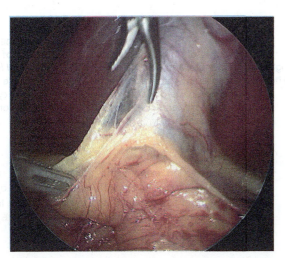

FIGURE 12 • Omental adhesions are stripped off from the gallbladder.

ideally, puts the cystic duct at a 90° angle to the common bile duct, minimizing the risk of inadvertent injury to the hepatic or common bile ducts.
- The peritoneum is then bluntly dissected off the gallbladder to expose the infundibulum–cystic duct junction. This is done by stripping the peritoneum at the lateral edge of the gallbladder just below where the infundibulum is grasped (FIGURE 14).

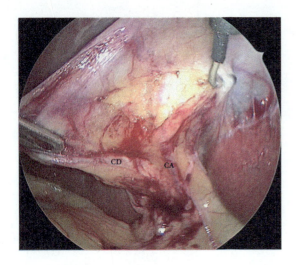

FIGURE 14 • The peritoneum is dissected off the gallbladder and the structures are becoming visible, exposing the triangle of Calot. Notice the dissection is carried high along the body of the gallbladder so that injury to the hepatic or common bile duct is avoided. CA, cystic artery; CD, cystic duct.

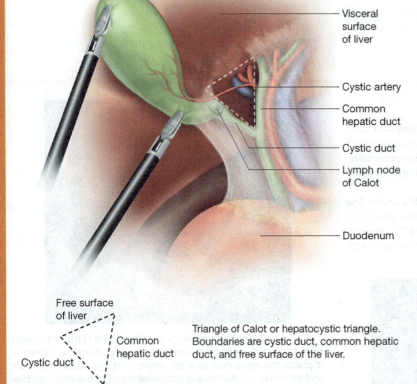

FIGURE 15 • Schematic drawing showing the triangle of Calot, its borders and the content of the triangle, and the cystic artery. The *interrupted lines* represent the borders of the triangle. Notice the lymph node of Calot, immediately above the cystic artery. It can act as landmark for identification of the cystic artery.

- As the peritoneum is dissected from the gallbladder wall, the lymph node of Calot is also often identified. The lymph node often overlies the cystic artery and thus can be a useful landmark. Peritoneal attachments around the node of Calot can be taken with hook electrocautery in order to minimize bleeding.

- This initial dissection exposes the triangle of Calot, also known as the hepatocystic triangle, bounded by the cystic duct, the common hepatic duct, and the edge of the liver. The cystic artery is contained within the triangle (FIGURE 15) (▶ Video 1).

Chapter 1 LAPAROSCOPIC CHOLECYSTECTOMY

EXPOSURE OF THE REVERSE TRIANGLE

- The reverse side of the hepatocystic triangle is bordered by the cystic duct, the inferior lateral border of the gallbladder, and the right lobe of the liver.
- In order to expose the reverse triangle, the infundibulum is retracted medially and superiorly and then peritoneal attachments are taken bluntly or with the hook electrocautery (**FIGURE 16**). Exposing the reverse triangle can aid in identification of the cystic duct and artery and facilitates circumferential dissection of these structures.
- Importantly, division of the posterior triangle peritoneum early in the dissection can dramatically impact exposure to the anterior triangle by facilitating retraction of the infundibulum away from other portal structures.

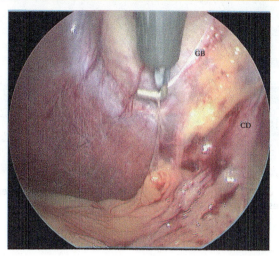

FIGURE 16 • Exposure of the reverse triangle. The gallbladder (GB) is retracted medially and the reverse triangle can be exposed by dissection of the peritoneum off the structures. CD, cystic duct.

THE CRITICAL VIEW

- It is of paramount importance to obtain "the critical view of safety" of the cystic duct and artery prior to clipping or dividing any structures. This view is obtained when both the cystic duct and cystic artery are circumferentially dissected and windows have been created between the two structures and medial to the cystic artery, so that the liver can be visualized through each of these windows (**FIGURE 17**). Ideally, the medial wall of the gallbladder is dissected up to the liver. This visualization minimizes the risk of dividing the hepatic or common bile duct or an aberrant branch of the right hepatic duct. The dissection medial to the cystic artery reduces the risk of injuring a meandering right hepatic artery that is also at risk for inadvertent injury.
- Should this dissection and exposure be limited by inflammation or other factors such as an intrahepatic gallbladder, a hypertrophied left lobe of the liver, or aberrant anatomy, a retrograde ("dome-down") dissection of the gallbladder as is classically done during an open cholecystectomy can be considered or the decision for conversion to an open procedure should be made.
- Utilization of indocyanine green (ICG) is a useful adjunct in identifying biliary structures intraoperatively. However, it requires a specialized laparoscopic camera to visualize the near infrared spectrum. ICG must also be injected prior to initiation of the case as it takes several hours for the liver

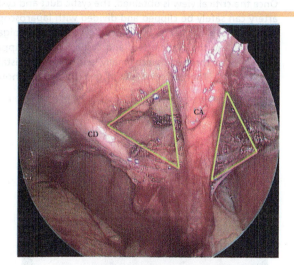

FIGURE 17 • The critical view. The two triangles show the windows that need to be formed between the cystic duct and the cystic artery and medial to the cystic artery. The surgeon should be able to see the visceral surface of the liver through these windows. CA, cystic artery; CD, cystic duct.

to excrete ICG into biliary ductal system. If using ICG, the patient should ideally be given 2.5 to 5 mg intravenously approximately 2 to 4 hours prior to surgery in order to provide a biliary to liver contrast ratio of >1 resulting in optimal visualization (**FIGURE 18**) (▶ Videos 2-3).[2,3]

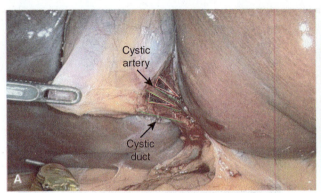

FIGURE 18 • Intraoperative imaging with Indocyanine green (ICG) outlining the cystic duct (black lines) and common bile duct (red lines).

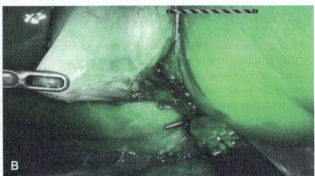

DIVISION OF THE CYSTIC DUCT AND CYSTIC ARTERY

- Once the critical view is obtained, the cystic duct and cystic artery can safely be clipped and divided with laparoscopic shears. A clip applier is introduced through the epigastric port, and the cystic artery and cystic duct are clipped with two to three clips proximally and one clip distally (FIGURE 19). The posterior jaw of the clip applier should be visualized across the structure to assure that the clip will traverse the entire lumen of each structure. Once both structures are divided, the clipped stumps of the two structures are inspected (FIGURE 20). An alternative approach for a large caliber cystic duct or friable tissues is the use of a laparoscopic endoloop or stapling device to control the duct.

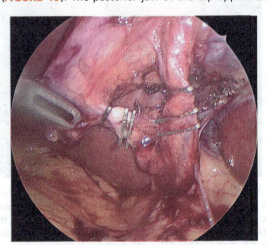

FIGURE 19 • Clipping of the cystic duct and cystic artery.

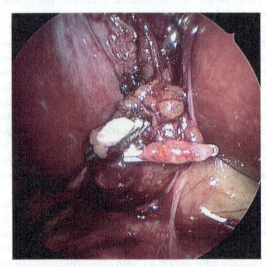

FIGURE 20 • Inspecting the clipped stumps of both structures.

DISSECTION OF THE GALLBLADDER OFF THE GALLBLADDER FOSSA

- Next, the gallbladder is dissected from attachments to the undersurface of the liver using hook and/or spatula electrocautery. The infundibulum is grasped and elevated toward the anterior abdominal wall and lateral to create tension and the body of the gallbladder is dissected off the gallbladder fossa (FIGURE 21). In order to dissect the lateral side of the gallbladder, the infundibulum is retracted medially and superiorly and again the hook electrocautery dissects the whole length of the lateral wall of the gallbladder (FIGURE 22). Prior to completely freeing the gallbladder, it can be used as a handle to lift the liver and inspect the operative bed for bleeding. The gallbladder is then completely separated from the liver (FIGURE 23).

Chapter 1 LAPAROSCOPIC CHOLECYSTECTOMY

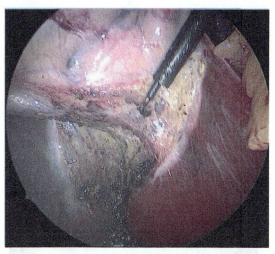

FIGURE 21 • Dissection of the gallbladder fossa with electrocautery.

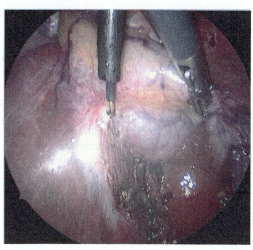

FIGURE 22 • Dissection of the lateral wall of the gallbladder off the gallbladder fossa.

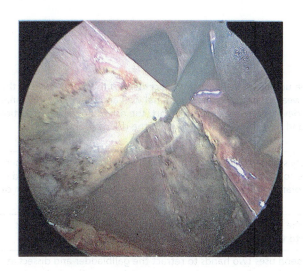

FIGURE 23 • The gallbladder is pulled away from the liver, and the tip of the fundus is divided from the liver to complete the gallbladder dissection.

EXTRACTION OF THE GALLBLADDER

- The gallbladder is now completely dissected off the liver. A 10-mm specimen bag is introduced through the epigastric port (or 10-12 mm port if placed in alternative location) and opened facing the camera. The gallbladder is placed in the specimen bag (FIGURE 24) and then extracted through the port site. If the gallbladder is too big or contains large stones, the port incision may need to be extended to accommodate the bigger gallbladder.
- The specimen is sent to pathology for histologic examination.

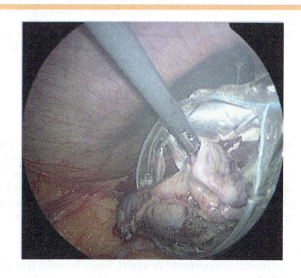

FIGURE 24 • The gallbladder is placed in an EndoCatch bag.

CLOSURE

- The epigastric port (or other ports 10 mm or greater) is closed at the fascial level with the use of a transfascial suture passer and 0 braided absorbable suture (FIGURE 25).
- The other ports are retrieved under direct vision to rule out hemorrhage at the port sites.
- Once hemostasis is confirmed at the port sites, the peritoneum is deflated and the skin incisions are closed with subcuticular 4-0 monofilament absorbable suture.

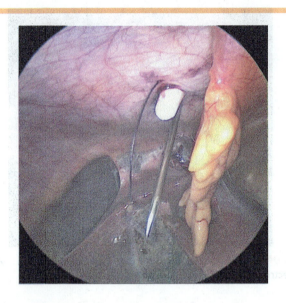

FIGURE 25 • The incision is reapproximated with a transfascial suture passer and 0 braided absorbable suture.

PEARLS AND PITFALLS

Placement of 12-mm port	■ Many authors place the 12-mm port in the umbilicus. We advocate placement of the 12-mm port in the epigastrium because the umbilicus is the weakest point of the abdominal wall and the risk of incisional hernia is higher. Furthermore, if a hernia develops at the epigastric port, the risk of bowel incarceration is very low because the port is very high and above the liver, minimizing the risk of strangulation or incarceration.
Intraoperative cholangiogram	■ A surgeon performing laparoscopic surgery should be facile and comfortable performing an intraoperative cholangiogram. We do not advocate routine performance of cholangiograms, but there should be a **very low threshold** for performing a cholangiogram in cases of questionable anatomy or suspicion of injury.
Dissection of triangle of Calot	■ Dissection of the peritoneum to identify the structures should be done *as close* to the gallbladder as possible. This minimizes the risk of injury to the hepatic or common bile duct which lies deeper.
Two-handed skills	■ In the above description, the primary surgeon uses two hands to retract the gallbladder and dissect at the same time. In a teaching institution, or when a laparoscopic novice is performing the cholecystectomy, two-hand laparoscopic cholecystectomy is a very good starting procedure to obtain bimanual dexterity before embarking on more complex laparoscopic cases.
Spilled stones	■ Every effort should be made to avoid perforation of the gallbladder and spillage of gallstones. If this happens, all gallstones should be retrieved to avoid associated complications such as postoperative granulomas or abscesses.

POSTOPERATIVE CARE

- The majority of laparoscopic cholecystectomies are performed as outpatient surgery and thus patients are discharged home on the same day. If the procedure is performed in the setting of resolved pancreatitis or choledocholithiasis on a patient who was already hospitalized, an overnight postoperative stay is the norm. A diet can be initiated immediately.

COMPLICATIONS

- The overall perioperative mortality varies between 0% and 0.3%.[4,5]
- The overall incidence of bile duct injuries requiring corrective surgery varies between 0.1% and 0.3%. Corrective surgery for bile duct injury carries its own risks including perioperative mortality (1%-4%), secondary biliary cirrhosis (11%), anastomotic stricture (9%-20%), and cholangitis (5%).[6,7]
- Other complications include the following:
  - Bile leak treated conservatively (0.1%-0.2%), radiologically (0%-0.1%), or endoscopically (0.05%-0.1%), or by operation (0%-0.05%).
  - Peritonitis requiring reoperation, typically from a missed, inadvertent enterotomy (0.2%)
  - Postoperative bleeding requiring operation (0.1%-0.5%)
  - Intra-abdominal abscesses requiring operation (0.1%)

REFERENCES

1. Keus F, Gooszen HG, van Laarhoven CJ. Open, small-incision, or laparoscopic cholecystectomy for patients with symptomatic cholecystolithiasis. An overview of Cochrane Hepato-Biliary Group reviews. *Cochrane Database Syst Rev*. 2010;2010(1):CD008318.
2. Boogerd LSF, Handgraaf HJM, Huurman VAL, et al. The best approach for laparoscopic fluorescence cholangiography: overview of the literature and optimization of dose and dosing time. *Surg Innov*. 2017;24(4):386-396.
3. Ambe PC, Plambeck J, Fernandez-Jesberg V, Zarras K. The role of indocyanine green fluoroscopy for intraoperative bile duct visualization during laparoscopic cholecystectomy: an observational cohort study in 70 patients. *Patient Saf Surg*. 2019;13(2):1-7.
4. Duca SS, Bălă OO, Al-Hajjar NN, et al. Laparoscopic cholecystectomy: incidents and complications. A retrospective analysis of 9542 consecutive laparoscopic operations. *HPB*. 2003;5(3):152-158.
5. Giger UF, Michel JM, Opitz I, et al. Risk factors for perioperative complications in patients undergoing laparoscopic cholecystectomy: analysis of 22,953 consecutive cases from the Swiss Association of Laparoscopic and Thoracoscopic Surgery database. *J Am Coll Surg*. 2006;203(5):723-728.
6. Sicklick JK, Camp MS, Lillemoe KD, et al. Surgical management of bile duct injuries sustained during laparoscopic cholecystectomy: perioperative results in 200 patients. *Ann Surg*. 2005;241(5):786-785.
7. Schmidt SC, Settmacher U, Langrehr JM, et al. Management and outcome of patients with combined bile duct and hepatic arterial injuries after laparoscopic cholecystectomy. *Surgery*. 2004;135(6):613-618.

Chapter 2 Open Cholecystectomy

Erin L. Vanzant, Martin D. Rosenthal, and Alicia M. Mohr

DEFINITION
- Removal of the gallbladder for benign disease using an open technique when the laparoscopic technique is not prudent.

DIFFERENTIAL DIAGNOSIS OVERLAPS WITH INDICATIONS FOR LAPAROSCOPIC CHOLECYSTECTOMY
- Acute cholecystitis
- Symptomatic biliary colic
- Acalculous cholecystitis
- Mirizzi syndrome
- Emphysematous or gangrenous cholecystitis
- Gallstone pancreatitis
- Choledocholithiasis
- Biliary dyskinesia
- Diseases that can present similarly and are not treatable by simple cholecystectomy include peptic ulcer disease, hepatitis, pancreatitis, cholangitis, gallbladder cancer, nephrolithiasis, colitis, irritable bowel syndrome, pyogenic or amebic liver abscesses, and atypical appendicitis

PATIENT HISTORY AND PHYSICAL FINDINGS
- Biliary colic (symptomatic cholelithiasis) is typically a right upper quadrant (RUQ) or epigastric postprandial sharp crampy pain. Symptoms classically start 30 to 90 minutes after eating and typically are associated with high-fat meals. Nausea and bloating are common. Pain can often radiate to the right scapula. The symptoms typically will resolve within 6 hours. Pain lasting more than 6 hours and/or fever is suggestive of acute cholecystitis.
- On physical examination, tenderness will usually be present in the RUQ. The presence of a Murphy sign (inspiratory pause with deep RUQ palpation) is suggestive of acute cholecystitis.
- Additional findings may be seen with obstructive jaundice as sludge or stones originating in the gallbladder can terminate in the common bile duct or sphincter of Oddi culminating in elevated bilirubin on liver function tests. This results in scleral icterus and if elevated enough clinical jaundice.

IMAGING AND OTHER DIAGNOSTIC STUDIES
- A fasting RUQ ultrasound is the first test of choice for the diagnosis of gallstones and is frequently the only imaging necessary to diagnose acute cholecystitis. Gallstones are identified as echogenic foci with posterior shadowing (**FIGURE 1**). Cholecystitis is suggested by gallbladder wall thickening (>3 mm), pericholecystic fluid, or inspiratory pause elicited by placement of the ultrasound probe directly over the gallbladder (a sonographic Murphy sign). The sensitivity and specificity of ultrasound for calculous cholecystitis are around 82%.[1] In critically ill patients with acalculous cholecystitis, the specificity drops significantly.
- The other common imaging study used to diagnose gallbladder pathology is a nuclear medicine test called either hepatobiliary scintigraphy or a hepatobiliary iminodiacetic acid scan (commonly referred to as a HIDA scan). In this test, a radiolabeled substrate is intravenously administered, taken up by the liver, and excreted into the biliary tree (**FIGURE 2**). Normally, the gallbladder will fill within 30 minutes. If the radiotracer uptake is absent by 4 hours, the sensitivity for acute cholecystitis is 96%.[1] An HIDA scan will also provide information about obstruction of the common bile duct, as substrate will be seen accumulating in the duodenum if the duct is not obstructed. In the setting of hepatic failure, prolonged fasting states, or cholestasis, this study is not useful, as the liver often will not take up enough substrate to allow an adequate study. Gallstones are not revealed with this study, but rather, the presence or absence of cholecystitis is

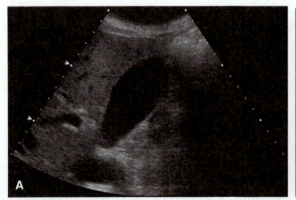
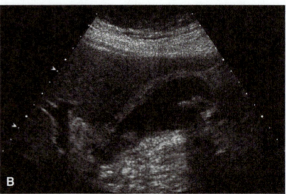

FIGURE 1 • Gallbladder ultrasound. **A,** The normal ultrasound appearance of the gallbladder. **B,** The presence of gallstones, thickening of the gallbladder wall, and gallbladder wall edema are suggestive of acute cholecystitis.

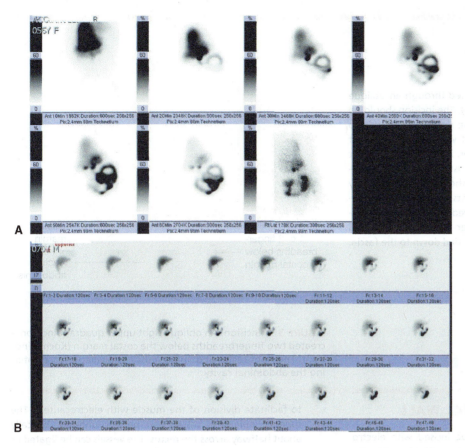

FIGURE 2 • Hepatobiliary iminodiacetic acid scintigraphy. **A,** Tracer promptly fills the gallbladder and duodenum, demonstrating normal gallbladder physiology and a nonobstructed biliary system. **B,** Nonfilling of the gallbladder at 1 hour following substrate injection is consistent with acute cholecystitis.

determined by assessing patency of the cystic duct regardless of the etiology. HIDA scintigraphy is generally performed if the clinical findings and ultrasound are inconclusive for calculous cholecystitis or in critically ill patients with suspected acalculous cholecystitis.[2]

SPECIAL PATIENT POPULATIONS

Pregnancy
- Open cholecystectomy is associated with increased fetal, maternal and surgical complications, and increased hospital length of stay. Laparoscopic cholecystectomy is the preferred approach to biliary pathology regardless of trimester.[3]

Liver Cirrhosis
- Open cholecystectomy has increased postoperative complications and longer hospital length of stay in patients with symptomatic cholelithiasis. Laparoscopic cholecystectomy is felt to be a safer alternative to the open approach in Child A and B cirrhosis. Currently, nonoperative approaches are recommended in Child C cirrhosis.[4]

Gallbladder Cancer
- Laparoscopic cholecystectomy is curative for Tis and T1a gallbladder cancers (those confined to the gallbladder mucosa). Current guidelines recommend the open approach for known more advanced cancer and in those that require re-resection after initial laparoscopic approach.[5]

SURGICAL MANAGEMENT

Preoperative Planning
- The vast majority of patients will be appropriate candidates for a laparoscopic cholecystectomy. Conversion from laparoscopy due to variable anatomy or severe inflammation is the most common indication for the open procedure. Indications for open cholecystectomy include any previously accepted contraindications to laparoscopic procedures. Rare patients in whom a primary open cholecystectomy should be considered are the following:
  - Septic patients on vasoactive agents for hemodynamic support when percutaneous drainage options are not available or who have failed percutaneous drainage.
  - Patients with complicated anterior abdominal walls and/or severe adhesions. Specifically, if there are large pieces of prosthetic mesh in the umbilical and epigastric areas and/or prior RUQ surgery, laparoscopic completion of a cholecystectomy can be challenging.
  - The need for concomitant open common bile duct exploration when laparoscopic exploration is not feasible.
  - Patients with severe untreated coagulopathy.

Positioning
- The patient is positioned supine. Arms should be preferentially tucked by the side or extended out at right angles to the bed. An oral or nasal tube for gastric decompression is placed.

TECHNIQUES (▶ Video 1)

INCISION

- The gallbladder is most easily accessed through an oblique or subcostal RUQ incision (FIGURE 3). The incision should be placed two fingerbreadths below the right costal margin to facilitate fascial closure on a patient without insufflation if conversion from laparoscopic to open is necessary. A patient who is not marked for an open incision prior to attempting laparoscopy will tend to place the incision erroneously high on the costal margin. In patients with significant hepatomegaly, the incision may be moved inferiorly to two fingerbreadths below the palpable liver edge, but this should rarely be necessary. The incision is carried down to the fascia.

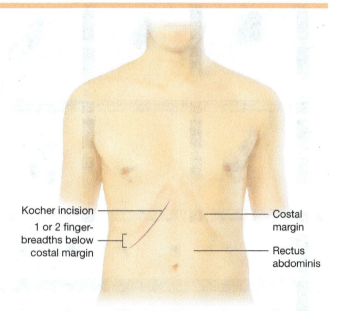

FIGURE 3 • Incision. An oblique right upper quadrant incision is created two fingerbreadths below the costal margin (Kocher incision). The right rectus abdominis muscle is divided before entering the abdominal cavity.

OPENING OF THE ABDOMINAL WALL

- The anterior rectus fascia should be incised with electrocautery. A Kelly or other large clamp is placed under the lateral border of the rectus muscle, retracting it anteriorly, to facilitate division of the muscle with electrocautery. The superior epigastric vessels can be encountered, typically about halfway across the rectus. The vessels can be ligated or cauterized, or they can be reflected medially and preserved with the medial half of the rectus.

PLACEMENT OF RETRACTORS

- This step is the key to a successful operation. Safely keeping the bowel out of the operative field and delivering the gallbladder to the center of the wound will make the remainder of the case straightforward with proper exposure. A Bookwalter fixed retractor or another table-mounted retractor should be used (FIGURE 4). In cases of dense adhesions to the gallbladder, start with body wall retractors placed inferiorly and superiorly. In cases of minimal adhesions or after some initial adhesiolysis, use moist laparotomy pads to push the transverse colon and duodenum inferior and medial, respectively, away from the gallbladder. Malleable or long right-angled retractors for the Bookwalter should be placed inferomedially and inferolaterally to hold these lap pads away from the gallbladder. A deep body wall retractor may be required inferiorly to adequately open the space between the duodenum and gallbladder. Superomedially, a flat deep retractor, such as a Harrington (or *Sweetheart*) or medium-sized right-angled retractor, should be placed against the liver to pull it to the superior aspect of the wound. A superolateral body wall retractor can be progressively exchanged for deeper retractors as the gallbladder is progressively dissected from the gallbladder bed to elevate the liver and separate it from the gallbladder. A Kelly or large clamp is then placed on the infundibulum of the gallbladder to facilitate moving it within the space created.

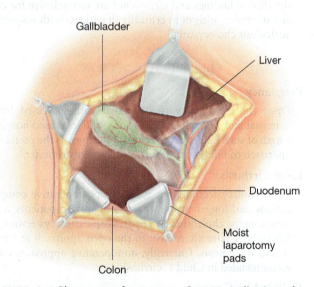

FIGURE 4 • Placement of retractors. Correct application of a fixed retracting device (Bookwalter) is the key to a successful and safe open cholecystectomy. Inferiorly, moist laparotomy pads are carefully placed behind deep retractors to exclude the duodenum, colon, and small bowel from the operative field. Superiorly, additional retractors are placed to retain the liver. As the gallbladder is dissected free from its bed, the more lateral superior retractor can be progressively exchanged for deeper retractors placed over the dissected bed to improve visualization.

INCISION OF THE VISCERAL PERITONEUM

- The peritoneum is incised just off the liver edge at the most anterior point of the gallbladder to start a traditional dome-down approach (**FIGURES 5** and **6**). A tonsil or other fine-tipped dissector is used to enter the plane between the peritoneum and the gallbladder. Electrocautery is then used to open the peritoneum. This is repeated for the other side of the gallbladder.

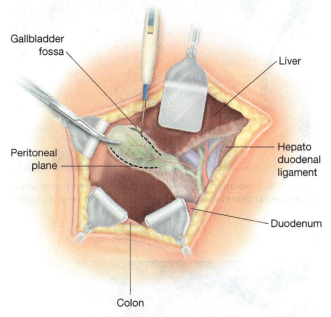

FIGURE 5 • Incision of the peritoneum and dissection of the gallbladder from the gallbladder fossa. The infundibulum is grasped with a large clamp (Kelly) to facilitate mobilization. The peritoneum (serosa of the gallbladder) is incised 3 to 5 mm from the interface with the substance of the liver and the areolar tissue between the gallbladder and the liver is divided with electrocautery. The gallbladder is dissected in a top-down fashion toward the porta hepatis.

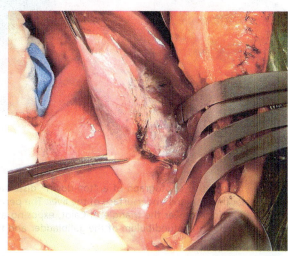

FIGURE 6 • Ligation of the cystic duct and cystic artery. After the gallbladder has been dissected free from its bed, a combination of blunt and sharp dissection is used to isolate the cystic duct and cystic artery. Dissection should be directed from the gallbladder toward the portal structures to avoid injury. Both structures are divided separately between ligatures. Care should be taken to not apply electrocautery when in proximity to the colon, duodenum, or portal structures.

RETROGRADE DISSECTION OF THE GALLBLADDER OFF OF THE GALLBLADDER FOSSA

- Electrocautery is then used to dissect the gallbladder free from the liver. This is performed in a dome-down fashion, starting anteriorly and continuing until the gallbladder is suspended from its pedicle.

LIGATION OF THE CYSTIC DUCT AND ARTERY

- After the gallbladder has been dissected free from its bed, a combination of sharp and blunt dissection is performed around the pedicle until the artery and duct are dissected free (**FIGURES 7-9**). Tracing the cystic duct until its intersection with the common bile duct is not necessary if the duct is confirmed to be headed directly out of the gallbladder. Because the most common indication for an open cholecystectomy is the presence of severe inflammation, unnecessary dissection in the porta hepatis can be unsafe and should be avoided if possible. Simple ligation of the cystic duct and artery is accomplished with separate ties, clips, endoloops, or even

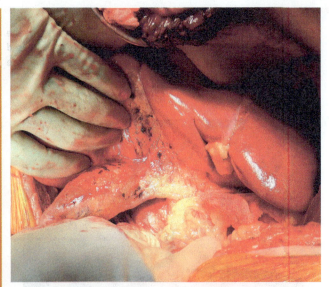

FIGURE 7 • Operative photograph of a "top-down" dissection of the gallbladder from the undersurface of the liver. The peritoneum has been incised over the triangle of Calot, exposing adipose tissue around the infundibulum of the gallbladder and the key portal structures.

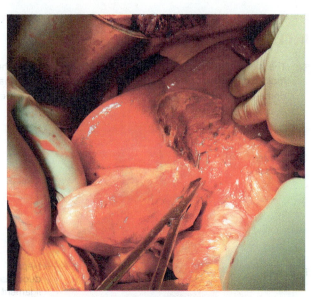

FIGURE 8 • Isolation of the cystic artery. Inferior and lateral retraction facilitates identification of the cystic artery as shown.

stapling devices if necessary. The authors recommend that if a stapling device is necessary one should consider performing a cholangiogram to truly identify correct anatomy. The gallbladder is then excised free. If the gallbladder or cystic duct appears necrotic, a drain should be placed to control a bile leak should one occur.

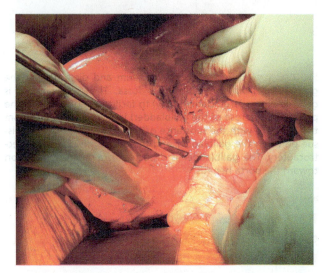

FIGURE 9 • Isolation of the cystic duct. Once the cystic artery has been ligated and divided, the cystic duct is circumferentially dissected.

ALTERNATIVE: SUBTOTAL CHOLECYSTECTOMY

- Open cholecystectomy is usually reserved for cases with severe inflammation. In some patients, the inflammation may be so severe that dissection around the neck of the gallbladder to identify the cystic duct becomes unsafe. If the cystic duct cannot be safely identified and dissected free due to adhesions, a subtotal cholecystectomy may be performed.

In this case, the gallbladder neck is dissected to the region where inflammation prohibits further dissection. The gallbladder is then transected at that point and the internal opening of the cystic duct is ligated with suture after confirming no retained gallstones (FIGURE 10). If a significant portion of the gallbladder wall remains, the remainder of the gallbladder should be fulgurated and then the edges of the walls are sewn closed with a running absorbable monofilament suture. In these cases, a drain should be left, as the

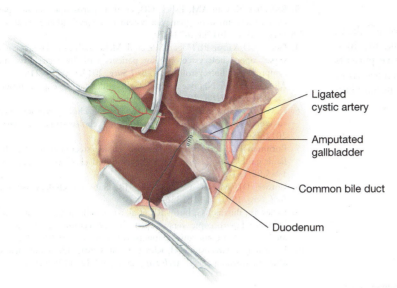

FIGURE 10 • Subtotal cholecystectomy. In cases where severe inflammation is encountered, dissection to the cystic duct may be unsafe. In such case, the infundibulum of the gallbladder can be amputated at the junction where dissection must be stopped and the cystic duct opening closed with suture ligature. When a cuff of gallbladder remains, it is fulgurated with electrocautery and closed with a running absorbable monofilament suture.

incidence of bile leak after subtotal cholecystectomy can be in excess of 20%.[6] It is for this reason that a complete cholecystectomy is performed whenever the cystic duct can be safely identified.

- If significant bleeding from the liver is encountered, such as in unsuspected portal hypertension, the back wall of the gallbladder can be left adherent to the liver.[7,8] Fulguration of any viable mucosa is advised.

CLOSURE

- The posterior and anterior fascia should be closed in separate layers. The skin is closed with staples or left open due to the clean-contaminated nature of the procedure.

PEARLS AND PITFALLS

Electrocautery	■ To avoid injury, electrocautery should be avoided when dissecting near the duodenum, colon, biliary structures, or porta hepatis.
Visualization	■ If the colon or duodenum is crowding the operative space, consider a deeper blade for the retractor, ie, "toed in" slightly on laparotomy pads.
Common bile duct injury	■ If the inflammation is so severe that it is difficult to dissect the cystic duct at the neck of the gallbladder, consider a subtotal cholecystectomy. In this circumstance, leave a drain.
Bleeding	■ During surgery for acute cholecystitis, inflammatory bleeding is often encountered from the gallbladder fossa during top-down dissection. When present, this can usually be best controlled with a laparotomy sponge and pressure applied directly to the raw surface following separation of the gallbladder from its liver bed. Often, a deeper retractor blade can be placed between the gallbladder and its bed to maintain pressure while also improving visualization.

POSTOPERATIVE CARE

- Ileus is unusual after open cholecystectomy, so diet can be rapidly advanced. Narcotic requirements will be higher than for laparoscopic cholecystectomy and a 2- to 3-day hospital stay may be necessary for adequate pain control.[9] If a cystic duct leak occurs, it will often not be clinically apparent for several days after the original operation (an average of 2.3 days).[10] Therefore, if drains were placed due to a high-risk cystic duct stump, they should be left for several days before being removed.

OUTCOMES

- Long-term outcomes after cholecystectomy are excellent. Short-term morbidities include cystic duct leak, the incidence of which averages about 0.4% for elective patients and threefold higher for emergent cholecystectomies. After subtotal cholecystectomy, issues from the remnant gallbladder are rare.[7,8]

COMPLICATIONS

- Cystic duct leak
- Common bile duct injury (<1/1000)
- Hepatic artery injury
- Wound infection
- Hemorrhage from the liver
- Injury to duodenum or transverse colon
- Retained common bile duct stone

REFERENCES

1. Kiewiet JJ, Leeuwenburgh MM, Bipat S, et al. A systematic review and meta-analysis of diagnostic performance of imaging in acute cholecystitis. *Radiology.* 2012;264(3):708-720.
2. Puc MM, Tran HS, Wry PW, et al. Ultrasound is not a useful screening tool for acute acalculous cholecystitis in critically ill trauma patients. *Am Surg.* 2002;68(1):65-69.
3. Sedaghat N, Cao AM, Eslick GD, et al. Laparoscopic versus open cholecystectomy in pregnancy: a systematic review and meta-analysis. *Surg Endosc.* 2017;31:673-679.
4. Goede BD, Klitsie PJ, Hagen MS, et al. Meta-analysis of laparoscopic versus open cholecystectomy for patients with liver cirrhosis and symptomatic cholecystolithiasis. *Br J Surg.* 2013;100:209-216.
5. Aloia TA, Jarufe N, Javle M, et al. Gallbladder cancer: expert consensus statement. *HPB.* 2015;17(8):681-690.
6. Davis B, Castaneda G, Lopez J. Subtotal cholecystectomy versus total cholecystectomy in complicated cholecystitis. *Am Surg.* 2012;78(7):814-817.
7. Bornman PC, Terblanche J. Subtotal cholecystectomy: for the difficult gallbladder in portal hypertension and cholecystitis. *Surgery.* 1985;98(1):1-6.
8. Cottier DJ, McKay C, Anderson JR. Subtotal cholecystectomy. *Br J Surg.* 1991;78(11):1326-1328.
9. Kelley JE, Burrus RG, Burns RP, et al. Safety, efficacy, cost, and morbidity of laparoscopic versus open cholecystectomy: a prospective analysis of 228 consecutive patients. *Am Surg.* 1993;59(1):23-27.
10. Eisenstein S, Greenstein AJ, Kim U, et al. Cystic duct stump leaks: after the learning curve. *Arch Surg.* 2008;143(12):1178-1183.

Chapter 3 | Radical Cholecystectomy

Richard J. Bold

DEFINITION

- Radical cholecystectomy is defined as the resection of the gallbladder and the hepatic parenchyma of the gallbladder fossa and is usually combined with a supraduodenal lymphadenectomy for the treatment of gallbladder cancer.[1] The extent of the hepatic resection may include nonanatomic parenchymal resection of the gallbladder fossa to a standard segment IVb/V resection (**FIGURE 1**), with data suggesting superior survival from segment IVb/V resection over standard cholecystectomy.[2] The goal of the resection is complete resection of all histopathologic disease, which may necessitate resection of the common hepatic duct/common bile duct (described elsewhere) if clearance of all disease cannot be obtained by division at the cystic duct/common hepatic duct junction.

DIFFERENTIAL DIAGNOSIS

- A variety of other conditions may mimic adenocarcinoma of the gallbladder. These include benign intraluminal polyps (due to the mass appearance on imaging), adenomyomatosis (due to the mucosal thickening), chronic cholecystitis especially xanthogranulomatous cholecystitis (due to the collapse of the lumen and associated mural thickening due to chronic inflammation), or hepatic masses within the gallbladder fossa (due to the presence of a hepatic mass adjacent to the gallbladder).[3] While [18]FDG PET-CT may be useful for staging (see discussion later), due to the inability to distinguish malignancy from chronic inflammation in cholecystitis, it has limited utility in the diagnostic evaluation of potential gallbladder malignancy.[4]

PATIENT HISTORY AND PHYSICAL FINDINGS

- The majority of early-stage gallbladder cancers are clinically silent and will not be diagnosed preoperatively but instead will be recognized on final pathology following cholecystectomy performed for other conditions, such as symptomatic cholelithiasis or cholecystitis.[5,6] Approximately 50% of all gallbladder cases are incidental with the diagnosis made after laparoscopic cholecystectomy; conversely due to the frequency of laparoscopic cholecystectomy performed, approximately only 0.4% of all laparoscopic cholecystectomy operations will yield gallbladder cancer.[7]
- Occasionally, polypoid gallbladder cancers will present with right upper quadrant pain similar to cholecystitis, presumably from the intraluminal mass effect or the obstruction of the fundus/cystic duct. In addition, should the tumor extend down the cystic duct to the common hepatic duct, patients may present with painless jaundice.
- Symptoms of abdominal bloating and/or weight loss should be concerning for the presence of malignant ascites due to the peritoneal metastasis, which is a common site of spread. The liver is the most other common site of metastasis.
- The incidence of gallbladder cancer is three times higher in women than in men.[8]
- Hispanics, American Indians, and Mexican Indians have been identified as high-risk groups for gallbladder cancer.[8]
- Large, multiple gallstones have an increased association with gallbladder cancer; gallstones are present in 60% to 80% of patients with gallbladder cancer.[3]
- Once thought to be associated with an extremely high risk of gallbladder cancer, the risk of an associated gallbladder cancer with a porcelain gallbladder is only 2% to 10%.[9]
- Obesity is a risk factor for both gallstones and gallbladder cancer; furthermore, obesity increases the risk for the development of nonalcoholic liver disease, particularly nonalcoholic steatohepatitis, which may impact the suitability for radical cholecystectomy.[10]
- Radical cholecystectomy involves a partial hepatic resection and therefore risk factors for cirrhosis (eg, alcohol abuse, chronic hepatitis virus infection, etc) are important aspects of the patients' history and evaluation for tolerability of hepatic resection.[11]
- Early-stage gallbladder cancer is usually not apparent on physical examination. Physical findings suggesting advanced disease include the presence of ascites (peritoneal metastasis), painless jaundice (either direct extension into the common hepatic duct or bulky portal adenopathy causing

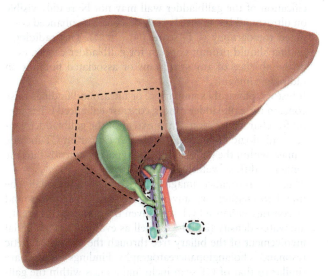

FIGURE 1 • Schematic representation of radical cholecystectomy by resection of hepatic segments IV/V (*dotted lines*), the gallbladder, and the lymphatics of the porta hepatis.

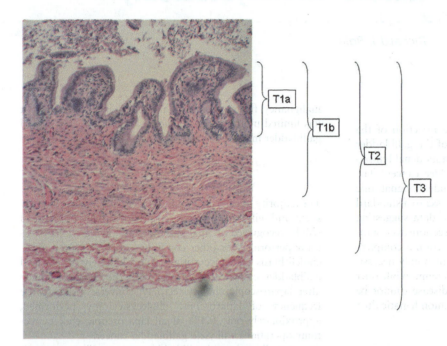

FIGURE 2 • Histology of the gallbladder wall with corresponding extent of T1a, T1b, T2, and T3 carcinoma of the gallbladder.

external biliary dilation), and a nontender, palpable gallbladder (concerning for extensive mural involvement). In addition, physical findings of end-stage liver disease raise the suspicion of underlying cirrhosis and therefore preclude radical cholecystectomy.

IMAGING AND OTHER DIAGNOSTIC STUDIES

- Radical cholecystectomy is appropriate only for those patients with T1b, T2, or T3 (primary tumor thickness), and N0 or N1 gallbladder cancer (**FIGURE 2**, **TABLE 1**).[12-17] The benefit of surgical resection has been redemonstrated in the current era of chemotherapy.[18,19]

Table 1: American Joint Commission on Cancer Staging System for Gallbladder Cancer

Primary Tumor (T)	Histopathologic Characteristics
TX	Primary tumor cannot be assessed
T0	No evidence of primary tumor
Tis	Carcinoma in situ
T1a	Tumor invades lamina propria
T1b	Tumor invades muscle layer
T2	Tumor invades the perimuscular connective tissue; no extension beyond serosa or into the liver
T3	Tumor perforates serosa and/or directly invades into the liver and/or one other adjacent organ or structure
T4	Tumor invades main portal vein or hepatic artery or involves multiple extrahepatic structures
Regional lymph nodes (N)	
NX	Regional lymph nodes cannot be assessed
N0	No regional lymph node metastasis
N1	Regional lymph node metastasis

Used with the permission of the American College of Surgeons. Amin MB, Edge SB, Greene FL, et al. (eds.) AJCC Cancer Staging Manual, 8th ed. Springer; 2017.

- The majority of patients will undergo an initial ultrasound for evaluation of right upper quadrant pain and suspected cholelithiasis. The presence of a gallbladder polyp within the lumen raises the suspicion for gallbladder cancer (**FIGURE 3**). Given the intraluminal aspect of any polyp, percutaneous biopsy is not usually feasible in the absence of any invasive features beyond the gallbladder wall.[20]
- There is only a weak association between patients with a calcified gallbladder ("porcelain gallbladder") and an underlying gallbladder cancer, such that prophylactic cholecystectomy may no longer be routinely advocated.[9] The calcification of the gallbladder wall may not be readily visible on ultrasound but is clearly seen on contrast-enhanced computed tomography (CT) scans (**FIGURE 4**). This radiologic finding should prompt concern for gallbladder cancer, even in the absence of any symptoms or associated findings on radiologic imaging.[9]
- If history, physical examination, or ultrasound findings raise concern for gallbladder cancer, contrast-enhanced CT is useful for characterization of the extent of the gallbladder cancer. Radiologic findings of gallbladder cancer on CT include a mass within the gallbladder that typically extends into the lumen or diffuse wall thickening (**FIGURE 5**).[20,21]
- Magnetic resonance imaging (MRI) may additionally be useful to characterize any mass seen on either ultrasound or contrast-enhanced CT scan given the ability to differentiate water–density (ie, bile) as well as evaluate any potential involvement of the biliary tree through the use of magnetic resonance cholangiopancreatography. Findings on MRI are similar to that of CT scan including a mass within the gallbladder lumen, focal or diffuse thickening of the gallbladder wall, or a mass replacing the gallbladder. In addition, contrast enhancement may demonstrate a difference from the density of the hepatic parenchyma and therefore useful for the determination of direct hepatic invasion (**FIGURE 6**).[22]

Chapter 3 RADICAL CHOLECYSTECTOMY   21

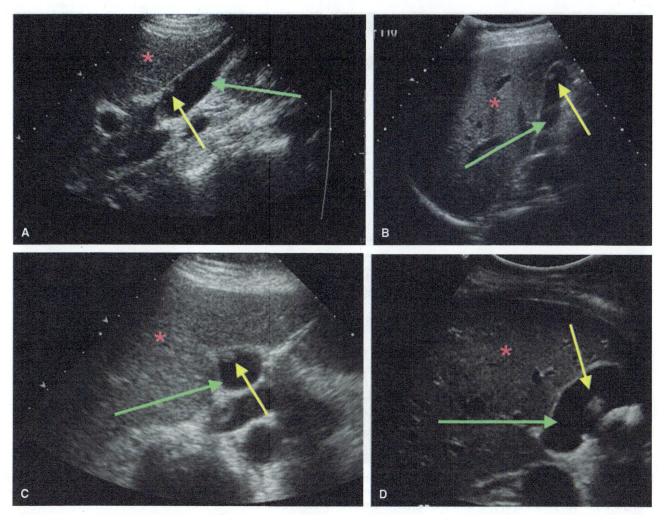

FIGURE 3 • Longitudinal (**A** and **B**) and transverse (**C** and **D**) ultrasonographic imaging of the gallbladder. A polypoid mass (*yellow arrow*) is seen within the gallbladder lumen (*green arrow*). The relationship of the polypoid mass to the liver (*red asterisk*) can be roughly determined as in (**A–C**) likely adjacent to the hepatic fossa, or (**D**), likely on the peritoneal/free aspect of the gallbladder.

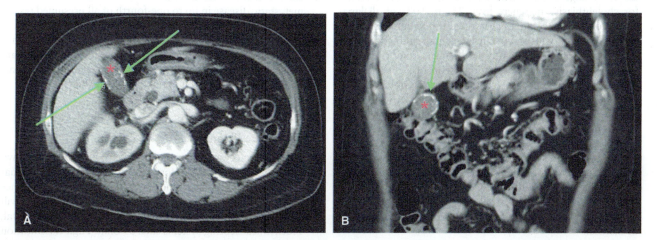

FIGURE 4 • Axial (**A**) and coronal (**B**) contrast-enhanced computed tomography findings of porcelain gallbladder. The calcification of the gallbladder wall (*green arrow*) is seen as a diffuse process, outlining the lumen of the gallbladder (red asterisk).

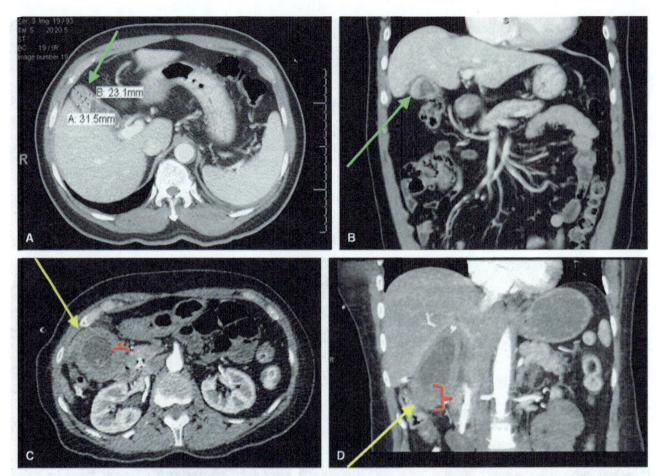

FIGURE 5 • Axial (**A** and **C**) and coronal (**B** and **D**) contrast-enhanced computed tomography findings of gallbladder cancer. Typical appearance may include that of a mass with intraluminal extension (*green arrow*; panels **A, B**), or diffuse thickening of the gallbladder wall (*yellow arrow*; panels **C, D**) with a measured wall thickness in excess of 2 mm.

- Unfortunately, many gallbladder cancers are not diagnosed preoperatively but identified in the final pathology specimen for early-stage disease after laparoscopic cholecystectomy for cholelithiasis; anywhere from 2% to 10% of all laparoscopic cholecystectomies performed for benign conditions as cholelithiasis will harbor an incidental gallbladder cancer.[9,23] Additionally, some advanced staged tumors may be mistaken for chronic cholecystitis preoperatively and only identified in the operating room. These tumors will have preoperative imaging of a contracted gallbladder with thickened walls. Intraoperatively, these tumors are clearly identified as malignant, with laparoscopic findings of nonpliable tissue, extremely thickened gallbladder wall, and often invasion into adjacent structures (eg, omentum, liver, duodenum, hepatic flexure of the colon, etc) (**FIGURE 7**).
- The tumor markers CEA and CA 19-9 may be elevated in patients with gallbladder cancer but are neither sensitive nor specific for diagnostic purposes or correlation with extent of disease.[24]
- Although patients may not have been noted to have any metastatic disease at the time of laparoscopic cholecystectomy, all should undergo imaging with at least a contrast-enhanced CT scan prior to definitive resection. Furthermore, there is early evidence that a [18]FDG PET-CT may identify occult metastatic disease in up to one-fourth of all presumed resectable patients.[25]
- The role of adjuvant chemotherapy in resectable gallbladder cancer is well established, though there is a lack of data with regard to neoadjuvant chemotherapy with clinical trials ongoing to establish the optimal regimen and timing.[26,27]

SURGICAL MANAGEMENT

Preoperative Planning

- Radical cholecystectomy may involve resection of up to two segments (IVb/V). Therefore, careful preoperative evaluation of hepatic function and the evaluation for the presence of cirrhosis is critical in determining whether the patient will have suitable hepatic reserve following parenchymal removal. Biochemical scoring systems such as Child-Pugh classification or the Model for End-Stage Liver Disease (MELD) can be useful for predicting morbidity and mortality following resection

Chapter 3 RADICAL CHOLECYSTECTOMY

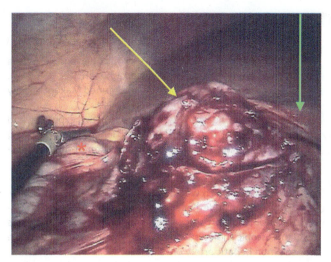

FIGURE 7 • Laparoscopic identification of a gallbladder cancer with diffuse firm, nodular thickening of the gallbladder wall (*yellow arrow*) with direct invasion of the hepatic flexure of the colon (*red asterisk*) as well as the hepatic parenchyma (*green arrow*).

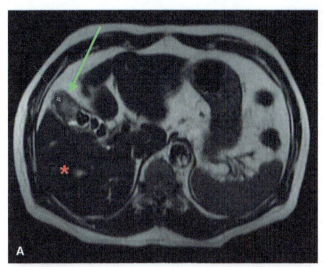

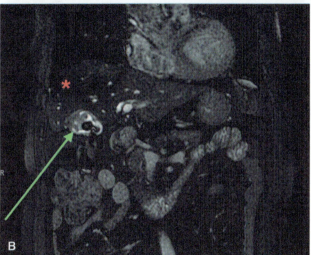

FIGURE 6 • Axial (**A**) and coronal (**B**) contrast-enhanced magnetic resonance imaging findings of gallbladder cancer. A focal thickening of the gallbladder wall is noted (*green arrow*) adjacent to the normal hepatic parenchyma (red asterisk).

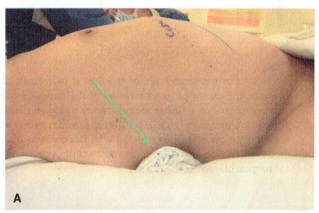

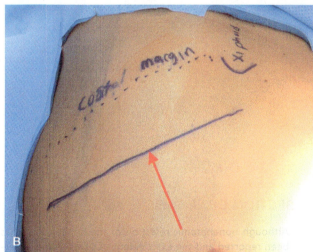

FIGURE 8 • Patient position for a radical cholecystectomy with a lateral view (panel **A**) demonstrating a rolled sheet (*green arrow*) under the back to allow flexion of the patient, which may be combined with flexing of the operative table, and the planned right subcostal (Kocher) incision (*red arrow*, panel **B**) approximately 2 finger breadths below the costal margin.

in cirrhotic patients. In addition, functional tests such as indocyanine green clearance can be a useful functional test, which can be used with computer software to preoperatively estimate the amount of resected hepatic tissue.[11,28-30]

- Although infections are uncommon following hepatic resection, prophylactic antibiotics should be administered to cover skin flora. If the patient has had recent biliary instrumentation, including the presence of a decompressive biliary stent, antibiotics should include coverage of intestinal flora.

Positioning

- Radical cholecystectomy is performed through a right subcostal incision. To facilitate exposure of the inferior aspect of the liver, the operative table may be slightly extended or a roll can be placed transversely under the patient's lower thoracic region (**FIGURE 8A**). These maneuvers elevate the costal margin and increase operative exposure of the liver.

SECTION I SURGERY OF THE BILIARY SYSTEM

TECHNIQUES

INCISION AND EXPOSURE

- A right subcostal incision offers excellent exposure of the gallbladder, hepatic fossa, and porta hepatic (**FIGURE 8B**). Alternatively a J-shaped incision (also termed Makuuchi) may offer broader exposure of the portal triad.
- The falciform ligament is divided to allow exposure and mobilization of the anterior hepatic lobes. A self-retaining retractor is placed that allows for retraction of the right costal margin and inferior abdominal wall (**FIGURE 9**).
- Exploration of the abdomen is performed to exclude metastatic disease which would preclude radical cholecystectomy. This would include hepatic metastasis, peritoneal metastases (including port site disease if the patient had a previous laparoscopic cholecystectomy), or lymph node disease of the common hepatic artery or celiac axis.
- The lesser omentum (also termed the gastrohepatic ligament) is divided to allow exposure of the common hepatic artery as well as the medial aspect of the porta hepatis. The porta hepatis is encircled with an umbilical tape that can be used as Rummel tourniquet during a Pringle maneuver if vascular inflow occlusion is desired.

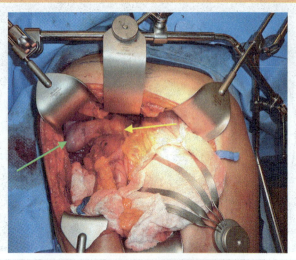

FIGURE 9 • Exposure of the gallbladder with placement of a self-retaining retractor to allow complete exposure of the gallbladder (*green arrow*) as well as the porta hepatic (*yellow arrow*). Costal margins are retracted superiorly as well as the hepatic flexure of the colon inferiorly.

INTRAOPERATIVE ULTRASOUND

- Ultrasound of segments IVb/V of the liver is performed to evaluate any extent of direct invasion of the hepatic fossa by the malignancy. A T-shaped linear array transducer with a broad frequency range (eg, 4-10 MHz) provides excellent resolution, especially when coupled with Doppler scanning mode to facilitate identification of vascular inflow structures for surgical planning (**FIGURE 10**).

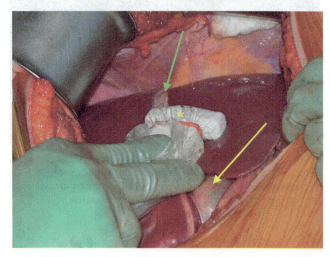

FIGURE 10 • Intraoperative ultrasound is performed using a T-shaped linear array transducer (asterisk) to allow interrogation of the hepatic parenchyma after the falciform ligament (*green arrow*) has been divided, as well as evaluation of the hepatic inflow vascular, and the possible extent of the cancer from the gallbladder (*yellow arrow*) into the hepatic fossa.

RESECTION OF SEGMENT IVB/V

- Although nonanatomic resection of the hepatic fossa has been reported and the exact extent of parenchymal resection remains a point of controversy, formal resection of segments IVb (inferior aspect of segment IV) and V has traditionally been considered the appropriate segments of resection for radical cholecystectomy (see Chapter 15, Figure 2).
- The hepatic parenchymal transection can be performed using a variety of techniques including clamp-crushing technique, ultrasonic dissection, thermal sealing devices (eg, LigaSure,

Chapter 3 RADICAL CHOLECYSTECTOMY

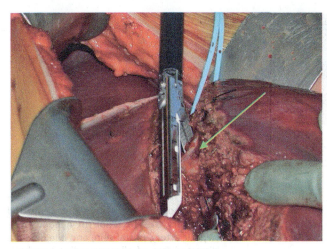

FIGURE 11 • Following division of the hepatic parenchyma to segments IVb/V, a vascular stapler can be used to divide the portal venous branch (*green arrow*) to segment IVb/V.

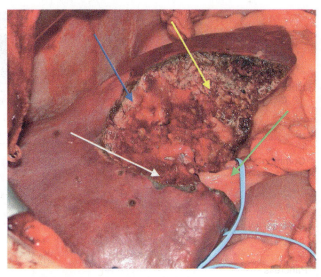

FIGURE 12 • Completed radical cholecystectomy with raw surface of the boundary of resection. The margin between segments III and IVb (*yellow arrow*), segments IVa and IVb (*blue arrow*), and segments V and VI (*white arrow*) define a resected radical cholecystectomy. The porta hepatis (*green arrow*) can be controlled with a vessel loop (blue vessel loop).

Harmonic), radiofrequency sealing devices (TissueLink), bipolar sealing devices (Aquamantys), or water jet dissection (see Chapter 19).
- Major hepatic vasculature can be ligated with either traditional suture ligation or stapling devices utilizing vascular staple loads (FIGURE 11).
- Should significant bleeding be encountered, the Rommel tourniquet can be used for temporary vascular inflow control (Pringle maneuver) to allow direct suture ligation or hemoclip application to ensure hemostasis.
- Following removal of segments IVb/V, the specimen should be oriented for the pathologist with intraoperative gross assessment of the margins if there is concern of significant tumor ingrowth into the hepatic fossa.
- The hepatic parenchymal surface is inspected for hemostasis and any evidence of biliary leak (FIGURE 12). Hemostasis can be obtained with either hemoclips or suture ligations; open biliary radicals should be directly suture ligated. The role of fibrin sealants may facilitate achieving hemostasis, but has not been shown to reduce the incidence of bile leakage.[31,32]
- An omental flap should be mobilized from the hepatic flexure of the colon and placed into the parenchymal cavity. This may facilitate the closure of small bile leaks. A closed suction drain is then placed into the abdomen over the omental flap ensuring that it provides drainage for the full extent of the hepatic parenchymal raw surface.

PORTAL LYMPHADENECTOMY AND OPTIONAL RESECTION OF THE EXTRAHEPATIC BILIARY TREE

- The lymphatic drainage of the gallbladder is primarily along the cystic duct/lymph node of Calot into the lymphatics surrounding the portal triad. Resection of these lymph nodes not only provides staging information for predicting survival but also appears to confer an improved outcome.[33]
- If the cystic duct margin status is unable to be assessed or positive, or biliary obstruction is present, excision of the extrahepatic biliary tree is indicated.
- Lymphadenectomy should be performed regardless but may lead to ischemia to the extrahepatic biliary tree, resulting in delayed presentation of biliary stricture. Thus, some surgeons advocate routine excision of the extrahepatic biliary tree as a fundamental component of radical cholecystectomy.
- The peritoneum of the porta hepatis is circumferentially incised just below the liver plate and at the level of the first portion of the duodenum (FIGURE 13).
- The hepatic artery and the portal vein are circumferentially dissected of associated lymphatics and splanchnic nerves. Ligation or bipolar electrocautery should be employed as these structures are rich in vascular supply. Care is taken to include the hepatic lymph nodes (FIGURE 13) in this dissection. Note that the majority of the portal lymph nodes are posterior and lateral to the preserved structures.
- If indicated, the common bile duct is divided as it enters the pancreatic parenchyma. The distal lumen should be oversewn with a running, monofilament suture of absorbable material. Assessment of this margin intraoperatively is controversial.

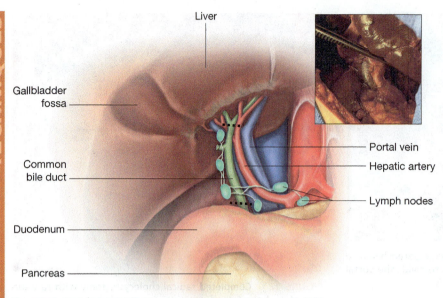

FIGURE 13 • Schematic representation of the portal lymph node dissection and the biliary tree resection (if needed). The hepatic artery, portal vein, and bile duct are dissected free of all surrounding lymphatic tissue. Completed portal lymph node dissection with skeletonization of the common hepatic/common bile duct as well as the hepatic artery (inset).

- The proximal hepatic duct is divided just distal to the confluence of the right and left hepatic ducts. An assessment of the proximal margin intraoperatively may be reasonable if an additional margin is feasible.
- Reconstruction of the biliary tree via Roux-en-Y hepaticojejunostomy is reviewed in detail in Chapter 14.

- The soft tissue of the porta hepatic and all lymph nodes should be resected from the hilar plate inferiorly to the pancreatic head/duodenal sweep. Care should be taken in the skeletonization of the bile duct to avoid injury (FIGURE 13 inset).

PEARLS AND PITFALLS

Indications	Preoperative abnormalities on ultrasound should be further evaluated with contrast-enhanced CT scans to rule out advanced/unresectable disease.
	Liver function should be carefully and thoroughly evaluated to ensure tolerability of hepatic bisegmentectomy.
	Gallbladder cancers diagnosed on postoperative pathology from laparoscopic cholecystectomy should be reimaged with contrast-enhanced CT scans to rule out advanced disease not identified at laparoscopy.
Placement of incision	Right subcostal incisions should be placed approximately 2 cm below the costal margin to ensure sufficient exposure yet allow adequate fascia for closure.
	If the gallbladder cancer is diagnosed following laparoscopic cholecystectomy, consideration should be given to excising the previous port site incisions.
Parenchymal transection	Care should be taken during parenchymal transection (independent of the method used) to seal major biliary radicals to reduce the incidence of a postoperative biliary leak.
	Marking of the planned lines of parenchymal transection can facilitate complete resection of segments IVb/V, especially posteriorly at the porta hepatic.
Vascular control	Preresection intraoperative ultrasound can be useful to identify the major vascular inflow to ensure ligation at the initiation of parenchymal transection.
	An umbilical tape around the porta hepatic can be a useful adjunct to allow rapid initiation of a Pringle maneuver to allow for hemostasis; care should be taken to minimize the time of vascular inflow clamping.
Closure	The closed suction drain should be placed to allow complete drainage of the hepatic operative bed, but not placed directly adjacent to the parenchyma but instead over the transposed omental flap.

POSTOPERATIVE CARE

- Adequate pain control is critical to the postoperative recovery of patients undergoing major hepatic resection. Thoracic epidural catheters may be beneficial in environments with sufficient expertise for placement and care.
- Laboratory assessment of coagulation profile should be routine checked and treated if abnormal to ensure adequate hemostasis.
- Elevated serum bilirubin levels can be a harbinger of bile leak, hepatic insufficiency, or vascular thrombosis. A contrast-enhanced CT scan should be used to differentiate the three etiologies.
- The fluid effluent from the closed suction drain can be evaluated for bilirubin content to evaluate for a bile leak. The drain should be removed as soon as there is no concern for a postoperative bile leak.

OUTCOMES

- Long-term hepatic function should not be adversely affected if the patient had normal preoperative hepatic function.
- Hepatic and peritoneal sites are the most common location for recurrent gallbladder cancer; outcomes are dependent on the initial TNM stage. Early-stage disease (ie, Stage I) may be associated with 60% to 80% 5-year survival rates, whereas advanced stage disease (ie, Stage III) is associated with <20% 5-year survival.

COMPLICATIONS

- Hemorrhage
- Bile leak
- Abscess formation
- Delayed stricture of the common hepatic duct/common bile duct due to devascularization associated with portal lymphadenectomy

REFERENCES

1. Marsh RDW, Alonzo M, Bajaj S, et al. Comprehensive review of the diagnosis and treatment of biliary tract cancer 2012. Part II: multidisciplinary management. *J Surg Oncol*. 2012;106:339-345.
2. Pilgrim C, Usatoff V, Evans P. A review of the surgical strategies for the management of gallbladder carcinoma based on T stage and growth type of the tumour. *Eur J Surg Oncol*. 2009;35:903-907.
3. Marsh RDW, Alonzo M, Bajaj S, et al. Comprehensive review of the diagnosis and treatment of biliary tract cancer 2012. Part I: diagnosis-clinical staging and pathology. *J Surg Oncol*. 2012;106:332-338.
4. Bo X, Chen E, Wang J, et al. Diagnostic accuracy of imaging modalities in differentiating xanthogranulomatous cholecystitis from gallbladder cancer. *Ann Transl Med*. 2019;7(22):627. doi:10.21037/atm.2019.11.35
5. Konstantinidis IT, Deshpande V, Genevay M, et al. Trends in presentation and survival for gallbladder cancer during a period of more than 4 decades: a single institution experience. *Arch Surg*. 2009;144:441-447.
6. Kiran RP, Pokala N, Dudrick SJ. Incidence pattern and survival for gallbladder cancer over three decades-an analysis of 10301 patients. *Ann Surg Oncol*. 2007;14:827-832.
7. Kellil T, Chaouch MA, Aloui E, et al. Incidence and preoperative predictor factors of gallbladder cancer before laparoscopic cholecystectomy: a systematic review. *J Gastrointest Cancer*. 2021;52(1):68-72. doi:10.1007/s12029-020-00524-7
8. Siegel RS, Miller KD, Fuchs HE, Jemal A. Cancer Statistics 2021. *CA Cancer J Clin*. 2021;71(1):7-33. doi:10.3322/caac.21654
9. Khan ZS, Livingston EH, Huerta S. Reassessing the need for prophylactic surgery in patients with porcelain gallbladder: case series and systematic review of the literature. *Arch Surg*. 2011;146(10):1143-1147.doi:10.1001/archsurg.2011.257
10. Vucenik I, Stains JP. Obesity and cancer risk: evidence, mechanisms, and recommendations. *Ann NY Acad Sci*. 2012;1271:37-43.
11. Schneider PD. Preoperative assessment of liver function. *Surg Clin North Am*. 2004;84:355-373.
12. Coburn NG, Cleary SP, Tan JCC, Law CHL. Surgery for gallbladder cancer: a population-based analysis. *J Am Coll Surg*. 2008;207:371-382.
13. Downing SR, Cadogan K-R, Ortega G, et al. Early-stage gallbladder cancer in the surveillance, epidemiology, and end results database. *Arch Surg*. 2011;146:734-738.
14. Duffy A, Capanu M, Abou-Alfa GK, et al. Gallbladder cancer (GBC): 10-year experience Memorial Sloan-Kettering Cancer Centre (MSKCC). *J Surg Oncol*. 2008;98:485-489.
15. Foster JM, Hoshi H, Gibbs JF, et al. Gallbladder cancer: defining the indications for primary radical resection and re-resection. *Ann Surg Oncol*. 2007;14:833-840.
16. Jensen EH, Abraham A, Jarosek S, et al. A critical analysis of the surgical management of early-stage gallbladder cancer in the United States. *J Gastrointest Surg*. 2009;13:722-727.
17. Mayo SC, Shore AD, Nathan H, et al. National trends in the management and survival of surgically managed gallbladder adenocarcinoma over 15 years: a population-based analysis. *J Gastrointest Surg*. 2010;14:1578-1591.
18. Xu L, Tan H, Liu X, et al. Survival benefits of simple versus extended cholecystectomy and lymphadenectomy for patients with T1b gallbladder cancer: an analysis of the surveillance, epidemiology, and end results database (2004 to 2013). *Cancer Med*. 2020;9(11):3668-3679. doi:10.1002/cam4.2989
19. Chen M, Cao J, Xiang Y, et al. Hepatectomy strategy for T2 gallbladder cancer between segment IVb and V resection and wedge resection: a propensity score-matched study. *Surgery*. 2021;169(6):1304-1311. doi:10.1016/j.surg.2020.12.039
20. Pilgrim CHC, Groeschl RT, Pappas SG, Gamblin TC. An often overlooked diagnosis: imaging features of gallbladder cancer. *J Am Coll Surg*. 2013;216:333-339.
21. Ganesha D, Kambadakone A, Nikolaidis P, et al. Current update on gallbladder carcinoma. *Abdom Radiol (NY)*. 2021;46(6):2474-2489. doi:10.1007/s00261-020-02871-2
22. Ogawa T, Horaguchi J, Fujita N, et al. High b-value diffusion-weighted magnetic resonance imaging for gallbladder lesions: differentiation between benignity and malignancy. *J Gastroenterol*. 2012;47:1352-1360.
23. Choi SB, Han HJ, Kim CY, et al. Incidental gallbladder cancer diagnosed following laparoscopic cholecystectomy. *World J Surg*. 2009;33:2657-2663.
24. Rana S, Dutta U, Kockhar R, et al. Evaluation of CA 242 as a tumor marker in gallbladder cancer. *J Gastrointest Cancer*. 2012;43:267-271.
25. Goel S, Aggarwal A, Iqbal A, et al. 18-FDG PET-CT should be included in preoperative staging of gallbladder cancer. *Eur J Surg Oncol*. 2020;46(9):1711-1716. doi:10.1016/j.ejso.2020.04.015
26. Yua K, Sakat J, Hiros Y, et al. Outcome of radical surgery for gallbladder carcinoma according to TNM stage: implications for adjuvant therapeutic strategies. *Langenbeck's Arch Surg*. 2021;406(3):801-811. doi:10.1007/s00423-020-02068-7
27. Khan TM, Verbus EA, Hong H, et al. Perioperative versus adjuvant chemotherapy in the management of incidentally found gallbladder cancer (OPT-IN). *Ann Surg Oncol*.2021;29(1):37-38. doi:10.1245/s10434-021-10277-7
28. Hsu KY, Chau GY, Lui WY, et al. Predicting morbidity and mortality after hepatic resection in patients with hepatocellular carcinoma: the role of Model for End-Stage Liver Disease score. *World J Surg*. 2009;33:2412-2419.

29. Lang H, Radtke A, Hindennach M, et al. Impact of virtual tumor resection and computer-assisted risk analysis on operation planning and intraoperative strategy in major hepatic resection. *Arch Surg.* 2005;140:629-638.
30. Manizate F, Hiotis SP, Labow D, et al. Liver functional reserve estimation: state of the art and relevance for local treatments—the Western perspective. *J Hepatobiliary Pancreat Sci.* 2010;17:385-388.
31. de Boer MT, Boonstra EA, Lisman T, Porte RJ. Role of fibrin sealants in liver surgery. *Dig Surg.* 2012;29:54-61.
32. Hanna EM, Martinie JB, Swan RZ, Iannitti DA. Fibrin sealants and topical agents in hepatobiliary and pancreatic surgery: a critical appraisal. *Langenbeck's Arch Surg.* 2014;399(7):825-835. doi:10.1007/s00423-014-1215-5
33. Maegawa FB, Ashour Y, Hamadi M, et al. Gallbladder cancer surgery in the United States: lymphadenectomy trends and the impact on survival. *J Surg Res.* 2021;258:54-63. doi:10.1016/j.jss.2020.08.041

Chapter 4

Endoscopic Retrograde Cholangiopancreatography

Shailendra S. Chauhan and Dennis Yang

DEFINITION

- Endoscopic retrograde cholangiopancreatography (ERCP) is an endoscopic technique whereby a specialized side-viewing upper endoscope (duodenoscope) is passed through the mouth to the major papilla in the second portion of the duodenum.
- Using various instruments through the working channel of the duodenoscope, access can be gained into the bile and pancreatic ducts and a variety of complex interventions can be performed. The ducts are usually visualized with x-ray after injection of a contrast medium into the ducts. Alternatively, direct visualization of the ducts is also possible via smaller scopes usually passed through the working channel of the duodenoscope or directly into the ducts without use of the duodenoscope.
- ERCP allows for minimally invasive management of pancreatic and biliary disorders, but it can be a challenging technique to learn and has higher potential for complications than other standard endoscopic procedures.

DIFFERENTIAL DIAGNOSIS

- ERCP should be performed with a therapeutic intent and not for routine diagnostic purposes only.
- The endoscopist should obtain diagnostic information from patient history and physical, imaging, and laboratory parameters to carefully select those patients who will benefit most from therapeutic ERCP.
- ERCP is commonly performed for the evaluation and management of various pancreaticobiliary obstructive processes. These can generally be broadly divided into benign and malignant etiologies as outlined in **TABLE 1**.

PATIENT HISTORY AND PHYSICAL FINDINGS

- Prior to ERCP, a thorough patient history and physical examination should be performed to select appropriate laboratory and imaging studies for workup. These preprocedural studies will enable the proper selection of patients to benefit most from ERCP. A careful history of pancreatic and biliary symptoms and previous endoscopic and surgical therapy of the biliary tree or pancreas is essential. In addition, previous intestinal surgery may make ERCP technically difficult or impossible (such as a previous Roux-en-Y gastric bypass). Finally, complicating medical conditions can be elicited, which might impact the safety of anesthesia or increase the risk of complications of ERCP (such as anticoagulation).
- ERCP is indicated for patients with a variety of biliary tract and pancreatic disorders.[1,2] For patients with such disorders, specific symptoms may include abdominal pain (location, character, frequency, duration, alleviating and exacerbating factors), nausea and vomiting, jaundice, change in color of stools and urine, pruritus, steatorrhea, weight loss, and hyper or hypoglycemia. Physical examination should evaluate for jaundice, detailed abdominal examination, and signs of malnutrition or cachexia, which may suggest underlying chronic disease or malignancy.
- Key aspects of social history include tobacco use and alcohol. In those patients with suspected malignancy, it is important to elicit any family history of similar malignancies.

IMAGING AND OTHER DIAGNOSTIC STUDIES

- Specific laboratory work obtained to decide the need for ERCP usually includes liver enzymes (transaminases, alkaline phosphatase, direct and indirect bilirubin) and pancreatic enzymes (amylase and lipase). In suspected malignancy, certain tumor markers such as carbohydrate antigen 19-9, carcinoembryonic antigen, and α-fetoprotein may be obtained as deemed appropriate. Typically, coagulation parameters (platelets, prothrombin time, international normalized ratio, and partial thromboplastin time) are not obtained unless the patient is on anticoagulation or history suggests coagulopathy.
- Imaging studies for suspected biliary and pancreatic disease may include transabdominal ultrasound; high-quality, cross-sectional imaging such as abdominal computed tomography (CT) scan; or magnetic resonance imaging (MRI) or magnetic resonance cholangiopancreatography (MRCP). Transabdominal ultrasound is typically not adequate for accurate visualization of the entire pancreas. Endoscopic ultrasound (EUS), however, can provide valuable information about pancreatic ductal and parenchymal anatomy and biliary anatomy for proper selection of patients for ERCP.

SURGICAL MANAGEMENT

- ERCP has evolved from a diagnostic to an almost exclusively therapeutic procedure.[1,2] Imaging studies that have been described in the previous section (transabdominal ultrasound, CT, MRI/MRCP, intraoperative cholangiography, EUS) should provide diagnostic information for proper selection

Table 1: Common Causes of Pancreaticobiliary Obstruction

Benign etiologies	Malignant etiologies
Choledocholithiasis	Ampullary adenoma/carcinoma
Choledochal cyst	Gallbladder cancer
Mirizzi syndrome	Cholangiocarcinoma
Duodenal diverticulum	Pancreatic cancer
Acute and chronic pancreatitis	Lymphoma
Benign biliary stricture	Extrabiliary malignancies
Ampullary stenosis	
Biliary atresia	
Benign infectious/ischemic/inflammatory cholangiopathy	

of patients requiring therapeutic ERCP. In general, a careful assessment of pancreatic ductal and biliary anatomy by one of these techniques is required prior to considering ERCP. ERCP should almost never be used for diagnostic purposes only, as the risk of ERCP outweighs the benefit in this circumstance.
- ERCP is not indicated in the evaluation of abdominal pain of obscure origin in the absence of other objective findings suggesting biliary tract or pancreatic disease.[1,2]
- ERCP is indicated in patients with various pancreaticobiliary disorders. Specific biliary indications include therapy for choledocholithiasis, management of benign and malignant biliary strictures (including tissue sampling, stricture dilation, stenting), and evaluation and treatment of bile leaks.[1,2]
- Pancreatic diseases that can be evaluated and treated with ERCP include recurrent acute pancreatitis, management of pain in patients with chronic pancreatitis with obstruction of pancreatic duct due to stones and/or strictures, pancreatic duct leaks, drainage of fluid collections that communicate with the pancreatic duct, and pancreatic cancer causing pancreatic duct and/or bile duct obstruction.[1,2]
- Other specific conditions that can be evaluated and treated with ERCP include ampullary stenosis, sphincter of Oddi dysfunction (SOD), type III biliary cysts (choledochocele), pancreas divisum causing recurrent acute pancreatitis, and treatment of ampullary cancers and adenomas.[1,2]
- **TABLE 2** outlines indications for therapeutic ERCP.

Table 2: Indications for Therapeutic Endoscopic Retrograde Cholangiopancreatography

Biliary
- Choledocholithiasis
  - High preoperative probability
  - Intraoperatively diagnosed
  - Definitive diagnosis prior to surgery
- Strictures
  - Benign
  - Malignant
- Postoperative bile leaks
- Choledochocele (type III biliary cyst)
- Biliary sphincter of Oddi dysfunction
  - Type I
  - Type II

Pancreatic
- Chronic pancreatitis
  - Stricture
  - Stones
  - Both
- Pancreatic duct disruption
- Transpapillary pseudocyst drainage
- Strictures
  - Benign
  - Malignant
- Acute pancreatitis
  - Acute biliary pancreatitis
  - Recurrent acute pancreatitis
  - Pancreas divisum causing recurrent acute pancreatitis
- Pancreatic sphincter of Oddi dysfunction
  - Type I
  - Type II

Other
- Ampullary cancer or adenoma

Reprinted from Pannu DS, Draganov PV. Therapeutic endoscopic retrograde cholangiopancreatography and instrumentation. Gastrointest Endosc Clin N Am. 2012;22(3):401-416. Copyright © 2012 Elsevier. With permission.

Preoperative Planning

- ERCP is usually performed as an outpatient procedure, but postprocedural observation may be prolonged due to the potential complexity of the procedure as compared with other standard endoscopic procedures.
- Prior to initiation of the procedure, the endoscopist should be absolutely certain of the indication of the procedure taking into account all of the preprocedural workup. The importance of having a well-defined therapeutic goal for the procedure cannot be overemphasized. ERCP should not be performed for diagnostic purposes only.
- Informed consent should be obtained, explaining all the potential benefits, risks, and alternatives. This should include a discussion of the risk to that individual patient, taking into account the patient and procedural factors that influence the rate of postprocedure complications.
- **TABLE 3** details risk factors for overall complications of ERCP.
- Patients are kept NPO overnight prior to the procedure. Antibiotics with broad-spectrum coverage should be considered periprocedurally in only limited circumstances of biliary ductal obstruction or transpapillary pancreatic pseudocyst drainage.

Positioning

- The patient lies in a left semiprone position on the fluoroscopy table with both arms at their side. The right chest/shoulder is usually propped up slightly so that the head faces the endoscopist (**FIGURE 1**). A plain radiograph (scout film) is usually taken to ensure the field is clear of any radiopaque material such as monitoring wires and to document the presence/absence of any devices such as drains, stents, and feeding tubes.
- Sedation can be either conscious sedation (combination of benzodiazepine and opiate) administered under the supervision of the endoscopist or monitored anesthesia care (MAC). Most units now use either MAC or general anesthesia, depending on patient and case specifics.

Table 3: Risk Factors for Overall Complications of Endoscopic Retrograde Cholangiopancreatography

Definite	Possible	No
Sphincter of Oddi dysfunction	Young age	Comorbid illness
Cirrhosis	Pancreatic contrast injection	Small-diameter CBD
Difficult cannulation	Failed biliary drainage	Female sex
Precut sphincterotomy	Trainee involvement	Billroth II anatomy
Lower case volume	Periampullary diverticulum	
Percutaneous biliary access		

CBD, common bile duct.
Reprinted from Freeman ML. Complications of endoscopic retrograde cholangiopancreatography: avoidance and management. Gastrointest Endosc Clin N Am. 2012;22(3):567-586. Copyright © 2012 Elsevier. With permission.

Chapter 4 **ENDOSCOPIC RETROGRADE CHOLANGIOPANCREATOGRAPHY**

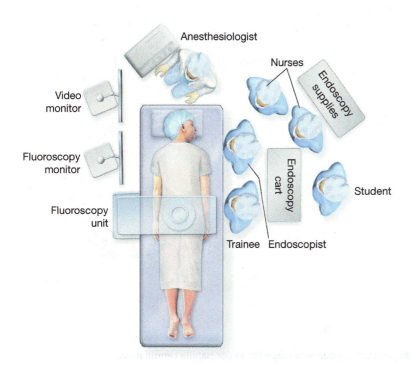

FIGURE 1 • Positioning of patient for ERCP.

- Depending on the indications, various maneuvers may be performed during ERCP. However, passage of the scope to the major papilla in the duodenum and selective cannulation of the desired duct is essential to every successful ERCP.

INTUBATION OF ESOPHAGUS AND PASSAGE OF SCOPE TO DUODENUM

- Because the duodenoscope is a side-viewing instrument, passage through the oropharynx and esophagus is more by feel than direct visualization. Before intubation, ensure that instrument is in proper working order. The up-and-down and lateral movement dials should be unlocked and the elevator checked to ensure proper functioning; the elevator should be in a relaxed (down) position during insertion. The light source and attachments to the scope, that is, irrigation, suction, insufflation should be checked. Once the patient is adequately sedated, the back of the scope is lubricated (taking care not to smear over the lens) and the scope is guided over the patient's tongue to the upper esophageal sphincter. With gentle pressure, the scope should pass into the patient's esophagus and down to the stomach. If any abnormal resistance is encountered while intubating the esophagus, the scope should not be forced. It may need to be removed and the anatomy reviewed with a forward-viewing gastroscope.
- Once the scope enters the stomach, slight air insufflation may be required to orient the tip toward the antrum. The scope is then passed along the greater curvature toward the pylorus. Once the exact location of the pylorus is determined, the scope tip is angled upward and advanced through the pylorus. Because of the side-viewing nature of the scope, the pylorus will not be seen as the scope passes through it.
- The scope is then passed carefully under direct vision to the level of the second portion of the duodenum. Full forward vision is not possible with this scope, and duodenal perforation is possible if an attempt is made to obtain a full forward view of the lumen. At this point, the scope is usually in a "long position." A shortening maneuver is performed by torquing the scope shaft clockwise and pulling the scope out of the patient's mouth while the right wheel is locked in a full rightward position. This usually leads to paradoxical forward motion of the scope tip such that the scope ends up in the preferred "short position" (FIGURE 2). From this position, small adjustments can be made with a combination of movement of up-and-down and lateral movement dials as well as the endoscopist changing their stance slightly left or right. These motions ultimately bring the major papilla into an adequate en face cannulating position. At this point, depending on endoscopist preference, the scope dials may be locked for a more stable position.

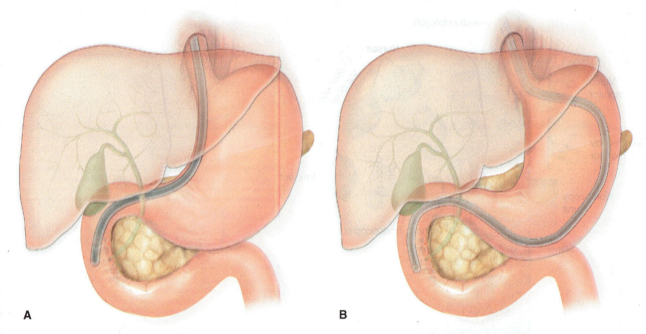

FIGURE 2 • Short **(A)** and long **(B)** positions of duodenoscope for major papilla cannulation.

MAJOR PAPILLA CANNULATION

- Selective cannulation of the desired duct is the most important and most difficult skill to master for successful ERCP. Knowledge of normal papillary anatomy is essential, as is adequate training and experience. The most common reason for failure is inability to cannulate the duct of interest. Studies suggest that 180 to 200 cases in training are necessary before even moderate rates of cannulation are achieved.[3] Furthermore, it has been suggested that it takes about 1000 cannulations to become truly comfortable with the technique and several thousand more to become expert.[4] Various cannulation techniques have been described, but all involve the use of catheters and guidewires. Typically, catheters with cutting wires (sphincterotomes) and preloaded guidewires are used for therapeutic ERCP. Another general principle is to avoid too much contrast injection until the endoscopist is reasonably sure that the cannulating device is at least superficially in the desired duct. This serves to avoid too much fluoroscopic exposure, avoid submucosal injection, and reduce the risk of post-ERCP pancreatitis.
- Selective biliary cannulation is initially achieved by superficially probing the major papilla usually at the 10- to 12-o'clock position, thereby staying superior to the intraductal septum and aiming the catheter upward (**FIGURE 3**). Once the catheter tip has advanced slightly into the duct orifice, either the guidewire can be advanced further or contrast can be injected to confirm position. If inadvertent pancreatic duct cannulation is achieved, it is important to avoid or limit any contrast injection (unless pancreatic duct cannulation is desired). Once superficial biliary cannulation is confirmed, the guidewire is advanced further proximally into the duct followed by catheter advancement to achieve deep cannulation.
- Selective pancreatic cannulation is achieved by approaching the papilla generally at its center but aiming at the 2-o'clock position. This usually aligns the catheter tip axis below the

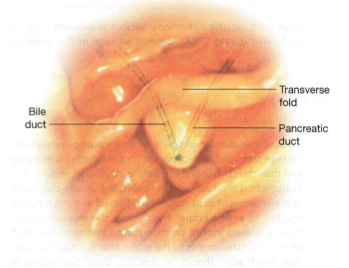

FIGURE 3 • Approach to major papilla for selective cannulation of bile and pancreatic ducts.

septum toward the pancreatic duct orifice (**FIGURE 3**). Using a combination of guidewire and catheter advancement, deep cannulation can be achieved. An important aspect is to limit contrast injection to small amounts so as to avoid acinarization of the pancreas, thereby decreasing the potential for post-ERCP pancreatitis.

- In certain instances where selective cannulation of the desired duct may not be easily achieved due to abnormal or pathologic anatomy (such as periampullary diverticulum, malignancy, postsurgical anatomy), special techniques and/or devices may need to be used. These may include performance of a "precut" or "access" sphincterotomy, use of rotatable cannulating devices, placement of a pancreatic stent (to facilitate biliary cannulation and reduce risk of post-procedure pancreatitis), and the use of specific guidewires that may differ in caliber or hydrophilic nature. In certain cases of postsurgical anatomy, ERCP may be impossible with duodenoscopes. In these instances, enteroscopes (device or nondevice assisted) may be required, which can make the procedure more technically challenging. Patients who have undergone bariatric surgery in whom the stomach and proximal small bowel is bypassed pose a special challenge. In such patients, the procedure can be attempted with enteroscopes, but alternate strategies, including laparoscopic-assisted ERCPs (with the assistance of a surgical team)[5] or EUS-directed transgastric ERCP[6] have gained traction in clinical practice.

- In patients in whom biliary cannulation is initially unsuccessful, the procedure can be reattempted in a day or two if the clinical situation allows. Referral to a center with expertise in ERCP is also reasonable. However, if delay is not feasible, patients generally proceed to percutaneous biliary catheter placement by interventional radiology. Depending on case specifics and endoscopist expertise, EUS-guided biliary access can be performed too.
- Pancreas divisum anatomy poses specific cannulation challenges because the major drainage of the pancreas is via the duct of Santorini via the minor papilla. These cases can be challenging since they may require a "long" scope position, use of smaller-caliber catheters and guidewires, and possibly even a pancreatic secretagogue such as secretin, which may allow for the opening of the ductal orifice.

SPHINCTEROTOMY

- Once deep access of the desired duct is obtained, biliary and/or pancreatic sphincterotomy is generally required to perform further therapeutic manipulations. The most common type of device for this maneuver is a traction-type sphincterotomes in which the cutting wire carries the electrosurgical current and bends the tip of the sphincterotome. These are used when deep guidewire access of the desired duct has been attained. Such sphincterotomes may be rotatable (depending on manufacturer) and can be especially helpful in postsurgical anatomy. In addition, a "needle-knife" sphincterotome may be required in difficult cannulation cases. Occasionally, needle-knife sphincterotomes can be used to perform an over-the-stent sphincterotomy. Electrosurgical current for sphincterotomy generally uses a blend current (mixture of cutting and coagulation), and it is commonplace to use an electrosurgical generator with pulse cutting so as to avoid inadvertent longer than desired or too rapid cuts ("zipper cuts").
- Biliary sphincterotomy is performed when deep biliary access has been achieved and the guidewire is passed into the proximal biliary tree. Once the scope and sphincterotome are in a stable position, the sphincterotome tip is bowed such that the cutting wire is aiming in the 11-o'clock position. It is important to keep as little of the wire in contact with the tissue so as to get a precise cut and avoid coagulation, which causes more of a charring effect. Using the shaft of the scope, the cut is guided toward the 11-o'clock position, taking care to not cut past the transverse fold (FIGURE 3). The size of

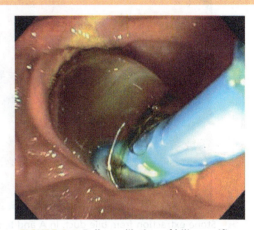

FIGURE 4 • Balloon dilation of biliary orifice.

the sphincterotomy generally depends on the therapeutic maneuver planned. In general, large biliary sphincterotomies are only required for removal of large biliary stones. Furthermore, if an adequate sphincterotomy has been performed but passage of stones is still difficult, balloon dilation of the biliary orifice can be performed (FIGURE 4).
- Pancreatic sphincterotomy is performed with a technique similar to biliary sphincterotomy, but the cutting wire aims at the 2-o'clock position. In general, pancreatic sphincterotomies should be smaller in length compared with biliary. Some endoscopists prefer to initially place a pancreatic stent as a guide and perform an over-the-stent cut using a needle-knife sphincterotome.

STONE EXTRACTION

- Stones are typically extracted using balloon catheters or baskets. Factors that influence success of stone extraction include their size and shape (especially in relation to duct size) and absolute number. In addition, pancreatic stones can be much harder to remove compared with biliary ones due to associated strictures and inflammation from chronic pancreatitis. An adequate sphincterotomy is essential prior to extraction. Occasionally, balloon dilation of the ductal orifice can be performed if the

sphincterotomy is deemed to be adequate but further cutting could cause bleeding or perforation (FIGURE 4).
- Typically, balloons are used first line, but if this fails, metal baskets are used to capture stones for removal (FIGURE 5) (▶ Video 1). Occasionally, the baskets may become impacted with a stone and difficult to remove due to stone shape and/or ductal anatomy. In this case, mechanical lithotripsy with various accessories can be performed. If complete stone removal is not possible in a single ERCP session, a stent is inserted to ensure ductal drainage prior to next ERCP.

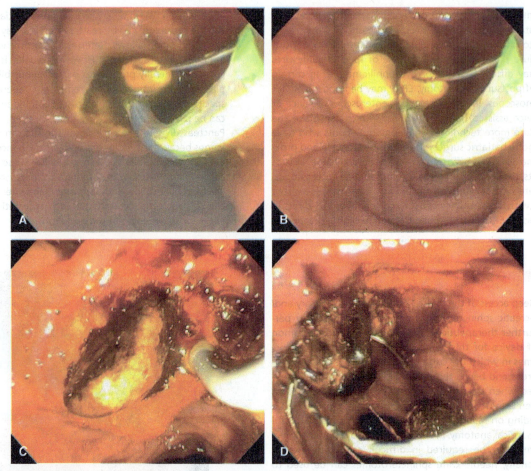

FIGURE 5 • Stone extraction from bile duct. In **A** and **B**, small stones may pass spontaneously after adequate biliary sphincterotomy. In **C**, a balloon extraction catheter is deployed proximal to a stone and the stone is being extracted. In **D**, an expanding wire basket has been deployed, enveloping the stone, and then withdrawn back into the duodenum leading to crushing and/or removal of the calculus.

- In cases of failed stone extraction or mechanical lithotripsy, other techniques such as electrohydraulic lithotripsy, holmium laser lithotripsy, or extracorporeal shock wave lithotripsy may be employed (▶ Video 2). Surgical removal of biliary stones is rarely required. For failed pancreatic stone extraction, surgery may be indicated to improve patient symptoms from chronic pancreatitis.

STRICTURE DILATION

- Devices for biliary and pancreatic stricture dilation are available. Stricture dilation is indicated for both benign and malignant indications. The general principle is that the dilating device is passed through the working channel of the scope over the preplaced guidewire until it is positioned across the stricture. Dilation is usually performed under fluoroscopic guidance to ensure that the device does not slip proximal or distal to the strictured area.
- Cylindrical-shaped balloon dilation catheters that exert radial force are typically used for dilation of biliary strictures. The balloons can be filled with contrast material and hence are visible on fluoroscopy as the balloon is inflated while ensuring the balloon is centered on the strictured area. The typical balloon diameter sizes for biliary dilation range from 4 to 10 mm. The lengths of the balloons are typically 2 to 4 cm.

- Dilation of pancreatic strictures can be performed using similar balloon dilation catheters as biliary strictures. However, owing to the smaller size of the pancreatic duct, the sizes of the balloons used are smaller. In addition, smaller graduated bougie-type dilators are also available for dilating smaller and tighter pancreatic duct strictures. These dilators provide axial force in addition to radial force and can be quite helpful in patients with chronic pancreatitis and resultant fibrotic strictures.
- Occasionally, larger-diameter dilators are required for biliary indications. In cases where the bile duct is dilated proximal to a stricture or dilation of a biliary sphincterotomy orifice is needed for large stone passage, graduated esophageal balloon dilators can be used. In principle, these devices, designed for esophageal strictures, work similarly to dedicated biliary and pancreatic balloon dilators.

Chapter 4 ENDOSCOPIC RETROGRADE CHOLANGIOPANCREATOGRAPHY 35

STENT INSERTION

- Various biliary and pancreatic stents are available, and they differ in terms of material (plastic or metal), diameter, length, and design. Whereas the practice of plastic stent insertion has not changed much over the years, the use of metal stents has expanded greatly (FIGURE 6). Previously, metal mesh stents were used for palliation of malignancy, but newer, covered metal stents are available. Such stents are easily removable and hence are being used for benign indications. The general purpose of stents is to serve as a conduit for duct drainage across an obstruction. Stents can be placed temporarily for benign indications or as a bridge to definite therapy. In addition, they can be

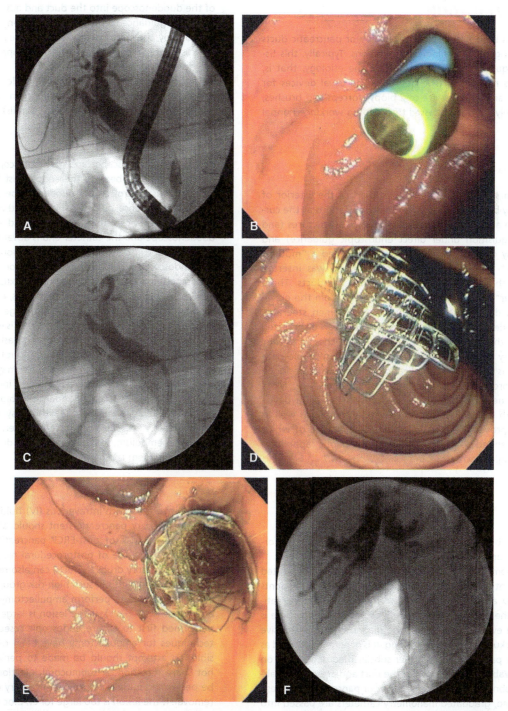

FIGURE 6 • Endoscopic and fluoroscopic views of plastic and metal biliary stents. **A,** Fluoroscopic view of a biliary stricture. **B,** Endoscopic image of a deployed plastic biliary stent. **C,** Radiographic appearance of a plastic biliary stent. **D** and **E,** Endoscopic views of a well-positioned metal biliary stent. **F,** Fluoroscopic appearance of a metal biliary stent.

- permanently placed for palliation in the setting of nonoperable malignancy.
- The general technique for stent insertion is over a guidewire advanced deeply into the desired duct (▶ Video 3). While keeping guidewire access, the stent is deployed using endoscopic and fluoroscopic guidance through the duodenoscope using a pushing catheter. It is important to keep the scope tip close to the papilla, making sure the stent is aiming in the axis of the desired duct as it is being deployed. If too much of the stent is exposed into the duodenal lumen, it can lead to bowing of the stent and difficulty in passage. This is especially important in trying to pass stents across tight strictures. Whether or not to dilate strictures prior to stent deployment depends on stricture characteristics and endoscopist preference.

TISSUE ACQUISITION

- Tissue can be acquired from the biliary or pancreatic ducts for histologic and cytologic examinations. Typically, this tissue is acquired from strictures when the etiology, that is, benign vs malignant, is in question. The usual devices for histology and cytology are cold biopsy forceps and brushes, respectively. These are passed through the working channel of the duodenoscope into the duct and advanced under fluoroscopic guidance to the area in question. Under real-time fluoroscopy, the endoscopist can then take biopsy specimens or brushings, which are then sent to the appropriate laboratory for analysis.
- Occasionally, specimens can be taken under direct visualization of the interior of the duct during choledochoscopy or pancreatoscopy (see next section for details).

CHOLANGIOSCOPY AND PANCREATOSCOPY

- In certain situations, direct visualization of the interior of ducts may be required. The two main indications at the current time are visualization of indeterminate strictures (and tissue acquisition under direct endoscopic guidance) and lithotripsy of large stones. Older systems used a "mother-daughter" system in which a smaller scope was inserted through the duodenoscope directly into the ducts. These "daughter" scopes were prone to damage from the elevator of the duodenoscope. Disposable, multilumen, steerable catheter devices are presently used. These can be inserted through the duodenoscope channel into the pancreatic and biliary ducts. Through these catheters, a reusable optical fiber is passed for visualization and specially designed biopsy forceps can be used for tissue acquisition. More recently, newer single-operator systems have been developed with better suction and irrigation abilities as well as vastly improved high-resolution digital optics, all of which have expanded both diagnostic and therapeutic capabilities of cholangiopancreatoscopy.[7]
- Usage of cholangioscopes and pancreatoscopes can be technically challenging because the endoscopist has to maintain simultaneous control of the duodenoscope and the smaller scope. Usually, once guidewire access of the desired duct is achieved, the device with its control dial end is attached to the duodenoscope and the catheter end is advanced through the duodenoscope into the duct. Using both fluoroscopic guidance and endoscopic visualization of the interior of the duct, the endoscopist can evaluate for presence or extent of malignant-appearing lesions, obtain biopsy specimens, examine the duct for any stones, or perform lithotripsy of large stones.
- In specific situations when the duct caliber is very large, it may be possible to insert a forward-viewing gastroscope directly into the biliary or pancreatic ducts (without the use of a duodenoscope). Although such procedures may be technically challenging, the potential advantages include improved visualization, ability to pass standard-size biopsy forceps, and capture/removal or mechanical lithotripsy of large stones under direct view. This procedure has been associated with air venous embolism, so the use of carbon dioxide (CO_2) as an insufflating agent is required.

SPECIAL SITUATIONS

- ERCP can be used in special situations such as SOD, performance of ampullectomy, or in the pediatric setting.
- SOD is a somewhat controversial topic but has been implicated as a potential cause of pancreatic or biliary disease. Patients with SOD are especially high risk for post-ERCP pancreatitis, and the procedure should only be undertaken if there is objective evidence to support the diagnosis or an extensive prior workup has been unrevealing. It is generally classified as biliary or pancreatic and further subclassified depending on presence/absence of dilation of the duct and presence of laboratory abnormalities (elevated liver or pancreatic enzymes). Specialized, graduated manometry catheters are passed into the ductal orifices and pressure is measured. A sustained pressure over 40 mm Hg is considered abnormal and is an indication for sphincterotomy. Postprocedurally, patients should be well hydrated with intravenous (IV) fluids and a prophylactic, temporary pancreatic stent should always be placed to reduce the risk of post-ERCP pancreatitis. Newer data suggest that the use of postprocedural rectal, nonsteroidal anti-inflammatory drugs (NSAIDs) can also reduce the risk of post-ERCP pancreatitis in such high-risk groups.[8]
- ERCP can be used to perform ampullectomy for obstructing adenomas (FIGURE 7). If the lesion is large, EUS should be performed first to ensure endoscopic resectability. Various techniques for ampullectomy have been described; if possible, an attempt should be made to perform an en bloc hot snare resection. A submucosal injection of saline may be performed initially to provide a cautery cushion prior to removal. If the lesion is too large for en bloc resection, piecemeal ampullectomy with cauterization of the edges of the resection base can be performed (▶ Video 4). Placement of a prophylactic pancreatic stent and biliary sphincterotomy

Chapter 4 **ENDOSCOPIC RETROGRADE CHOLANGIOPANCREATOGRAPHY**

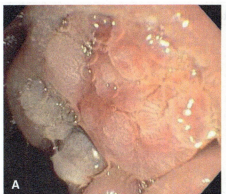
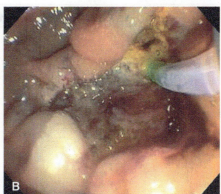
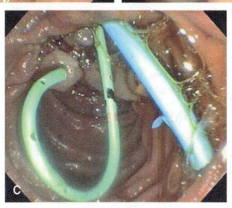

FIGURE 7 • Pre- and postampullectomy endoscopic images. **A,** Endoscopic visualization of a sessile, ampullary polyp. **B,** Endoscopic ampullectomy has been performed, and catheter access to pancreatic duct is achieved. The biliary orifice is seen above. **C,** Protective stents in both the bile duct **(right)** and pancreatic duct **(left)** are an essential component of endoscopic ampullectomy.

are recommended to reduce the risk of postprocedure pancreatitis and cholangitis, respectively.

- ERCP is less common in the pediatric population but is usually performed for biliary stone extraction. For small children, a specialized pediatric duodenoscope is used. It is limited by the small-sized accessory devices, which can be accommodated through its working channel. For older children and adolescents, generally, the standard duodenoscope with accessories can be used. Other less common indications could include postoperative strictures, traumatic or postoperative bile or pancreatic leaks, or chronic pancreatitis due to a genetic etiology.

PEARLS AND PITFALLS

Indications	■ ERCP should be performed with a therapeutic intent and not for diagnostic purposes only. ■ The endoscopist should obtain diagnostic information from patient history and physical, imaging, and laboratory parameters to carefully select those patients who will benefit most from therapeutic ERCP.
Intubation of esophagus	■ Owing to the side-viewing nature of scope, passage through oropharynx and esophagus is mostly by feel and not by direct visualization. ■ If patient's history suggests abnormal or postsurgical anatomy or any difficulty is encountered with the duodenoscope, the anatomy should be evaluated with a forward viewing scope.
Cannulation	■ Selective cannulation of the desired duct is the key to successful ERCP and requires expertise and patience. ■ Successful cannulation is achieved by knowledge of normal papillary anatomy, proper scope position, and aligning the cannulating device to the axis of the duct of choice. ■ The cannulating device should never be forced into the duct.
Post-ERCP complications	■ Patients who are highest risk for post-ERCP complications (especially pancreatitis) are often the ones who do not have a firm indication for the procedure. ■ In those with high risk for pancreatitis, ensure that they receive adequate intra- and postprocedure IV fluids, placement of temporary pancreatic stent, and/or rectal NSAIDs. It may be wise to admit these patients postprocedurally for observation. ■ If complication is suspected or confirmed, admit the patient and treat accordingly. Keep patient and family fully informed of patient progress.

Table 4: Complications of Endoscopic Retrograde Cholangiopancreatography
Post-ERCP pancreatitis (1.5%-20%)
Hemorrhage (0.1%-2.0%)
Perforation (<1%)
Infection (<1%)
Cardiopulmonary (1%)
Miscellaneous
Stent-related (migration, occlusion, perforation, acute cholecystitis, biliary or pancreatic duct injury)
Ileus
Hepatic abscess
Pneumothorax/pneumomediastinum
Duodenal hematoma
Portal venous air
Impaction of therapeutic devices (stone retrieval baskets)
Perforation of colonic diverticula

ERCP, endoscopic retrograde cholangiopancreatography.
Reprinted from ASGE Standards of Practice Committee; Anderson MA, Fisher L, Jain R, et al. Complications of ERCP. Gastrointest Endosc. 2012;75(3):467-473. Copyright © 2012 American Society for Gastrointestinal Endoscopy. With permission.

POSTOPERATIVE CARE

- Generally, ERCP can be done as an outpatient procedure; however, patients may need to be observed longer than those undergoing standard endoscopic procedures. High-risk patients (such as those with SOD) or those with difficult cannulation have higher rates of post-ERCP pancreatitis and may be prophylactically admitted to the hospital for observation.
- Once patients recover from the procedure, they can resume their normal activities, medications, and diet. In patients who need to restart anticoagulation, it is generally safe to resume postprocedurally.

OUTCOMES

- ERCP itself has high procedural success rates when performed by skilled endoscopists, but patient outcomes ultimately depend on the indications of the procedure.
- For biliary indications, the procedure has excellent immediate success rates for stone clearance, reestablishing bile flow in benign and malignant strictures, and resolution of bile leaks.
- ERCP in patients with chronic pancreatitis should be in well-selected patients who are maximized on medical therapy. In such patients, it has potential for good short-term results, but due to the nature of the disease, patients may ultimately need surgical therapy. In patients with pancreatic malignancy causing biliary obstruction, ERCP can reestablish immediate bile flow, but ultimate outcome will depend on the clinical stage of the disease.

COMPLICATIONS

- See **TABLE 4**.

REFERENCES

1. Adler DG, Baron TH, Davila RE, et al. ASGE guideline: the role of ERCP in diseases of the biliary tract and the pancreas. *Gastrointest Endosc*. 2005;62(1):1-8.
2. Adler DG, Lieb JG II, Cohen J, et al. Quality indicators for ERCP. *Gastrointest Endosc*. 2015;81(1):54-66.
3. Jowell PS, Baillie J, Branch MS, et al. Quantitative assessment of procedural competence. A prospective study of training in endoscopic retrograde cholangiopancreatography. *Ann Intern Med*. 1996;125(12):983.
4. Baillie J. Advanced cannulation technique and precut. *Gastrointest Endosc Clin N Am*. 2012;22(3):417-434.
5. Abbas AM, Strong AT, Diehl DL, et al. Multicenter evaluation of the clinical utility of laparoscopy-assisted ERCP in patients with Roux-en-Y gastric bypass. *Gastrointest Endosc*. 2018;87(4):1031-1039.
6. Kochhar GS, Mohy-UD-Din N, Grover A, et al. EUS-directed transgastric endoscopic retrograde cholangiopancreatography versus laparoscopic-assisted ERCP versus deep enteroscopy-assisted ERCP for patients with RYGB. *Endosc Int Open*. 2020;8(7):E877-E882.
7. Shah RJ, Neuhaus H, Parsi M, et al. Randomized study of digital single-operator cholangioscope compared to fiberoptic single-operator cholangioscope in a novel cholangioscopy bench model. *Endosc Int Open*. 2018;6(7):E851-E856.
8. Elmunzer BJ, Scheiman JM, Lehman GA, et al. A randomized trial of rectal indomethacin to prevent post-ERCP pancreatitis. *N Engl J Med*. 2012;366(15):1414-1422.

Chapter 5

Laparoscopic Cholangiography, Common Bile Duct Exploration, and Endobiliary Stent Placement

Tyler John Loftus

DEFINITION

- Laparoscopic common bile duct exploration involves laparoscopic-assisted fluoroscopic and endoscopic techniques and direct laparoscopic instrumentation for the diagnosis and management of common bile duct stones and sludge (microlithiasis).
- Endobiliary stent placement across the ampulla of Vater promotes decompression of the biliary tree into the duodenum and allows for primary closure of the common ductotomy after transcholedochal exploration.

PATIENT HISTORY AND PHYSICAL FINDINGS

- History and physical examination focus on signs and symptoms of cholecystitis with or without biliary obstruction with obstructive jaundice.
- The examiner elicits contraindications to laparoscopic cholecystectomy and common bile duct exploration, including severe cholangitis with septic shock, pancreatitis, and pancreatic or biliary tumor.

IMAGING AND OTHER DIAGNOSTIC STUDIES

- Right upper quadrant ultrasound
  - Assess for cholecystitis and measure common bile duct diameter
  - Patients with common duct obstruction and history of cirrhosis or biliary tree inflammation and fibrosis may not develop biliary ductal dilation
- Liver function tests
  - Direct hyperbilirubinemia suggests extrahepatic biliary obstruction
- Serum lipase
  - If elevated then consider computed tomography of the abdomen
  - Defer cholecystectomy until resolution of pancreatitis and perform endoscopic retrograde cholangiopancreatography or percutaneous transhepatic biliary drain placement as needed
- If unexplained weight loss, cachexia, painless jaundice, chronic pancreatitis, or family history of pancreatic or biliary tumor then measure carcinoembryonic antigen and CA 19-9
  - If pancreatic or biliary tumor is suspected then perform staging

SURGICAL MANAGEMENT

Preoperative Planning

- For patients with prior Roux-en-Y gastrojejunostomy, laparoscopic-assisted endoscopic retrograde cholangiography may become necessary if common bile duct exploration fails.

Positioning

- The patient is positioned supine with the left arm tucked to facilitate fluoroscopy via C-arm from the patient's left side while the surgeon performs laparoscopic and endoscopic interventions standing on the patient's right side, in line with the cystic duct (**FIGURE 1**).
- Reverse Trendelenburg position with the right side of the table tilted up exposes the target anatomy.

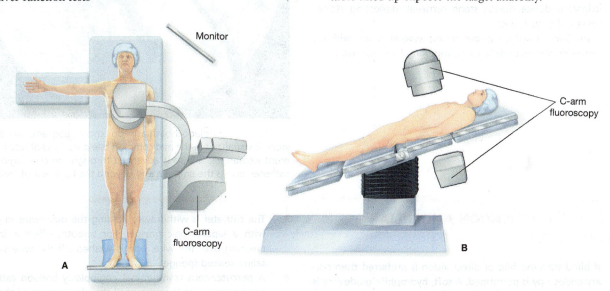

FIGURE 1 • **A,** The patient is positioned supine with the left arm tucked. A footboard is placed. The C-arm fluoroscopy unit is positioned to the patient's left, with the monitor readily visible to the operating surgeon who is on the patient's right. **B,** The patient must be positioned with respect to the pedestal of the operating table so that there is adequate room for the C-arm.

TROCAR PLACEMENT

- Trocar arrangements for laparoscopic cholecystectomy are usually adequate for laparoscopic common bile duct exploration.
- If inflammation is extensive or the gallbladder is intrahepatic then an additional 5-mm trocar is placed at the mid-clavicular line 1 to 2 cm caudal to the costal margin for ergonomic instrumentation of the biliary tree while instruments through other trocars provide retraction, exposure, and direct manipulation of the choledochoscope with a padded grasper as needed.

CHOLANGIOGRAPHY

- The infundibulum is mobilized, Calot triangle is dissected, and a critical view of safety is obtained.
- The cystic duct is clipped at its insertion on the infundibulum. A cystic ductotomy is created on the distal cystic duct, minimizing the cystic duct length that must be traversed during biliary endoscopy while preserving adequate length for clip or endoloop placement.
- A 5-Fr catheter is saline flushed to evacuate air bubbles that mimic stones on fluoroscopy, inserted through the cystic ductotomy, and secured with a laparoscopic clamp or nonocclusive clip. Low-osmolar, radiopaque contrast is mixed 1:1 with saline to reduce viscosity and the probability that small, nonocclusive stones are obscured by high-density contrast.
- When cholangiography reveals biliary tree filling defects or nonfilling of the duodenum refractory to power flushing and glucagon administration to relax the Sphincter of Oddi and allow passage of small stones, common bile duct exploration is indicated (See also ▶ Video 1).

TRANSCYSTIC EXPLORATION

- Some advocate for blind trawling of the biliary tree with stone retrieval baskets or Fogarty balloons. The basket or balloon is inserted through the cholangiogram catheter, gently advanced with or without fluoroscopic guidance to the ampulla of Vater, opened, and retrieved (FIGURE 2).
- Stones can migrate into the common hepatic duct. With adequate biliary tree dilation, a skilled endoscopist can retroflex the endoscope into the common hepatic duct (ie, wiper blade technique[1]) and clear it.
- To prevent stone migration into the common hepatic duct during blind trawling, extrinsic compression is applied to the proximal hepatic duct with a laparoscopic grasper or suction-irrigation device during stone retrieval, deflecting stones toward the cystic duct.
- Once blind trawling is performed several times without retrieving stones or debris, cholangiography is repeated.

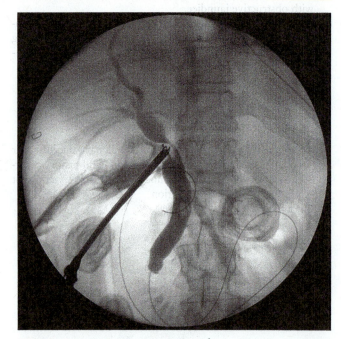

FIGURE 2 • Choledocholithiasis on cholangiogram. An 8-mm stone is visualized in the mid common bile duct. To facilitate instrument exchanges, a wire is advanced through the cholangiogram catheter, across the ampulla and beyond the ligament of Treitz.

CYSTIC DUCT DILATION AND BILIARY ENDOSCOPY

- If blind trawling fails or direct vision is preferred then biliary endoscopy is performed. A soft, hydrophilic guidewire is inserted through the cholangiogram catheter and advanced across the ampulla of Vater under fluoroscopy, leaving 10 to 20 cm of wire outside of the patient for instrument exchanges.
- The catheter is withdrawn, holding the guidewire in place with a laparoscopic grasper. For smooth, efficient instrumenting over the wire, bile is washed off the wire with a saline-soaked sponge.
- A percutaneous transluminal angioplasty balloon catheter is advanced over the wire until the distal aspect of the balloon is within the common bile duct. The cystic duct is dilated approximately 2 mm beyond its original diameter, disrupting the spiral valves of Heister.

- After withdrawing the balloon, the choledochoscope is inserted with or without wire guidance. A 10-mm padded grasper allows atraumatic manipulation of the choledochoscope.
- Continuous irrigation through the endoscope maintains visualization. High-pressure (180 mm Hg) irrigation may be adequate to clear impacted sludge. Stones are encircled with a stone extraction basket under direct vision and cleared by withdrawing the endoscope.

TRANSCHOLEDOCHAL EXPLORATION

- The conditions listed in **TABLE 1** indicate early transition to transcholedochal exploration.
- A longitudinal incision is made on the ventral surface of the mid-distal common bile duct, avoiding the 3- and 9-o'clock blood supply and preserving enough length on the proximal common bile duct for reconstruction with hepaticojejunostomy if necessary (**FIGURE 3**).
- The biliary tree is cleared with endoscopic stone retrieval or direct laparoscopic instrumentation (**FIGURE 4**).

Table 1: Indications for Early Transition to Transcholedochal Exploration

Conditions indicating transcholedochal exploration

- The cystic duct diameter is 3 mm or less (compare with the shaft diameter of a laparoscopic instrument)
- The cystic duct inserts on the common bile duct in a medial or distal position
- The cystic duct inserts on the right hepatic duct
- Large stone size precludes transcystic extraction
- Numerous (more than five) stones render transcystic extraction inefficient
- Stones are cephalad to the cystic duct insertion and endoscopic retroflexion (ie, wiper blade technique[1]) and retrieval is not feasible

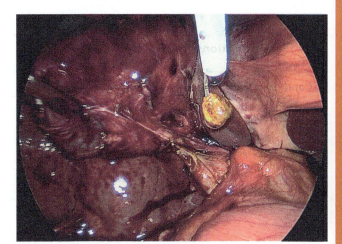

FIGURE 4 • Stone capture. An extracted stone captured within a basket. The gallbladder dome and infundibulum are retracted to expose the cystic ductotomy and align the biliary tree and endoscope trajectory during stone retrieval.

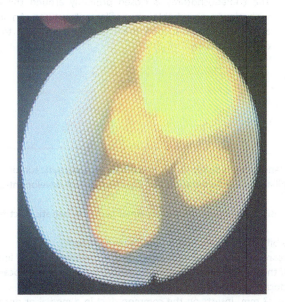

FIGURE 3 • Choledocholithiasis on biliary endoscopy. Several small stones are visualized in the distal common bile duct, amenable to retrieval with the single deployment of a meshed basket.

ENDOBILIARY STENT PLACEMENT

- The conditions listed in **TABLE 2** indicate endobiliary stent placement. A plastic, double-flanged endobiliary stent is gently advanced over a wire across the ampulla under fluoroscopic guidance. Cholangiography confirms appropriate stent position and contrast flow into the duodenum (**FIGURE 5**).
- After stent deployment, completion cholangiography confirms contrast flow into the duodenum. The choledochotomy is primarily closed with slowly absorbable, monofilament suture. Cholecystectomy is completed.

Table 2: Indications for Endobiliary Stent Placement

Conditions indicating endobiliary stent placement

- The biliary tree cannot be cleared and early endoscopic retrograde cholangiography is unavailable
- Cholangitis (adequate biliary tree drainage is paramount)
- Difficult guidewire passage across the ampulla of Vater, suggesting sphincter of Oddi spasm or edema, which may worsen after instrumentation
- Transcholedochal exploration was performed and primary choledochotomy closure is preferred over T-tube placement

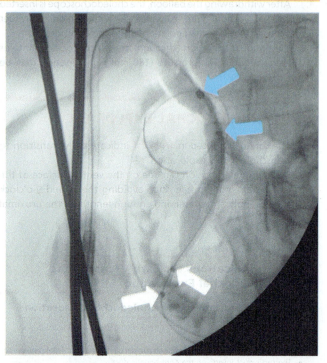

FIGURE 5 • Endobiliary stent placement. The stent is advanced over a wire until the distal radiographic markers (*white arrows*) and corresponding flange are in the duodenum and the proximal markers (blue arrows) and corresponding flange are in the common bile duct.

T-TUBE PLACEMENT

- If a choledochotomy is created and endobiliary stent placement is not feasible then a T-tube is placed through the choledochotomy.
- The choledochotomy is closed primarily around the tube with slowly absorbable, monofilament sutures. An intra-abdominal closed-suction drain is placed adjacent to the choledochotomy.

PEARLS AND PITFALLS

- The initial patient assessment must exclude pancreatitis, severe cholangitis with septic shock, and biliary or pancreatic tumor.
- Patients with common duct obstruction and history of cirrhosis or biliary tree inflammation and fibrosis may not develop intra- or extrahepatic ductal dilation.
- If performing blind trawling of the common duct then apply extrinsic compression of the proximal common hepatic duct to prevent stone migration into the hepatic ducts.
- For smooth, efficient instrumenting over the wire, wash the viscous bile off the wire with a saline-soaked sponge.
- If inflammation is extensive or the gallbladder is intrahepatic then consider an additional 5-mm trocar at the midclavicular line 1 to 2 cm below the costal margin for ergonomic instrumentation of the biliary tree while graspers placed through other trocars provide retraction, exposure, and direct manipulation of the choledochoscope.
- Transition to transcholedochal exploration early if the cystic duct is ≤3 mm, inserts on the common duct in a medial or distal position, inserts on the right hepatic duct, or large stone size precludes transcystic extraction.
- Perform choledochotomy on the mid-distal common bile duct, preserving common duct length in case hepaticojejunostomy becomes necessary.
- Consider endobiliary stent placement when biliary tree clearance fails, the patient has cholangitis, sphincter of Oddi spasm or edema prevents biliary tree decompression, or primary closure of a choledochotomy is preferred over T-tube placement.
- Endobiliary stents are usually retrievable with a forward-viewing upper endoscope and snare; stents migrating proximally require retrieval by endoscopic retrograde cholangiography.

Chapter 5 LAPAROSCOPIC CHOLANGIOGRAPHY, COMMON BILE DUCT EXPLORATION, AND ENDOBILIARY STENT PLACEMENT   43

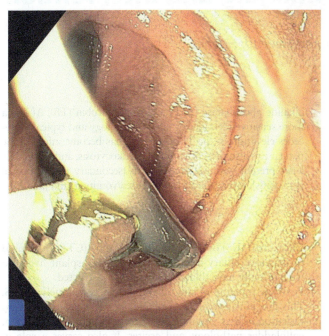

FIGURE 6 • Stent retrieval. Plastic endobiliary stent retrieval with a standard, forward-viewing upper endoscope and grasper. The stent is grasped and advanced into the duodenum until clearing the ampulla before withdrawing the endoscope.

POSTOPERATIVE CARE

- Routine postoperative admission and observation is unnecessary after uncomplicated laparoscopic common bile duct exploration.
- For endobiliary stent placement, stent retrieval is performed 2 to 6 weeks after surgery. Before retrieval, an abdominal radiograph confirms that the stent remains in situ. A stent migrating distally may pass the gastrointestinal tract entirely, obviating retrieval. A stent migrating proximally into the common bile duct requires retrieval by endoscopic retrograde cholangiography. Absent migration, the stent is retrieved with a standard forward-viewing upper endoscope and grasping instrument or snare (FIGURE 6).
- For T-tube placement, cholangiography is performed approximately 2 weeks after surgery. Retained stones are retrieved by image-guided extraction through the T-tube. After T-tube removal, an adjacent closed-suction, intra-abdominal drain remains until the biliary fistula seals.

OUTCOMES AND COMPLICATIONS

- TABLE 3 lists outcomes and complications for laparoscopic common bile duct exploration and cholecystectomy vs two-stage endoscopic retrograde cholangiography plus laparoscopic cholecystectomy.

ACKNOWLEDGMENT

We gratefully acknowledge the past contributions by the previous edition authors, Chasen A. Croft and Dawood G. Dalaly, as portions of that chapter were retained in this revision.

Table 3: Outcomes and Complications for Laparoscopic Common Bile Duct Exploration and Cholecystectomy vs Two-Stage Endoscopic Retrograde Cholangiography Plus Laparoscopic Cholecystectomy

Outcomes and complications	Laparoscopic common bile duct exploration and cholecystectomy	Two-stage endoscopic retrograde cholangiography plus laparoscopic cholecystectomy
Stone clearance	88.1%-90.2%[2,3]	82.2%-85.7%[2,3]
Recurrent common duct stones	2.1%[4]	9.5%[4]
T-tube complications[a]	13.8%[5]	Not applicable
Pancreatitis[b]	3.9%-4.5%[6,7]	7.2%-15.1%[c,8,9]
Severe pancreatitis[d]	0.2%-0.3%[6,7]	0.4%-1.0%[c,8,9]
Hospital length of stay (days, mean ± standard deviation)	4.9 ± 1.6[2]	6.5 ± 3.4[2]
Overall morbidity	13.9%-15.4%[2,3,10]	12.5%-14.6%[2,3]
Mortality	0.3%-0.7%[2,3,10]	0.9%-2.3%[2,3,10]

[a]Dislodgement, biliary peritonitis, prolonged biliary fistula, or bile duct stricture.
[b]Amylase three to four times higher than serum in the presence of abdominal pain.
[c]Reported for all diagnostic and therapeutic endoscopic retrograde cholangiopancreatography, not specific to patients undergoing two-stage endoscopic retrograde cholangiography plus laparoscopic cholecystectomy.
[d]Pancreatic necrosis, pancreatic pseudocyst, critical illness, hospitalization prolonged for more than 10 days, hemorrhagic pancreatitis, or a need for secondary intervention.

SUGGESTED READINGS

1. Cheng CL, Sherman S, Watkins JL, et al. Risk factors for post-ERCP pancreatitis: a prospective multicenter study. *Am J Gastroenterol*. 2006;101(1):139-147.
2. Czerwonko ME, Pekolj J, Uad P, et al. Acute pancreatitis after laparoscopic transcystic common bile duct exploration: an analysis of predisposing factors in 447 patients. *World J Surg*. 2018;42(10):3134-3142.
3. Dasari BVM, Tan CJ, Gurusamy KS, et al. Surgical versus endoscopic treatment of bile duct stones. *Cochrane Database Syst Rev*. 2013;2013(12):CD003327. doi:10.1002/14651858.CD003327.pub4. PMID: 24338858; PMCID: PMC6464772.
4. Ding GQ, Cai W, Qin MF. Single-stage vs. Two-stage management for concomitant gallstones and common bile duct stones: a prospective randomized trial with long-term follow-up. *J Gastrointest Surg*. 2014;18(5):947-951.
5. Nassar AHM, Gough V, Ng HJ, Katbeh T, Khan K. Utilisation of laparoscopic choledochoscopy during bile duct exploration and evaluation of the wiper blade manoeuvre for transcystic intrahepatic access. *Ann Surg*. 2021. doi:10.1097/SLA.0000000000004912.
6. Paganini AM, Feliciotti F, Guerrieri M, et al. Laparoscopic common bile duct exploration. *J Laparoendosc Adv A*. 2001;11(6):391-400.
7. Singh AN, Kilambi R. Single-stage laparoscopic common bile duct exploration and cholecystectomy versus two-stage endoscopic stone extraction followed by laparoscopic cholecystectomy for patients with gallbladder stones with common bile duct stones: systematic review and meta-analysis of randomized trials with trial sequential analysis. *Surg Endosc*. 2018;32(9):3763-3776.
8. Vandervoort J, Soetikno RM, Tham TC, et al. Risk factors for complications after performance of ERCP. *Gastrointest Endosc*. 2002;56(5):652-656.
9. Wills VL, Gibson K, Karihaloo C, Jorgensen JO. Complications of biliary T-tubes after choledochotomy. *ANZ J Surg*. 2002;72(3):177-180.
10. Zhu HY, Xu M, Shen HJ, et al. A meta-analysis of single-stage versus two-stage management for concomitant gallstones and common bile duct stones. *Clin Res Hepatol Gastroenterol*. 2015;39(5):584-593.

Chapter 6: Percutaneous Transhepatic Biliary Imaging and Intervention

Brian S. Geller and Steven J. Hughes

DEFINITION

- Cholangiography is the term used to describe the evaluation of the biliary system by fluoroscopy after injection of radiopaque material (contrast). The introduction of contrast can be performed either in a retrograde (via endoscope) or an antegrade manner.
- The antegrade introduction of contrast requires percutaneous transhepatic access into the biliary system. A percutaneous transhepatic cholangiogram (PTC) is commonly performed when a magnetic resonance cholangiopancreatography (MRCP) and endoscopic retrograde cholangiopancreatography (ERCP) were inconclusive or unable to be performed.
- When an obstruction of the biliary system cannot be managed by endoscopic means, a drainage catheter can be placed. This procedure is known as percutaneous transhepatic drainage (PTHD).
- Numerous biliary pathologies are routinely managed by the percutaneous route: stone/debris removal, stricture dilation, long-term catheter drainage, and metallic stent placement.

PATIENT HISTORY AND PHYSICAL FINDINGS

- A PTC is an invasive procedure and as such, non- or less invasive imaging of the biliary system should be attempted; these include MRCP and ERCP. If these options fail to make the diagnosis or cannot be performed due to the patient's anatomy, then a PTC should be performed.
- Indications for cholangiography include biliary stenosis or obstruction, or bile leak. The underlying pathology includes stones, malignancy, infection, inflammation, fibrosis/scarring, and iatrogenic complications.
- Patients with biliary obstruction or moderate- to high-grade stenosis usually present jaundiced with elevations of the alkaline phosphatase (ALP) and total bilirubin (TB). ALP is a more sensitive identifier of biliary pathology and typically precedes elevation of the TB. If the bile has become infected, the patient can also present with fever, leukocytosis, and sepsis. Bile leaks present with abdominal pain (secondary to a chemical peritonitis), fever, leukocytosis, nausea/vomiting, and jaundice.

IMAGING AND OTHER DIAGNOSTIC STUDIES

- Ultrasound (US) or computed tomography (CT) can be used to diagnose biliary dilation. Note: Posttransplant livers do not normally have dilated ducts when obstructed.
- First-line imaging of the biliary system is routinely an US. This modality is readily available, inexpensive, and uses no radiation. US is optimal for detection of biliary dilation, gallbladder pathology, and ascites. It also serves a role in the identification and characterization of hepatic masses and Doppler mode provides information regarding potential vascular pathology (**FIGURE 1**).
- When a broader view of the abdomen is needed, a CT scan can be performed. Intravenous contrast is routinely administered, and due to the nature of the examination, the patient will be exposed to radiation (equivalent of ~100 chest X-rays) (**FIGURES 2** and **3**).
- MRCP can also be performed to evaluate the biliary system and surrounding liver parenchyma. The nature of the MR protocol that is required to optimally visualize the biliary system does not fully assess surrounding structures, thus limiting the evaluation of non-biliary pathology. (**FIGURE 4**).

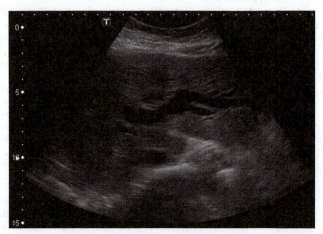

FIGURE 1 • Axial ultrasound image of the liver demonstrating marked intrahepatic biliary ductal dilation.

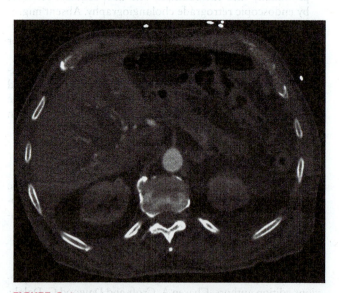

FIGURE 2 • Axial CT image with marked intrahepatic biliary ductal dilation and pancreatic ductal dilation.

Chapter 6 PERCUTANEOUS TRANSHEPATIC BILIARY IMAGING AND INTERVENTION

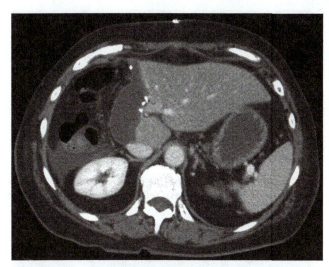

FIGURE 3 • Contrast enhanced axial CT image with biloma and free fluid. The patient was status-post right hepatectomy.

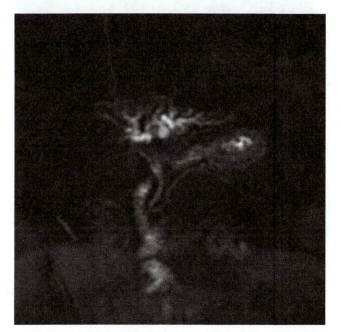

FIGURE 4 • Coronal image from a MRCP demonstrating dilation of the right anterior and left hepatic ducts. The right posterior, common hepatic, and pancreatic ducts are of normal caliber.

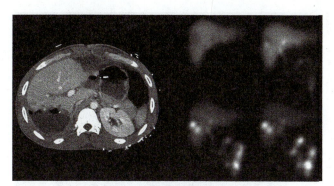

FIGURE 5 • Images from a hepatobiliary iminodiacetic acid (HIDA) scan (four images on right) of a trauma patient with a liver laceration. There is tracer accumulation in the region of the right hepatic lobe, which corresponds to an increasing fluid collection on CT.

- When evaluating for a bile leak, cholescintigraphy (also known as a hepatobiliary iminodiacetic acid [HIDA] or diisopropyl iminodiacetic acid [DISIDA] scan) can be performed. The radiopharmaceutical is taken up by the liver and excreted into the bile. When the tracer is seen accumulating outside of the liver, or in intrahepatic cavities, the diagnosis of leak can be confirmed (FIGURE 5).

SURGICAL MANAGEMENT

Preprocedure Planning

- All related imaging to the patient's condition should be reviewed. A PTC/PTHD can be performed either under conscious sedation or with general anesthesia (preferred). Thus, the patient ideally will be NPO for at least 6 hours prior to the procedure.
- For any procedure that manipulates the biliary system, there is an increased risk of septicemia and endotoxemia. The patient should receive antibiotics within 1 hour of start time. The mix of gastrointestinal flora should guide antibiotic choice (gram negatives and anaerobes). At our institution, piperacillin/tazobactam 3.375 g is routinely used. In patients who are penicillin allergic, ciprofloxacin 400 mg and metronidazole 500 mg are given.
- Unless the left-sided ducts are unilaterally dilated, a right-sided approach is routinely used, as this will drain a larger portion of the liver and will decrease radiation exposure to the interventionalist.

Positioning

- Biliary procedures are performed with the patient in the supine position, arms at the side.

PERCUTANEOUS TRANSHEPATIC CHOLANGIOGRAPHY

Immediate Preprocedure

- The patient's abdomen should be cleaned and prepped from the nipple line to the left midaxillary line to 5 cm below the umbilicus and beyond the right posterior axillary line.
- When right-sided access is warranted, a hemostat should be placed at the right midaxillary line at the selected access site during deep inspiration (FIGURE 6). This is used to verify that the entrance site is below the greatest diaphragmatic excursion. Access above this mark should *not* be attempted as it exposes the patient to the risk of violating the pleura, resulting in pneumothorax or biliary–pleural fistula.
- Local anesthetic should be used and a small incision (2-3 mm) made to facilitate needle passage.

Duct Cannulation

- Duct cannulation can be performed with a 15-cm, 21- or 22-gauge Chiba needle. These needles are relatively small (thereby reducing bleeding risk) and can accept a 0.018-in wire.

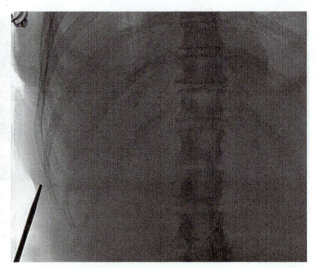

FIGURE 6 • Placement of hemostat to mark the entrance site.

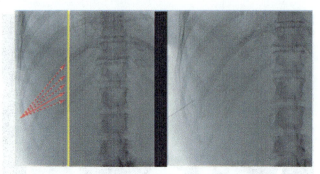

FIGURE 7 • Fan pattern of needle passes (*solid line*, initial pass; *dashed line*, subsequent passes). *Yellow* indicates midaxillary line.

- When left-sided access is required, US is routinely used to localize a relatively superficial duct. The duct is then cannulated under direct US guidance.
- Due to the overlying ribs, right-sided access is usually accomplished with a "blind" technique, which can either be subclassified into an antegrade or retrograde approach.
- When using the retrograde approach, the Chiba needle is advanced from the liver margin to the midaxillary line. The stylet is removed, and under fluoroscopy, a small amount of dilute contrast is injected as the needle is pulled back.
- When using the antegrade approach, the stylet is removed from the Chiba needle, and under fluoroscopic guidance, the needle is advanced while injecting dilute contrast until reaching the midclavicular line.
- Regardless of approach, multiple passes through the liver at different obliquities (cranial–caudal *and* anterior–posterior) are often required before a duct is cannulated (**FIGURE 7**). The technical challenge and number of passes required for successful cannulation is directly related to the extent of intrahepatic biliary dilation. This is particularly problematic in the setting of bile duct injury with a biliary tree that is fully decompressed into the peritoneal space.
- Peripheral cannulation is the goal. Cannulation of centrally located duct increases the risk of arteriobiliary or venobiliary fistula and hemorrhage.

Cholangiogram

- It is very easy for a well-placed needle to dislodge while the patient is breathing. To prevent this from occurring, a 0.018-in wire is placed through the Chiba needle and coiled within the biliary system. The needle is exchanged for a short 3 or 4 Fr

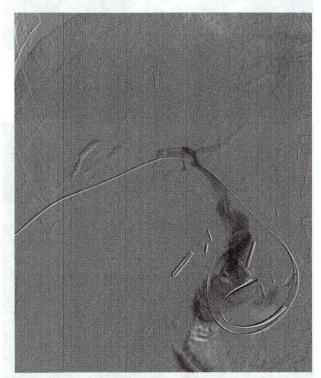

FIGURE 8 • PTC in a patient following liver transplant with history of hepaticojejunostomy stricture. Cholangiogram demonstrates no evidence of stricture. Intrahepatic ducts were normal on other images (not shown).

catheter. A Tuohy-Borst sidearm introducer is then placed over the wire and attached to the catheter, allowing for contrast injection without loss of wire access.
- While injecting dilute contrast, either an angiographic run or static images are obtained in multiple obliquities (**FIGURE 8**).
- Once adequate images are obtained, the catheter and wire are removed.

PERCUTANEOUS TRANSHEPATIC DRAIN

- If durable access to the biliary tree is indicated, once a 0.018-in wire is coiled within the biliary system, a stiff coaxial catheter is advanced into the biliary system. Once the wire and inner catheter are removed, the bowel is cannulated using a short angled catheter and hydrophilic wire.
- The hydrophilic wire is removed and exchanged for a stiff wire through the catheter. The tract is dilated to accommodate a biliary drainage catheter, which is positioned so the proximal side holes are draining the intrahepatic ducts and the distal pigtail is in the bowel (**FIGURE 9**).
- The catheter should then be sutured to the skin and placed to external drainage for 24 to 48 hours, after which it can be capped.

Chapter 6 PERCUTANEOUS TRANSHEPATIC BILIARY IMAGING AND INTERVENTION

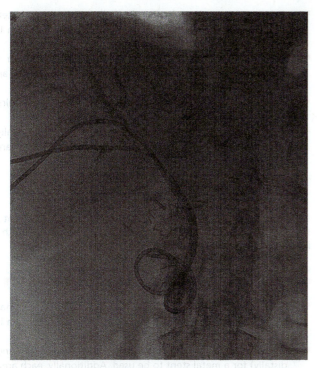

FIGURE 9 • Internal/external biliary drainage catheters in both the right anterior and posterior ducts.

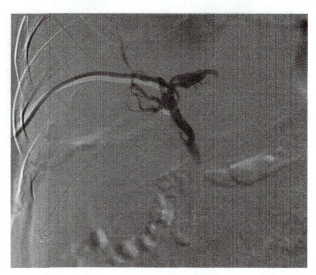

FIGURE 10 • Digital subtraction angiography image of an 8-Fr external drainage catheter within the main hepatic duct.

- If the area of stenosis cannot be crossed, an external drain can be placed with the pigtail coiled within the intrahepatic biliary ducts (FIGURE 10). This catheter must be kept to gravity bag drainage.

BALLOON DILATION

Dilations

- Postsurgical or focal inflammatory scarring can routinely be treated with serial balloon dilation.
- With a stiff wire in place, serial dilations, starting with balloons 1 to 2 mm smaller than the area of stenosis and then 2 to 3 mm larger than normal ducts, are performed. The length of the balloon can be either 2 or 4 cm in length, depending on the area of stenosis.
- When a regular balloon is not adequate, a scoring balloon or a cutting balloon can be used in certain (FIGURE 11).
- After dilation a larger internal/external biliary drain is usually placed.
- Dilations are performed every 2 to 3 weeks, for a total of three dilations.

Challenge

- When the patient returns 2 to 3 weeks after the third dilation, a TB is drawn preoperatively.
- If the cholangiogram shows that the area of stenosis is patent, an external drainage catheter is placed with the pigtail peripheral to the area in question and capped (FIGURE 10).

Success or Failure

- The patient returns in 1 to 2 weeks after challenge. A TB is drawn preoperatively.

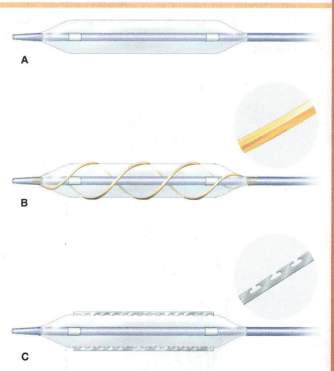

FIGURE 11 • A, Standard noncompliant balloon. B, A modified balloon allows for the scoring of the ductal walls, which has shown to increase the chances of successful dilation. C, A cutting balloon for extremely difficult stenoses. Due to the risk of perforation, great care should be taken when using this balloon.

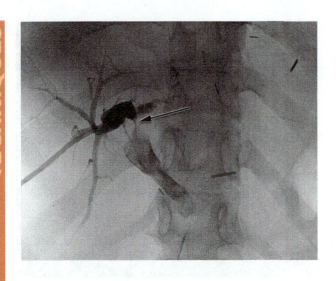

- A cholangiogram is performed through the existing catheter. If the area in question remains patent and the bilirubin is normal, the catheter is removed.
- If either the cholangiogram is abnormal or the bilirubin is elevated, the external drainage catheter is replaced with an internal/external catheter (FIGURE 12).
- Until definitive surgical management, the patient will require routine (every 3 months) changes of this catheter.
- Alternatively, if anatomically feasible, an endoscopically retrievable stent can be placed until definitive surgical management (see following discussion of "Stent Placement").

FIGURE 12 • Arrow indicates residual high-grade anastomotic stricture after challenge. Patient required replacement of the internal/external drainage catheter.

STENT PLACEMENT

Evaluation

- Only until recently, metallic stents were permanent and reserved for those patients with a life expectancy of less than 6 months, as there is a 50% occlusion rate at this interval.[1] With introduction of the covered metal stents that can be endoscopically exchanged, patients with longer life expectancies can benefit from indwelling metallic stents (FIGURE 13). However, in patients whose biliary systems are not endoscopically accessible, these stents cannot be changed.

- Once a PTHD has been performed and the biliary system has had time to drain (24-72 hours), a formal cholangiogram is performed.
- There must be an adequate landing zone (proximally and distally) for a metal stent to be used. Additionally, each area of stenosis will usually require a stent. In most situations, a single central area of stenosis of the right, left, and/or main hepatic ducts are amendable to stent placement. Patients with Klatskin tumors, who present with multiple areas of stenosis, are typically not candidates (FIGURE 14).

Placement

- Over a stiff wire, a properly sized stent is advanced and deployed (FIGURE 15).

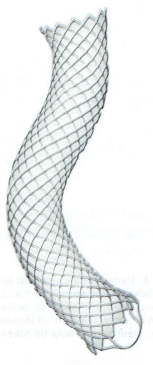

FIGURE 13 • A covered, self-expanding metal biliary stent.

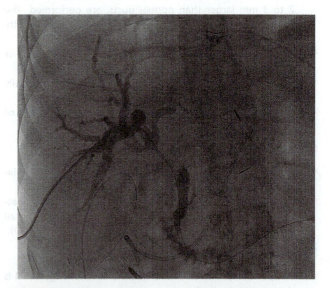

FIGURE 14 • Cholangiogram demonstrating multiple central intrahepatic biliary strictures as well as a long-segment stricture of the peripheral common bile duct consistent with a Klatskin tumor. Due to the number of strictures, this patient was not a stent candidate.

Chapter 6 **PERCUTANEOUS TRANSHEPATIC BILIARY IMAGING AND INTERVENTION**   49

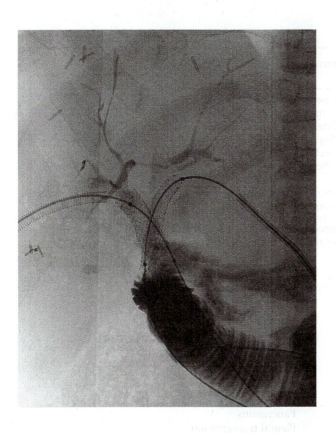

- If the stenosis involves the distal common bile duct, a short segment of stent (1-2 mm) should extend into the small bowel. When there is an associated duodenal stricture that also requires stenting, a longer segment of the biliary stent should extend into the bowel, alongside the duodenal stent.
- A small catheter should remain across the stent for 24 to 72 hours.

Follow-up

- The patient should return for a cholangiogram in 24 to 72 hours to determine if the stent remains patent. If the stent is patent, the catheter can be removed.
- If the stent is occluded, an internal/external catheter should be placed. The patient should return for routine catheter changes every 3 months.

FIGURE 15 • With sheaths and wires through both the right and left biliary ducts, self-expanding stents were deployed. In each stent is an angioplasty balloon, which will be inflated simultaneously to prevent one from crushing the other.

MISCELLANEOUS BILIARY INTERVENTIONS

Brushings/Biopsy

- Once a PTHD has been performed, the area of stenosis crossed and the biliary system has had time to drain, and any associated blood that is invariably present after the initial access procedure had cleared, biopsies can be performed. Both brushings and a forceps biopsy are routinely performed to increase in the likelihood of diagnosis (**FIGURE 16**).
- To obtain brushings, a sheath must be placed across the stenosis, through which the brush system is advanced. The sheath is pulled back to expose the brush system. The brush is advanced out of its catheter multiple times to collect the cells. The brush is removed and placed in cytology solution.
- When performing a forceps biopsy, the sheath is placed just proximal to the lesion and two to three samples are obtained and placed in formalin.

Stone and Debris

- After adequate drainage, a sheath is placed through which a noncompliant angioplasty balloon is advanced to dilate any common bile duct stricture, if present.
- Using a compliant balloon, debris and small stones are swept into the common duct and then pushed into the bowel.
- When the stone is too large to be pushed into the bowel, a stone-crushing basket can be used to break the stone into smaller pieces.

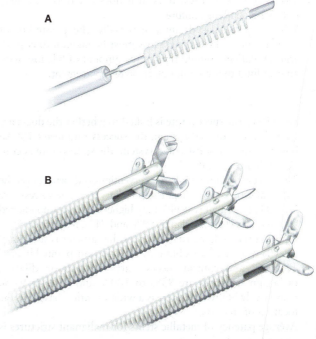

FIGURE 16 • **A**, Biliary brush. **B**, Biliary introducer forceps.

PEARLS AND PITFALLS

Patient history and physical findings	• Biliary dilation does not normally occur in posttransplant livers.
Operative technique	• Defining maximum inspiration is important to prevent pleural transgression. • To prevent septicemia and endotoxemia, dilated biliary systems should be drained for 24 to 72 hours after catheter placement. Further intervention should be delayed. • Crossing the midclavicular line during duct cannulation increases the risk of a left-sided cannulation as well as traversing central vessels in the porta hepatis. • Minimizing the ductal entry angle allows for a proper force vector when dilating the tract and advancing the catheter. • Each puncture of the liver capsule increases the risk of bleeding. When redirecting the needle, care should be made not to remove it completely from the liver.
Postoperative care	• Upper endoscopy should not be performed for up to 6 weeks after PTHD to prevent lethal air embolus from possible biliary to hepatic vein fistula.

POSTOPERATIVE CARE

- Drainage catheters should be flushed twice a day with 10 mL of sterile 0.9% saline.
- Patients with internal/external biliary catheters that are capped should be instructed to uncap the catheter and place it to gravity bag drainage if they experience abdominal pain, fevers, leakage, or pruritus. They should be evaluated in the next 24 to 48 hours.
- During the process of a "challenge," it is not uncommon for there to be some leakage around the biliary catheter; this should resolve in a few days. If it does not resolve, it may indicate a challenge failure.
- When a patient is draining externally, the possibility of dehydration and electrolyte loss must be taken into consideration. Patients should replace the amount of bile loss with an oral fluid that contains electrolyte replacement.

OUTCOMES

- For a PTC, the success rate is linked to whether the ducts are dilated. For a dilated system, the success rate nears 100%; however, in a nonobstructed system, the success rate is considerably lower (65%).[2]
- The success rate for all biliary interventions is dependent on the technical success of cannulating the biliary tree. The success rate for a dilated system is significantly higher than for a nondilated system (including transplants), 99% and 74%, respectively.[2,3]
- Once cannulated, internalization of the catheter is successful in 78% of native livers but only 59% in transplanted livers.[4]
- Technical and clinical success rates for balloon dilation of benign strictures are 93% to 100% and 75% to 94%, respectively.[5] However, there is a wide variation based on the location of stenosis.[6]
- Average patency of metallic stents for malignant strictures is about 6 months.[1]

COMPLICATIONS

- The risk of all complications is <3%[7] and include
  - Hemorrhage
  - Bile leak
  - Bile peritonitis
  - Sepsis
  - Pancreatitis
  - Pleural transgression
  - Contrast reaction
  - Death

REFERENCES

1. Gordon RL, Ring EJ, LaBerge JM, et al. Malignant biliary obstruction: treatment with expandable metallic stents—follow-up of 50 consecutive patients. *Radiology*. 1992;182:697-701.
2. Jander HP, Galbraith J, Aldrete JS. Percutaneous transhepatic cholangiography using the Chiba needle: comparison with retrograde pancreatocholecystography. *South Med J*. 1980;73(4):415-421.
3. Mueller PR, Harbin WP, Ferrucci Jr JT, et al. Fine-needle transhepatic cholangiography: reflections after 450 cases. *AJR Am J Roentgenol*. 1981;136:85-90.
4. Morita S, Kitanosono T, Lee D, et al. Comparison of technical success and complications of percutaneous transhepatic cholangiography and biliary drainage between patients with and without transplanted liver. *AJR Am J Roentgenol*. 2012;199(5):1149-1152.
5. Kucukay F, Okten RS, Yurdakul M, et al. Long-term results of percutaneous biliary balloon dilation treatment for benign hepaticojejunostomy strictures: are repeated balloon dilations necessary? *J Vasc Interv Radiol*. 2012;23:1347-1355.
6. Citron SJ, Martin LG. Benign biliary strictures: treatment with percutaneous cholangioplasty. *Radiology*. 1991;178:339-341.
7. Saad WEA, Wallace MJ, Wojak JC, et al. Quality improvement guidelines for percutaneous transhepatic cholangiography, biliary drainage, and cholecystostomy. *J Vasc Interv Radiol*. 2010;21:789-795.

Chapter 7

Surgically Assisted Endoscopic Retrograde Cholangiopancreatoscopy

Crystal N. Johnson-Mann and Steven J. Hughes

DEFINITION

- Surgical assistance to successfully perform endoscopic retrograde cholangiopancreatography (ERCP) is necessary when intestinal continuity has been surgically modified precluding standard endoscopic access to the ampulla of Vater from the mouth.
- Prior gastric bypass history is the surgical procedure that commonly leads to the need for laparoscopic-assisted ERCP, given the Roux-en-Y anatomy.
- The presence of a gastric remnant is essential to the performance of laparoscopic-assisted endoscopic retrograde cholangiopancreatography (LA-ERCP).
- Rarely, a clinical scenario may arise where surgical access to a gastric remnant may be indicated to facilitate endoscopic ultrasound.
- As magnetic resonance cholangiopancreatography provides a noninvasive means to assess the pancreaticobiliary duct systems in most patients, ERCP is generally not indicated as a diagnostic modality. Therapeutic intent is the indication for ERCP, and this concept must be emphasized when considering LA-ERCP.

DIFFERENTIAL DIAGNOSIS

- Choledocholithiasis
- Biliary strictures
- Sphincter of Oddi dysfunction
- Bile leak following cholecystectomy
- Pathology involving the Ampulla of Vater or common bile duct (ie, ampullary tumors, cholangiocarcinoma)
- Intraductal papillary mucinous neoplasm
- Chronic pancreatitis
- Disrupted pancreatic duct syndrome

PATIENT HISTORY AND PHYSICAL FINDINGS

- Historically, LA-ERCP was initially reported as a novel method of accessing the common bile duct in patients with a history of Roux-en-Y gastric bypass.[1]
- Additional surgical history should be reviewed. If the gallbladder is in situ, a cholecystectomy is likely warranted as part of the LA-ERCP. In this rare clinical setting, intraoperative cholangiography should first be performed and justify proceeding to LA-ERCP.

SURGICAL MANAGEMENT

Preoperative Planning

- The potential need for serial ERCP procedures should be determined prior to LA-ERCP. A gastrostomy tube (G-tube) can be placed at the index procedure to facilitate subsequent endoscopic interventions, if indicated. Potentially affected patients should be prepared for this possibility.
- These operations require significant coordination between multidisciplinary teams. The authors highly recommend that these procedures be scheduled as the first case of the day.
- The procedure needs to be scheduled in a room that can accommodate both the surgical and gastroenterology teams, a C-arm fluoroscopy unit, and a mobile endoscopy cart.

Positioning

- The operative table should be configured so that C-arm fluoroscopy can be readily performed of the upper abdomen (FIGURE 1).

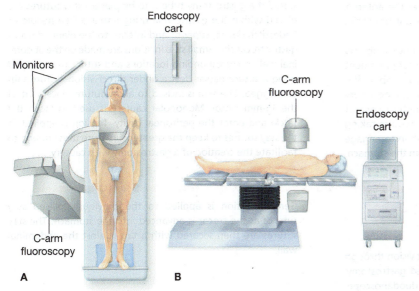

FIGURE 1 • The C-arm fluoroscopy unit is positioned on the patient's right, and the mobile duodenoscopy equipment on the patient's left.

- After induction of general anesthesia, a urinary bladder catheter is placed. An orogastric tube is rarely necessary.
- The patient is positioned supine, ideally with both arms tucked to facilitate access for both C-arm fluoroscopy and the endoscopy team. A footboard is placed. A fixed liver retractor can be positioned on either side of the patient if needed.
- Venous thromboembolism prophylaxis (both mechanical and pharmacologic) should be used. Antibiotics are administered within the guidelines of Surgical Care Improvement Program (SCIP) criteria for a clean-contaminated procedure.

- See ▶ **Videos 1** and **2**.

TROCAR PLACEMENT

- Trocar placement is depicted in **FIGURE 2**. Four to five trocars will be required for the procedure, depending on whether cholecystectomy is also performed.
- Initial trocar placement is performed in the left upper abdomen, midclavicular line, using an optical trocar and a 0° laparoscope with low insufflation flow. Once within the peritoneal cavity, insufflation is increased to high flow, the laparoscope is then exchanged to a 30°, and subsequent tracts are placed under direct vision.

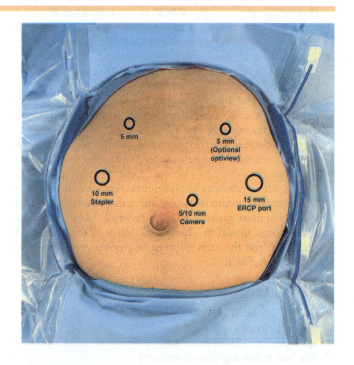

FIGURE 2 • Trocar placement for LA-ERCP. Pneumoperitoneum is established via the left upper abdominal incision. The far right abdominal 5-mm trocar is used for grasping and the bowel clamp. The right, midclavicular line port (12 mm) is used for suture and stapler placement. The left midabdominal 5-mm trocar is used for the camera, and the left port is used to provide access for the duodenoscope. It must be at least 15 mm in diameter.

GASTRIC PEXY

- The patient is placed in reverse Trendelenburg position, if needed, and the location of the transgastric trocar placement determined. Ideally, the trocar will enter the anterior gastric wall at the junction of the body and the antrum of the stomach along the greater curve.
- Determine the relationship of an antegastric Roux limb and the associated mesentery to the ideal location for placement of the transgastric trocar. Dissection of the Roux limb and/or its mesentery should be avoided unless absolutely necessary to avoid injury or vascular compromise. It is better to accept a more lateral target, including one that may require taking down some of the greater curve mesentery, than to engage in a significant dissection of the Roux limb from the stomach.
- Two stab wounds are placed around the planned site of the transgastric trocar (four if planning to also place a gastrostomy tube at the end of the procedure).
- Starting with the cranial suture, two (or four as previously stated if a gastrostomy tube is to be placed) stay sutures are placed within the gastric wall using either a free needle or Endostitch device, superior and inferior to the planned transgastric trocar site. Small stab incisions are made on the abdominal wall in corresponding locations and suture tails grasped using a suture passer device under direct vision. Suture tails are tagged. The skin is incised to allow future placement of the 15-mm trocar. Monopolar cautery is used to incise the fascia and enter the peritoneal cavity. Tension is applied to the stay sutures to keep the greater curvature taut enough to facilitate the creation of a gastrostomy with cautery.

PLACEMENT OF THE TRANSGASTRIC TROCAR

- A 15-mm trocar is then advanced under direct vision through the abdominal wall into the recently created gastrostomy. This allows for passage of the side-viewing duodenoscope.

Gentle traction is applied to the previously placed stay sutures as the trocar is advanced into the stomach. The stay sutures are then secured with a tag against the abdominal wall.

ATRAUMATICALLY CLAMP THE PANCREATICOBILIARY LIMB

- The omentum and transverse colon are reflected cephalad to expose the ligament of Treitz.
- The pancreaticobiliary limb is identified and an atraumatic bowel clamp is applied to occlude the lumen to prevent gaseous distention of the small bowel distally (**FIGURE 3**).

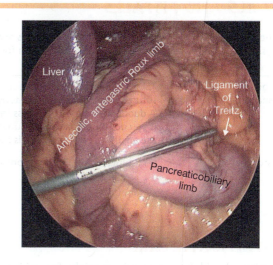

FIGURE 3 • The pancreaticobiliary limb is atraumatically clamped to prevent distention of the small bowel from insufflation required during the ERCP.

DRAPE THE OPERATIVE FIELD AND PERFORM ENDOSCOPIC RETROGRADE CHOLANGIOPANCREATOGRAPHY

- A small hole in the center of a large laparotomy sheet is created then positioned over the patient such that only the 15-mm trocar is visible.
- The gastroenterology team then proceeds with the ERCP. We advise that the surgical team remain in the room during this portion of the procedure.
- At completion of the ERCP, the stomach is desufflated via the transgastric trocar. The duodenoscope and the 15-mm trocar (no longer sterile) are removed before the second surgical drape is removed.

GASTROSTOMY CLOSURE OR TUBE PLACEMENT

- If proceeding with gastrostomy closure, the two existing stay sutures are left in place to facilitate stapled closure of the gastrostomy with either a green or blue stapler load using the EndoGIA stapler.
- Alternatively, all stay sutures are left in place and used to secure the stomach to the anterior gastric wall if a gastrostomy tube will be placed.
- If indicated, a large-caliber G-tube with an inflatable balloon is advanced through the abdominal wall and into the lumen of the stomach (**FIGURE 4**). The balloon is inflated, and the stay sutures are secured under direct vision if possible. Occasionally, the pneumoperitoneum will lead to excessive tension of these sutures, and securing them should be deferred until pneumoperitoneum is released.
- Consider placing a purse-string around the gastrostomy using monofilament suture. This will allow the caliber of the gastrostomy to equal that of the G-tube.

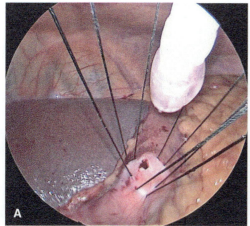 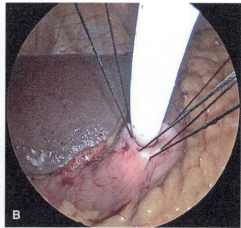

FIGURE 4 • **A** and **B**, Operative photographs of the laparoscopic placement of a G-tube. Inflate the balloon, release the pneumoperitoneum, and then tie the stay sutures.

PEARLS AND PITFALLS

Patient history and physical findings	▪ Be familiar with the patient's anatomy prior to this procedure. ▪ Depending on the indication for the procedure, ensure the patient has been appropriately counseled on risks.
Surgical management	▪ Take large, deep bites of the stomach with the stay sutures. The stomach is prone to laceration by the sutures given the significant tension that is typically applied during this procedure. ▪ A duodenoscope will not pass through a 12-mm trocar. Use a 15-mm trocar. ▪ If you do not effectively occlude the pancreaticobiliary limb with a bowel clamp, you will not be able to see anything once the ERCP is completed due to significant gaseous distention of the bowel.
Postoperative care	▪ If multiple future ERCP sessions are planned, leave a large-caliber, balloon-tipped, gastrostomy tube.

POSTOPERATIVE CARE

- Patients should be monitored overnight for evidence of complications.
- A liquid diet can usually be initiated the evening of surgery.
- If a gastrostomy tube has been placed, it should be left to gravity drainage overnight and can be clamped the morning of the first postoperative day prior to discharge.

COMPLICATIONS

- Devascularization or laceration to the Roux limb
- Posterior gastric wall injury
- Pancreatitis
- Other complications of ERCP (ie, retroduodenal perforation)

OUTCOMES

- LA-ERCP can be successfully completed in a high percentage of cases.[2]
- Outcomes should be equivalent to those reported for ERCP without the need for surgical access to a gastric remnant.

REFERENCES

1. Peters M, Papasavas PK, Caushaj PF, Kania RJ, Gagné DJ. Laparoscopic transgastric endoscopic retrograde cholangiopancreatography for benign common bile duct stricture after Roux-en-Y gastric bypass. *Surg Endosc.* 2002;16(7):1106. doi:10.1007/s00464-001-4180-3
2. AlMasri S, Zenati MS, Papachristou GI, et al. Laparoscopic-assisted ERCP following RYGB: a 12-year assessment of outcomes and learning curve at a high-volume pancreatobiliary center. *Surg Endosc.* Published online 2021. doi:10.1007/s00464-021-08328-x

Chapter 8 Roux-en-Y Choledochojejunostomy

Catalina Mosquera and Mark Bloomston

DEFINITION

- Choledochojejunostomy refers to an anastomosis between the common bile duct (CBD) and the jejunum. This anastomosis is used in the treatment of biliary tract disease; it provides continuity to the biliary flow and has significant use in traumatic, benign, and malignant processes (**FIGURE 1**).
- Roux-en-Y choledochojejunostomy is considered to have the lower incidence of postoperative cholangitis and recurrent stones compared to other choledochojejunostomy procedures.

DIFFERENTIAL DIAGNOSIS

- Restoring biliary flow following traumatic or iatrogenic injuries of the CBD.
- Re-creating bilioenteric anatomy following choledochal cyst excision (type I-II and III) and resection of biliary, ampullary, duodenal, or pancreatic lesions. In case of malignant disease, choledochojejunostomy is used following resection with curative intent or as palliation (ie, periampullary unresectable tumor, unresectable extrahepatic cholangiocarcinoma, or obstruction secondary to portal lymphadenopathy).
- Diverting biliary flow in the presence or impending development of biliary obstruction (ie, pancreatic adenocarcinoma).
- Reconstruction of biliary flow following orthotopic liver transplantation.

PATIENT HISTORY AND PHYSICAL FINDINGS

- A thorough history is relevant in determining the cause for biliary obstruction. Vague abdominal pain, nausea, and emesis may be the only presenting symptoms. However, symptoms like jaundice, acholic stools, tea-colored urine, and pruritus are consistent and more specific with biliary obstruction. These in association with fever, chills, and signs of hypoperfusion may be indicative of ascending cholangitis. Easy bruising, malnutrition, ascites, and changes in mental status may increase concern of associated hepatic dysfunction.
- On physical examination, patients may present with scleral icterus, jaundice, and tenderness to palpation of the right upper quadrant. In case of advanced malignant disease, patients may present with cachexia.
- Evaluation of abdominal scars and reviewing history of previous surgical interventions and operative notes are of paramount importance to determine etiology of the disease and for surgical planning.
- The patient's overall health should be taken into consideration when determining surgical candidacy.

IMAGING AND OTHER DIAGNOSTIC STUDIES

- Preoperative imaging is of imperative importance in understanding the disease process and helping plan the surgical approach.
- Ultrasonography should be used as the first evaluation tool when concerned about biliary obstruction. Presence of stones, inflammatory changes of the biliary tree/gallbladder, and intra/extrahepatic biliary duct dilation may be reported.
- Contrast-enhanced computed tomography and magnetic resonance imaging are the best image modalities to evaluate anatomy and determine the presence of any aberrant biliary or arterial anatomy. Imaging will aid in elucidating the possible etiology of obstruction, its extent, and/or site of injury. Magnetic resonance cholangiopancreatography is specifically useful for evaluating biliary and pancreatic ductal anatomy (**FIGURE 2**).
- Endoscopic retrograde cholangiopancreatography (ERCP) and endoscopic ultrasound are useful for relieving

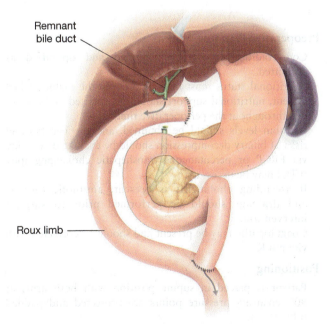

FIGURE 1 • Illustration of a Roux-en-Y choledochojejunostomy.

SECTION I SURGERY OF THE BILIARY SYSTEM

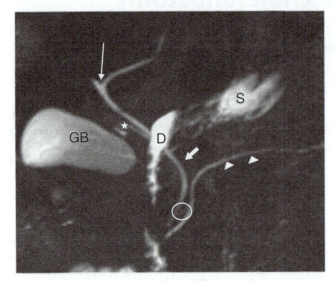

FIGURE 2 • Magnetic resonance cholangiopancreatography image depicting normal biliary anatomy. *S*, stomach; *D*, duodenum; *GB*, gallbladder; *arrowheads*, pancreatic duct; *thin arrow*, confluence of the right and left hepatic ducts; *thick arrow*, common bile duct; *star*, cystic duct; *white circle*, accessory pancreatic duct.

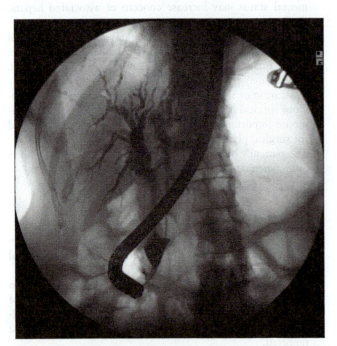

FIGURE 3 • Endoscopic retrograde cholangiopancreatography image reveals dilated intrahepatic and extrahepatic ducts, with the common bile duct dilated at 17 mm and narrowing of the distal portion at the ampulla in a patient with ampullary cancer.

- obstruction and further defining biliary anatomy and allow for tissue biopsy, respectively (**FIGURE 3**).
- Intraoperative cholangiogram allows for real-time evaluation of the biliary tree and may be helpful in identifying iatrogenic injuries (**FIGURE 4**).

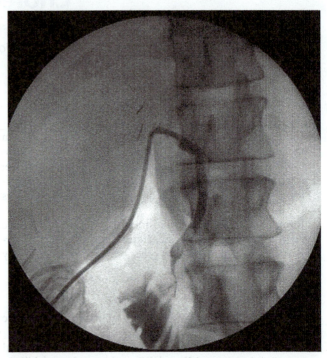

FIGURE 4 • Intraoperative cholangiogram image with identification of an iatrogenic duct injury occurring during an attempted laparoscopic cholecystectomy for acute cholecystitis. Surgical clips are noted. Contrast is seen with antegrade flow into the duodenum, but no retrograde flow is appreciated, indicating iatrogenic occlusion of the proximal bile duct.

SURGICAL MANAGEMENT

Preoperative Planning

- Comorbidities should be identified and optimized as permitted.
- Nutritional status must be evaluated. In the malnourished patient, nutritional support should be initiated and continued throughout the perioperative time.
- Bilirubin levels should be obtained, and the benefits and risks of biliary decompression should be evaluated. Stenting via ERCP or percutaneous transhepatic cholangiography (PTC) may be necessary.
- If ascending cholangitis is present, antibiotic therapy and drainage should be performed prior to surgical intervention.
- Coagulopathy may be present and should be corrected with vitamin K.

Positioning

- Patient is placed in supine position with both arms at 90°, ensuring pressure points are protected and padded (**FIGURE 5**).
- We use a bilateral post, framed retractor system (**FIGURE 6**) to maximize exposure via a bilateral subcostal incision.

Chapter 8 ROUX-EN-Y CHOLEDOCHOJEJUNOSTOMY   57

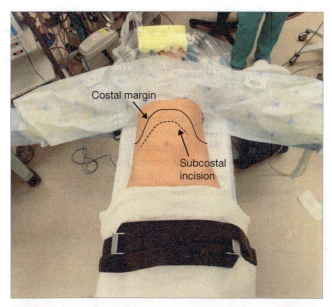

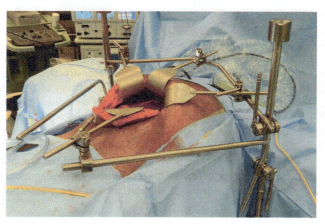

FIGURE 6 • Bilateral subcostal incision with a bilateral post retractor system in place to maximize exposure.

FIGURE 5 • Proper patient positioning with arms at 90° and placement of an airflow warming device over the patient's upper body to prevent hypothermia. *Solid line* denotes the costal margin. *Dotted line* depicts planned placement of bilateral subcostal incision.

PLACEMENT OF INCISION AND OPERATIVE EXPOSURE

- A bilateral subcostal incision provides optimal exposure. Once the peritoneum is entered, adhesions are cleared if present, and the falciform ligament is divided between ties or with an energy device. This further exposes the operative field and permits retractor placement (**FIGURE 6**).
- The abdomen is explored and all peritoneal surfaces are palpated if malignancy is suspected. The root of the mesentery is palpated early to assess for foreshortening due to tumor infiltration, inflammation, or previous surgery, which may impact the ability to develop a Roux limb for reconstruction.
- Exposure of the porta hepatis is begun by mobilizing the hepatic flexure of the colon, as necessary.
- Mobilization (Kocher maneuver) of the duodenum provides optimal exposure of the distal CBD.
- The gallbladder, if present, is removed in a top-down fashion. If the porta hepatis is involved in acute and/or chronic inflammation, the cystic duct should be traced to locate the common hepatic duct (CHD) and the CBD.
- Meticulous dissection of the porta hepatis is necessary to identify essential structures to prevent inadvertent injury. Care should be taken to search for and prevent injury to aberrant or replaced anatomic variations. A replaced right hepatic artery arising from the superior mesenteric artery will lie to the right and deep to the CBD and can be injured during CBD transection if not anticipated. The right hepatic artery commonly courses behind the CHD, but on occasion, the artery may lie anterior to the CHD. Biliary anatomic variations should also be expected (see Chapter 15, Figure 17). The absence of aberrant anatomy on preoperative imaging should not usurp careful dissection with anticipation of variance.
- Dissection and exposure of the CBD may be difficult in the face of inflammatory changes resulting from prior surgeries, radiation exposure, and/or preoperative placement of a biliary stent. At times, intraoperative ultrasound may be helpful in proper identification of the structures within the porta hepatis. Another method to identify the CBD when dissection is difficult is to use a small-gauge needle and aspirate looking for bile.
- With proper identification and dissection of the CBD, the site of transection is selected proximal to the location of injury or obstruction. It should be noted that the arterial supply to the bile duct runs along the lateral and medial aspects of the CBD and CHD, and care should be taken to avoid extensive dissection or mobilization that may compromise this blood supply. When transection of the bile duct with end-to-side reconstruction is planned, the predominant blood supply will come from the right hepatic artery near the liver hilum. Thus, a higher point of transection is desired to optimize blood supply to the anastomosis. The margin of resection should be submitted for pathological assessment in the clinical setting of malignancy.
- With the transection site selected, the CBD is divided sharply. If a stent has been placed preoperatively, it is removed at this point. Cultures of the bile are advised, particularly if the biliary tree has been instrumented. The proximal duct should be probed to ensure patency and confirm ductal anatomy—the probe should be guided up both the left and right hepatic ducts. Cholangioscopy can be undertaken if there is concern for proximal obstruction or hepatolithiasis. To control bile spillage and facilitate hemostasis, the proximal stump is temporarily closed with an atraumatic vascular bulldog clamp.

CREATION OF THE ROUX LIMB

- Although choledochoduodenostomy and choledochojejunostomy using a loop of jejunum are reconstructive options that may be appropriate in the clinical setting of a short life expectancy or a particularly hostile abdomen due to adhesions, a defunctionalized segment of jejunum using a Roux-en-Y technique is preferred due to superior outcomes. Beginning at the ligament of Treitz, the jejunum is examined to the first point at which a loop can easily be brought up through a defect in the proximal transverse mesocolon to the divided CBD without tension. The transection point is based upon the length of the mesentery and the vascular arcades as determined by transillumination of the mesentery. A gastrointestinal anastomosis stapler is used to divide the jejunum at this point. The mesentery is then carefully divided, preserving the vascular arcades, down to its base using ligatures for hemostasis. Care must be taken to maintain proximal and distal orientation of the divided jejunum. A defect is created in the transverse mesocolon, to the right of the middle colic vessels, and the Roux limb is brought up in a retrocolic orientation to serve as the defunctionalized biliary-enteric limb and placed without tension near the divided CBD.

CHOLEDOCHOJEJUNOSTOMY ANASTOMOSIS

- The choledochojejunostomy is created in a single-layer, interrupted fashion using 4-0 or 5-0 polydioxanone monofilament absorbable suture. Nonabsorbable and/or braided sutures should be avoided to minimize risk of stone formation.
- Stenting across the anastomosis is also avoided, even in the case of a normal-sized duct.
- An end-to-side anastomosis provides for ease of exposure during the reconstruction. Electrocautery is used to create an enterotomy on the antimesenteric side of the Roux limb approximately 1 to 2 cm from the stapled end to minimize a potential reservoir and associated bacterial overgrowth. The enterotomy is sized smaller than the transected CBD width, in anticipation of "enterotomy stretch" that occurs during suturing.
- The CBD is reopened, bile flow is again confirmed, and the duct cleared as necessary. The duct is trimmed as needed with Potts scissors, allowing for maximal diameter; sharp, crisp edges; and identification of good vascularity. Small figure-of-8 sutures of 5-0 polydioxanone may be necessary to manage hemorrhage from the arterial supply.
- The jejunum is placed near the transected CBD, positioned so as to limit redundancy and kinking of the jejunum. Lateral traction sutures are placed full thickness out-to-in on the jejunum and in-to-out on the bile duct, left untied, and placed on hemostats under gentle lateral traction.
- The posterior row sutures are placed approximately every 2 to 3 mm apart, taking full-thickness bites of the duct and jejunum, working from one lateral corner to the other. Be certain that the jejunal mucosa is incorporated into the stitch. Sutures are placed in-to-out on the jejunum and out-to-in on the duct, such that when tied the knot will be within the lumen (**FIGURE 7**). Gentle upward traction on the anterior wall of the bile duct provides nice exposure of the lumen to ensure proper suture placement through the posterior wall. The sutures are tagged and left untied to allow the Roux limb to be manipulated freely to maximize exposure.
- Great care is taken to maintain orientation of the sutures. Suture order must be preserved to prevent overlapping, and thus narrowing of the anastomosis when the posterior row is complete and the knots tied. Small hemostats should be used to tag each suture and place them in the proper orientation and order on a sponge clamp (**FIGURE 8**).

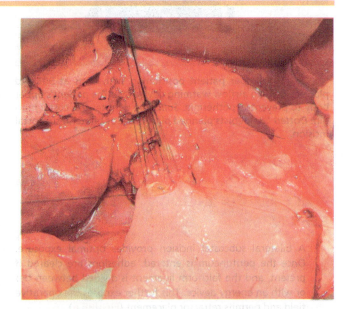

FIGURE 7 • Creation of the choledochojejunostomy anastomosis. Corner sutures placed to permit lateral traction and orientation of the posterior and anterior rows. Posterior row of monofilament sutures are placed in such a way that the knots will lay within the lumen.

- Once all of the posterior row sutures are placed, tie each suture in order from one corner to the other, carefully laying the knots to ensure optimal intervals along the way. If an interval is determined to be too large (>3-4 mm), an additional suture is placed, tied, and then the remainder of the row sutures are tied (**FIGURE 9**). The corner sutures are left untied to allow mobility and maximum exposure of the entire back row while placing the anterior row of sutures. Suture tails are then cut short and the anterior row is addressed.
- The anterior row sutures are placed in an out-to-in fashion on the jejunum and an in-to-out fashion on the duct so that the suture knots will be outside the lumen (**FIGURE 10**). Again, intervals are assessed and additional sutures placed as needed.
- Once complete, the anastomosis is inspected for evidence of a bile leak (**FIGURE 11**). Absence of tension on the anastomosis is confirmed. The surgical field is dried, ensuring good hemostasis, a clean, white surgical sponge is carefully packed around the anastomosis, and attention is turned to creating the jejunojejunal anastomosis.

Chapter 8 ROUX-EN-Y CHOLEDOCHOJEJUNOSTOMY 59

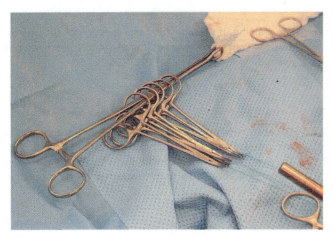

FIGURE 8 • Sutures placed during creation of the posterior and anterior rows are left untied, tagged with hemostats, and their orientation and order maintained by arranging them on a sponge forceps clamped to a laparotomy sponge. This is placed above the retractor system on the drapes and optimizes efficiency when tying the sutures.

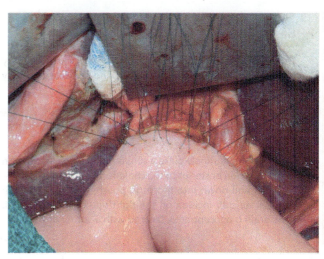

FIGURE 10 • The anterior row sutures have been placed. Visual inspection confirms proper interval placement of the sutures. The sutures are ready to be tied to complete the choledochojejunostomy anastomosis.

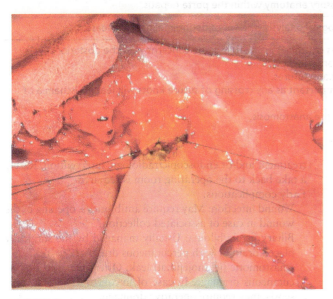

FIGURE 9 • The choledochojejunostomy posterior row sutures have been tied and the row inspected. The previously placed lateral traction sutures are left untied in preparation for placement of the anterior row sutures. Gentle downward traction on the Roux limb enhances exposure as shown in the picture.

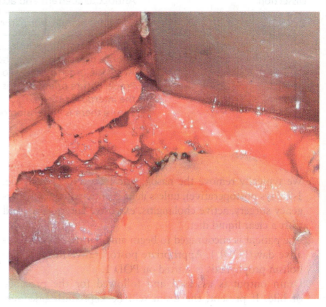

FIGURE 11 • The anterior row sutures have been tied, and the choledochojejunostomy anastomosis is carefully inspected for any bile leak. A small, clean, white gauze (not pictured) is placed posterior to the anastomosis to aid in evaluation of a biliary leak.

JEJUNOJEJUNAL ANASTOMOSIS

- Intestinal continuity is reestablished by a Roux-en-Y anastomosis. The proximal biliopancreatic limb is anastomosed to the biliary-enteric Roux limb approximately 45 to 65 cm downstream from the choledochojejunostomy anastomosis to minimize enteric reflux. We prefer to create a side-to-side, functional end-to-end anastomosis using a linear stapling device, and then closing the common enterotomy with a single row of interrupted 3-0 silk sutures.
- The small bowel mesenteric defect is closed at the Roux-en-Y anastomosis using interrupted silk sutures.
- The mesocolic defect is closed, incorporating a seromuscular bite of the passing jejunum, with 3-0 silk sutures to prevent the possibility of limb migration and/or internal herniation. Every attempt should be made to ensure that this closure does not impinge upon the bowel.

PREPARING FOR CLOSURE

- Returning to the choledochojejunostomy, the previously placed sponge is carefully removed and inspected for any bile staining. If present, further inspection of the anastomosis is warranted and additional sutures are placed as needed.

CLOSURE

- The authors routinely place a single fluted surgical drain on closed suction posterior to the choledochojejunostomy anastomosis and down into Morrison pouch, then out through a separate stab incision on the right side of the abdomen. The drain is appropriately secured with a suture at the skin.
- The abdominal fascia is closed in two layers (posterior fascia and anterior fascia) with 1-0 polydiaxonone.
- The skin is reapproximated with buried, deep dermal, interrupted, 3-0 absorbable braided sutures. The skin is closed with surgical glue.

PEARLS AND PITFALLS

Indications	A thorough history and physical examination with good preoperative imaging is important in anticipating the extent of the procedure.
Dissection	Anticipate aberrant and accessory anatomy within the porta hepatis.
Excision	Send CBD margins for pathological analysis when considering malignant disease.
Choledochojejunostomy	Meticulous suture technique is critical. There should be no concerns with the posterior row prior to proceeding with the anterior row.
	Avoid the urge to place too many sutures.
	Proper suture orientation is important as any crossing of suture knots will lead to ischemia of the interposed tissue.
	Ensure there is no tension on the anastomosis.

POSTOPERATIVE CARE

- We typically remove the nasogastric tube (NGT) early (ie, 1-2 days postoperative), unless ileus is anticipated (eg, emergency surgery, active cholangitis, extensive enterolysis), and start a clear liquid diet.
- The patient is encouraged to begin ambulating on postoperative day (POD) 1. Appropriate postoperative thromboembolism prophylaxis is started on POD 1.
- Drain output is assessed and followed for the presence of bile. If present, the drain will be kept until bile output has cleared, as it almost always will do so on its own. If drain output is serous, then the drains can be pulled with little concern for volume of output. Drains are pulled after the patient is tolerating a diet and usually prior to discharge.
- Postoperative laboratory studies are followed on a daily basis to include a complete blood count, serum chemistry, and liver function tests.

OUTCOMES

- Long-term survival rates after choledochojejunostomy are dependent on the underlying indication for the procedure.

COMPLICATIONS

- Complications are reported up to 40% of the time. Most of the time, these can be managed with pharmacologic treatment and/or endoscopic/radiologic intervention. Rarely a take back to the operating room is required.
- Early complications:
  - Wound infection: May require antibiotics ± opening of the wound in case of associated collection.
  - Biliary fistula/biloma: Usually managed by the surgically placed drain or with percutaneous drainage.
  - Anastomotic (jejunojejunal) leak: Often managed by percutaneous drainage. In case of uncontrolled drainage or sepsis, may require operative drainage.
  - Cholangitis: Generally indicates reflux from ileus; it can be managed with NGT decompression and antibiotics; PTC may be used to decompress Roux limb specifically if NGT is ineffective.
- Late complications:
  - Biliary stricture: Can occur up to 10 or more years after surgery—heralded by rising alkaline phosphatase; often can be treated with PTC and balloon dilation but may require surgical revision of the anastomosis.

SUGGESTED READINGS

1. Morris-Stiff G, Tamijmarane A, Tan YM, et al. Pre-operative stenting is associated with a higher prevalence of post-operative complications following pancreatoduodenectomy. *Int J Surg*. 2011;9(2):145-149. doi:10.1016/j.ijsu.2010.10.008
2. Sicklick JK, Camp MS, Lillemoe KD, et al. Surgical management of bile duct injuries sustained during laparoscopic cholecystectomy: perioperative results in 200 patients. *Ann Surg*. 2005;241:786-792.

Chapter 9

Minimally Invasive Choledochojejunostomy

Eugene P. Ceppa and C. Max Schmidt

DEFINITION

- Hepaticojejunostomy is the operative formation of an anastomosis between the biliary tree and the jejunum. Biliary obstruction secondary to benign and malignant strictures is the primary indication for biliary bypass.

DIFFERENTIAL DIAGNOSIS

- Benign
  - Bile duct injury
    - Iatrogenic
    - Traumatic
  - Chronic pancreatitis
  - Choledochal cyst
  - Mirizzi syndrome
- Malignant
  - Cholangiocarcinoma (mid-bile duct)
  - Periampullary tumors (palliative)
  - Portal lymphadenopathy (palliative)

PATIENT HISTORY AND PHYSICAL FINDINGS

- History
  - Weight loss
  - Fevers/chills
  - Yellow eyes/skin
  - Tea-colored urine
  - Acholic stools
  - Right upper quadrant pain
- Physical examination
  - Temporal wasting
  - Scleral icterus
  - Jaundiced skin
  - Right upper quadrant tenderness
  - Courvoisier's sign—painless, palpable gallbladder with jaundice

IMAGING AND OTHER DIAGNOSTIC STUDIES

- Ultrasonography
  - Fast and inexpensive
  - Gallbladder
    - Stones
    - Cholecystitis
  - Biliary tree
    - Extrahepatic duct dilatation
    - Intrahepatic duct dilatation
- Cross-sectional imaging
  - Computed tomography abdomen/pelvis with IV contrast—triple phase (CT A/P)
    - Determine location of hepatic arteries
    - Location of right hepatic artery relative to bile duct
    - Presence of replaced right or common hepatic artery
    - Presence of portal/splenic/superior mesenteric thrombosis
  - Magnetic resonance imaging/cholangiopancreotography with IV contrast
    - Location of biliary stricture visualization superior to CT
- Cholangiography
  - Endoscopic retrograde cholangiopancreatography
    - Gold standard
    - Diagnostic by identifying level of obstruction/anatomy
    - Sample obstruction for brushings and cytology
    - Therapeutic by placement of biliary endoprosthesis to decompress biliary tree
  - Percutaneous transhepatic cholangiography
    - Second option
    - Transhepatic approach less desirable
    - Diagnostic by identifying level of obstruction/anatomy
    - Sample obstruction for brushings and cytology
    - Percutaneous biliary drain left proximal to stricture for biliary decompression

SURGICAL MANAGEMENT

- The bulk of surgical treatment should be discussed in the Techniques section. Here, consider indications and other more general concerns, such as:

Preoperative Planning

- Cardiopulmonary disease
  - Increased risk relative to the laparoscopic approach primarily as a function of length of anesthetic time and ability to clear carbon dioxide from the pneumoperitoneum
  - Obstructive sleep apnea and chronic obstructive pulmonary disease can be exacerbated as a result of a prolonged anesthetic
- Past surgical history
  - Peritoneal access
  - Port placement
  - Roux limb reach to porta hepatis
  - Small bowel adhesions
- Obesity
  - Distinct instrumentation for reach to the right upper quadrant
  - Fine motor movement limitations with suturing and intracorporeal knot tying
  - Mobilization of the hepatic flexure and a Kocher maneuver are made more difficult when the transverse mesocolon and omentum contain more fat and organs are larger in size overall
- High body mass index (>50 kg/m^2) patients
  - Large, friable livers as a result of fatty liver disease and are prone to lacerations (hemorrhage within the operative field significantly impairs image brightness)

- Patients are placed on a preoperative liquid diet with protein supplementation (7 days prior) to diminish the water weight of the liver, resulting in a temporary reduction in liver size to optimize the intraoperative exposure and minimize surrounding tissue injury
- Intravenous indocyanine green administration
  - Commercially available laparoscopic and robotic optical systems allow for fluorescent imaging to be displayed either in place or superimposed on white light images during surgery
- A 2.5 mg/mL injection (0.5 mL push with 10 mL saline flush to follow) 1 hour prior to surgery in the preoperative area allows the indocyanine green to be present in the biliary system (liver and biliary ducts; weakly in the pancreatic parenchyma as well). This may allow the surgeon improved recognition of the extrahepatic bile duct at the time of surgery

Positioning

- Supine; arms out

LAPAROSCOPIC CHOLEDOCHOJEJUNOSTOMY

First Step

- Port placement (FIGURE 1)

Second Step

- To create the Roux limb, start in the supine position and the ligament of Treitz is identified at the base of the transverse mesocolon.

Third Step

- The small bowel is divided using a laparoscopic stapler with a 3.5-mm staple load approximately 50 cm distal to the ligament of Treitz after a window is created between the vasa rectae of the small bowel.

Fourth Step

- Use the tissue-sealing device to divide the mesentery evenly in order not to encroach on the arterial arcade on either side of the divided bowel (optional). This will give you a slightly longer reach to the bile duct and less undue tension. The bowel proximal to the staple line is the alimentary limb; an additional 50 cm of small bowel distal to the staple line is measured and referred to as the Roux limb.

Fifth Step

- A side-to-side jejunojejunostomy is fashioned:
  - Two 3-0 absorbable stay sutures are placed 6 to 10 cm apart.
  - Enterotomies are created with cautery.
  - An articulating 60-mm long, 2.5-mm staple load is introduced into the bowel via the enterotomies. This load is generally more hemostatic than the typical 3.5 mm load used commonly for small bowel anastomoses. The bowel is manipulated so that the mesentery is outside the staple load.
  - The anastomosis between the alimentary and Roux limbs is created with the stapler.
  - The common enterostomy is oversewn with a 3-0 absorbable running suture.

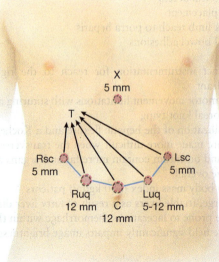

Rsc = Right subcostal port
Ruq = Right upper quadrant port
Luq = Left upper quadrant port
Lsc = Left subcostal port
C = Camera port
X = Liver retractor port
T = Target
— <8-cm width acceptable
— Instrument length and direction

FIGURE 1 • Laparoscopic access ports. The surgeon is positioned on the patient's right. The liver is retracted anterior with a fixed retractor. The first assistant on the patient's left facilitates the procedure by maintaining tension on the running suture at all times and assisting in the positioning of the Roux limb to facilitate accurate placement of sutures.

- The jejunojejunostomy mesenteric defect is closed with a running 2-0 nonabsorbable suture to prevent internal hernia. Avoid full-thickness bites across the bowel mesenteric edge that was previously sealed with an energy device; this can lead to unnecessary hemorrhage, ischemia, or hematoma near your anastomosis, rather suture the peritoneum superficially together.
- Visualize the Roux limb mesenteric edge and travel down toward the root of the mesentery to ensure the mesentery is not twisted.
- Create a defect in the transverse mesocolon to the patient's right of the right branch of the middle colic artery. Preserve the left space in case a future pancreatic Roux limb is needed.
- Mark the Roux limb staple line with a stich or a Penrose drain/colored tourniquet to make passing the bowel through the mesenteric defect to the porta hepatis atraumatic (optional).

Sixth Step

- Mobilization of the common bile duct within the hepatoduodenal ligament
    - If no cholecystectomy has been performed previously, use this to identify the cystic duct and travel proximally toward the common hepatic–bile duct junction; if not then, start with a lateral to medial approach to the soft tissues of the hepatoduodenal ligament. Typically, there is a station 12p lymph node just cephalad to the duodenum along the lateral border of the ligament to mark the location of the distal common bile duct.
    - Incise the peritoneum anterior to ligament to expose the bile duct and hepatic arterial supply. The bile duct will be lateral to the proper hepatic artery. Be mindful of variant anatomy and that the right hepatic artery travels anterior to the common hepatic duct in 15% of patients.
    - Mobilize the ligament further by incising the peritoneum laterally down toward the inferior vena cava to open near the shared border of the common bile duct and portal vein. This will allow for less resistance when dissecting medial to lateral just posterior to the bile duct.
    - Encircle the bile duct with a vessel loop or Penrose drain; use metallic clips to secure both tails together for retraction purposes.
    - Pass a blunt instrument posterior to the bile duct and use the cautery to divide the bile duct. The cautery or fine absorbable sutures can be used to obtain hemostasis at the 3- and 9-o'clock arterial supply at the cut edge of the bile duct. The bile duct should bleed briskly; if it does not, then consider shortening the bile duct proximally to better-perfused tissue.
    - If a biliary endoprosthesis or percutaneous biliary drain is across the bile duct, it can be used to stent your anastomosis. Preferably, stents are removed at this point as they may make the anastomosis more difficult and/or require additional procedures for removal.
- A laparoscopic bulldog clamp can be used to control the proximal cut edge of the bile duct to minimize biliary effluent contamination and hemorrhage.

Seventh Step

Biliary-Enteric Anastomosis

- The authors prefer the Trendelenburg position at the time of an intracorporeal handsewn choledochojejunostomy to take tension off the anastomosis by way of the small bowel mesentery using gravity to bring the Roux limb closer. Reverse Trendelenburg position is useful in obese patients by using gravity to retract the hepatic flexure away from the porta hepatis. The Roux limb is usually supported with a grasper from one of the assistant port sites in either scenario.
- For larger bile ducts, tie two separate 4-0 absorbable sutures together leaving it double-armed. Each suture is cut to a shorter length prior typically 15 to 20 cm each in length but can be adjusted based on the size of the bile duct. For small bile ducts, interrupted 4-0 absorbable sutures are used for the posterior and anterior rows.
- An enterotomy is made on the anterior aspect (ie, bowel side closest to the camera) of the antimesenteric border of the Roux limb.
- A stay suture is placed at 12 o'clock on the bile duct for retraction of the anterior wall during creation of the posterior row.
- The "double-armed" suture that was created is introduced into the peritoneum; one arm is passed "outside-in" on the bowel and the other "outside-in" on the bile duct (starting at 3 o'clock). Thus, both needles are "inside" and the knot is "outside" (**FIGURE 2**).
- The posterior row is created first by taking the suture "inside" the bowel and going "inside-out" on the bile duct, then "outside-in" on the bowel, then end-over-end across entire posterior row. Special attention is necessary during the first bite with the suture, as most leaks will occur posteriorly on the bile duct side after the initial anchoring of the double-armed suture.
- Upon completion of the posterior row, a bulldog clamp is placed on the remainder of the posterior row stitch to maintain tension preventing a loss of appropriate tension and apposition of the posterior row (**FIGURE 3A** and **B**).
- The 12-o'clock stay suture is removed.
- If desired, placement of an 8 French biliary stent is now placed, ensuring the distal aspect traverses the ampulla of Vater.
- Again, the anterior row is completed by taking the suture "inside" the bile duct and going "inside-out" on the bile duct, then "outside-in" on the bowel, then end-over-end across entire anterior row (**FIGURE 4A** and **B**).
- The anastomosis is completed by tying the two sutures on the outside at the 9-o'clock position.
- After completion of the ack through the mesocolon defect toward the jejunojejunostomy, which is thought to prevent biliary stasis in the Roux limb. Furthermore, the limb is secured directly to the peritoneum at the mesenteric defect with 3-0 nonabsorbable suture to prevent future herniation.
- Surgical drainage of the anastomosis is by surgeon preference.

64 SECTION I **SURGERY OF THE BILIARY SYSTEM**

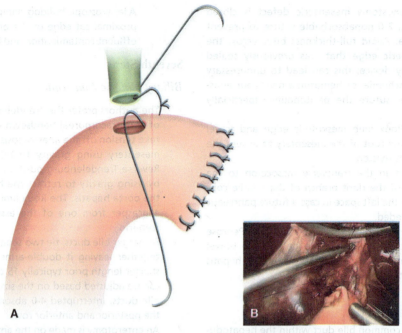

FIGURE 2 • **A,** The initial suture is placed in the 3-o'clock position, such that the knot used to form the double-armed suture is external to the planned anastomosis. **B,** Intraoperative photograph of the 3-o'clock suture.

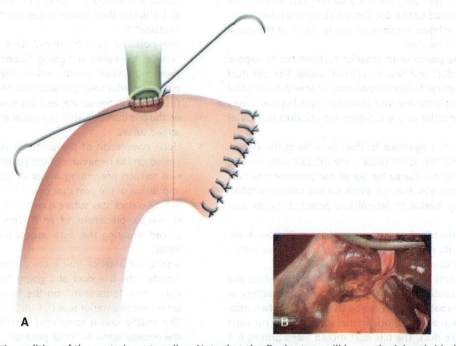

FIGURE 3 • **A,** Artist's rendition of the posterior suture line. Note that the final suture will be on the jejunal side (outside the bowel) to facilitate tying this arm to the anterior suture row arm. **B,** Intraoperative photograph of the anastomosis at the completion of the posterior suture line.

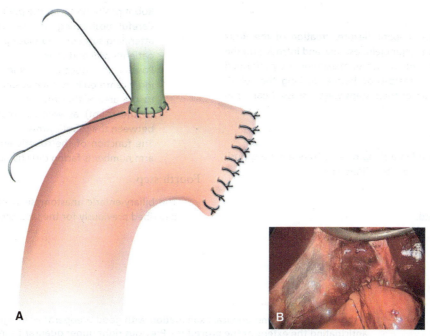

FIGURE 4 • **A,** Artist's rendition of the complete anastomosis prior to tying the two arms of suture. **B,** Intraoperative photograph of the anastomosis at the completion of the anterior suture line. This arm of the suture will finish on the outside of the bile duct.

ROBOTIC CHOLEDOCHOJEJUNOSTOMY

- Overall technique is similar to that of the laparoscopic choledochojejunostomy.

First step

- Port placement for robotic choledochojejunostomy is as seen in **FIGURE 5**.
- Port placement is set further away from the target of dissection due to the long robotic instruments and inability of the robot to optimally articulate when the arms approach >90° angle to the patient.
- Additionally, the robotic ports should be placed wider than the laparoscopic ports. This helps avoid "conflict" or collisions between the robotic arms.

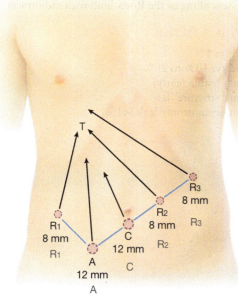

R1 = Robotic operative port (horizontal)
R2 = Robotic operative port (horizontal)
R3 = Robotic retraction port (horizontal)
A = Assistant port (horizontal)
C = Camera port (vertical)
T = Target
— 8-cm width (handbreadth)
— Instrument length and direction

Gray letters shown if distance between xiphoid and umbilicus is <16 cm

FIGURE 5 • Robotic access ports. R1 serves as the surgeon's left hand and R2 serves as their right hand. R3 provides liver retraction. The assistant provides tension on the running suture or provides additional exposure via retraction of the jejunal limb.

Second step

- Mobilization of the hepatic flexure, creation of the Roux limb, creation of the jejunojejunostomy, and introducing the Roux limb through the transverse mesocolon are performed with conventional laparoscopy before docking the robot. The technical details of these steps were discussed earlier in the chapter.

Third step

- The patient is placed in a steep reverse Trendelenburg position with the right side tilted slightly up.

Fourth step

- The robot is docked.
- Robot positioned over the patient's right shoulder.
- Careful positioning of the robot supervised by the attending surgeon and placing of a foam pad over the patient's arm and face.
- Position the robot correctly in terms of both maintaining it centered in its "sweet spot" (the arrow must point to the area within the blue stripe visible on the front of the robot) as well as creating sufficient distance between the robotic arms.
- The function of the robotic arms is optimal when the arm number is facing directly out.

Fourth step

- The biliary-enteric anastomosis is performed robotically as described previously for the laparoscopic approach.

PEARLS AND PITFALLS

Indications	A thorough history and physical examination with good preoperative imaging is important in anticipating the extent of the procedure. Previous right upper quadrant surgery or extensive prior abdominal surgical history may preclude a minimally invasive approach.
Dissection	Anticipate aberrant and accessory anatomy within the porta hepatis.
Excision	Send CBD margins for pathological analysis when considering malignant disease.
Choledochojejunostomy	Meticulous suture technique is critical. There should be no concerns with the posterior row prior to proceeding with the anterior row. Ensure there is no tension on the anastomosis.

POSTOPERATIVE CARE

- Dependent on bowel function
- Assess for biliary fistula
  - Fevers
  - Tachycardia
  - Right upper quadrant pain
  - Leukocytosis

OUTCOMES

- Biliary-enteric reconstruction patency rate
  - Open: 70% to 90%
  - Minimally invasive: limited data; no long-term follow-up to date
- Follow-up
  - Four weeks postoperatively with laboratory studies (CBC, CMP)
  - 12 weeks with a right upper quadrant ultrasound to examine for dilated intrahepatic ducts or postoperative fluid collections
  - 24 weeks with a ^{99m}Tc Choletech scan in nuclear medicine to assess filling of the Roux limb with radiotracer

COMPLICATIONS

- Mortality: 1%
- Morbidity: 10% to 20%
  - Biliary fistula (early)
  - Biliary stricture (late)
  - Jejunojejunostomy leak (<1%)

Chapter 10 Choledochoduodenostomy

Katherine A. Morgan and David B. Adams

DEFINITION

- Choledochoduodenostomy (CDD) describes an anastomosis between the extrahepatic biliary tree and the duodenum undertaken to provide internal drainage of an obstructed distal common bile duct (CBD).

DIFFERENTIAL DIAGNOSIS

- Choledocholithiasis
- Autoimmune-induced biliary strictures
- Chronic pancreatitis
- Periampullary malignancy

PATIENT HISTORY AND PHYSICAL FINDINGS

- The primary indications for CDD are benign causes of biliary obstruction including chronic pancreatitis and distal biliary stricture related to choledocholithiasis. In the current era of endoscopic retrograde cholangiography, the frequency of operative biliary bypass has decreased; nonetheless, CDD remains an important part of the general surgeon's armamentarium.
- Patients with distal biliary obstruction will typically present with right upper quadrant abdominal pain and associated jaundice. If cholangitis is attendant, fever and chills (Charcot triad) or, in more severe cases, hypotension and altered mental status (Reynolds pentad) may be evident.
- Elevated serum hepatic chemistries are essential to the diagnosis of significant biliary obstruction. Total and direct bilirubin, alkaline phosphatase, and gamma-glutamyltransferase are elevated preferentially to the hepatic transaminases in cases of biliary obstruction as contrasted to intrinsic hepatic disease.
- Patients with chronic pancreatitis who present with biliary obstruction may have a reversible component to the inflammatory obstruction and thus are often best managed initially with endoscopic stenting. In cases with persistent biliary obstruction due to constricting fibrosis in the pancreatic head, marked by elevated serum hepatic chemistries and a dilated CBD, surgical intervention is warranted. In patients with an accompanying inflammatory pseudotumor in the head of the pancreas or a concern for malignancy, pancreatic head resection may be indicated. When resection is not indicated, CDD is an excellent means of biliary bypass while minimizing perioperative morbidity and preserving pancreatic parenchyma.
- Patients with a terminal biliary stricture due to long-standing choledocholithiasis do well with CDD. Common indications include a dilated CBD (>1.5 cm); multiple CBD stones; and primary, recurrent, or recalcitrant choledocholithiasis.

IMAGING AND OTHER DIAGNOSTIC STUDIES

- Right upper quadrant ultrasound is the frontline test for biliary obstruction, visualized as dilated intrahepatic and extrahepatic biliary ducts. It is highly sensitive, noninvasive, inexpensive, and readily available and requires no radiation.
- Contrast-enhanced computed tomography (CT) is a useful modality to evaluate abdominal pain. CT will demonstrate a dilated biliary tree and can help in the evaluation for causative-associated pathology including choledocholithiasis, chronic pancreatitis, and periampullary malignancy.
- Magnetic resonance cholangiopancreatography (MRCP) can give detailed information about biliopancreatic ductal anatomy and pathology (T2-weighted images) and soft tissue abnormalities related to pancreatitis or neoplasm (T1-weighted images). MRCP is an important tool for assessment of biliary obstruction because of the advanced ductal imaging capability.
- Endoscopic retrograde cholangiopancreatography (ERCP) is the primary initial therapeutic approach to biliary obstruction in the current era. ERCP can be both diagnostic and therapeutic in the management of biliary obstruction. It can be used to identify stones and apply a variety of maneuvers that facilitate stone clearance:
  - Sphincterotomy
  - Balloon cholangioplasty and sweeping
  - Basket retrieval
  - Lithotripsy
- Strictures can be dilated and stented endoscopically. Even with alternative strategies (metal stents, multiple plastic stents), endoscopic stenting lacks durability in the management of chronic, longer-segment CBD strictures due to chronic pancreatitis and stone disease, and CDD is often employed in these cases.
- Endoscopic ultrasound (EUS) can be helpful in the careful evaluation of the terminal biliary tree for the diagnosis or exclusion of malignant obstruction and the assessment for occult cholelithiasis. EUS has also been more recently used for an endoscopic-directed choledochoduodenal stent.
- Percutaneous transhepatic cholangiography (PTC) is undertaken to study the biliary tree and allow for biliary drainage in cases where endoscopic transampullary access is not possible. Maturation and dilation of the tract after PTC can allow for percutaneous instrumentation to be used under radiographic guidance to clear stones from the biliary tree.

SURGICAL MANAGEMENT

- CDD is indicated in patients with a benign terminal biliary stricture, with an associated dilated CBD (>1.5 cm diameter), most commonly due to chronic pancreatitis or

- choledocholithiasis. CDD has been effectively used in the management of malignant biliary obstruction.
- When planning a biliary bypass procedure, a neoplastic cause for biliary obstruction should be sought out and recognized, as a malignant (or potentially malignant) process may call for a divergent operative approach.
- When biliary bypass is indicated in unresectable periampullary malignancy, CDD may be selected as an alternative to hepaticojejunostomy.
- Classically, the CDD anastomosis is performed in a side-to-side fashion but may also be performed with an end (bile duct) to side (duodenum) technique, particularly when using a laparoscopic approach. Both methods are presented.

Preoperative Planning

- CDD is best undertaken in an elective setting. Acute pancreatitis should be allowed to settle, and cholangitis should be properly treated. Often, endoscopic stenting can be helpful to temporize patients and allow for medical optimization.
- Particular attention should be taken to the nutritional status of the patient, as patients with chronic inflammation are often malnourished. Enteral or parenteral supplementation may be appropriate to condition the patient for surgery.
- Hepatic function should also be assessed prior to surgery, as it may be compromised in patients with long-standing biliary obstruction. Vitamin K supplementation, in particular, may be useful.
- Patients with terminal biliary stenosis due to chronic pancreatitis may have associated duodenal stenosis, pancreatic ductal obstruction and dilation, or splanchnic venous obstruction, which may require operative management and should be confirmed with preoperative evaluation.
- Patients with terminal biliary stenosis and cavernous transformation of the portal vein may undergo CDD safely, although additional emotional and physical work is demanded in the conduct of the procedure.

TECHNIQUES

CHOLEDOCHODUODENOSTOMY, SIDE TO SIDE

Incision and Exposure

- An upper midline incision or a right subcostal incision may be used for this operation (**FIGURE 1**). The abdomen is explored for unexpected findings including evidence for distant malignancy. Caudal mobilization of the hepatic flexure of the colon is undertaken to aid in adequate duodenal exposure.
- Use of self-retaining retractors facilitates exposure of the terminal bile duct and the first and second portions of the duodenum (**FIGURE 2**).
- An extensive Kocher maneuver is performed to optimally mobilize the duodenum. This mobilization is a critical step for the success of a tension-free anastomosis. The pancreatic head and terminal bile duct are palpated and examined to assess for extent of disease and unexpected findings.
- If the gallbladder remains in place, a cholecystectomy is performed (**FIGURE 3**).

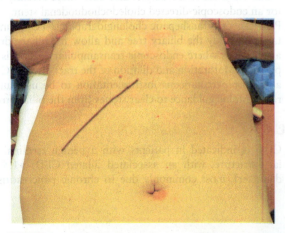

FIGURE 1 • The authors favor a right subcostal incision.

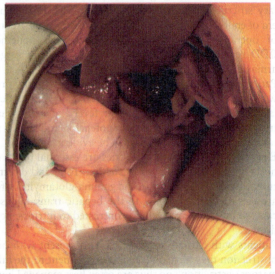

FIGURE 2 • A fixed retractor facilitates exposure.

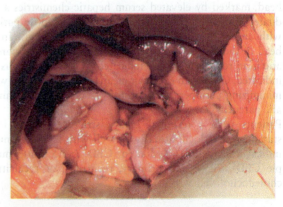

FIGURE 3 • When present, retrograde dissection of the gallbladder facilitates identification of the cystic duct confluence and distal CBD.

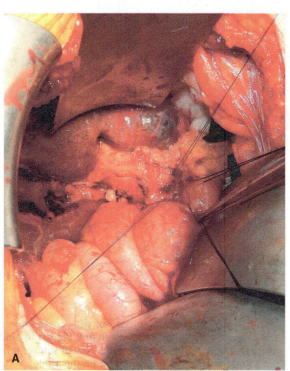 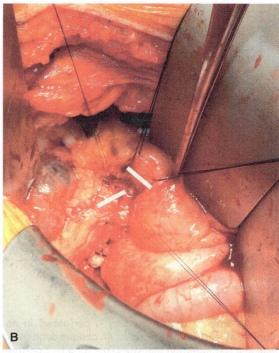

FIGURE 4 • **A,** After caudal mobilization of the duodenum, stay sutures are placed in the distal CBD (fine monofilament sutures) and the duodenum (larger braided sutures) to facilitate exposure. **B,** Additional view from the patient's right further demonstrates how this mobilization facilitates an anastomosis free of tension. Planned ductotomy and duodenotomy *(white lines).*

- The porta hepatis is examined and the CBD clearly identified for the course of greater than 3 cm along its anterior wall. In cases with significant inflammation and fibrosis, the anatomy can be distorted. Palpation of the hepatic artery can be helpful in orientation, as can palpation of an intraductal biliary stent or aspiration of bile with a fine needle and syringe.
- Incision of the peritoneum at the cephalad aspect of the first portion of the duodenum can facilitate the establishment of a plane between the posterior wall of the duodenum and the anterior wall of the CBD, providing additional length and improving the proximity of the planned ductotomy and duodenotomy sites, thus reducing potential tension on the anastomosis (**FIGURE 4**).

Choledochoduodenal Anastomosis

- Identification of the CBD is confirmed by aspiration with a 21-gauge needle.
- An anterior ductotomy is made sharply, typically with a no. 11 blade at the site of the needle aspiration, large enough to permit entrance into the duct with the tip of a fine hemostat. An anterior longitudinal choledochotomy is then extended with scissors or electrocautery for 1.5 cm in length. The ductotomy is made on the distal CBD as close as safely possible to the duodenum. Arterial bleeding on the distal ductotomy means "far enough."
- The distal CBD and common hepatic duct should be irrigated with an 8-Fr catheter to clear the duct of stones and sludge. If ductal lithiasis is present, choledochoscopy should be undertaken to confirm clearance of the duct of stones. Residual stones may require balloon catheter or basket extraction.
- When cavernous transformation of the portal vein is present, the venous network surrounding the common duct will require a combination of suture ligation, coaptive electrocautery, and argon beam coagulation to achieve hemostasis.
- The mobility of duodenum is assessed to determine where an anastomosis will most suitably lie without tension. A duodenotomy is then made with electrocautery, with cutting current in the postbulbar duodenum. The angle of the duodenotomy will vary from patient to patient, depending on the underlying disorder and variation from normal anatomy. In pancreatitis, the mobility of the duodenum varies with the underlying peripancreatic fibrosis so the location of the duodenotomy will vary accordingly. The duodenotomy is usually an oblique incision, with the goal of a comfortable anastomosis without distortion of the duodenal flow. The duodenotomy should be cut at a length of about 1.0 cm as it will always stretch more than expected (**FIGURE 5**).
- If a preoperative prograde or retrograde stent has been placed, it may be prudent to leave it in place to serve as a postoperative stent, particularly in the difficult anastomosis in the presence of severe peripancreatic fibrosis, recognizing the risk of stent-induced postoperative biliary sepsis related to the sialomucin stent biofilm harboring gram-negative bacteria.
- A single layer of interrupted sutures with fine 4-0 or 5-0 monofilament absorbable suture is used for this anastomosis. Full-thickness corner sutures are placed through the duodenum and then the bile duct at either end of the anastomosis such that the tails are outside the lumen. They are marked with a hemostat and act for exposure and for conceptual planning (**FIGURE 6**).
- The posterior row of sutures is placed with the tails on the inside of the lumen, beginning with the middle suture to aid in spatial planning. This suture will be at the end

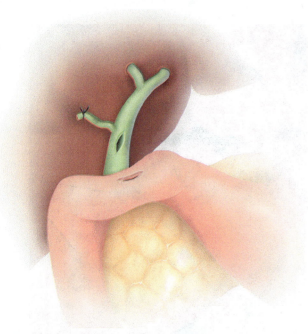

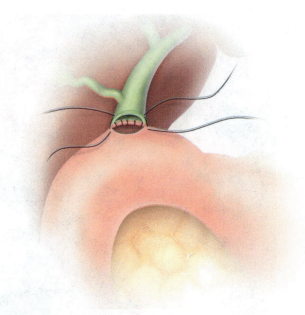

FIGURE 5 • An anterior choledochotomy is performed in an oblique manner, at least 1.5 cm in length. An oblique duodenotomy is made in a configuration that will allow for a tension-free anastomosis without distortion of the duodenum, approximately 1.0 cm in length as it will stretch.

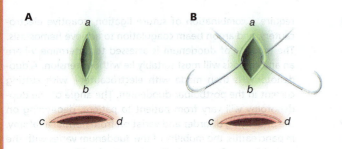

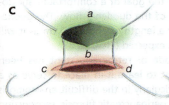

FIGURE 6 • Schematic drawing of how the two ostomies are oriented for the anastomosis. **A,** Depiction of the ostomies as they lie perpendicular to one another. **B,** Stay sutures are placed on both sides of the midpoint of the choledochotomy (halfway between *a* and *b*). **C,** These stay sutures are then used to take full-thickness bites of the duodenum at the ends of the duodenotomy. This aligns the structures for placement of the posterior suture line.

FIGURE 7 • Anatomic depiction of the corner sutures that are placed with tails outside the lumen and tagged to aid for exposure and spatial planning. The back row of sutures is performed in an interrupted fashion, with tails on the inside.

of the choledochotomy and at the middle of the duodenotomy. The individual sutures are tagged and then tied down at the completion of the posterior row, except the corner stitches, which remain untied to aid in exposure (**FIGURE 7**).

- The anterior row of sutures is then placed, beginning with the middle suture, with the tails on the outside of the anastomotic lumen. All remaining sutures are then tied securely in place (**FIGURE 8**).
- When the anatomy is favorable, particularly with a thickened bile duct, a large anastomosis, and easy duodenal mobility, the anastomosis can be constructed with continuous sutures.
- A closed suction drain is placed near the anastomosis.

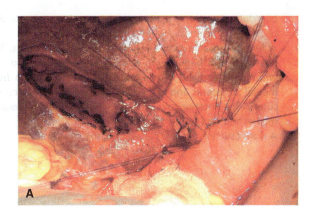
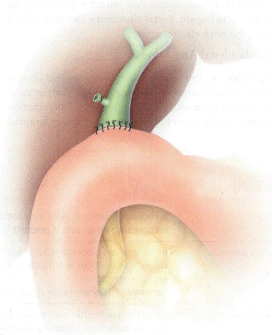

FIGURE 8 • **A,** The anterior row of sutures is then placed in an interrupted fashion, with tails on the outside of the lumen, and tied in turn to complete the anastomosis. **B,** Schematic drawing of the completed anastomosis.

CHOLEDOCHODUODENOSTOMY, END TO SIDE

Incision and Exposure Including Portal Dissection

- The incision and exposure are similar to that for the side-to-side technique, including an extensive Kocher maneuver to mobilize the duodenum. In the end-to-side technique, however, circumferential dissection of the CBD is necessary. In cases with severe inflammation and fibrosis of the porta hepatis, a side-to-side technique may be prudent to avoid vascular injury. Medial-to-lateral dissection of the posterior CBD away from the hepatic artery and portal vein is the safest technique. Once the CBD has been encircled, it is divided as distally as possible, with attention to precise control of the radial blood supply of the duct, avoiding excessive use of cautery. The distal end of the divided bile duct is then oversewn in a running fashion using an absorbable suture.

Choledochoduodenal Anastomosis, End to Side

- A longitudinal incision is made in the second portion of the duodenum near where the divided bile duct is located. A single layer of fine (4-0) absorbable suture is also used for this anastomosis. Full-thickness corner sutures first through the bowel, then through the bile duct, are placed at either end of the anastomosis for exposure and spatial planning.
- If an anastomosis with interrupted suture is planned, the conduct of the anastomosis is identical to that of the side-to-side technique. If an anastomosis with a running suture is planned, the corner sutures are tied and left long with needle in place. On one end, the needle is passed to the inside and run along the posterior wall inside the lumen and tied to the other corner's tail. The other suture is then run along the anterior wall and tied to the other corner's tail.
- A closed suction drain is placed near the anastomosis.

LAPAROSCOPIC CHOLEDOCHODUODENOSTOMY

Patient Positioning and Port Placement

- The patient is positioned supine and in reverse Trendelenburg with a left side down tilt.
- Laparoscopic port sites are placed in an arc above the level of the umbilicus with a right-sided bias. Port site placement is similar to that of a laparoscopic cholecystectomy.

Initial Dissection

- The conduct of the operation is similar to that for the open technique, including mobilization of the hepatic flexure of the colon and an extensive Kocher maneuver to mobilize the duodenum. A laparoscopic liver retractor is necessary to expose the porta hepatis. Portal dissection is carried out with care using the hook electrocautery.

Choledochoduodenal Anastomosis

- When possible, an end-to-side technique is favored laparoscopically, as this anastomosis without tension is often technically easier to perform. In cases with severe inflammation and fibrosis of the porta hepatis, however, circumferential bile duct dissection may be treacherous and a side-to-side technique is favored.
- A fine absorbable suture is used for the anastomosis. The anastomosis is begun with corner sutures placed and tied without cutting the needle. The posterior row is run from medial to lateral and tied to the tail of the other corner suture. The anterior row is then similarly run, now lateral to medial and tied to the other corner's tail.
- A closed suction drain is placed near the anastomosis.

PEARLS AND PITFALLS

Indications	■ A thorough preoperative evaluation of the cause for biliary obstruction is important, specifically recognizing neoplasia if present to allow for proper operative decision making.
Preoperative planning	■ Inflammation associated with acute pancreatitis and infection and inflammation related to cholangitis on presentation should be properly treated and allowed to resolve prior to proceeding with this elective operation. ■ Patient nutritional status should be optimized prior to surgery to minimize morbidity.
Incision and exposure	■ An extensive Kocher maneuver should be performed to mobilize the duodenum and minimize tension potentially leading to anastomotic failure.
Choledochoduodenal anastomosis	■ The choledochotomy and duodenotomy should be configured in a way so as to minimize anastomotic tension and duodenal distortion. Careful intraoperative planning and an oblique bias to the incisions are useful. ■ The anastomosis should be greater than 1.5 cm in length to avoid stenosis resulting in cholangitis, hepatic abscess, stones, and potentially sump syndrome.

POSTOPERATIVE CARE

- Nasogastric decompression should be undertaken in the initial postoperative period.
- The closed suction drain is removed once diet is tolerated and there is no evidence of anastomotic leak.

OUTCOMES

- Outcomes following CDD are limited to small, retrospective, single-institution case series, including both open and laparoscopic approaches. Postoperative morbidity following CDD is reported as 9.8% to 28%, with the most common complications being wound infection and anastomotic leak.
- A phenomenon known as "sump syndrome" has been described following CDD where food debris or stones accumulate in the terminal portion of the CBD, resulting in episodes of abdominal pain, fever, and cholangitis. The incidence of sump syndrome after CDD appears to be relatively uncommon, reported as 0% to 9% in case series, and presents in a delayed fashion, typically years after the procedure. Anastomotic stenosis has been implicated as the cause for sump syndrome as well as for the rare occurrence of recurrent stones, cholangitis, and hepatic abscess, and therefore, generous anastomotic girth is encouraged to prevent these complications.

COMPLICATIONS

- Intraoperative hemorrhage from portal vein or proper hepatic artery
- Anastomotic leak, duodenal fistula
- Anastomotic stricture
- Cholangitis
- Hepatic abscess
- Choledocholithiasis or intrahepatic ductal stones
- Sump syndrome

SUGGESTED READINGS

1. Blankenstein J, Terpstra O. Early and late results following choledochoduodenostomy and choledochojejunostomy. *HPB Surg*. 1990;2:151-158.
2. de Almeida AC, dos Santos NM, Aldeia FJ. Choledochoduodenostomy in the management of common duct stones or associated pathology—an obsolete method?. *HPB Surg*. 1996;10:27-33.
3. Escudero-Fabre A, Escallon A Jr, Sack J, et al. Choledochoduodenostomy: analysis of 71 cases followed for 5 to 15 years. *Ann Surg*. 1991;213:635-642.
4. Khajanchee TS, Cassera MA, Hammill CW, et al. Outcomes following laparoscopic choledochoduodenostomy in the management of benign biliary obstruction. *J Gastrointest Surg*. 2012;16:801-805.
5. Leppard WM, Shary TM, Adams DB, et al. Choledochoduodenostomy: is it really so bad?. *J Gastrointest Surg*. 2011;15:754-757.
6. Pitt HA, Kaufman SL, Coleman J, et al. Benign postoperative biliary strictures: operate or dilate? *Ann Surg*. 1989;4:417-425.
7. Stuart M, Keo T, Hermann RE, et al. Palliation of malignant obstruction of the common bile duct by side to side choledochoduodenostomy. *Am J Surg*. 1971;121:505-509.

Chapter 11
Resection of Hilar Cholangiocarcinoma

Ryan T. Groeschl and T. Clark Gamblin

DEFINITION
- Hilar cholangiocarcinoma (HC), also referred to as Klatskin tumor, is an extrahepatic cancer of biliary epithelial origin near the confluence of the right and left hepatic ducts. The hepatic artery and portal vein are in close proximity to the bile duct, and vascular involvement is common. Given the limited effectiveness of other therapies, margin-negative resection is the optimal treatment. Although multimodal therapy combined with transplantation is also a potential approach to HC,[1] this chapter focuses on the resection technique for this biliary disease.

DIFFERENTIAL DIAGNOSIS
- Growth patterns for HC may be exophytic, infiltrative, polypoid, or any combination thereof (FIGURE 1). The differential diagnosis includes pathologies that may mimic any of these appearances.
  - Papilloma—composed of vascular connective tissue and covered with columnar epithelium; low-grade malignant potential
  - Adenoma—glandular tissue surrounded by fibrous stroma; low-grade malignant potential
  - Benign biliary stricture from recurrent pyogenic cholangitis, primary sclerosing cholangitis, choledocholithiasis, Mirizzi syndrome, previous surgery, or trauma

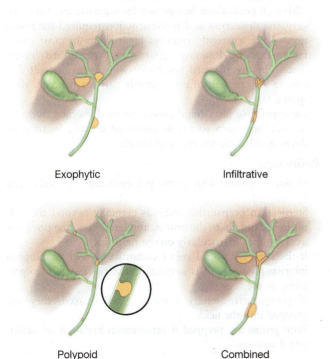

FIGURE 1 • Various growth patterns of extrahepatic cholangiocarcinoma.

PATIENT HISTORY AND PHYSICAL FINDINGS
- Successful hepatectomy must maintain an adequately healthy liver remnant. Initial assessment of the patient must focus not only on the malignancy itself but also on general liver function. Underlying liver dysfunction (due to chronic alcohol exposure, viral hepatitis, fatty liver disease, etc) may alter operative planning and the minimum remnant required.
- History
  - Symptoms: jaundice, itching, unintentional weight loss, abdominal pain
  - Broader aspects of patient history: gallstones, cholangitis, primary sclerosing cholangitis, ulcerative colitis, previous surgery or trauma, viral hepatitis, cirrhosis, alcohol consumption, international travel, obesity, diabetes, hyperlipidemia, bruising, immune deficiency
- Physical examination
  - Jaundice or scleral icterus; muscle wasting may be present.
  - If disease occludes cystic duct, gallbladder may be palpable (Courvoisier sign).
- Assess for stigmata of cirrhosis, portal vein thrombosis, or portal hypertension: ascites, encephalopathy, spider angiomata, skin telangiectasias, palmar erythema, bruising

IMAGING AND OTHER DIAGNOSTIC STUDIES
- Transabdominal ultrasound
  - May identify duct dilation and large hilar tumors, but primarily functions as a screening tool.
  - Doppler may identify narrowing or thrombosis of the hepatic artery or portal vein.
- Cross-sectional imaging: computed tomography and magnetic resonance
  - Good visualization of mass lesions and ductal dilation.
  - Staging: may identify intra-abdominal lymphadenopathy and/or metastases.
  - Contrast enhancement allows assessment of vascular involvement and identification of anomalous hepatic inflow, which are critical to operative planning.
  - Signs of cirrhosis or portal hypertension may be present: irregular hepatic capsule, caudate hypertrophy, cavernous transformation, hypersplenism, ascites, recanalized umbilical vein.
- Cholangiography
  - Magnetic resonance cholangiopancreatography
    - Noninvasive; allows visualization and three-dimensional reconstruction of ductal anatomy
    - Does not provide opportunity to sample tissue
  - Endoscopic retrograde cholangiography
    - Allows visualization of ductal anatomy, provides opportunity for brushing or biopsy, and allows stenting in case of biliary obstruction
    - Invasive; risk of procedure-induced pancreatitis

- Cholangiography via percutaneous catheters
  - If percutaneous biliary drainage catheters have been placed, contrast can be used to delineate ductal anatomy and also allow brushings.
  - Ideally, such catheters are placed in the future remnant liver or bilaterally.
- Endoscopic ultrasound
  - Allows evaluation of the duct and regional lymph nodes, which may also be sampled with fine needle aspiration or core biopsy when available (19 to 22 gauge).
  - Intraductal fiberoptic direct visualization (with biopsy) and intraductal ultrasonography are available at some centers.
- Positron emission tomography
  - Fluorodeoxyglucose (FDG) avidity is typically limited to mass lesions greater than 1 cm but provides poor quality for identifying cancers with infiltrative growth; hence, limited use beyond standard cross-sectional imaging for assessing primary tumor.
  - May identify occult metastatic disease.
- Laboratory evaluation
  - Cholestasis may be indicated by elevated bilirubin, alkaline phosphatase, and gamma-glutamyltransferase levels.
  - Albumin and prothrombin time evaluate synthetic function.
  - Aspartate and alanine aminotransferase levels are often normal.
  - Low platelet levels may reflect hypersplenism due to portal hypertension.
  - Elevations in carbohydrate antigen 19-9 (CA 19-9) or carcinoembryonic antigen may be elevated in patients with HC.
    - CA 19-9 may be spuriously elevated in the setting of jaundice.
    - When workup reveals tumor marker elevation, these levels may be followed after resection to assess for disease recurrence.

SURGICAL MANAGEMENT

Preoperative Planning

- Patients with jaundice should be drained either endoscopically or percutaneously to optimize liver remnant function.
- Operations for HC involve the dissection of critical structures, biliary and vascular reconstruction, and adaptation to intraoperative findings. Expertise in hepatobiliary anatomy and surgical technique is essential. In particular, familiarity with common patterns of anomalous ductal and arterial hilar anatomy (**FIGURE 2**) will prevent injury to unintended structures. Features of unresectability are shown in **TABLE 1**.
- When a diminutive liver remnant is anticipated, preoperative angioembolization of the contralateral (tumor-supplying) portal vein should be pursued in an attempt to hypertrophy the potential remnant.
- The Bismuth-Corlette classification is used to describe the extent of right and left duct involvement (**FIGURE 3**). Careful review of cholangiography and cross-sectional imaging will identify resectable patients and aid in operative planning.

Table 1: Liver-Specific Criteria for Unresectable Klatskin Tumors

Tumor extension to bilateral secondary branches of hilar structures
  Portal vein
  Hepatic artery
  Bile duct
In patients with normal background liver
  Future remnant liver <25%
  Inability to preserve two adjacent segments
In cirrhotic patients
  If resection is considered, preservation of a large remnant is essential to prevent postoperative liver failure.
  These patients can be considered for transplantation in the context of an established multimodal treatment protocol or clinical trial.

- Right hepatectomy or trisectionectomy is generally indicated for types II and IIIa tumors.
- Left hepatectomy, and especially left trisectionectomy, is uncommonly performed and often carries a higher complication rate. This type of resection is usually reserved for type IIIb tumors or those cases where the future left-sided remnant would be inadequate for type II tumors.
- Type IV tumors are unresectable unless a full sectoral branch is uninvolved and free of tumor.
- Type I HC may occasionally be amenable to local biliary resection alone; however, R0 rate and thus survival have been directly linked to the use of hepatic resection.[2]
- Apparent invasion of the portal vein or vena cava does not preclude resection. Large tumors can narrow adjacent vessels on imaging; however, this may be a mass effect and not necessarily represent invasion.
- Contraindications to resection include distant metastatic disease and bilobar liver involvement.
- Although enthusiasm has grown for laparoscopic liver surgery, the dissection and reconstruction required for resection of HC currently requires laparotomy in most cases. However, a preliminary laparoscopy (performed immediately before planned resection) will identify occult disease in at least half of unresectable patients, who are then spared laparotomy.[3]
- Intraoperative ultrasound should be used liberally throughout the operation to assess extent of disease, location of ducts, and location/patency of vessels.

Positioning

- Supine position with arms perpendicular to body axis (**FIGURE 4**).
- Sterile skin preparation extends cranially beyond the nipple line, caudally to the groins, and laterally to the posterior axillary lines (particularly on the right side).
- If the need for portal vein reconstruction with autologous internal jugular vein is suspected, a sterile field is also prepared at the neck.
- If preoperative biliary catheters were placed, they are prepped into the field.
- Both groins are prepped if venovenous bypass is an anticipated strategy.

Chapter 11 RESECTION OF HILAR CHOLANGIOCARCINOMA   75

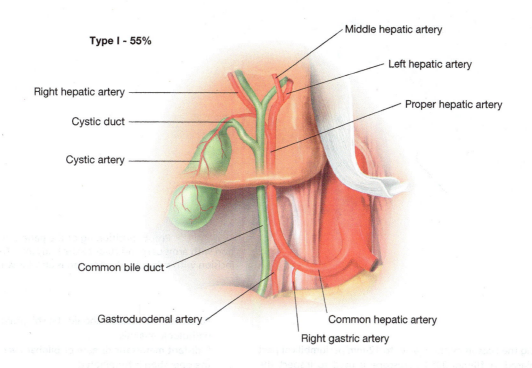

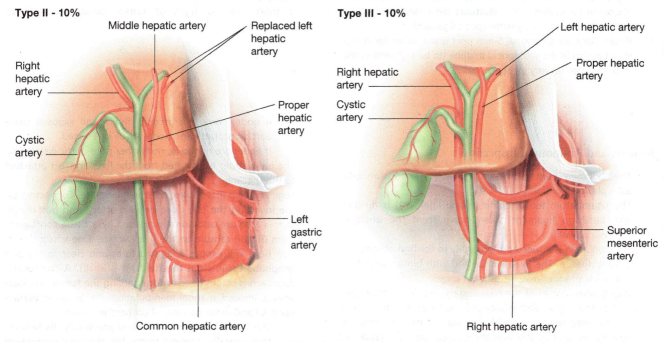

FIGURE 2 • Common variations of hilar arterial anatomy. Although the usual course of the right hepatic artery is from the common hepatic artery and crossing laterally posterior to the bile duct confluence, a replaced (or accessory) right artery may originate from the superior mesenteric artery. A replaced (or accessory) left artery may be found in the gastrocolic ligament originating from the left gastric artery.

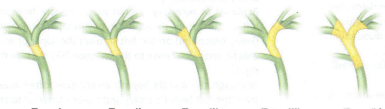

FIGURE 3 • Bismuth-Corlette classification of Klatskin tumors.

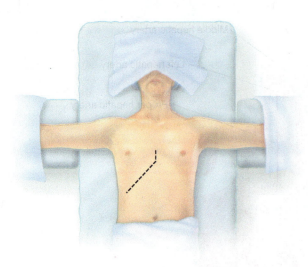

FIGURE 4 • Proper positioning of the patient in the supine position with arms perpendicular to the body axis. The right subcostal incision with subxiphoid extension is also shown.

TECHNIQUES

PRELIMINARY LAPAROSCOPY

- Using the Hasson method, a 10- to 12-mm periumbilical port is placed. A 10-mm 30° laparoscope is used to inspect the abdomen for evidence of metastases: peritoneal cavity, liver surface, porta hepatis, gastrohepatic ligament.
- If necessary, an additional 5-mm port is placed under direct visualization in the subxiphoid midline (to be included in the potential laparotomy incision).
- Potential metastases should be biopsied for immediate pathologic analysis.
- If distant metastatic disease or bilobar liver disease is noted, the operation is terminated.
- If there are no signs of unresectability, proceed to laparotomy.

LAPAROTOMY

Incision and Abdominal Inspection

- The abdomen is entered with a right subcostal incision with subxiphoid extension (FIGURE 4).
- The ligamentum teres hepatis (round ligament) is divided and falciform ligament taken down from the anterior abdominal wall.
- The abdomen is inspected thoroughly to confirm absence of distant disease. The liver is inspected with bimanual palpation and intraoperative ultrasonography.
- Along with control of the hilar vessels, circumferential control of the supra- and infrahepatic vena cava with a tape can be used selectively, which allows for nearly complete vascular control of the liver should venovenous bypass be necessary.

Para-Aortic Node Assessment and Biliary Dissection

- The omentum is freed from the transverse colon, allowing access to the omental bursa.
- The hepatic flexure of the colon is mobilized and rotated medially until the duodenum and vena cava are identified.
- A Kocher maneuver is performed, retracting the duodenum to the left until the aortocaval groove is exposed.
- Firm or enlarged para-aortic nodes are sampled for immediate pathologic examination.
    - If nodes are grossly positive, the operation is terminated.
    - If nodes show microscopic disease, all exposed para-aortic fibrofatty and nodal tissue is resected.
    - If nodes are negative, no further para-aortic dissection.
- The gallbladder is dissected from the liver and left attached to the specimen via the cystic duct.
- Segment 4b is lifted to expose the hilar plate. Connective tissue investing the bile duct, hepatic artery, and portal vein in this area are additionally covered by a tissue confluence from Glisson capsule on the liver surface. Fine scissor dissection here will expose hilar structures and clear fascial and lymphatic tissue from the field (FIGURE 5). A "no-touch" approach is recommended for handling the tumor and hilar vessels. Instead, manual manipulation should target periadventitial and other noncritical connective tissues.
    - The hepatic artery is identified proximally. Its bifurcation typically is caudal to the bile duct and portal vein confluences. The right hepatic artery most often courses posterior to the proximal common bile duct. Careful examination of high-quality cross-sectional imaging should allow the surgeon to anticipate the course of the artery and protect it.
    - Replaced or accessory arteries may originate from the left gastric artery through the gastrohepatic ligament (lesser omentum) on the left or from the superior mesenteric artery posterior to the common bile duct on the right.
    - Although the middle hepatic artery most often arises from the left hepatic artery and crosses anterior to the left duct, its origin and orientation are highly variable.

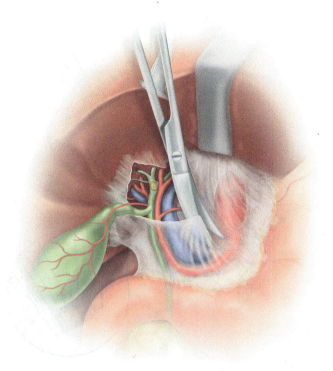

FIGURE 5 • Dissection of the hilar plate begins with proximal identification of the bile duct and hepatic artery, which lie anterior to the portal vein. The gallbladder has been removed from the base of the liver and is used for retraction. A no-touch technique should be observed when dissecting near the tumor.

- The proximal extent of tumor is determined by caudal retraction of the bile duct and gallbladder. This step is critical as it will determine whether right or left hepatectomy is undertaken. Some liver parenchyma may need to be transected to adequately assess either duct. Dividing connective tissue between the base of segment 4 and the bile duct confluence (tumor) will often facilitate lowering the hilar plate.
  - To adequately inspect the left hepatic duct, the narrow bridge of liver parenchyma under the umbilical fissure can be divided. The left duct has a longer extrahepatic course and lies perpendicular to the common duct before entering the liver parenchyma at the base of the umbilical fissure. The length of the extrahepatic portion of the left duct is the primary reason that a right liver resection is most often performed in pursuit of an R0 resection.
  - The extrahepatic right hepatic duct is typically shorter and rapidly ascends laterally into the parenchyma. In nearly one-fourth of patients, a right segmental duct will cross Cantlie line to join the main left hepatic duct. Owing to its short length and orientation, the right duct is prone to inadvertent injury. Intraoperative cholangiogram serves as a valuable tool to clarify the anatomy.
  - If gross disease extends to all four hepatic sectional ducts, the tumor is unresectable and further operative exploration is not warranted.
- The right gastric artery is ligated and divided at its origin from the common hepatic artery.
- The posterior superior pancreaticoduodenal artery (PSPD) crosses the common bile duct near the superior aspect of the pancreatic head. The common bile duct will be ligated and transected in this area:
  - If no tumor involvement nearby, the PSPD may be left in situ.
  - If adherent to tumor, the PSPD should be ligated and resected en bloc with tumor specimen.
  - If tumor extends into the pancreatic head but the PSPD is not involved, then the PSPD is divided and retracted to allow dissection of tumor inferiorly into pancreatic parenchyma. In rare cases of HC, a pancreaticoduodenectomy may be necessary for margin-negative resection.
- The distal common bile duct is transected just above the pancreas and a distal margin sent for immediate pathologic assessment.
  - The distal peripancreatic stump is oversewn with running 5-0 Prolene.
  - If biliary drainage catheters are in place, they are retracted into the hepatic parenchyma, allowing for the proximal duct to be tied off and retracted superiorly.
- Caudate resection is recommended.[4,5] Exploration commences by exposing the inferior vena cava posterior to the liver. The most inferior hepatic veins are ligated and divided to allow posterior exposure of the caudate.
  - Veins less than 5 mm in diameter can be divided with standard suture ligation or clips.
  - Commonly, there will be at least one vein greater than 5 mm in diameter behind the caudate. Such veins should be controlled with a Satinsky clamp on the vena cava, tie ligated at the caudate aspect, divided, and the caval stump oversewn with running 5-0 Prolene suture (**FIGURE 6**).
  - Figure-of-eight stay sutures placed in the caudate are a useful means of retracting the caudate off the vena cava (**FIGURE 7**).
  - The left aspect of the hepatocaval ligament may have to be divided to allow visualization.
- Portal vein involvement is assessed by retracting the bile duct anterior and cranial.
- Caudate preservation is only possible if sufficient biliary outflow can be spared. Although variability exists, the caudate will typically have at least two ducts, which most often drain to the main left duct, the main right duct, or the right posterior sectional branch.

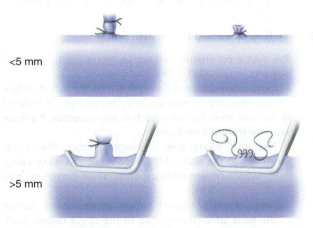

FIGURE 6 • Technique of dividing short hepatic veins from segment 1, 4, 5, or 8.

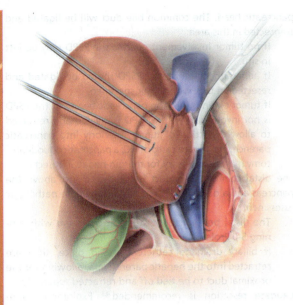

FIGURE 7 • To assist with caudate retraction, figure-of-eight stay sutures can be placed in the caudate parenchyma and gently retracted.

- If caudate resection is performed, then small portal vein branches (posterior aspect of both right and left main portal veins) must be ligated and divided.
- Caudate mobilization is assisted by approaching from both the right side and left side of the vena cava.

Hepatectomy

- As previously described, the choice of hepatectomy is directly related to the extent of ductal, portal venous, and hepatic arterial involvement.
  - Right hepatectomy is described in Chapter 21.
  - Left hepatectomy is described in Chapter 23.
  - Right trisegmentectomy is described in Chapter 27.
  - Left trisegmentectomy is described in Chapter 28.
- Portal vein considerations are unique during hepatectomy for HC, however, and described here.
- En bloc hepatic arterial resection and reconstruction is rarely needed, as this extent of tumor is generally deemed unresectable.

Biliary Resection and Reconstruction

- The duct is cut sharply without cautery artifact. Periductal bleeding is controlled with digital pressure.
- Frozen section pathologic analysis guides the extent of biliary resection into the remnant liver. Stay sutures (5-0 Prolene) in the duct allow further retraction and dissection if a more proximal margin is necessary.
- A Roux-en-Y jejunal limb is brought through the colonic mesentery to the right of the middle colonic vessels (retrocolic), with sufficient mobilization to allow for tension-free hepaticojejunostomy.
- An enterotomy is created on the antimesenteric border of the Roux limb, size-matched to the target hepatic duct. When practical, multiple adjacent ductal branches can be incorporated en masse to the anastomosis (**FIGURE 8**).

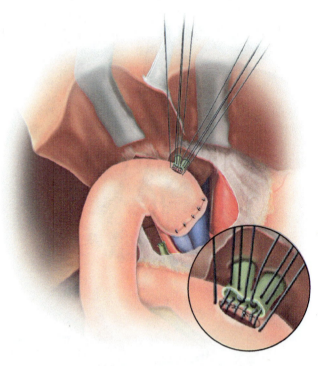

FIGURE 8 • Hepaticojejunostomy.

- Interrupted, double-armed 5-0 Prolene sutures are initially placed in the anterior wall of the duct and gently retracted with shods to facilitate exposure.
- Anastomosis begins along the posterior wall, where a single layer of 5-0 Prolene sutures incorporate the full-thickness wall of both the duct and Roux limb. Knots are tied once all posterior sutures are successfully placed.
- If already present, percutaneous transhepatic stents are advanced and left in place across the bilioenteric anastomosis.
- As an alternative, a 4- to 6-Fr transanastomotic tube can be placed through the antimesenteric wall of the Roux limb with the Witzel technique, placed proximally into the remnant biliary tree, brought out through the abdominal wall, and connected to a drainage bag. This allows access to the biliary tree without placing retrograde biliary catheters through the liver (**FIGURE 9**).
- The previously shod-retracted anterior ductal 5-0 Prolene sutures are incorporated into the bowel wall and tied to complete the anastomosis.
- The final hilar margin should be marked with clips (or gold fiducial markers) to guide subsequent needs for external beam radiation.
- Closed suction drains are placed adjacent to the bilioenteric anastomosis and under the right diaphragm before abdominal closure.

Division of Portal Vein

- If the portal vein is free of tumor, then the portal vein is divided in standard fashion as for routine hepatectomy.
- If the right or left portal vein transection plane encroaches into the confluence due to tumor involvement (**FIGURE 10**).
  - Clamp the main and contralateral portal vein branch separately and transect the vein as necessary to achieve tumor-free margins.

Chapter 11 RESECTION OF HILAR CHOLANGIOCARCINOMA

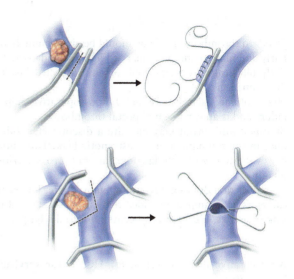

FIGURE 10 • Various approaches to portal vein resection. When complete tumor resection encroaches on the portal vein confluence, closure should be performed in a transverse fashion, as longitudinal suture lines may cause stenosis of the remaining vessel.

- Portal vein resections of up to 3 cm can be repaired primarily.
  - Clamp the main and contralateral portal vein, and excise the portal vein en bloc with tumor. Heparin is administered systemically prior to clamping the main portal vein and is reversed at the completion of the operation.
  - After ensuring proper mobilization of remaining vein, running 6-0 Prolene suture is used to approximate ends.
- Portal vein resections greater than 3 cm in length typically require interposition autograft (the authors prefer either left renal vein or internal jugular vein).

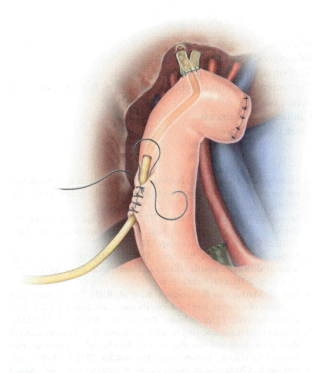

FIGURE 9 • Alternative placement of transanastomotic tube.

- Close the portal defect in a transverse orientation with running 6-0 Prolene. Longitudinal closure results in unnecessary narrowing and skewing of the remaining portal vein.
- If tumor involves the portal confluence, vein resection and reconstruction is performed later in the operation (after liver parenchyma has been fully transected and left hepatic duct dissected).

PEARLS AND PITFALLS

Indications	▪ Multidetector cross-sectional imaging should accurately stage most patients and will often reveal anomalous hilar vascular anatomy. Careful preoperative review of these images is essential.
Skeletonizing the hepatoduodenal ligament	▪ Observe a no-touch technique when mobilizing the tumor, ducts, and arteries. ▪ Grasping adjacent connective tissue (such as periadventitium or neural plexus) will avoid iatrogenic injury and tumor capsule violation.
Variable anatomy	▪ Complexity of ductal and vascular dissection increases with the presence of tumor bulk and infiltration in the hilum. ▪ Review of imaging and knowledge of common anatomic variants will expedite a safe operation.
Caudate resection	▪ Should be routinely performed and can be approached from either side. ▪ The caudate and right posterior section should be divided by parenchymal transection toward the right caval edge.

POSTOPERATIVE CARE

- Standard thromboprophylaxis should be given immediately.
- Early ambulation and pulmonary toilet are mandatory.
- Early ultrasound is a vital tool for any suspected insult to the remnant liver.
- High-volume ascites may signify postoperative hepatic failure and is an early sign of portal thrombosis.
- Bilious drain output may indicate a disconnected biliary duct in the remnant or an anastomotic leak. This should be evaluated with cholangiogram and cross-sectional imaging.
- Closed suction drains are typically removed after biliary tree catheters are clamped, provided there is no substantial bile leak or ascites. This typically occurs prior to discharge.

OUTCOMES

- After curative intent resection for HC, 5-year survival is 25% to 30%.[6]
- Rate of R0 resection is typically 64% to 71%.
- Postoperative morbidity and mortality rates range up to 50% and 10%, respectively.
- Bile leaks may occur in up to 20% of resected patients.
- Left liver resection (particularly left trisectionectomy) is associated with greater morbidity and a higher rate of positive margins.

COMPLICATIONS

- Bile leak
- Bilioenteric anastomotic stricture
- Torsion of liver remnant
- Thrombosis of portal vein, hepatic vein, hepatic artery, or vena cava
- Cholangitis or abscess
- Liver failure

REFERENCES

1. Heimbach JK, Gores GJ, Haddock MG, et al. Liver transplantation for unresectable perihilar cholangiocarcinoma. *Semin Liver Dis*. 2004;24(2):201-207.
2. Jarnagin WR, Fong Y, DeMatteo RP, et al. Staging, resectability, and outcome in 225 patients with hilar cholangiocarcinoma. *Ann Surg*. 2001;234(4):507-517. discussion 517-519.
3. Weber SM, DeMatteo RP, Fong Y, et al. Staging laparoscopy in patients with extrahepatic biliary carcinoma: analysis of 100 patients. *Ann Surg*. 2002;235(3):392-399.
4. Endo I, Matsuyama R, Taniguchi K, et al. Right hepatectomy with resection of caudate lobe and extrahepatic bile duct for hilar cholangiocarcinoma. *J Hepatobiliary Pancreat Sci*. 2012;19(3):216-224.
5. Uesaka K. Left hepatectomy or left trisectionectomy with resection of the caudate lobe and extrahepatic bile duct for hilar cholangiocarcinoma (with video). *J Hepatobiliary Pancreat Sci*. 2012;19(3):195-202.
6. Friman S. Cholangiocarcinoma—current treatment options. *Scand J Surg*. 2011;100(1):30-34.

Chapter 12 Intrahepatic Biliary-Enteric Anastomosis

Reid B. Adams and Victor M. Zaydfudim

DEFINITION

- Intrahepatic biliary-enteric anastomosis is defined as biliary reconstruction at the level of the hepatic hilum (biliary confluence) or more proximal bile ducts.
- Intrahepatic biliary-enteric anastomoses are indicated for definitive treatment of hilar biliary strictures; rarely, they may be indicated for palliation of malignant hilar obstruction.

DIFFERENTIAL DIAGNOSIS

- Biliary strictures at the hepatic hilum can be due to benign or malignant processes. Common malignant etiologies include hilar cholangiocarcinoma and gallbladder carcinoma; benign strictures typically are a result of prior biliary tract surgery or intervention.
- Uncommon benign etiologies include inflammatory or autoimmune diseases such as primary sclerosing cholangitis or IgG4 immune-mediated sclerosis.

PATIENT HISTORY AND PHYSICAL FINDINGS

- The most common presentation is jaundice. Associated symptoms may include pruritus, cholangitis, or less commonly, pain. If the patient has had biliary surgery, they may present with an acute abdomen or sepsis due to cholangitis, biloma, or biliary fistula.
- In the absence of prior biliary surgery, stone disease should be suspected.
- If a history of prior biliary surgery or instrumentation is present, a benign stricture should be suspected. Postoperative strictures present within the first 6 months in approximately 70% of patients. However, benign strictures can present years after biliary surgery.
- In the absence of stone disease and prior biliary surgery, a malignant stricture should be suspected.
- A complete history and physical examination is required to ensure the patient does not have evidence of infection or symptoms suggestive of metastatic disease. This assessment also should assess whether the patient is a candidate for major surgery.

IMAGING AND OTHER DIAGNOSTIC STUDIES

- A fundamental knowledge of biliary anatomy and the adjacent vascular structures is critical for success, both in deciding whether operative intervention is indicated, and if so, the type of procedure and an approach to ensure it is safe and effective. Biliary anomalies are frequent and should be expected; imaging studies should clearly define these structures and their relationship to each other. Hepatic vasculobiliary anatomic details are reviewed in Chapter 15.
- The aim of the diagnostic evaluation is to define the anatomy for restoration of biliary-enteric continuity in patients with benign strictures or plan appropriate palliative care in patients with malignant disease not amenable to curative resection. Magnetic resonance cholangiopancreatography (MRCP) is the initial diagnostic study of choice in patients with obstructive jaundice thought to be due to stone disease. Otherwise, magnetic resonance imaging (MRI) with intravenous contrast and MRCP is the initial study of choice for patients with obstructive jaundice due to a stricture (**FIGURE 1**). Ideally, it should be performed prior to any biliary interventions such as endoscopic retrograde cholangiography (ERC) or percutaneous transhepatic cholangiography (PTC). However, most patients come for referral with prior invasive studies or biliary stents in place; these can make image interpretation challenging and/or lead to cholangitis in obstructed segments.
- MRI/MRCP gives a detailed view of the biliary tract and the level or type of obstruction when a stricture is the cause (**FIGURE 2**). The vascular phases allow assessment of hepatic artery and portal vein involvement in the case of malignant processes and whether the hepatic arteries are intact and patent in cases of benign strictures related to prior biliary surgery. Finally, it allows for the assessment of direct hepatic involvement or metastatic disease.
- When contrast for MRI cannot be given or the vascular anatomy is not adequately assessed, B-mode and Doppler ultrasonography (US) is highly accurate in assessing vascular patency and/or involvement.[1,2] It is important to note whether lobar atrophy is present, as this dictates treatment options.

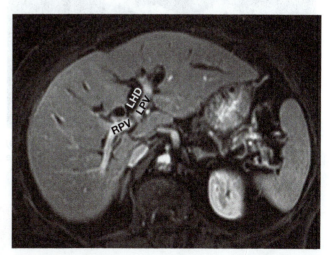

FIGURE 1 • MRI during the portal venous phase showing the right portal vein *(RPV)* and left portal vein *(LPV)*. The dilated left hepatic duct (LHD) lies anterior and superior to the LPV.

- ERC and PTC are supplementary techniques for defining the anatomy of the biliary tract and the extent of a stricture when these are not clear from the MRCP. Either or both may be used to obtain a tissue diagnosis in unresectable patients or for stent placement to treat symptoms and/or for preoperative preparation. There is considerable debate as to which technique is optimal for treating hilar biliary strictures, and this discussion is beyond the scope of this chapter.
- To effectively relieve jaundice, approximately 30% of the functioning liver volume must be drained.[3] The functioning and proposed drained volumes can be estimated using calculated liver volumes from preoperative cross-sectional imaging (computed tomography [CT] or MRI).[4] Conversely, drainage of an atrophied hepatic lobe or segment is not effective.

SURGICAL MANAGEMENT

- Issues associated with repair of benign strictures are discussed separately from malignant strictures.
- Intrahepatic biliary-enteric anastomoses are complex procedures that require experienced, multidisciplinary, hepatobiliary team care. If this is not available at your institution, the patient should be referred to an appropriate institution for definitive repair.
- All procedures are done with 2.5× magnification using loupes. This allows for meticulous surgical technique and allows precise dissection and reconstruction.
- It is important to establish a standardize approach for biliary-enteric anastomoses. Use this each time, and the high intrahepatic anastomosis will be easier to perform.

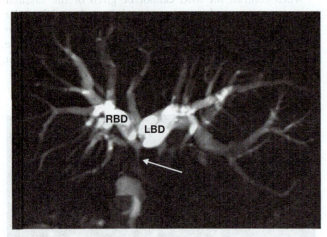

FIGURE 2 • This MRCP shows a dilated right biliary duct (*RBD*) and left biliary duct (*LBD*), leading to a type II hilar stricture at the proximalmost common hepatic duct (*white arrow*).

Preoperative Planning

Benign Stricture

- The goal for benign strictures is definitive restoration of biliary-enteric continuity. The type of stricture will dictate the nature of the biliary-enteric anastomosis (**FIGURE 3**).[5] Types E1 to E3 strictures are amenable to a Hepp–Couinaud approach.[6] E4 and E5 strictures require a modified Hepp–Couinaud approach and generally two separate anastomoses to reconstruct the right and left ducts separately.[7]
- Prior to undertaking surgery, sepsis and biliary fistulae must be resolved and all the biliary segments drained. Biliary drainage usually requires a PTC for hilar (high) strictures or injuries.
- In the clinical setting of sepsis, operative repair should not be undertaken until a minimum of 6 to 12 weeks have passed. This waiting period allows for resolution of active inflammation and evolution of any ischemic injury. Both of these are critical issues, as repair prior to resolution of these processes will decrease the success of the repair.
- Prior to operative repair, each isolated segment of the biliary system ideally should have a PTC placed. Just prior to surgical repair, the PTC drain(s) is exchanged such that the tip is guided into the distal most part of the intubated duct(s) to intraoperatively facilitate localization.

Malignant Stricture

- For this group, the preoperative evaluation focuses on whether the patient is a candidate for potentially curative resection. If so, they are approached as outlined in Chapter 11.
- With unresectable disease, current percutaneous and endoscopic techniques (drainage with plastic or expandable metallic stents and intraductal photodynamic therapy or radiofrequency ablation) provide excellent palliation; thus, there is little to no role for a planned palliative intrahepatic biliary-enteric bypass.
- Consequently, intrahepatic biliary-enteric anastomosis generally is reserved for patients with biliary obstruction found to be unresectable at the time of exploration and who are expected to survive more than 6 months. Otherwise, the morbidity and mortality associated with bypass is not justified. For instance, patients with unresectable gallbladder carcinoma have a median survival of 20 weeks. Thus, stenting is a better choice for palliation. On the other hand, the median survival for unresectable hilar cholangiocarcinoma is 52 weeks and a bypass may be reasonable under these circumstances.[8] Even this circumstance is questionable, as there appears to be no survival advantage between surgical and nonsurgical drainage approaches and the morbidity and mortality for surgical approaches are significant in comparison.[9]

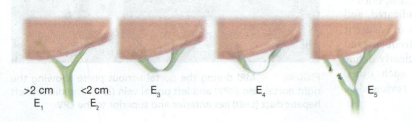

FIGURE 3 • Strasberg classification of biliary strictures.

- Other intrahepatic biliary-enteric anastomotic approaches are not included in this discussion as they are primarily of historical interest. These include the Longmire approach, mucosal graft operation, and right duct approaches. Current alternatives provide better palliation with lower risks.
- This discussion, therefore, is limited to the segment 3 bypass (round ligament or ligamentum teres approach) as the primary practical option for these patients. Although a right sectorial duct bypass can be done, the circumstances where it might be applicable are quite limited and the results relatively poor.[8] As such, it has little practical value and the best palliation for these patients is stenting and possibly tumor ablation to prevent liver failure and cholangitis.
- Patients eligible for a segment 3 bypass are limited to those with unresectable Bismuth type I, II, or IIIa strictures without atrophy of the left hepatic lobe; to be effective, at least 30% of the functioning liver volume must be drained. Types IIIb and IV lesions are not effectively drained by a segment 3 approach. Of importance, there is no role for this bypass if the right ductal system has been contaminated by prior right duct intubation, as these patients will require continued right duct drainage to prevent cholangitis.

Positioning

- The patient is placed in the supine position with both arms extended (**FIGURE 4**).
- The percutaneous drains are aseptically prepped but positioned out of the field as much as possible (ie, under additional sterile draping) and ideally left to drain. The catheters will need freedom of movement from within the abdominal cavity during the procedure; thus, extreme care must be taken to ensure that this is feasible without undue risk of inadvertent dislodgement of the drains.

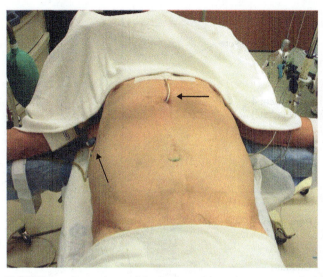

FIGURE 4 • Operative positioning is supine with arms extended. Position the percutaneous transhepatic catheters *(black arrows)*, leaving them intact during the procedure. Sterilely prep those portions left in the field and cover them with an adherent drape.

HILAR HEPATICOJEJUNOSTOMY (HEPP–COUINAUD APPROACH)

Preparation

- This approach takes advantage of the extrahepatic course of the left hepatic duct as it runs along the base of segment 4 for approximately 2 to 3 cm from the biliary confluence to the umbilical fissure (**FIGURE 5**). It is the anterior–superior most structure in the hilum, and this position facilitates its exposure and the anastomosis while minimizing injury to the portal vein and hepatic artery (**FIGURES 6** and **7**).

Incision

- A right subcostal incision allows access to the hepatic hilum. Often, a midline extension facilitates full exposure (**FIGURE 8**).

Exposure

- Identify, doubly clamp, and divide the falciform ligament. Ligate each end and leave a long tie on the superior side to use as a handle. Divide the falciform ligament superiorly to the superior edge (diaphragm) of the liver. When the patient has extensive adhesions, the ligamentum teres is an invaluable guide to locating the umbilical fissure. During dissection, follow it posteriorly to locate the umbilical fissure; this assists in identifying the anterior surface of the hepatoduodenal ligament.

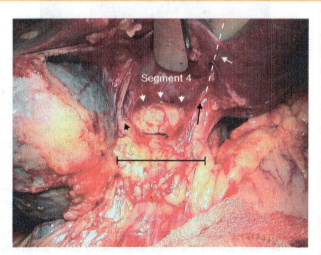

FIGURE 5 • The left hepatic duct runs in the hilar plate. Find it just posterior to the base of segment 4 *(white arrowheads)* at its junction with the hepatoduodenal ligament *(black line)*. The base of the gallbladder fossa is shown *(black arrowhead)* as well as the base of the umbilical fissure *(black arrow)*. The left hepatic duct runs approximately 1 to 2 cm to the patient's left of the base of the gallbladder fossa to the base of the umbilical fissure. The umbilical fissure *(dotted white line)* runs between segment 4 and the segments 2 and 3 of the left lobe. A bridge of liver tissue *(white arrow)* between segment 4 and segment 3 frequently covers a portion of the umbilical fissure.

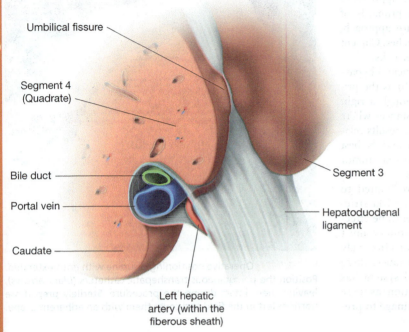

FIGURE 6 • This oblique sagittal section shows the relationship of the left hepatic duct and portal vein in the hilar plate (superiormost portion of the hepatoduodenal ligament) and the plate's relationship to segment 4 (quadrate lobe). The base of segment 4 covers the anterior–superiormost portion of the hilar plate. At this location, the left hepatic duct lies anterior–superior to the left portal vein. The left hepatic artery usually is not present at this site as it runs along the left lateral edge of the hepatoduodenal ligament and joins these structures at the base of the umbilical fissure. As segment 4 lies over the anterior hilar plate, this necessitates incising Glisson capsule at this site to push segment 4 superiorly and anteriorly, thereby exposing the hilar plate and the left hepatic duct.

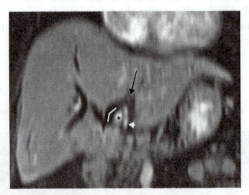

FIGURE 7 • Coronal MRI showing the relationship between the left hepatic duct *(bent white line)* and the left portal vein *(asterisk)*. The duct lies anterior–superior to the left portal vein at the base of segment 4. The left hepatic artery *(white arrowhead)* runs along the left side of the hepatoduodenal ligament and joins the duct and vein at the base of the umbilical fissure *(black arrow)*.

- Take down adhesions to the inferior surface of the liver and the anterior surface of the hepatoduodenal ligament to expose the gallbladder fossa and the base of segment 4 (**FIGURE 9**). It is easiest to work from the right edge of the liver back toward the hilum when taking down adhesions. There often is a free space at the right edge of the liver that allows access posteriorly around the lateral edge of the adhesions.
- Place a clamp behind the usually present liver bridge joining segments 4 and 2 or 3, and divide it with electrocautery. This exposes the umbilical fissure and facilitates exposure of the left hepatic duct (**FIGURE 10**).
- Carry the dissection to the base (posterior aspect) of segment 4 and its junction with the hepatoduodenal ligament (**FIGURE 5**). Retract the base of segment 4 superiorly

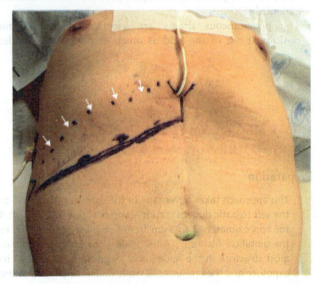

FIGURE 8 • A right subcostal incision *(solid line)* often allows sufficient exposure to the hepatic hilum. If not, a midline extension to the xiphoid facilitates access to the hilum and superior liver. The right subcostal incision typically is two fingerbreadths (~4 cm) below the right costal margin *(white arrows/dotted line)*. This image shows the two PTC tubes secured off the field except at the level of the xiphoid process (solid "V").

and anteriorly with a malleable retractor if necessary for exposure.
- Caution is warranted if the patient has right hepatic lobe atrophy and left lobe hypertrophy. The hepatoduodenal ligament anatomy often is distorted with the bile duct complex and hepatic arteries rotated to the right and posteriorly. Consequently, the main portal vein often is the anteriormost structure in the ligament in this situation.

Chapter 12 **INTRAHEPATIC BILIARY-ENTERIC ANASTOMOSIS** 85

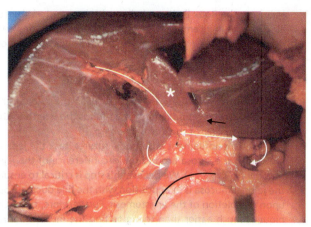

FIGURE 9 • Incise adhesions to expose the inferior surface of the liver and anterior surface of the hepatoduodenal ligament *(white double-headed arrow)*. This exposes the gallbladder fossa *(curved white line)*. The base of segment 4 is not apparent in this image, as an exophytic lobe of segment 4 *(asterisk)* covers it. The bridge of liver tissue connecting segment 4 with segment 3 *(black arrow)* limits access to the base of segment 4. The foramen of Winslow *(curved arrow, patient's right)* allows access posterior to the hepatoduodenal ligament. Opening the gastrohepatic ligament to the left of the hepatoduodenal ligament *(curved arrow, patient's left)* connects with the space posterior to the ligament and superior to the duodenum *(curved black line)*.

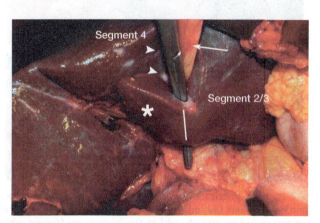

FIGURE 10 • To open the bridge of liver connecting segment 4 and segment 2 or 3 *(white line)*, place a clamp between it and the ligamentum teres *(white arrow)*. This can be divided with electrocautery because there are rarely vessels of any size within this structure. This opens the umbilical fissure exposing portal structures for segment 4 *(white arrowheads)*. This patient has an exophytic portion of segment 4 *(asterisk)*. A small portal pedicle connected this exophytic lobe. It was divided and the lobe removed to facilitate exposure to the base of segment 4.

Lower the Hilar Plate

- Incise Glisson capsule at its junction with the hepatoduodenal ligament at the base of segment 4. This leads to entry into the hepatic parenchyma adjacent to the hilar plate (**FIGURE 11**). Venous bleeding will occur; it is easily controlled with pressure. Once the base of segment 4 is released, it is retracted further superiorly and anteriorly, exposing the hilar plate and providing access to the left hepatic duct (**FIGURE 11**). This is the Hepp–Couinaud approach or "lowering the hilar plate" to expose the left and right hepatic ducts.[6]

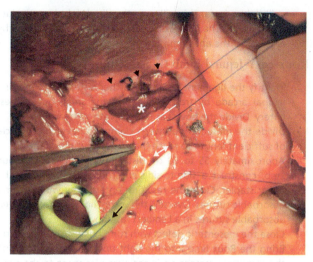

FIGURE 11 • At its junction with the hepatoduodenal ligament, incise Glisson capsule *(black arrowheads)* to expose the hepatic parenchyma *(asterisk)* superior to the hilar plate *(curved white line)*. The anterior surface of the left hepatic duct *(white double-headed arrow)* is incised longitudinally, exposing the PTC tube within the duct. Pull the PTC from within the duct and place a nylon suture through the straight portion of the tube *(black arrow)* to manipulate the tube during the procedure.

Locate the Left Hepatic Duct

- Palpate the stent in the left duct to locate it within the fibrous sheath of the hepatic plate. Intraoperative ultrasound can help locate the stent within the duct. Likewise, aspiration of bile using a 25-gauge needle and syringe can assist in locating the duct and verifying its position.

Incise the Hepatic Ducts

- Once located, make a longitudinal incision in the anterior surface of the duct until the lumen is entered (**FIGURE 11**). The lumen will be evident from the stent within it. The stent serves as a guide, delineating the lumen and course of the duct. Use a blunt probe to explore the left and right hepatic ducts and identify the confluence of the two.

- Grasp the stent and pull it out of the duct. Place a monofilament suture through the straight portion of the stent above the curved end (**FIGURE 11**). Cut the stent just distal to the suture, thus removing the self-retaining end of the stent. The suture through the stent serves as a "handle" to move the stent in and out of the opened duct. Allow it to retract above the distal left duct (**FIGURE 12**). Removing the distal end of the stent facilitates probing and opening of the duct. Having the stent out of the opened duct makes suture placement easier during the anastomosis.

- With a right-angled instrument, the stent, or a probe within the duct as a guide, use a knife to sharply open the duct a minimum of 1 cm for the anastomosis; open it longer if the patient's anatomy allows. Alternatively, angled (eg, Potts) scissors can be used to open the duct. The duct is opened toward the patient's left to the base of the umbilical fissure or just to the right of the segment 4 (middle) hepatic artery, which often lies along the right edge of the umbilical fissure. This artery runs anterior to the left hepatic duct; take care to avoid injury to it. Reverse the direction of the incision and open the duct to the patient's right to the base of the gallbladder fossa. This will open the distal right hepatic duct (**FIGURE 13**). The goal is exposure of viable duct and healthy mucosa for the anastomosis.

Roux-en-Y Jejunal Limb Construction

- Identify the ligament of Treitz. Further distally, find the first jejunal arcade by transilluminating the small bowel mesentery. Divide the bowel at this site with a linear stapler.
- Divide the mesentery between clamps to develop a pedicle of sufficient length to reach the right upper quadrant.
- Approximately 55 to 60 cm distal to the end of the Roux limb, construct a side-to-side enteroenterostomy with the linear stapler. Close the resulting enterotomy with running absorbable sutures. Oversew this suture line with interrupted absorbable sutures in a Lembert fashion.
- Close the mesenteric defect with running absorbable suture.
- Bring the Roux limb into the right upper quadrant through the transverse mesocolon in the avascular space to the right of the middle colic vessels. This results in a retrocolic Roux limb that passes anterior to the second portion of the duodenum.

- Imbricate the Roux limb staple line with interrupted absorbable sutures in a Lembert fashion (**FIGURE 14**). This prevents dense adhesions to the staple line in the event reoperation is necessary.

Hepaticojejunostomy

- Make an antimesenteric jejunotomy near the end of the Roux limb that is approximately two-thirds the length of the longest diameter of the ductal opening.
- Using 6-0 monofilament absorbable sutures, tack the jejunal mucosa to the serosa around the circumference of the jejunotomy (**FIGURE 14**). We believe this step is critical to ensure the jejunal mucosa is in apposition with the bile duct mucosa upon completion of the anastomosis. Furthermore, this technique is much easier than trying to find the mucosa during each stitch of the anastomosis, especially if the duct is small or it is difficult to see well in the depth of the field. This technique is particularly helpful to ensure the mucosa is incorporated in the anterior layer when placing the anterior row of sutures in the bowel after the posterior layer has been tied.
- If two separate ducts are present and they are close enough to be joined into a single anastomosis, this is desirable. Interrupted absorbable monofilament sutures are used to approximate the ducts (**FIGURE 15**).

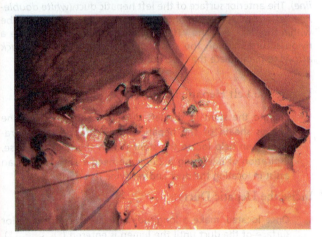

FIGURE 12 • Cut the PTC tube distal to the nylon suture, allowing it to retract above the site of the anastomosis. The left duct orifice is shown (*white arrowhead*).

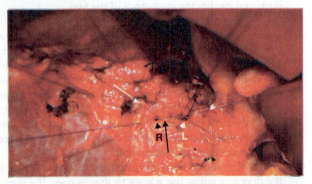

FIGURE 13 • Incising the duct toward the base of the umbilical fissure (*white arrowhead*) exposes a portion of the left hepatic duct (between *black arrow* and *white arrowhead*, L) along the base of segment 4. Incising the duct toward the base of the gallbladder fossa (*white arrow*) opens the very short extrahepatic portion of the right hepatic duct exposing its orifice (*black arrowhead*, R). The septum between the right and left ducts (*black arrow*) is shown illustrating the longer extrahepatic course of the left hepatic duct. The left duct orifice is shown (*white arrowhead*, L).

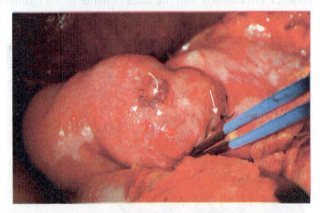

FIGURE 14 • Imbricate the staple line (*white arrow*) of the Roux limb in a Lembert fashion. Tack the jejunal mucosa to the edge of the serosa (*white arrowheads*) at the jejunotomy (*curved white arrow* indicating the lumen) to ensure a mucosal-to-mucosal anastomosis with the bile duct.

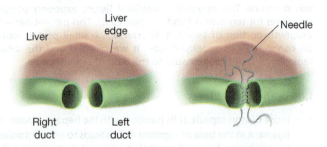

FIGURE 15 • When two separate duct openings are in close approximation, a single lumen is constructed as this facilitates a single biliary-enteric anastomosis. Use fine (5-0 or 6-0) absorbable suture to approximate the adjacent bile duct walls to form a common septum. The corner sutures are tied on the outside, and the remaining sutures are tied in the interior.

Chapter 12 **INTRAHEPATIC BILIARY-ENTERIC ANASTOMOSIS** 87

- Typically, 5-0 or 6-0 (depending on duct size, thickness/friability of the tissue) interrupted monofilament absorbable sutures on a small needle are used for the anastomosis. Place the corner sutures in the bile duct first (9- and 3-o'clock positions) such that the knot will be tied on the outside of the anastomosis. Place the anterior row sutures through the bile duct next such that the knot will be tied on the outside of the anastomosis (**FIGURE 16**). Place sutures approximately 4 to 5 mm apart. Leave the needle on and secure each suture with a fine clamp, placing it on moderate tension. It is essential to establish a system to keep the sutures organized (**FIGURE 17**). Placing the anterior row first and keeping it under tension opens the duct to facilitate the remaining portions of the anastomosis and ensure precise suture placement.
- In the event two anastomoses are required, treat them as one and place all the anterior sutures first. Trying to perform each anastomosis separately makes construction of the second one very difficult. When two anastomoses are required, place the anterior sutures into the first duct in a similar fashion to that described previously. Once they are laid out under tension, place a white towel over these sutures and clamps. Place the anterior row sutures in the second duct. Using this method, the two sets of sutures will not get confused when it is time to complete the anterior row sutures.
- Keep the bowel and bile duct apart while placing the posterior row sutures. It is easier to precisely place each suture using this technique. Start by placing the corner sutures through each corner of the jejunotomy, then place a clamp on the suture and put it under tension (**FIGURE 18**). To start the posterior row, place a suture through the posterior wall of the jejunotomy and then the posterior duct halfway between each corner stitch, thereby bisecting the distance between the two. This places the posterior row sutures so the knots will be tied on the inside of the anastomosis. Place this suture and each subsequent one on a clamp and organize the sutures as done for the anterior row to prevent tangling. Complete the right half of the posterior row by placing sutures to sequentially bisect the remaining distance between the right corner and middle sutures until there are no gaps of more than 4 to 5 mm. Complete the left half of the posterior row in a similar fashion.
- Slide the bowel to the bile duct while keeping each of the sutures taut. Tie the corner suture furthest from the surgeon first. Sequentially tie each next suture, working from the tied corner to the other corner suture. The assistant can use

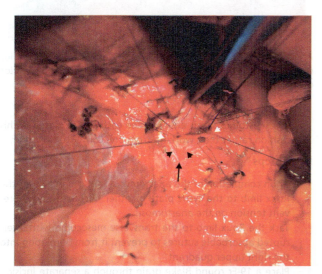

FIGURE 16 • Place the corner sutures initially in the bile duct *(white arrowheads)* so they will be tied on the exterior. Place the remaining anterior sutures such that they will be tied on the exterior. Place the first suture to bisect the distance between the corners. Then place the remaining sutures to bisect each half until the sutures are 4 to 5 mm apart. The scarred and obstructed proximal common hepatic duct *(black arrow)* is seen at its junction *(black arrowheads)* with the left and right hepatic ducts.

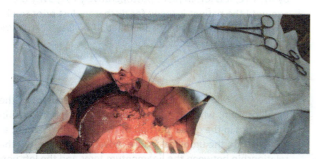

FIGURE 17 • After each anterior suture is placed in the bile duct, attach a fine clamp and organize each suture to prevent tangling. Placing each suture under moderate tension and arranging them on white towels as shown facilitates this. The white towels make the sutures easier to see on the field.

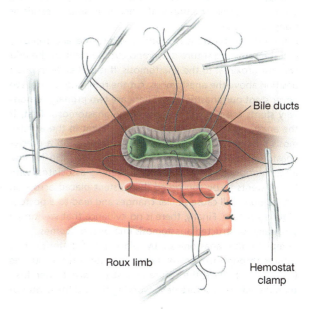

FIGURE 18 • Place the posterior suture row by placing each corner suture in the corresponding corner of the jejunotomy. Place each of these under tension as shown in **FIGURE 17**. Keep the bowel and bile duct separated by 5 to 10 cm while placing the remaining posterior sutures. Place the remaining sutures so they will be tied on the interior. The first suture is placed to bisect the distance between the corner sutures. Next, the right half sutures are placed, again by bisecting the distance between the corner and the middle suture. This is done until the distance is 4 to 5 mm between the sutures. Finish the posterior row by placing the left half sutures.

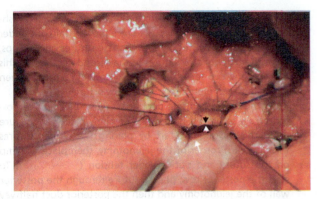

FIGURE 19 • Tie the posterior row sutures by pushing the bowel into apposition with the bile duct. Start by tying the corner furthest from the surgeon, tying each next suture in succession. Forceps retracting the anterior edge of the jejunotomy *(white arrow)* allow examination of the posterior wall of the anastomosis to ensure a mucosal-to-mucosal anastomosis (opposing *black* and *white arrowhead*).

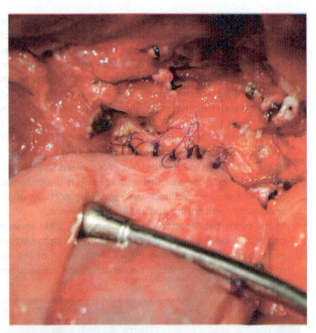

FIGURE 20 • Complete the anastomosis by placing the anterior row sutures through the bowel and tying them on the exterior of the anastomosis.

forceps to hold the anterior lip of the bowel inferiorly, opening the anastomosis and allowing the surgeon to observe each suture as it is tied, thus ensuring apposition of the bowel and bile duct mucosa (**FIGURE 19**).
- Once the posterior row sutures are tied, place a right-angle clamp into the lumen of the jejunotomy and gently open the clamp. This ensures that none of the anterior mucosa is trapped in the posterior sutures while tying them. This prevents webs or strictures in the anastomosis as a result of trapped mucosa.
- If the intraductal stent is protruding into the anastomosis, pull the retaining suture down and cut the stent so the end will rest proximal to the anastomosis. If it is already in good position above the anastomosis, cut the retaining suture. We never stent our anastomoses. There are two primary reasons why stents are not left traversing the anastomosis. First, if the anastomosis is done as described, a stent in the anastomosis provides no technical advantage in assuring a precise anastomosis. Second, one only has to observe the intense inflammation, tissue injury, and thickening associated with biliary stents to be concerned that a stent placed across an anastomosis will cause similar changes and lead to a postoperative stricture. Finally, there is no evidence that stenting a surgically constructed anastomosis improves outcomes.
- Complete the anastomosis by placing the anterior row sutures through the bowel, tying the knots on the outside (**FIGURE 20**). Place the suture closest to each corner first, then the adjacent suture next, working toward the center of the anastomosis. It is easier to see each suture placed in this fashion rather than working from one corner to the other.

Final Steps

- Upon completion of the anastomosis, use sutures to tack the Roux limb to the cystic plate or other fibrous tissue to prevent tension on the anastomosis.
- Tack the Roux limb to the transverse mesocolon with interrupted absorbable sutures to prevent it from herniating into the right upper quadrant.
- Place a 19-Fr round Blake drain through a separate incision and place the end in the subhepatic space.
- If the PTC tubes were manipulated and the fibrous sheath around them was disrupted, place a silk purse string in the liver and tie it around the tube at the exit site to prevent bile leakage.
- After closing the incision, suture the PTC to the skin to prevent dislodgement. Although the anastomosis is not stented by the PTC, it is left in place postoperatively to gravity drainage until the patient is ready for discharge. Just prior to discharge, a cholangiogram is completed. If no leak or stricture is seen, the tube is removed.

SEGMENT 3 HEPATICOJEJUNOSTOMY (LIGAMENTUM TERES OR ROUND LIGAMENT APPROACH)

Preparation

- This approach takes advantage of the position of the segment 3 duct, which lies cranial to the left portal vein (**FIGURE 21**) at the anterior–inferior aspect of the umbilical fissure (**FIGURE 22**). The ligamentum teres (remnant of the umbilical vein, which joined the terminal left portal vein in utero) runs in the dorsal portion of the falciform ligament as it passes into the umbilical fissure. Advantage is taken of the relationship between the ligamentum teres and the left portal vein to facilitate identification of the segment 3 bile duct.
- Contraindications to the segment 3 approach include an isolated right ductal system that is infected or has been instrumented by an endoscopically or percutaneously placed drain,

Chapter 12 INTRAHEPATIC BILIARY-ENTERIC ANASTOMOSIS   89

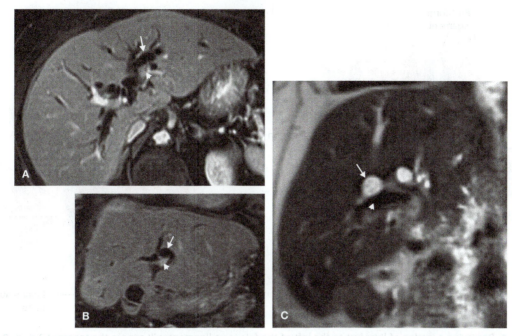

FIGURE 21 • The segment 3 duct *(white arrowhead)* is located cranial to the left portal vein *(white arrow)* within the umbilical fissure. **A,** Axial contrast-enhanced portal phase MRI. **B,** Coronal contrast-enhanced portal vein phase MRI. **C,** Sagittal T2-weighted MRI.

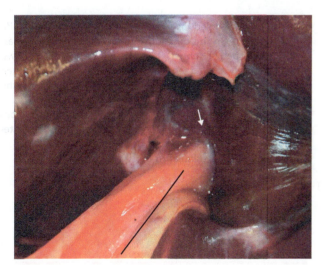

FIGURE 22 • The ligamentum teres *(black line)* runs in the dorsal portion of the falciform ligament and its junction with segment 3 *(white arrow)* helps locate the approximate position of the segment 3 duct.

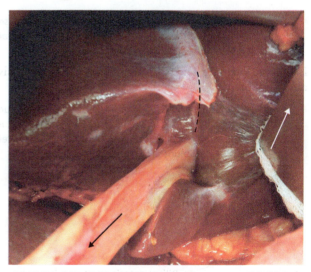

FIGURE 23 • Retracting the ligamentum teres *(black arrow)* inferiorly and to the right while retracting the lateral segment of the liver *(white arrow)* superiorly and anteriorly opens the umbilical fissure and facilitates exposure to the segment 3 portal pedicle. The liver is divided just to the left of the falciform ligament *(dotted black line)* to access the segment 3 duct.

atrophy of the left hepatic lobe, metastatic disease, or tumor involvement of the secondary bile ducts of the left lobe or posterior to the base of the umbilical fissure.

Locate the Segment 3 Duct

- The initial steps including positioning, incision, exposure, and construction of the Roux limb are the same as described in the prior section. Likewise, constructing the hepaticojejunostomy follows the principles outlined earlier.
- Retraction of the ligamentum teres inferiorly and to the right while retracting the adjacent liver superiorly and anteriorly facilitates exposure to the segment 3 duct (**FIGURE 23**).

- Divide the liver just to the left of the falciform ligament starting superior to the umbilical fissure and incise the liver inferiorly and posteriorly toward the junction of the left portion of the ligamentum teres with segment 3 of the liver (**FIGURE 23**). If necessary, remove a small wedge of hepatic parenchyma to expose the segment 3 duct (**FIGURE 24**). This approach avoids dividing the portal vein branches to segment 3. Avoid dissection of more than the anterior surface of the duct to avoid devascularization of the duct.

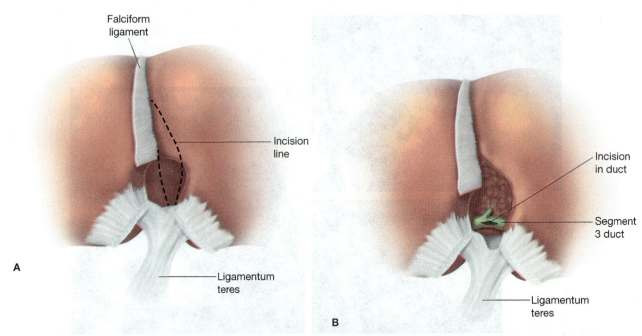

FIGURE 24 • **A,** Removing a wedge of liver just to the left of the falciform ligament will expose the segment 3 duct. **B,** Once the segment 3 duct is exposed, place stay sutures superior and inferior to the proposed ductotomy and longitudinally incise the duct. Once the lumen is identified, probe the duct in each direction and open the duct for a minimum of 1 cm for the anastomosis.

- Intraoperative ultrasound can help locate the duct. Likewise, aspiration of bile using a 25-gauge needle and syringe can assist in locating the duct and verifying its position.

Incise the Hepatic Ducts, Biliary-Enteric Anastomosis, and Final Steps

- Once located, place fine stay sutures in the anterior duct wall, elevate them, and make a longitudinal incision in the exposed surface of the duct until the lumen is entered (FIGURE 24). Use a blunt probe to explore the duct.
- With a right-angled instrument inside the duct, use a knife to sharply open the duct a minimum of 1 cm for the anastomosis; open it longer if the patient's anatomy allows. Alternatively, angled (eg, Potts) scissors can be used to open the duct. Reverse the direction of the incision and open the duct to the patient's right to the extent feasible.
- The biliary-enteric anastomosis to the Roux limb is constructed as described in the previous section. Place the anterior row sutures first followed by the posterior row.
- The final steps are similar to those described previously.

PEARLS AND PITFALLS

Indications	• Biliary-enteric anastomosis may be necessary for benign or malignant disease. • The stricture etiology (benign or malignant) dictates the anastomotic location and options.
Preoperative evaluation	• MRCP/MRI is the initial imaging study of choice. • Endoscopic/percutaneous cholangiography is a supplementary study for defining biliary anatomy. Biliary stenting often is necessary for preoperative preparation.
Benign	• Allow 6 to 12 weeks following resolution of sepsis and/or control of biliary fistulae before proceeding with repair. • Ensure all ducts are accounted for and each isolated biliary segment has a PTC within it.
Malignant	• Nearly all patients with unresectable disease can be effectively palliated without a biliary-enteric anastomosis. • A segment 3 bypass is reasonable for patients with malignant hilar obstructions that do not extend to the secondary radicles of the left hepatic duct.
Identifying the hilar bile duct	• At the base of segment 4 and its junction with the hepatoduodenal ligament, incise Glisson capsule at this junction to "lower" the hilar plate. • The left hepatic duct lies anterior and superior in the hilar plate.

Segment 3	• Identify the duct at the superior–posterior portion of the segment 3 portal triad by ultrasound or aspirating bile. • The duct lies cranial to the left portal vein in the anterior–inferior portion of the umbilical fissure. • Incise the liver just to the left of the falciform ligament and carry this inferiorly to the superior portion of the ligamentum teres. Remove a small wedge of liver if necessary. • Incise the duct longitudinally.
Constructing the biliary-enteric anastomosis	• Tack the mucosa to the serosa at the jejunotomy site. • Cut the PTC tube(s) above the level of the anastomosis. • Place each corner suture first in the bile duct and then the anterior row so the sutures will be tied on the exterior. • Place a clamp in the intestinal portion of the anastomosis and open to ensure the anterior mucosa is not trapped.
Final steps	• Tack the Roux limb to the hilar plate and transverse mesocolon. • Secure any PTC tube to the liver to prevent a bile leak. • If present, perform a cholangiogram through the PTC prior to discharge. If no leak or stricture, remove the PTC.

POSTOPERATIVE CARE

- If a preexisting PTC is left in place following biliary reconstruction, leave it to gravity drainage. Just prior to discharge, perform a cholangiogram. If there is no leak and the anastomosis is patent, remove the PTC prior to discharge.
- If no bile is present in the Blake drain, remove it prior to discharge. Otherwise, leave it until the leak has ceased.
- Long-term follow-up is necessary to assess for early and late anastomotic stricture. This includes symptom assessment for pruritus, jaundice, or cholangitis and serial serum liver studies (liver function tests). Liver tests typically are done every 4 months in the first year, every 6 months in years 2 and 3, and if stable, annually for life.

OUTCOMES

- Approximately 80% to 90% long-term excellent results are reported for hilar hepaticojejunostomy. The more complex the injury (E4, E5), the lower the success rate.
- Approximately 70% of anastomotic strictures occur in the first 3 years following surgery and 80% within the first 5 years. Follow-up longer than 5 years is important as late strictures may develop in up to 5% of patients even after more than 12 years.[10] A recent study confirmed improved results in recent patient cohorts undergoing biliary-enteric anastomosis.[11]
- Modest serum liver test elevations are seen following biliary-enteric anastomosis in patients with excellent results. Caution is warranted when interpreting these tests and trends over time are more useful than individual data points.[12] Rising values, particularly in the alkaline phosphatase, should lead to investigation for an anastomotic stricture.

COMPLICATIONS

- Bile leak, fistula, or biloma
- Cholangitis
- Anastomotic stricture
- Infection—organ space or wound abscess

REFERENCES

1. Bloom CM, Langer B, Wilson SR. Role of US in the detection, characterization, and staging of cholangiocarcinoma. *Radiographics*. 1999;19(5):1199-1218.
2. Looser C, Stain SC, Baer HU, et al. Staging of hilar cholangiocarcinoma by ultrasound and duplex sonography: a comparison with angiography and operative findings. *Br J Radiol*. 1992;65(778):871-877.
3. Jarnagin WR. Cholangiocarcinoma of the extrahepatic bile ducts. *Semin Surg Oncol*. 2000;19(2):156-776.
4. Chun YS, Ribero D, Abdalla EK, et al. Comparison of two methods of future liver remnant volume measurement. *J Gastrointest Surg*. 2008;12(1):123-128.
5. Strasberg SM, Hertl M, Soper NJ. An analysis of the problem of biliary injury during laparoscopic cholecystectomy. *J Am Coll Surg*. 1995;180(1):101-125.
6. Hepp J. Hepaticojejunostomy using the left biliary trunk for iatrogenic biliary lesions: the French connection. *World J Surg*. 1985;9:507-511.
7. Strasberg SM, Picus DD, Drebin JA. Results of a new strategy for reconstruction of biliary injuries having an isolated right-sided component. *J Gastrointest Surg*. 2001;5:266-274.
8. Jarnagin WR, Burke E, Powers C, et al. Intrahepatic biliary enteric bypass provides effective palliation in selected patients with malignant obstruction at the hepatic duct confluence. *Am J Surg*. 1998;175:453-460.
9. Singhal D, van Gulik TM, Gouma DJ. Palliative management of hilar cholangiocarcinoma. *Surg Oncol*. 2005;14:59-74.
10. Pitt HA, Miyamoto T, Parapatis SK, et al. Factors influencing outcome in patients with postoperative biliary strictures. *Am J Surg*. 1982;144:14-21.
11. Pitt HA, Sherman S, Johnson MS, et al. Improved outcomes of bile duct injuries in the 21st century. *Ann Surg*. 2013;258(3):490-499.
12. Fialkowski EA, Winslow ER, Scott MG, et al. Establishing "normal" values for liver function tests after reconstruction of biliary injuries. *J Am Coll Surg*. 2008;207(5):705-709.

Chapter 13 Operative Management of Choledochal Cyst

Charles S. Cox Jr. and Michael Collins Scott

DEFINITION

- Choledochal cyst represents a spectrum of cystic abnormalities of the extrahepatic biliary tree. It is not an isolated defect of the choledochus, rather, it also includes a constellation of abnormalities of the pancreaticobiliary system/junction.
- The classification of the cystic structural abnormalities (types I - V) as originally described by Alonso-Lej[1] and modified by Todani[2] is typically used (**FIGURE 1**).

- Type I is the predominant type of cyst (90%-95% of cases) and is a fusiform, solitary dilation of the common bile duct (CBD) and hepatic duct. Type I is further subdivided into a, b, and c subtypes.
- Type II is a cystic diverticulum of the CBD.
- Type III (subtypes 1 and 2) is called a choledochocele and is a cystic dilation of the duct at the junction with the duodenum (intraduodenal subtype 1), with the

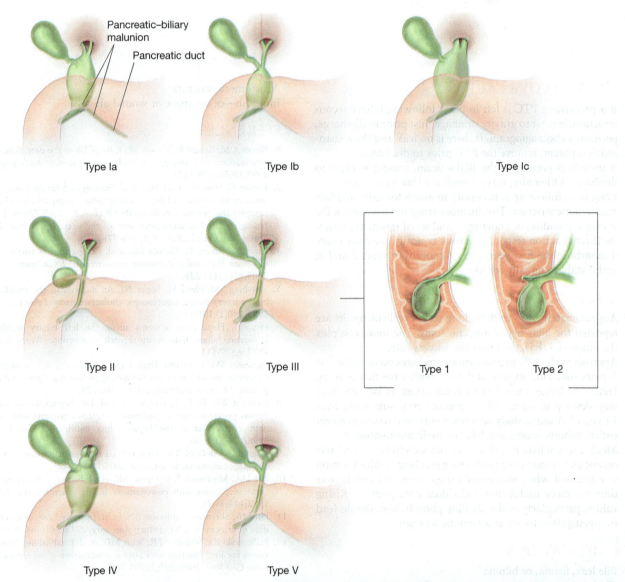

FIGURE 1 • The five major classifications of choledochal cysts are shown in schematic drawing. The classification and delineation of anatomic type has significant impact on surgical planning. Previously, these anatomic images were displayed clinically via ultrasound and/or cholangiography (intraoperative in neonates and endoscopic retrograde cholangiopancreatography in older children). More recently, magnetic resonance cholangiopancreatography has demonstrated greater anatomic detail in a noninvasive manner.

CBD and pancreatic duct entering the intraduodenal choledochocele separately and draining into the duodenum via a stenotic/inflamed opening; and rarely, the intrapancreatic subtype 2, the choledochocele, is a diverticulum of the CBD at the level of the ampulla of Vater.
- Type IV is a combined dilation of the intrahepatic and extrahepatic biliary tree and is the second most common type of cyst.
- Type V is also known as Caroli disease and is single or multiple intrahepatic cyst(s).
■ In symptomatic infants, the distal CBD often has a stenotic opening, whereas in older patients, the distal CBD has a patent communication. Types II, III, and V are all very rare, representing only a few percent of the total number of cysts.

DIFFERENTIAL DIAGNOSIS

■ The differential diagnosis of choledochal cyst is age-dependent.
■ In infants, the differential of most concern is cystic variants of biliary atresia; other abdominal cysts, including renal, are in the infant differential.
■ For older children, cystic lesions of the pancreas, hepatic tumors, rhabdomyosarcoma of the biliary tree, and cystic neuroblastoma are considerations. Most of these are distinguished on more advanced imaging, once the issue is raised with ultrasound.

PATIENT HISTORY AND PHYSICAL FINDINGS

■ Patients with choledochal cysts are usually characterized as either infantile (now includes fetal or in utero diagnoses) or noninfantile forms.
■ Infantile (in utero): The infantile patient with an in utero diagnosis is an increasing cohort of patients; the cystic mass adjacent to the liver is usually noted on prenatal ultrasound in midgestation. There have been reports of cystic lesions visualized as early as 15 weeks, but most are in the 20 to 24 weeks of gestation range. The antenatal abnormality should be confirmed by ultrasound postnatally. The issue that arises is timing of surgical intervention, as even the infantile forms are often asymptomatic for months.
■ Infantile forms that are not in utero diagnoses are by definition symptomatic—abdominal pain/mass, jaundice with mixed hyperbilirubinemia, acholic stools, and/or signs and symptoms of pancreatitis or cholangitis. In general, the infantile forms do not present with an abdominal mass or other signs of inflammation, rather, these patients are increasingly identified in utero with prenatal ultrasound and/or on postnatal ultrasound as part of the initial evaluation for mixed hyperbilirubinemia. Other presentations include failure to thrive and vomiting with mixed hyperbilirubinemia.
■ Noninfantile forms: Symptoms and signs of the noninfantile forms of choledochal cyst are classically described as right upper quadrant pain, jaundice (direct hyperbilirubinemia), and a mass. Pain and jaundice are the major symptoms, and it is rare that a right upper quadrant mass is palpable. The triad is present in fewer than 10% of patients. This presentation likely results from a delayed diagnosis/referral. The most likely cause is either misdiagnosis of mixed hyperbilirubinemia as hepatitis or an incomplete evaluation of an episode of pancreatitis or hyperamylasemia with abdominal pain. Rarely, children can present with cyst rupture; there is no correlation between cyst size and risk of rupture.

IMAGING AND OTHER DIAGNOSTIC STUDIES

■ Ultrasound is the initial imaging study of choice. Ultrasound is the least invasive and most cost-effective method of investigating the biliary tree after an episode of pancreatitis or abnormal elevations in liver enzymes in association with abdominal pain (with or without jaundice). This modality will suffice in the setting of calculus disease, but additional imaging with greater resolution is required when dilation of the biliary tree is identified.
■ Endoscopic retrograde cholangiopancreatography (ERCP) (**FIGURE 2**) vs magnetic resonance cholangiopancreatography (MRCP) (**FIGURES 3** and **4**): Both types of imaging of the biliary tree can be useful. ERCP was more frequently used in older children to obtain direct contrast injection into the extrahepatic biliary tree under fluoroscopic guidance. It provides excellent detail of the structural anatomy of the cyst but very little input into the relationship to structures other than the pancreatic duct. ERCP has the advantage over MRCP in that it can also be therapeutic in the setting of obstructive jaundice. MRCP provides a similar level of detailed imaging of the ductal relationships with 3D reconstruction of the anatomy of adjacent

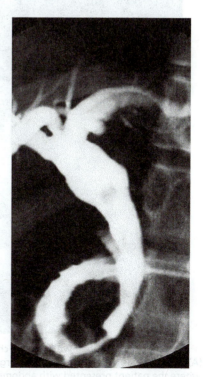

FIGURE 2 • Endoscopic retrograde cholangiopancreatography in an older child demonstrating a type I cyst with fusiform morphology and moderately dilated right and left hepatic ducts.

SECTION I SURGERY OF THE BILIARY SYSTEM

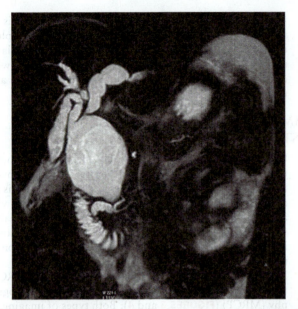

FIGURE 3 • Magnetic resonance cholangiopancreatography in an older child demonstrating a type I cyst. This image demonstrates a greater detail in the anatomic relationship of the pancreatic duct. This also shows how there is a relative continuum between type I and IV cysts.

structures as well. MRCP also has the advantage of being noninvasive and thus is associated with less risk. **FIGURE 5** shows an intraoperative cholangiogram of a type IV cyst that can be an adjunct to the other imaging modalities.

- Computed tomography (CT): CT imaging is most commonly used when investigating abdominal pain of an undetermined etiology and when the findings suggest a choledochal cyst. With the more advanced CT imaging and 3D reconstruction/multiplanar imaging now available, MRCP or ERCP is rarely required if a CT has been obtained.

SURGICAL MANAGEMENT

- The technique described in the following text represents the principal management of types I and IV cysts, which represents over 95% of choledochal cyst cases. Timing of intervention is debated. The debate between immediate (first 2 weeks of life) vs delayed (6 weeks to 3 months of age) surgical intervention hinges on whether there is a risk for progressive liver dysfunction developing in the interim time of waiting. There are no solid data to support either approach. The rationale for not waiting indefinitely is that it can be somewhat difficult to distinguish the cystic variant of biliary atresia from a choledochal cyst in infancy. Missing the window to surgically correct a

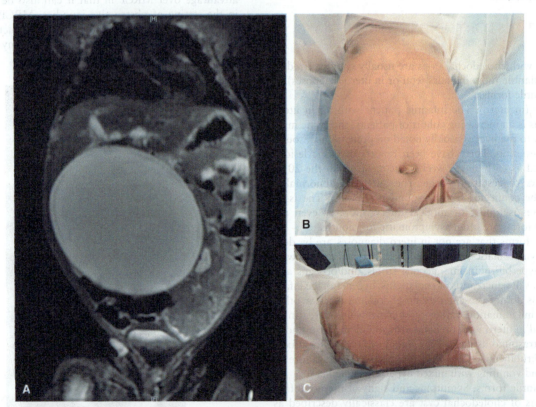

FIGURE 4 • Depicted here is a child with a type I choledochal cyst. The cyst is easily visible on magnetic resonance cholangiopancreatography **(A)** with obvious mass effect on other organs in the intra-abdominal cavity. This is consistent with his physical examination **(B** and **C)**, where the patient presented with abdominal distension.

Chapter 13 OPERATIVE MANAGEMENT OF CHOLEDOCHAL CYST 95

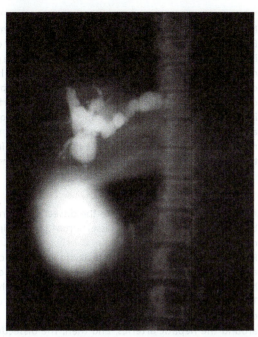

FIGURE 5 • Intraoperative cholangiogram demonstrating a type IV cyst with multiple proximal ductal cysts that have areas of narrowing between the dilated regions (as opposed to the type I cyst).

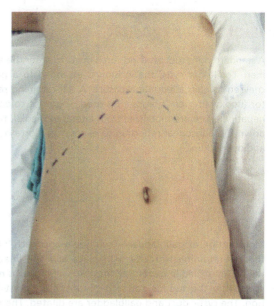

FIGURE 6 • The patient is placed supine on the operating table with the abdomen available for fluoroscopic imaging. A small towel bump is placed under the right flank. The right arm is at 90° and is the site for a radial arterial catheter for blood pressure monitoring/sampling.

patient with biliary atresia could lead to potentially devastating, although avoidable, outcomes. A reasonable intermediate approach is to follow the asymptomatic, anicteric patient serially with serum biochemical studies and ultrasound with a planned operation at 6 weeks of age to earlier if worsening. Symptomatic patients or patients with a mixed hyperbilirubinemia undergo early operation if other comorbidities are manageable. Older patients can undergo operation when physiologically stable. If these patients present with cholangitis/pancreatitis, they can typically be managed akin to an adult with gallstone pancreatitis. Once the acute inflammatory response has subsided, an operation is performed during that admission, as the risk of early recurrent pancreatitis is elevated.

Preoperative Planning

- We advise the use of an epidural catheter for perioperative pain management; this is placed after the induction of anesthesia. Two peripheral intravenous lines, radial arterial line, Foley catheter, and nasogastric tubes are routinely inserted under aseptic conditions. Any coagulopathy is corrected preoperatively (unusual), and 20 mL/kg body weight of packed red blood cell are crossmatched and available for the procedure. Preoperative cefoxitin (40 mg/kg body weight) is used as antibiotic prophylaxis and redosed at 4 hours if needed.

Positioning

- The patient is placed supine on the operating room table such that fluoroscopic cholangiography can be performed if needed. A small towel "bump" is placed under the right flank. The right arm is on an armboard at 90° (**FIGURE 6**).

- The rationale for total cyst excision is to minimize the risk of malignant degeneration in the future. Roux-en-Y cyst jejunostomy is favored over cyst duodenostomy because of poor long-term results associated with the latter, namely recurrent cholangitis and anastomotic stenosis leading to insidious biliary cirrhosis. We exclusively use an open laparotomy with total cyst excision for types I and IV lesions (over 95% of cases) with Roux-en-Y hepaticojejunostomy.

- The use of minimally invasive approaches has been described and is technically feasible. There are no long-term data on this approach; laparoscopic portoenterostomy for biliary atresia has been abandoned not due to technical issues but rather due to exacerbation of hepatic insufficiency that is thought to be due to either technical dissection of the portal plate or more recently a reduction of hepatic/portal blood flow for the time of operation.[3]

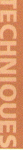

INCISION AND EXPOSURE

- A standard right subcostal incision is made to enter the abdomen. For larger cysts, the incision is extended to a partial chevron to gain adequate exposure. A self-retaining retractor (Bookwalter or Thompson) is used. The right colon and hepatic flexure are mobilized from lateral to medial, taking down the peritoneal reflection to expose the porta hepatis and duodenum.

- Next, the duodenum is fully mobilized (Kocher maneuver). Be prepared for the potential severe acute and/or chronic inflammation including saponification of these tissue planes, making dissection tedious, bloody, and potentially hazardous. If the anatomy is difficult to discern, an intraoperative cholangiogram can be very helpful. This can be performed in the usual manner at the cystic duct using Omnipaque 300 and fluoroscopy. A 5-Fr infant feeding tube is used to cannulate the cystic duct, and real-time fluoroscopy can identify the anatomy and help resolve any anatomic questions.

GALLBLADDER AND ARTERIAL DISSECTION

- Mobilization of gallbladder—"top-down approach": Once the self-retaining retractor is in place and the anatomic field is identified in general terms, the gallbladder is mobilized from the fundus down to the cystic duct/cyst junction. The cystic duct and gallbladder are dilated. The cystic artery is identified and traced back to the right hepatic artery (RHA) or its origin. The gallbladder is then available for traction and can be rotated medially to facilitate exposure and identification of the portal vein (PV), posteriorly.

- FIGURES 7 and 8 demonstrate the dissection of the gallbladder and circumferential dissection of the cyst in separate patients.

- RHA identification and further dissection of hepatic artery and left hepatic artery: Once the RHA is identified, the hepatic arterial anatomy can be dissected off of the cyst. The ease of this dissection is dependent on the degree of pericystic inflammation. Vessel loops can be placed around the hepatic arteries, and then, the dissection can proceed directly on the cyst wall anterior and lateral to the artery.

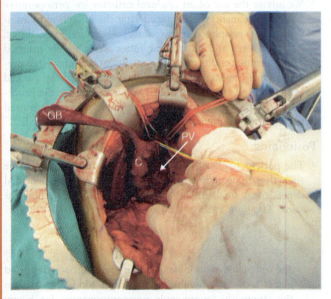

FIGURE 7 • This intraoperative photograph (type I cyst magnetic resonance cholangiopancreatography in **FIGURE 3**) demonstrates the circumferential dissection of the cyst (yellow vessel loop, *C*), with the right hepatic artery (RHA) and left hepatic artery (LHA) looped (*red*). The gallbladder (*GB*) has been completely mobilized and the duodenum Kocherized. The cyst is partially dissected posteriorly from the portal vein (*PV*).

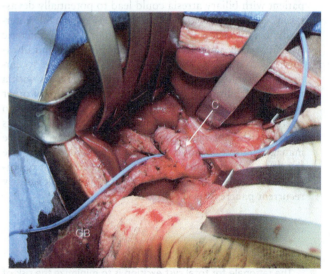

FIGURE 8 • This intraoperative photograph of another type I cyst (*C*) demonstrates using the same operative approach of gallbladder (*GB*) mobilization and circumferential dissection of the cyst cephalad to the cystic duct confluence (blue vessel loop). The duodenum is completely Kocherized and under the retractor/laparotomy pad. There is minimal inflammation in this case.

Chapter 13 OPERATIVE MANAGEMENT OF CHOLEDOCHAL CYST 97

CIRCUMFERENTIAL DISSECTION OF CYST

- Typical approach: The goal of the dissection is a radical excision of the complete cyst from the level of the confluence of the hepatic ducts to the junction with the pancreatic ducts distally. To achieve this, the arterial anatomy is isolated anteriorly as described in the previous text, and then the back wall of the cyst is dissected free from the PV. Identify the PV just before it bifurcates, and circumferentially dissect on the undersurface of the cyst until the cyst is encircled with an umbilical tape or vessel loop. Dividing the cyst at the confluence of the right and left ducts allows anterior traction on the cyst and provides exposure of the anterior aspect of the PV as the dissection is carried distally toward the superior mesenteric vein. Once the cyst is off of the PV and divided proximally, then the biliary tree is retracted anteriorly as dissection directly on the cyst wall toward the junction with the pancreatic duct.
- Alternative approach: In the setting of extensive pericystic inflammation that obscures the anatomy and precludes safe circumferential dissection, Lilly[4] described an alternative approach of intramural dissection that leaves the posterior wall in place, akin to abdominal aortic aneurysm repair. The cyst is opened transversely, and the plane within the cyst wall that allows separation of the mucosa from the thinner exterior cyst wall is developed. There are numerous perforating small vessels that can be controlled with cautery. This dissection proceeds superiorly and inferiorly, leaving the back wall of the cyst in place and adherent to the PV. This approach allows removal of all of the potentially malignant mucosa and prevents the potential catastrophic complication of injury to the PV.

CYST EXCISION

- Level of distal resection: As the cyst is circumferentially dissected down toward the pancreas, it invariably tapers down to a narrow neck. Preoperative imaging provides guidance as to the site of the confluence with the pancreatic duct; it can be quite high in cases of pancreatic–biliary malunion. This dissection typically dives into the head of the pancreas and it is critical to stay directly on the cyst wall for the dissection and not inadvertently violate the pancreatic duct—a catastrophic error that invariably leads to pancreatic fistula. **FIGURE 9** demonstrates the upward traction on the divided extrahepatic biliary tree and dissection down to the distal end of the cyst. Once the distal extent of the cyst is determined, it is divided at this level and oversewn with monofilament suture (3-0 or 4-0 Prolene), using care to preserve the pancreatic duct. **FIGURE 10** depicts a type I choledochal cyst retracted out of the abdominal cavity into the surgical field.

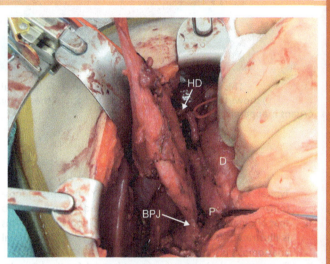

FIGURE 9 • This intraoperative photograph demonstrates the extrahepatic biliary tree retracted anteriorly, after the proximal cyst has been divided at the junction of the confluence of the hepatic ducts (*HD*), and the gallbladder is used as the point of traction. The duodenum (*D*) is fully Kocherized, exposing the posterior aspect of the pancreas (*P*), and the red vessel loop is on the left hepatic artery. Stay sutures are on the transected duct. The cyst is tapering down to the junction with the pancreatic duct in an intrapancreatic position (*BPJ*). The transition to an intramural dissection is noted on the anterior wall of the cyst halfway down the dissection.

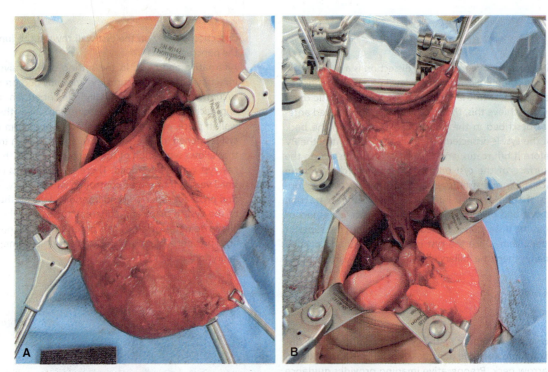

FIGURE 10 • This intraoperative photograph (type I choledochal cyst magnetic resonance cholangiopancreatography and examination **FIGURE 4**) shows the choledochal cyst retracted out of the wound into the surgical field **(A)**. Its size compared to other intra-abdominal organs is apparent **(B)**.

BILIARY–ENTERIC RECONSTRUCTION

- Typical approach: retrocolic Roux-en-Y hepaticojejunostomy—The standard approach is to create a 40-cm Roux limb that originates 10 cm from the duodenojejunal junction. This is illustrated in the drawings in **FIGURE 11** and the initial anastomosis is shown in photographs in **FIGURE 12**.
- Numerous techniques are commonly used for the jejunojejunostomy. Most pediatric surgeons prefer an end (proximal jejunum) to side (distal jejunum), two-layered, handsewn anastomosis in older children. The inner row of sutures is placed using 4-0 Vicryl and hemi-Connell technique and the outer row thrown using Lembert technique and using 3-0 silk. In infants/small children, a single-layer anastomosis of interrupted 5-0 or 4-0 Vicryl is most often employed.
- The end of the Roux limb is closed in two layers and then brought through a defect created in the transverse mesocolon, just to the right of the middle colic vessels. The antimesenteric side of the Roux limb is used for the anastomosis to the confluence of the hepatic ducts. Interrupted 4-0 or 5-0 polydioxanone or equivalent monofilament, absorbable sutures are placed to create a single-layer anastomosis. This should be tension free and care should be taken to ensure that the limb is not kinked or twisted in the final anatomic configuration. **FIGURE 13** demonstrates a completed anastomosis. The limb is secured to the mesocolic defect with interrupted sutures and the mesenteric defect of the jejunal anastomosis is closed as well.
- In cases that are complicated due to multiple previous bouts of pancreatitis and/or cholangitis, most surgeons prefer to leave a drain; in straightforward cases (usually the infantile

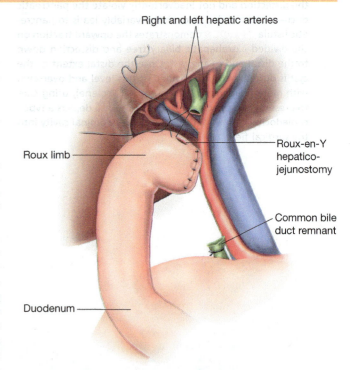

FIGURE 11 • This drawing is a schematic diagram of the Roux-en-Y hepaticojejunostomy. The side jejunotomy is matched to the size of the hepatic duct, leaving a small distance of "j" configuration to the limb. This is nothing left more than a few centimeters to prevent dumping of bile, as this will grow with the child.

Chapter 13 OPERATIVE MANAGEMENT OF CHOLEDOCHAL CYST 99

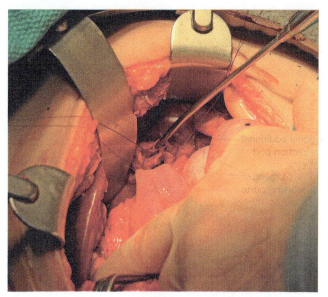

FIGURE 12 • This is an intraoperative photograph of the Roux limb on stay sutures at 3- and 9-o'clock positions and the suction tip in the hepatic duct confluence. The duct was irrigated with saline to ensure no debris/stones were in the proximal ducts. After the sutures were laid in the back wall of the anastomosis, it was "parachuted" down, and then the anterior row was completed.

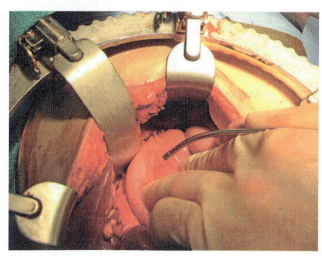

FIGURE 13 • The completed hepaticojejunostomy is in the proper anatomic orientation.

forms), most omit the drain. Admittedly, there are no data to support either approach.
- Alternative approach: hepaticoduodenostomy—The group at Children's Hospital of Philadelphia has presented an alternative to the Roux-en-Y reconstruction, using a direct hepaticoduodenostomy.[5] The rationale for this approach is that there is a more physiologic end point for bile drainage and a simpler reconstruction. In their hands, the operations were shorter by approximately 1 hour, and there were fewer complications requiring reintervention. The long-term follow-up is not yet available. Of note, these patients were selected and not randomized patients with hepaticoduodenostomy being used in those patients in whom there would not be a tension at the anastomosis.
- Other approaches: There have been a number of other reconstructive options forwarded by others, such as valved Roux limb conduits to the duodenum or use of the appendix as a pedicled graft.[6] These approaches are unnecessarily complex and in the case of the appendix, have worse long-term outcomes.

LAPAROSCOPIC APPROACH

- The laparoscopic approach to choledochal cyst excision and reconstruction has been described by numerous authors. Monitor positioning and port placement are shown in **FIGURE 14**.
- The laparoscopic technique is much more amenable to the patient who has not experienced multiple bouts of cholangitis/pancreatitis.
- Unlike the open procedure, the gallbladder is divided at the cystic duct and then it is used to retract cephalad to expose the cyst/porta hepatis; the gallbladder is removed at the conclusion of the procedure (**FIGURE 15**).
- The procedure is otherwise performed in the sequence of events as described in the previous text. The hepatic flexure is mobilized to facilitate a Kocher maneuver. The cyst dissection is as described for the open approach starting with cephalad, superior exposure of the cyst, and subsequent dissection of the vessels from proximal to distal (**FIGURE 16**).
- The jejunojejunostomy can be performed via an extended umbilical incision in infants to allow an extracorporeal jejunojejunal anastomosis.
- Early results are similar between open and laparoscopic cases.

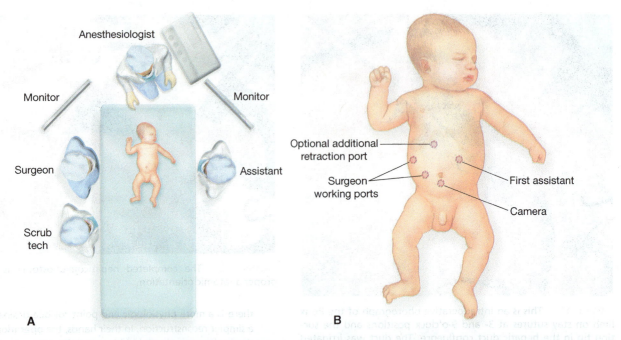

FIGURE 14 • Laparoscopic approach: display arrangement and port placement. **A,** The surgeon is positioned on the patient's right side with a monitor over the patient's left shoulder. **B,** A 5-mm umbilical port and 30° camera are employed. Two subsequent ports are placed in the right midabdomen as shown. Another left-sided port is placed in the midclavicular line above the umbilicus; this is the right-handed working port of the assistant. An optional retraction port is in the right upper quadrant, below the costal margin in the midaxillary line.

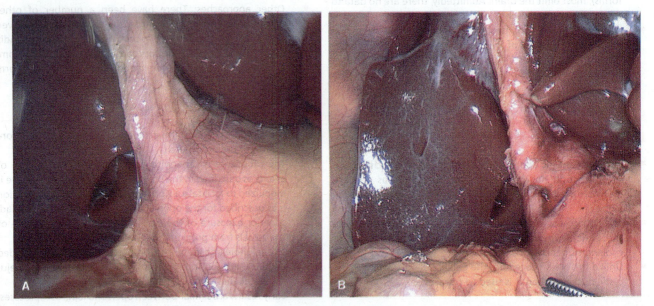

FIGURE 15 • These intraoperative images were taken during laparoscopic excision of a choledochal cyst. Laparoscopic excision is amenable to patients who have not experienced multiple bouts of cholangitis or pancreatitis, and likely developed numerous intra-abdominal adhesions making dissection more difficult. Excision of the cyst proceeds in a manner similar to the open operation. However, in the laparoscopic approach, the gallbladder is divided at the cystic duct and used for cephalad retraction, thus exposing the cyst and porta hepatis. The gallbladder is removed at the conclusion of the operation. Here, the laparoscopic view predissection of the gallbladder **(A)** and postdissection with cystic duct ligation **(B)** are depicted.

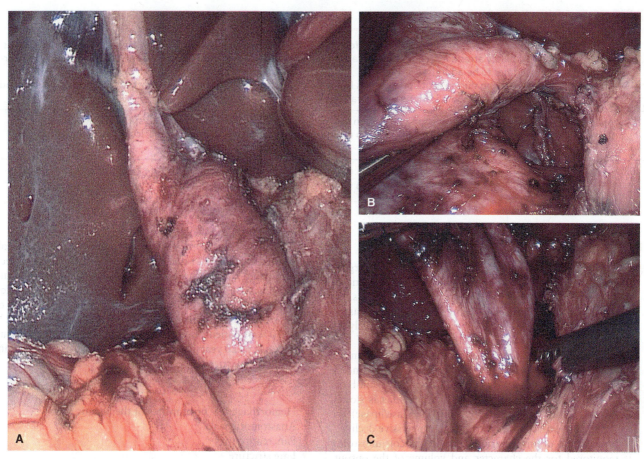

FIGURE 16 • After mobilization of the hepatic flexure and a Kocher maneuver, the cyst is exposed for further mobilization **(A)**. Dissection of the cyst is similar to the technique used in the open operation, by starting with cephalad, superior exposure near the hepatic surface **(B)**. As dissection and mobilization is carried down toward the pancreas **(C)**, it is important to remember that the cyst tapers to a narrow neck. It is critical to stay on the cyst wall and not violate the pancreatic duct.

OTHER CYST TYPES (II, III, V)

- Type II: The type II cyst is a diverticulum of the CBD. This configuration, especially with a long, narrow neck, is most amenable to a minimally invasive approach.[7] Most surgeons recommend removal of the gallbladder at the same operation.
- Type III: The type III cysts or choledochoceles are more complex procedures that are best addressed by transduodenal resection and sphincteroplasty. Once the duodenum is fully Kocherized, it is opened transversely along the antimesenteric border. The intraduodenal, stenotic ampulla is cannulated and opened. An intraoperative cholangiogram is useful, at times, and usually best done through the openings of the bile duct and pancreatic duct via the duodenum. Excision and then reapproximation of the duct to duodenal mucosa with 5-0 or 6-0 Vicryl is standard. This can be done over a calibrating stent of a 5-Fr to 7-Fr catheter. The intrapancreatic lesions should be managed with internal drainage, and conceivably, this could not be accomplished and require a pancreaticoduodenectomy. The gallbladder is traditionally removed at the same operation.
- Type V: Caroli disease is characterized by unilateral or bilateral cystic dilation of the intrahepatic biliary tree. This is surgically treated by lobectomy if there is disease isolated to a single anatomic lobe. Palliation is often done by interventional radiology by dilation of multiple strictures and stone retrieval. Liver transplantation may be required to effectively treat this problem.

PEARLS AND PITFALLS

Timing of operation	■ Delaying operation in the infantile form can potentially allow biliary cirrhosis to progress due to either stasis or biliary atresia misdiagnosis. Operation by 6 wk of age should mitigate this risk and allow any other comorbidities to be addressed. ■ Operating during acute pancreatitis in the noninfantile form can increase the difficulty of dissection and lead to increased complications such as vascular injury and anastomotic leak.
Cyst excision	■ Too distal of a dissection with a high union of the pancreatic duct to the CBD/cyst can result in pancreatic duct injury or ligation. Appreciation of preoperative imaging with the pancreaticobiliary malunion in mind can avoid this complication.
Biliary–enteric reconstruction	■ Ensure proper anatomic orientation of the Roux limb. Disorientation can create a loop of proximal jejunum–hepatic duct anastomosis or kinking of a properly corrected Roux limb.

POSTOPERATIVE CARE

- The postoperative care of the patient who undergoes resection of a choledochal cyst is similar to many patients undergoing major hepato-pancreato-biliary operations. As stated in the preoperative management, we use nasogastric decompression early in the perioperative period (usually 48 hours) and epidural analgesia with a combination of narcotic/local anesthetics. The postoperative pain management is augmented with scheduled intravenous Toradol and/or acetaminophen. No prophylactic, postoperative antibiotics are given. With return of bowel function, diet is slowly advanced. Serum chemistries (bilirubin, amylase/lipase) are followed in the first few days to ensure progressive decline.
- If present, the drain posterior to the hepaticojejunostomy is monitored for the character and volume of the output. Once the patient is tolerating a diet, and the drain effluent is serous, then the drain is removed prior to discharge.
- Some surgeons maintain these patients on suppressive antibiotics against cholangitis as with biliary atresia.
- Postoperative follow-up is at 2 weeks as part of routine care. Long-term follow-up is every 3 months for year 1, and then annually in asymptomatic patients. This includes monitoring of serum liver enzymes (aspartate aminotransferase [AST], alanine aminotransferase [ALT], γ-glutamyltransferase [GGT]), bilirubin, and amylase/lipase. Patients with elevations in their chemistries or clinical symptoms will undergo either a screening ultrasound with a focus on intrahepatic dilation or possibly a hepatobiliary iminodiacetic acid (HIDA) scan to evaluate functional bile excretion into the Roux limb. If there is a question about the Roux limb, a CT scan of the abdomen may be helpful. The long-term issue is related to anastomotic stricture and/or late stone formation as the etiology of the obstructive symptoms.

OUTCOMES

- The long-term outcomes for the surgical resection of choledochal cyst with Roux-en-Y hepaticojejunostomy are excellent (symptom-free and overall survival over 90%). The historical issue of malignancy and high rates of cholangitis/stones (90%) due to retained cysts has largely been eliminated due to the approach of complete excision and reconstruction, although there are rare cases after cyst excision. These cases probably represent incomplete excision of proximal or distal margins of the cyst. In broad terms, 2% to 10% of patients develop intrahepatic stones as follow-up goes out to 20 years. Stone formation can be associated with cholangitis, stricture, or both.

COMPLICATIONS

- Hemorrhage: PV or branches of the hepatic artery
- Anastomotic leak
- Pancreatitis
- Late stricture
  - Cholangitis
  - Recurrent stones
- Adhesive bowel obstruction

REFERENCES

1. Alonso-Lej F, Rever Jr WB, Pessagno DJ. Congenital choledochal cyst, with a report of 2, and an analysis of 94, cases. *Int Abstr Surg.* 1959;108:1-30.
2. Todani T, Watanabe Y, Narusue M, et al. Congenital bile duct cyst: classification, operative procedures and review of 37 cases including cancer arising from choledochal cyst. *Am J Surg.* 1977;134:263-269.
3. Wong KKY, Chung PHY, Chan KL, et al. Should open Kasai portoenterostomy be performed for biliary atresia in the era of laparoscopy? *Pediatr Surg Int.* 2008;24:931-933.
4. Lilly JR. The surgical treatment of choledochal cyst. *Surg Gynecol Obstet.* 1979;149:36-42.
5. Santore MT, Behar BJ, Blinman TA, et al. Hepaticoduodenostomy vs. hepaticojejunostomy for reconstruction after resection of choledochal cyst. *J Pediatr Surg.* 2011;46:209-213.
6. Cromblehome TM, Harrison MR, Langer JC, et al. Biliary appendicoduodenostomy: a nonrefluxing conduit for biliary reconstruction. *J Pediatr Surg.* 1989;24:665-667.
7. Liu DC, Rodriguez JA, Meric F, et al. Laparoscopic excision of a rare type II choledochal cyst: case report and review of the literature. *J Pediatr Surg.* 2000;35:1117-1119.

Chapter 14: Operative Treatment of Biliary Atresia

Charles S. Cox Jr. and Michael Collins Scott

DEFINITION

- Biliary atresia is an inflammatory process of unknown etiology that results in obliteration of the extrahepatic bile ducts in newborn infants. The incidence of biliary atresia is quoted as 1 per 10,000 live births, which in most US referral centers should translate into approximately 4 to 5 cases per year.
- The Japanese Society of Pediatric Surgeons has classified the anatomic configurations of biliary atresia (**FIGURE 1**). The most common pattern is obliteration of the ducts from the porta to the common bile duct (CBD) (type I).
- Other variants not shown include fibrotic ducts and porta with a patent gallbladder and distal CBD.
- The "surgically correctable" form of biliary atresia is rare (10% of cases). In this situation, there is patency of a proximal segment of hepatic and/or common duct.

DIFFERENTIAL DIAGNOSIS

- The differential diagnosis of a mixed hyperbilirubinemia in an infant includes the following:
  - Biliary atresia
  - Neonatal hepatitis
  - α1-Antitrypsin deficiency
  - Other metabolic deficiencies
  - Alagille syndrome (biliary hypoplasia, pulmonary stenosis, vertebral anomalies, and elfin facies)
  - Choledochal cyst

PATIENT HISTORY AND PHYSICAL FINDINGS

- Infants are usually referred at approximately 6 to 8 weeks of age, placing priority on rapid evaluation, diagnosis, and early operation. They typically present for evaluation of a mixed hyperbilirubinemia and the primary physical findings are jaundice and hepatomegaly. They also have acholic stools and dark urine.

IMAGING AND OTHER DIAGNOSTIC STUDIES

- Laboratory: The hallmark of the laboratory evaluation is a mixed hyperbilirubinemia. Investigations will be focused on excluding neonatal hepatitis, metabolic diseases, and α1-antitrypsin deficiency.
- Nuclear medicine: Technetium-based hepatobiliary scans are often used in the evaluation of infants with a mixed hyperbilirubinemia. Pretest preparation with phenobarbital for 3 to 5 days is useful. Visualization of the tracer in the duodenum/small intestine excludes biliary atresia. Slow uptake is indicative of a global hepatocyte dysfunction.
- Ultrasound: Imaging is usually supportive of the diagnosis of biliary atresia but is not definitively diagnostic. Usually, there is a thickened, contracted gallbladder and difficulty visualizing the extrahepatic biliary tree.
- Percutaneous liver biopsy: Recently, percutaneous needle biopsy has become one of the most definitive diagnostic tests in the evaluation of biliary atresia. The histologic appearance is that of any bile duct obstruction: portal tract edema and fibrosis, bile duct proliferation, and stasis. Mimics of biliary atresia are giant cell hepatitis, as it has some similar findings, most notably multinucleated giant cell infiltrates that can also occur with biliary atresia. Similar findings occur with Alagille syndrome, which is characterized by biliary hypoplasia. Other features of Alagille syndrome include a characteristic elfin facies, pulmonary stenosis, and vertebral anomalies.

SURGICAL MANAGEMENT

- In the surgical management of patients with biliary atresia, the timing of the operation is of great importance. In general terms, earlier is better. Outcomes are better if the operation is performed before the infant reaches 6 weeks of age. Portoenterostomy may be reasonable up to 120 days of age, recognizing that the prognosis declines rapidly with delayed intervention.

PREOPERATIVE PLANNING

- Ensure that there is no coagulopathy. If present, the patient must be treated with vitamin K (phytomenadione, 1 mg/d intramuscularly) and/or fresh frozen plasma replacement. Typically, a central vascular catheter or arterial line is not necessary. Epidural catheter anesthesia is a useful adjunct to intraoperative and postoperative pain management. A second-generation or third-generation cephalosporin should be administered prior to incision. Intravenous antibiotics should be continued until transition to oral cholangitis prophylaxis can be achieved.

POSITIONING

- The patient is placed in the supine position. A small towel roll is positioned transversely under the patient at the level of the lower chest/abdomen.

SECTION I SURGERY OF THE BILIARY SYSTEM

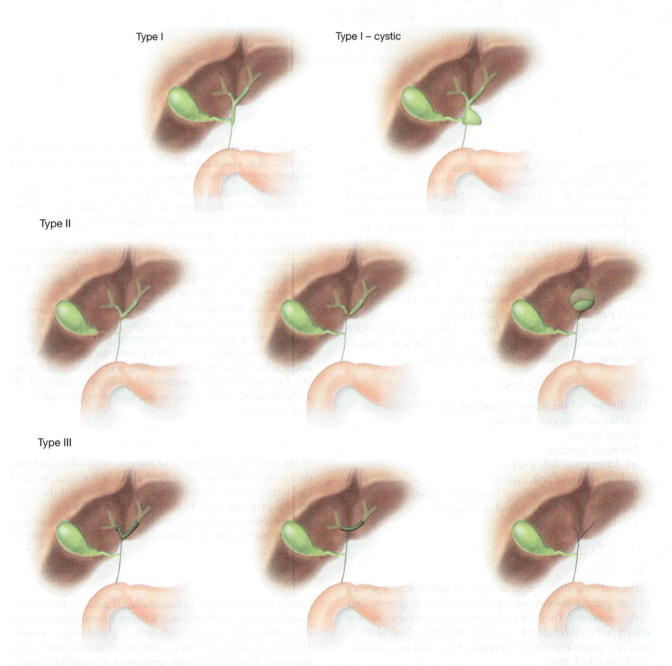

FIGURE 1 • Classification of biliary atresia. Type I is associated with atresia at the level of the common bile duct; in type II, the atresia is at the level of the hepatic duct; in type III, atresia occurs at the porta hepatis.

- The authors recommend proceeding directly to an open exploration and cholangiogram. If positive, a classic Kasai portoenterostomy biliary drainage procedure is performed.

The use of a laparoscopic approach has been associated with significantly worse outcomes.[1,2]

INCISION

- Initially, a small right-sided subcostal incision is made to perform the cholangiogram and then extended to facilitate the procedure once confirmation of the diagnosis has occurred (**FIGURE 2**).

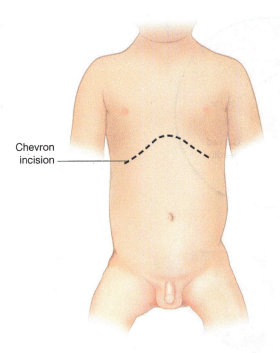

FIGURE 2 • Incision. A modified hemi-chevron incision is used. Some centers use a more limited right subcostal incision, but to fully mobilize the liver requires a larger incision.

CHOLANGIOGRAM

- The gallbladder is identified; it is usually small and contracted with clear or milky bile in the lumen. A purse-string suture of 5-0 silk on a TF needle (or equivalent) is used and a cholecystotomy is made of a size to admit a 5-Fr infant feeding tube (**FIGURE 3**). Nondiluted Omnipaque 300 is injected under fluoroscopic visualization. If there is no visualization of the intrahepatic biliary tree, the distal porta hepatis should be occluded to promote visualization of the proximal hepatic ducts. If there is nonvisualization of the intrahepatic biliary tree, this typically confirms the diagnosis of biliary atresia.

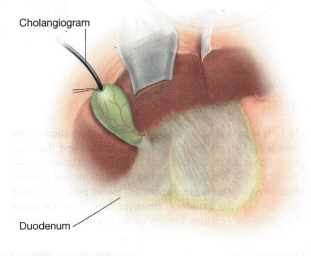

FIGURE 3 • Intraoperative cholangiogram. A 5-Fr infant feeding tube is used to cannulate the dome of the gallbladder via a purse-string suture. Omnipaque 300 is used as a full-strength contrast agent to visualize the extrahepatic biliary tree. Aspiration of clear bile usually is indicative of biliary atresia. It can be difficult to be certain that the cannula is truly within the lumen of the gallbladder.

LIVER BIOPSY

- With more liberal use of percutaneous biopsy, there is little need for a redundant biopsy at the time of portoenterostomy. However, a classic biopsy that provides a larger sample is often informative regarding degree of liver injury and is essential when a percutaneous biopsy has not been obtained. This is performed as depicted in **FIGURE 4**. Using a 2-0 chromic suture on an SH or equivalent needle, two mattress-type sutures are placed in a "V" configuration from which the wedge biopsy will be obtained. A no. 15 blade knife is used to excise a wedge of liver, and the bed is coagulated with the cautery. The tails of the chromic suture are left long and used to reapproximate the edges of the liver over a Gelfoam bolster that renders the field hemostatic. This should be done immediately after the cholangiogram to optimally ensure the site is hemostatic at the conclusion of the procedure and to prevent inadvertent omission of the biopsy following the main portion of the procedure—the portoenterostomy.

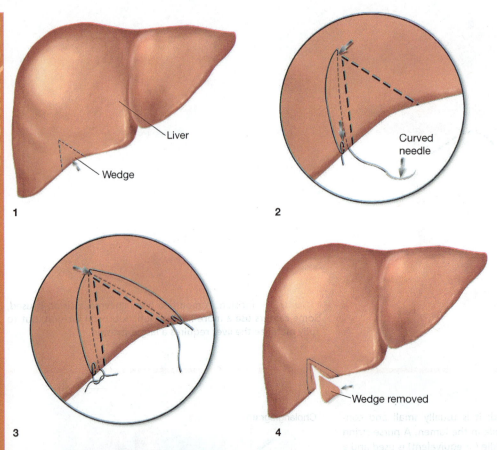

FIGURE 4 • Liver biopsy. A V-shaped incision is made between two mattress sutures of 2-0 chromic that are then tied together over a Gelfoam bolster for hemostasis.

HEPATIC MOBILIZATION

- To fully expose the porta hepatis, a full mobilization of the liver is performed. Both triangular ligaments and the falciform ligament are divided, and the liver is rotated up into the wound. This is far more effective in infants and children than in adults. Laparotomy pads are placed behind the liver to maintain the exposure. However, care must be taken to not allow excessive tension to be placed on the portal vascular structures. An assistant's hand can further splay open the porta during critical elements of the dissection. Some authors have advocated against this maneuver arguing that it increases retrohepatic scarring in case of future transplantation. The authors are of the opinion that the value of optimum exposure to provide the greatest precision of the portal dissection and anastomosis outweighs the additional dissection that will be required should liver transplant ultimately be required (FIGURE 5).

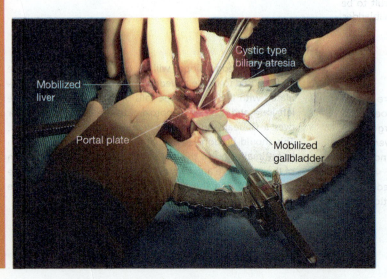

FIGURE 5 • Intraoperative photographs of the hepatic and gallbladder mobilization. The left and right triangular ligaments and the ligamentum teres are all divided up to the hepatic venous hilum. This allows complete mobilization of the liver up into the incision, thus providing excellent exposure of the porta hepatis. The gallbladder is mobilized after the cholangiogram and used for a traction "guide" to the atretic extrahepatic biliary tree. The veil of peritoneum overlying the portal structures is divided with cautery and the vascular structures are identified and separated from the atretic bile ducts.

PORTAL DISSECTION

- Identification of vascular structures: The gallbladder is mobilized in a retrograde fashion using electrocautery until the cystic artery is identified. This is then traced back to the right hepatic artery. Further antegrade dissection beginning near the celiac artery trifurcation first identifies the common hepatic artery and then origin of the left and right hepatic arteries. Aberrant arterial anatomy must be considered. Expect disproportionately enlarged lymph nodes in the region. The left and right hepatic arteries should be isolated with vessel loops or 0 silk suture. Posterior and left in the porta, the anterior aspect of the portal vein (PV) is exposed.
- Division of distal extrahepatic biliary tree: With the hepatic vessels identified, the gallbladder is used for traction to dissect the posterior aspect of the atretic extrahepatic biliary tree from the vessels (FIGURE 6A). This dissection is carried distally to the head of the pancreas. The distal segment is ligated and sharply divided. The dissection is then followed proximally revealing a cone of tissue in the porta (FIGURE 6B).
- Proximal dissection: The outline of the portal plate dissection is the crescent-shaped boundary of the PV and the right and left hepatic arteries from which the atretic, extrahepatic biliary tree exits the hepatic parenchyma. As dissection enters the liver, there should be a transition from fibrotic, atretic, pale structures to softer, darker liver.
- Portal transection: The critical element of the operation is the depth and boundaries of the portal dissection. The confluence of the PV must be retracted inferiorly and the left and right branches must be retracted laterally with small tributaries ligated or cauterized (bipolar electrocautery can be useful). The entire liver plate is sharply transected either with angled scissors or a beaver-blade knife (FIGURE 6C). The optimal level is to be just at but not into the liver parenchyma. The optimal level for the portoenterostomy is represented by the virtually translucent, thin layer that is left in place. Bleeding is controlled with 1:100,000 epinephrine-soaked Gelfoam and pressure using

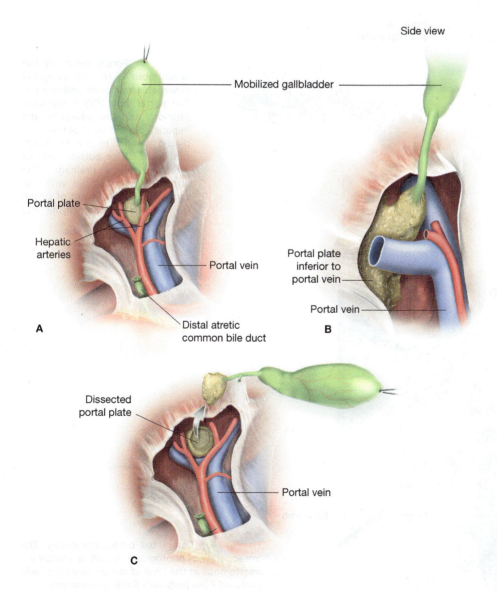

FIGURE 6 • Portal dissection. The portal dissection commences once the vascular and ductal structures are identified. The common bile duct is divided and ligated distally and then dissected up until the tissue fans out into a conical configuration bordered by the portal vein (PV) inferiorly and laterally. A, The gallbladder is mobilized and used as traction to expose the cone of tissue at the porta. B, Lateral view of the dissection showing how the cone of the portal plate dips inferior to the PV confluence and why retraction down on the PV to place the posterior row of sutures is important. C, The dissected portal plate is transected just at the level of the liver capsule.

SECTION I SURGERY OF THE BILIARY SYSTEM

cotton tip applicators. Very minimal needle tip/low-setting cautery can be used judiciously if absolutely necessary. The Gelfoam can be left in place and the liver returned to the abdomen as the Roux limb is created and the jejunojejunostomy performed.

Some surgeons send this proximal margin of the portal dissection for specific evaluation of ductal diameter to guide further dissection and/or prognosis; however, the authors have not found this to be particularly useful intraoperative information.

ROUX-EN-Y LIMB CREATION

- Retrocolic Roux-en-Y hepaticojejunostomy: The standard approach is to create a 40-cm Roux limb that originates 10 cm from the duodenojejunal junction. This is illustrated in the drawings in **FIGURE 7** and the initial anastomosis is shown in

FIGURE 8. Numerous techniques are commonly used for the jejunojejunostomy. The authors prefer an end (proximal jejunum) to side (distal jejunum), single-layer, handsewn anastomosis using interrupted 5-0 sutures. The end of the Roux limb is closed in two layers and then brought through a defect created in the transverse mesocolon to the right of the middle colic vessels.

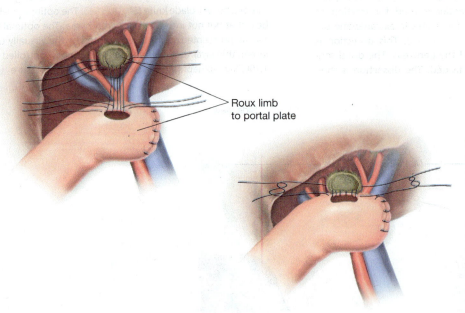

Roux limb to portal plate

FIGURE 7 • Portoenterostomy. The anastomosis is created using 5-0 absorbable monofilament sutures. The portal vein (PV) is retracted inferiorly and the sutures on the hepatic parenchyma/capsule are placed parallel to the PV. Knots can be inside or outside without affecting biliary drainage. The anterior row is placed with the same type of placement of suture on the hepatic parenchyma and knots on the outside.

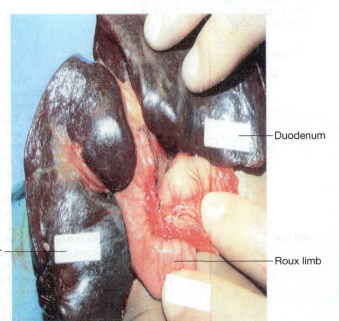

Duodenum

Mobilized liver

Roux limb

FIGURE 8 • Completed portoenterostomy. The intraoperative photograph shows a completed anastomosis at the level of the porta with a well-perfused Roux limb with a side anastomosis.

PORTOENTEROSTOMY

- The antimesenteric border of the Roux limb is used for the anastomosis to the portal plate. Absorbable 5-0 monofilament sutures are used to create an interrupted, single-layer anastomosis (see **FIGURE 7**). First, the posterior row of sutures is placed in the liver capsule parallel to the porta border while inferiorly retracting the PV. This retraction maneuver minimizes the risk of occluding the plate with the edge of the anastomosis/jejunal border. The critical elements of the anastomosis are designed to capture the biliary drainage from the regions adjacent to the PV branches; these are lateral in the portal plate. To accomplish this, the hepatic capsular sutures should be oriented parallel to the PV, retracting the PV to get as far back from the site of drainage so as not to occlude these ductules with the subsequent anastomosis. The anterior suture line is then completed. **FIGURE 8** demonstrates a completed anastomosis. The limb is secured to the mesocolic defect with interrupted sutures, and the mesenteric defect of the jejunal anastomosis is closed as well.

PEARLS AND PITFALLS

Interpretation of cholangiogram	- It is critical to occlude the distal CBD to ensure that potentially hypoplastic proximal ducts can fill. This avoids performing a Kasai for biliary hypoplasia.
Roux limb certainty	- Always double check Roux limb anatomy such that distally divided jejunum is used for the limb; an error can be made by erroneously bringing proximal jejunum to the porta. Also, ensure that there is not a redundant segment that can kink as the normal anatomic position of the liver is reestablished.
Portal dissection/ anastomosis	- The critical dissection is to divide the porta just at the liver capsule to a translucent layer, behind which is the hepatic parenchyma. Do not cut into the liver as it only bleeds and increases scarring. - Ensure lateral dissection at the zone into which one can imagine the bile ducts exiting the liver normally. Do not allow hepatic sutures to occlude the sites of drainage; place these sutures parallel to the vessels as the PV is retracted.
Vascular injury	- If the hepatic arteries are looped, do not allow them to stay on tension for any significant period of time; thrombosis has been reported.

POSTOPERATIVE CARE

- Standard: The postoperative care is routine. A nasogastric tube remains in place until the patient passes flatus (2-3 days). A small Jackson-Pratt drain can be left in Morrison pouch, but this could easily be omitted without consequence. If present, the drain is removed once the patient is on a diet and there is no bile in the drain. Pain control is heavily augmented by an epidural catheter and allows minimization of narcotics. Avoid the use of acetaminophen or other hepatotoxic drugs.
- The most important prognostic sign is the transition of the color of the stool with a green diaper representing an excellent day for the patient and team; pigmented stools suggest successful bile flow.
- Antibiotic prophylaxis for cholangitis: Intravenous antibiotics against gram-negative organisms are continued beyond the perioperative prophylaxis time period to minimize the risk of cholangitis. Once the patient has begun an oral diet (usually days 2-4), they can be transitioned to trimethoprim (TMP)-sulfamethoxazole at 2.5 mg/kg/d based on the TMP component.
- Nutritional supplementation: We routinely discharge patients with vitamins A, D, E, and K supplements.
- Steroids: The perioperative use of steroids is controversial. The rationale is that biliary atresia is a progressive inflammatory process and also has choleretic effects. Currently, approximately half of pediatric surgical centers use perioperative steroids. Davenport et al. reported a hastening of jaundice resolution without an effect on transplant-free survival.[3] Their regimen was 2 mg/kg/d of prednisolone from days 7 to 21 tapering to 1 mg/kg/d from days 22 to 28. Davenport et al. conducted a similar clinical trial in 2013 to their trial in 2007, but with the addition of a high-dose steroid group. At 6 months post-Kasai, patients in the high-dose steroid group had a greater bile clearance than those in the no steroid group.[4] A multicenter randomized clinical trial comparing low-dose to high-dose steroids from the Japanese Biliary Atresia Society found similar results supporting high-dose steroids. In their trial, the greatest benefit was to infants who underwent a Kasai portoenterostomy at less than 70 days of age.[5] Similar results supporting steroid use have been found in retrospective reviews.[6,7] The START trial was a randomized clinical trial in the United States comparing a postoperative 13-week steroid course to placebo in patients undergoing a Kasai procedure. In their trial of 140 patients, Bezerra et al. found that there was a higher percentage of patients in the steroid group with an improved biliary clearance, albeit this was not a statistically significant finding based on the power of the study.[8] A systematic review and meta-analysis by Chen et al. found that post-Kasai patients treated with moderate high-dose steroid therapy had improved bile clearance at 6 months after operation;

Table 1: Post-Kasai Steroid Pulse-Taper Dosing Schedule

Dose	Days	Postoperative day
10 mg/kg	1	1
8 mg/kg	1	2
6 mg/kg	1	3
4 mg/kg	1	4
2 mg/kg	1	5
1 mg/kg	7	6-12
0.5 mg/kg	7	13-19
0.3 mg/kg	7	20-26
0.2 mg/kg	7	27-33
0.1 mg/kg	7	34-40

this benefit was particularly noted in infants that underwent an operation within the first 70 days of life.[9] In comparison to Davenport's regimen, our postoperative steroid therapy utilizes a higher pulse dose and earlier start time according to the schedule noted in **TABLE 1**.

OUTCOMES

- Early, successful biliary drainage is defined as a total serum bilirubin less than 2.0 mg/dL in the first 3 months post-Kasai. In multiple studies, the postoperative resolution of jaundice ranges from 40% to 60%. The 1-year transplant-free survival in those patients with successful drainage was approximately 50%, thus early successful bile drainage is a strong indicator of a durable operative result.[10,11]

COMPLICATIONS

- Cholangitis: This complication typically presents with fever, an acute rise in the bilirubin, and return of acholic stools. This occurs more frequently in the first 6 months post portoenterostomy, and we aggressively treat this with parenteral antibiotics against gram negatives, a repeat steroid pulse/taper regimen, and occasionally, a brief course of phenobarbital as a choleretic. Repetitive bouts of cholangitis should be investigated with a hepatobiliary iminodiacetic acid (HIDA) scan to rule out an afferent limb obstruction as the etiology rather than failure of the portoenterostomy.
- Progressive hepatic failure/portal hypertension: Despite bile drainage, some patients develop progressive hepatic insufficiency with a normal bilirubin. Typically, this is first manifest by hepatosplenomegaly and platelet sequestration in the spleen. Ascites and growth failure typically ensue. Duplex imaging of the portal venous system should be performed to evaluate for thrombosis or hepatofugal flow in the PV. The complications of portal hypertension are usually long-term management issues (>10 years). Varices should be conventionally managed with sclerotherapy or banding as appropriate. Rarely is portosystemic shunting required, and this usually corresponds with the need for ultimate hepatic transplantation.
- Early cessation of bile flow: Portoenterostomy revision has traditionally been discouraged due to the successful results with hepatic transplantation and the assumption that reoperation would only increase the difficulty of ultimate transplantation. This issue has been recently challenged.[1] Candidates for revision of the portoenterostomy should be limited to those with initially satisfactory bile drainage or those with recurrent cholangitis and jaundice. Revision in a select group of patients (ie, good initial bile drainage, not primary failure of the portoenterostomy) converted these patients to similar long-term transplant-free survival as those patients with durable bile flow. It remains controversial but probably reasonable to revise the portoenterostomy in this select group of patients.

REFERENCES

1. Bondoc AJ, Taylor JA, Alonso MH, et al. The beneficial impact of revision of Kasai portoenterostomy for biliary atresia. An institutional study. *Ann Surg*. 2012;255:570-576.
2. Ure BM, Kuebler JF, Schukfeh N, et al. Survival with the native liver after laparoscopic versus conventional Kasai portoenterostomy in infants with biliary atresia: a prospective trial. *Ann Surg*. 2011;253:826-830.
3. Davenport M, Stringer MD, Tizzard SA, et al. Randomized, double blind, placebo-controlled trial of corticosteroids after Kasai portoenterostomy for biliary atresia. *Hepatology*. 2007;46(1):1821-1827.
4. Davenport M, Parsons C, Tizzard S, Hadzic N. Steroids in biliary atresia: single surgeon, single centre, prospective study. *J Hepatol*. 2013;59(5):1054-1058.
5. Japanese Biliary Atresia Society, Nio M, Muraji T. Multicenter randomized trial of postoperative corticosteroid therapy for biliary atresia. *Pediatr Surg Int*. 2013;29(11):1091-1095.
6. Meyers RL, Book LS, O'Gorman MA, et al. High-dose steroids, ursodeoxycholic acid, and chronic intravenous antibiotics improve bile flow after Kasai procedure in infants with biliary atresia. *J Pediatr Surg*. 2003;38(3):406-411.
7. Dong R, Song Z, Chen G, Zheng S, Xiao XM. Improved outcome of biliary atresia with postoperative high-dose steroid. *Gastroenterol Res Pract*. 2013;2013:902431.
8. Bezerra JA, Spino C, Magee JC, et al. Use of corticosteroids after hepatoportoenterostomy for bile drainage in infants with biliary atresia: the START randomized clinical trial. *JAMA*. 2014;311(17):1750-1759.
9. Chen Y, Nah SA, Chiang L, Krishnaswamy G, Low Y. Postoperative steroid therapy for biliary atresia: systematic review and meta-analysis. *J Pediatr Surg*. 2015;50(9):1590-1594.
10. Hays DM, Kimura K. *Biliary Atresia: The Japanese Experience*. Cambridge, MA: Harvard University Press; 1980:52-56.
11. Superina R, Magee JC, Brandt ML, et al. The anatomic pattern of biliary atresia identified at time of Kasai hepatoportoenterostomy and early postoperative clearance of jaundice are significant predictors of transplant-free survival. *Ann Surg*. 2011;254:577-585.

SECTION II: Surgery of the Liver

Chapter 15 Surgical Anatomy of the Liver

Jordan M. Cloyd and Timothy M. Pawlik

SIZE AND POSITION

- The human liver is the largest internal organ in the body. It is estimated to weigh 0.2% to 0.3% of ideal body weight or approximately 1400 to 2100 g in an otherwise healthy adult patient,[1] depending on age, sex, and various disease processes.
- The liver sits in the right upper quadrant of the abdomen, beneath the diaphragm, and is sheltered by the ribs.
- In broad terms, the liver extends from the right 5th intercostal space superiorly to the edge of the costal margin inferiorly. A liver palpable below the costal margin can be a sign of hepatomegaly.
- The left hemiliver extends beyond the midline and can reach as far left as midclavicular line.
- Its location relative to external landmarks is neither consistent nor static and can vary depending on patient position, individual anatomy, and respiratory cycle. This must be taken into account when performing percutaneous procedures; radiographic guidance is essential.
- Liver dimensions vary depending on age, gender, and disease states. Average dimensions are presented in **TABLE 1**.
- The right and left hemilivers are anatomically and spatially divided by Cantlie line, which runs from the fundus of the gallbladder to the suprahepatic inferior vena cava (IVC). Within the substance of the liver, the middle hepatic vein (MHV) courses along this same path and is the true division of the right and left hemilivers (**FIGURE 1**).

COUINAUD SEGMENTS

- In 1954, Couinaud[2] published his seminal work, *Le Foie: Études Anatomiques Et Chirurgicales*, in which he classified the liver into segments, each with their own inflow, outflow, and biliary drainage (**FIGURE 2**). He based his segments on the arborization of the portal vein within the liver. These segments begin with the caudate lobe (segment 1) and continue in a clockwise fashion from left to right.

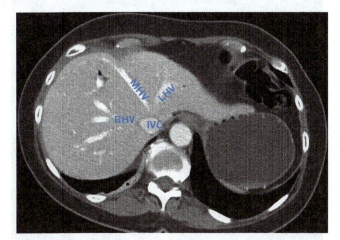

FIGURE 1 • Axial CT image showing the middle hepatic vein (*MHV*), which separates the right and left hemilivers. The inferior vena cava (*IVC*), left hepatic vein (*LHV*), and the branching of the right hepatic vein (*RHV*) are also shown.

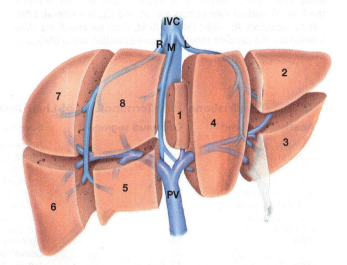

FIGURE 2 • Diagram showing the segments (numbered *1-8*) of the liver as described by Couinaud. The inferior vena cava (*IVC*) as well as the right (*R*), middle (*M*), and left (*L*) hepatic veins. The portal vein (*PV*) is also shown. (Reprinted from Blumgart LH, Schwartz LH, DeMatteo RP. Chapter 2 - Surgical and radiologic anatomy of the liver, biliary tract, and pancreas. In: Jarnagin WR. *Blumgart's Surgery of the Liver, Biliary Tract and Pancreas*. 6th ed. Elsevier; 2017:32-59.e1. Copyright © 2017 Elsevier Inc.)

Table 1: Average Dimensions of the Adult Liver

Direction	Length (cm)
Anterior to posterior	10.0-12.5
Right to left	20.0-25.5
Caudad to cephalad	15.0-17.5

Reprinted from Kennedy PA, Madding GF. Surgical anatomy of the liver. Surg Clin North Am. 1977;57:233-244. Copyright © 1977 Elsevier. With permission.

111

- Couinaud[3] further divided the liver based on sectors, which are based on the portal scissura that are marked by the hepatic veins (FIGURE 3).

GOLDSMITH AND WOODBURNE CLASSIFICATION

- Goldsmith and Woodburne[4] divided the liver into the caudate lobe and four distinct segments:
  - Left lateral (Couinaud segments 2 and 3)
  - Left medial (Couinaud segment 4)
  - Right anterior (Couinaud segments 5 and 8)
  - Right posterior (Couinaud segments 6 and 7)

BISMUTH CLASSIFICATION

- Bismuth divided the liver based on fissures: three vertical lines corresponding to the divisions made by the three major hepatic veins.[5]
- The fourth fissure, named the transverse fissure, is based on the level of the portal vein bifurcation within the liver and divides the "upper" liver from the "lower" liver.
- Bismuth identified eight subsegments:
  - Caudate lobe (Couinaud segment 1)
  - Left superior subsegment (Couinaud segment 2)
  - Left inferior subsegment (Couinaud segment 3)
  - Left medial subsegment (Couinaud segment 4)
  - Right anterior inferior subsegment (Couinaud segment 5)
  - Right posterior subsegment (Couinaud segment 6)
  - Right posterior superior subsegment (Couinaud segment 7)
  - Right anterior superior subsegment (Couinaud segment 8)

THE BRISBANE TERMINOLOGY OF LIVER ANATOMY AND RESECTION

- Due to the confusion between various classifications, the International Hepato-Pancreato-Biliary Association (IHPBA) formed a committee in 1998 to delineate an accepted and universal terminology to describe hepatic anatomy and, more specifically, hepatic resections.[6] In 2000, their terminology was published. In it, a nomenclature for anatomic terminology and that of surgical resection were clearly delineated and are widely accepted as the proper nomenclature for describing liver resections today (TABLE 2).

CAUDATE LOBE

- The caudate lobe is distinct in many ways. Because of its distinct inflow, outflow, and drainage, it is sometimes termed "the third lobe of the liver."

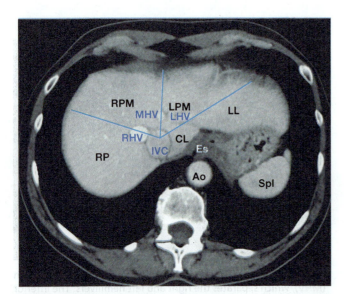

FIGURE 3 • Axial CT image, venous phase, showing the right hepatic vein (RHV), middle hepatic vein (MHV), and left hepatic vein (LHV) as they enter the inferior vena cava (IVC). *Blue lines* show approximate direction of hepatic veins as they traverse the liver. Individual liver sectors are labeled (*LL*, left lateral; *LPM*, left paramedian; *RL*, right lateral; *RPM*, right paramedian). Also labeled are the caudate lobe (*CL*), esophagus (*Es*), aorta (*Ao*), and spleen (*Spl*).

Table 2: The Brisbane 2000 Terminology of Liver Anatomy and Resections

Anatomical term[a]	Couinaud segments	Surgical resection term	Defined by
Right liver Right hemiliver	5-8	Right hepatectomy Right hemihepatectomy	Middle hepatic vein (Cantlie line)
Left liver Left hemiliver	2-4	Left hepatectomy Left hemihepatectomy	Middle hepatic vein (Cantlie line)
Right anterior section	5, 8	Right anterior sectionectomy	Between right hepatic vein and middle hepatic vein
Right posterior section	6, 7	Right posterior sectionectomy	Posterior to right hepatic vein
Left medial section	4	Left medial sectionectomy	Between middle hepatic vein and umbilical fissure
Left lateral section	2, 3	Left lateral sectionectomy	Lateral to umbilical fissure
Other	4-8	Right trisectionectomy Extended right hepatectomy	Right liver and left medial section
Other	2-5, 8	Left trisectionectomy Extended left hepatectomy	Left liver and right anterior section
Other	4, 5, 8	Central hepatectomy Mesohepatectomy	Between right hepatic vein and umbilical fissure

[a]Terms that include segment 1 should be stated as such (ie, left hepatectomy extended to segment 1). Any liver resection can also be defined by its third-order division (eg, segment 6 monosegmentectomy; segment 5-6 bisegmentectomy).

Adapted by permission from Springer: Strasberg SM. Terminology of liver anatomy and resections: the Brisbane 2000 terminology. In: Clavien PA, Sarr MG, Fong Y, eds. Atlas of Upper Gastrointestinal and Hepato-Pancreato-Biliary Surgery. Springer; 2007:313-317.

Chapter 15 SURGICAL ANATOMY OF THE LIVER   113

- Embryologically, it is derived from the right liver,[7] laying on the posterior surface of the right hemiliver, bordered on the left by the ligamentum venosum. It is bordered superiorly by the hepatic veins as they enter the IVC and posteriorly by the IVC itself. Inferiorly, it is bordered by the hilum of the liver and the bifurcation of the left and right portal veins.
- Anatomically, there are three portions to the caudate lobe (FIGURE 4), each based on the portal inflow[8]:
  - The Spiegelian lobe (or Spiegel lobe)
  - The paracaval portion (or Couinaud segment 9)
  - The caudate process
- Surgically, the caudate can be divided into two: segment 1 (Spiegel lobe) and so-called segment 9 (paracaval portion and caudate process) (FIGURE 5).
- The use of terminology related to Couinaud segment 9 is often dropped from the literature and this term is neither universally accepted nor used.
- The paracaval portion, which projects medially, can circumferentially wrap around the IVC.[9]
- The caudate derives its portal inflow from the left and right portal veins; venous drainage is directly into the IVC via multiple small caudate veins. Thus, in diseases of hepatic venous obstruction, such as Budd-Chiari syndrome, it will hypertrophy and provide alternate routes for obstructed hepatic venous flow.

SURFACE ANATOMY

- The liver is covered by a thin membrane called Glisson capsule. This epithelial layer is contiguous with internal anatomy of the liver as sheaths around the portal veins, hepatic arteries, and bile ducts (ie, portal pedicles).[10]
- Despite its rounded, pyramidal shape, the liver can be described as having two surfaces: visceral and diaphragmatic.
  - The visceral surface is inferior.
  - The diaphragmatic surface can be divided into anterior, posterior, superior, and lateral aspects.
    - The anterior aspect opposes the diaphragm and the abdominal wall. It is generally smooth and has few if any impressions.
    - The posterior aspect contains the bare area of the liver as well as the confluence of the hepatic veins prior to their entry into the IVC.
    - The lateral aspect opposes the right ribs 7 to 11, which often leave impressions on the liver surface.
    - The superior aspect is a continuation of the anterior surface and ends at the coronary ligament. It contains the cardiac impression and extends medially and laterally, sitting below the left and right lungs and pleura. This is clinically important, as neoplasms of the dome of the liver can manifest by sympathetic effusions and diaphragmatic splinting.
- The majority of the surface of the liver is free of peritoneum, but there are several attachments and reflections of

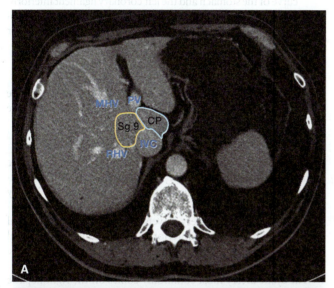

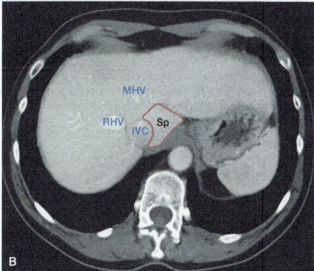

FIGURE 4 • **A**, Axial CT image showing the caudate lobe. The caudate process (*CP*) is bounded by the anterolateral surface of the inferior vena cava (*IVC*), the left portion of liver hilum, and the left hepatic vein (not shown). Segment 9 (*Sg 9*) is known as the paracaval process and is bounded by the anterior surface of the *IVC*, the middle hepatic vein (*MHV*), and the right hepatic vein (*RHV*). Also shown is the portal vein (*PV*). **B**, Axial CT image (slightly more caudal than in [**A**]) showing Spiegel lobe (*Sp*)—also known as segment 1—as it wraps around the medial aspect of the *IVC*.

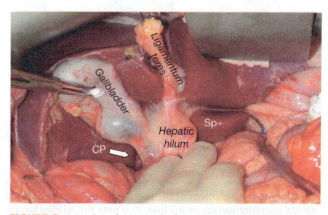

FIGURE 5 • In situ photograph showing Spiegel lobe (*Sp*) and the caudate process (*CP*) in relation to the hepatic hilum. Also shown are the gallbladder and the ligamentum teres.

peritoneum—referred to as ligaments—that suspend the liver in its position.
- Knowledge of these ligaments is important for mobilizing the liver as part of any liver resection.
- The falciform ligament is a folded extension of the peritoneum which envelops the ligamentum teres.
  - The ligamentum teres, or round ligament, is the remnant of the umbilical vein.
  - After enveloping the ligamentum teres, the peritoneum attaches anteriorly and superiorly to the posterior abdominal wall, tethering the liver slightly to the right of the midline.
  - Posteriorly and inferiorly, the ligamentum teres enters the liver between segments 3 and 4, whereas, in utero, the umbilical vein drains into the left portal vein.
  - Although technically obliterated early in life, the umbilical vein recanalizes in patients with portal hypertension and must be carefully controlled when divided.
- The ligamentum venosum, also known as Arantius ligament, contains the embryological remnant of the ductus venosus and lies between the caudate lobe (segment 1) and the left lateral section of the liver.
  - It forms a bridge between the left portal vein and the left hepatic vein (LHV). Division of the ligamentum venosum is generally required for dissection of the LHV during hepatic resection.
- The coronary ligament is the reflection of the visceral peritoneum as it attaches to the diaphragm. This creates a fibrous peritoneal ring or crown (Latin: *corona*) around the caudal posterior surface of the right hemiliver, encircling the bare area of the liver (**FIGURE 6**).
  - The bare area is so named because there is nothing between the liver and the diaphragm other than loose areolar tissue.
  - As the coronary ligament makes a sharp turn at the right posterior lateral edge of the liver, it creates an acute angle and is called the right triangular ligament.
- On the left, the anterior and posterior edges similarly combine to form the left triangular ligament, which is longer and suspends the left lateral liver from the diaphragm.
- Visceral ligaments include the hepatorenal, gastrohepatic, and hepatoduodenal ligaments (**FIGURE 7**).
  - The hepatorenal ligament reflects off of the right coronary ligament posteriorly and inferiorly and then again off the right adrenal gland and superior pole of the right kidney.
  - The hepatoduodenal ligament extends from the porta hepatis of the liver to the superior aspect of the duodenum and contains the hepatic arteries, portal vein, and bile duct.
  - The gastrohepatic ligament is a reflection off of the lesser curve of the stomach and the left coronary ligament inferiorly.
  - The gastrohepatic ligament is contiguous with the hepatoduodenal ligament and together they form the lesser omentum.

BLOOD SUPPLY

- The liver has a dual blood supply: portal vein supplies the liver with approximately 75% of its blood volume while the hepatic artery supplies the remainder.

Hepatic Arteries

- The common hepatic artery comes directly off the celiac trunk and gives rise to the right gastric and gastroduodenal arteries before becoming the proper hepatic artery (**FIGURE 8**).
- The proper hepatic artery travels within the hepatoduodenal ligament. It is spatially anterior to the portal vein and medial to the common bile duct. It divides into right and left hepatic arteries.
- The cystic artery most commonly comes off the right hepatic artery but can come off the proper hepatic artery or left hepatic artery, making misidentification of this structure a risk during cholecystectomy or other operations.

Right Hepatic Artery

- The right hepatic artery is generally longer than the left and follows a slightly more oblique angle, curving toward the neck of the gallbladder before arching again toward the posterior sector.[11]

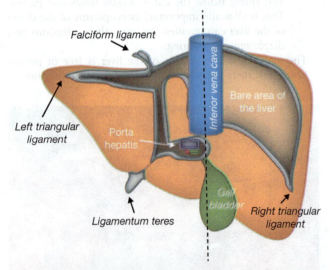

FIGURE 6 • Posterior view, depicting the peritoneal reflections constituting the ligaments of the liver. Note the bare area at the caudal posterior surface of the liver. Also note the relative length of the left triangular ligament as compared to the right triangular ligament. The *dotted line* represents Cantlie line, which divides the right and left hemilivers.

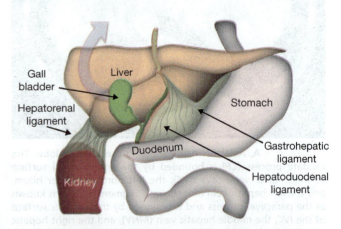

FIGURE 7 • Diagram showing the attachments of the gastrohepatic, hepatoduodenal, and hepatorenal ligaments. The free edge of the liver is rotated superiorly as depicted by the *arrow*. The gastrohepatic and hepatoduodenal ligaments are contiguous.

- The right hepatic artery generally courses posterior to the common hepatic duct (CHD) prior to entering the liver; however, in approximately 10% of patients, the right hepatic artery will cross anterior to the bile duct.
- Lateral to the bile duct, the right hepatic artery bifurcates into anterior (supplying segments 5 and 8) and posterior (supplying segments 6 and 7) sectoral branches. These, in turn, branch inferiorly and superiorly, to form the individual segmental branches.
- In up to 20% of patients, the right hepatic artery has a variable anatomy.[12,13] The most common variant is the replaced or accessory right hepatic artery (**FIGURE 9**), which originates from the superior mesenteric artery, traveling posterior to the portal vein.
- The pancreatobiliary surgeon must always be cognizant of this aberrant anatomy.

Left Hepatic Artery

- The left hepatic artery bifurcates early, into the medial (segment 4) and lateral (segments 2 and 3) sectoral branches. In some patients, the left hepatic artery does not exist, and the left medial sectoral branch arises from the right hepatic artery, crossing the midline passing posterior to the left lateral branch to supply segment 4.[14]
- A replaced or accessory left hepatic artery is less common, occurring in 10% to 15% of patients. When present, it arises from the left gastric artery, traveling in the gastrohepatic ligament (**FIGURE 10**).

Portal Veins

- The portal vein originates at the confluence of the splenic and superior mesenteric veins (**FIGURE 11**). It courses superolaterally into the hilum of the liver, posterior and medial to the proper hepatic artery and common bile duct (**FIGURE 12**). The portal vein then divides into right and left portal veins.

Right Portal Vein

- The right portal vein follows a more linear path and branches early into anterior (segments 5 and 8) and posterior (segments 6 and 7) branches. These, in turn, give off the individual superior and inferior segmental branches.
- The right portal venous anatomy is often variable and imaging is recommended prior to resection.

Left Portal Vein

- The left portal vein extends longer than the right. It makes an abrupt angle as it enters the liver from the hilum (**FIGURE 13**). The section of vein after the bifurcation and prior to the arborization of the left portal system is often referred to as the pars transversus.[13] This is important to identify when performing left hepatectomy.[15]

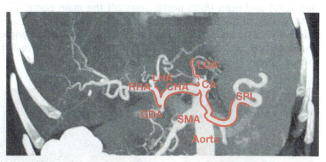

FIGURE 8 • CT angiogram showing classic arterial anatomy. The common hepatic artery (*CHA*) and splenic artery (*SPL*) come off of the celiac axis (*CA*). The CHA then gives off the gastroduodenal artery (*GDA*) and becomes the proper hepatic artery. This then divides into the right (*RHA*) and left (*LHA*) hepatic arteries. The *aorta* is also labeled, as is the left gastric artery (*LGA*) and the superior mesenteric artery (*SMA*).

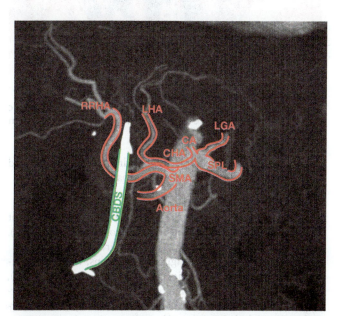

FIGURE 9 • A CT angiogram showing a replaced right hepatic artery (*RRHA*) arising from the superior mesenteric artery (*SMA*). A stent (*CBDS*) is seen in the common bile duct, which shows the anatomical relationship of the RRHA as it passes behind the common bile duct and portal vein (not shown).

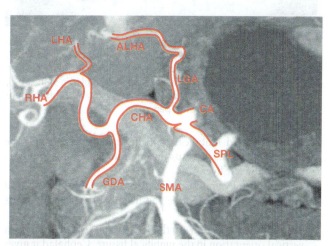

FIGURE 10 • CT angiogram showing an accessory left hepatic artery (*ALHA*) coming off of the left gastric artery (*LGA*). The right hepatic artery (*RHA*) is seen coming off in normal anatomic position, from the common hepatic artery (*CHA*) just after it gives off the gastroduodenal artery (*GDA*). The true left hepatic artery (*LHA*) is also seen, although it is far less pronounced than the ALHA which is the dominant arterial supply to the left hemiliver. Also shown are the following: superior mesenteric artery (*SMA*), celiac axis (*CA*), and splenic artery (*SPL*).

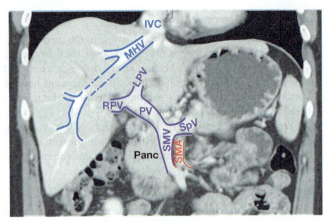

FIGURE 11 • Coronal CT demonstrating the confluence of the splenic vein (*SpV*) and the superior mesenteric vein (*SMV*) as they form the portal vein (*PV*). The left portal vein (*LPV*) makes a sharp angle from the *PV*, whereas the right portal vein (*RPV*) is more direct. Note the proximity of the *SMV* and the superior mesenteric artery (*SMA*) to the pancreatic head. Also shown are the inferior vena cava (*IVC*) and middle hepatic vein (*MHV*).

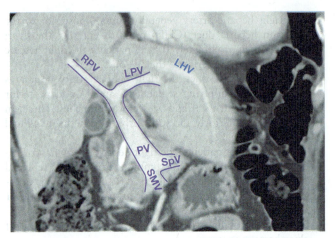

FIGURE 13 • Coronal CT demonstrating the branching of the left (*LPV*) and right (*RPV*) portal veins off the main portal vein (*PV*), which originates at the confluence of the superior mesenteric vein (*SMV*) and the splenic vein (*SpV*). Note the acute angle made by the *LPV* as it enters the liver. Also shown is the left hepatic vein (*LHV*).

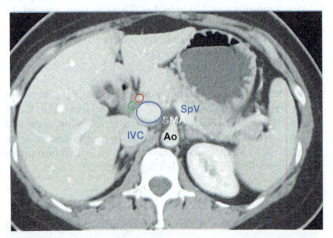

FIGURE 12 • Axial CT demonstrating the normal anatomic relationship of the bile duct (*green circle*), hepatic artery (*red circle*), and portal vein (*blue circle*). And they enter the hilum of the liver. Also labeled are the inferior vena cava (*IVC*), splenic vein (*SpV*), aorta (*Ao*), and superior mesenteric artery (*SMA*). This patient had a mass in the head of the pancreas.

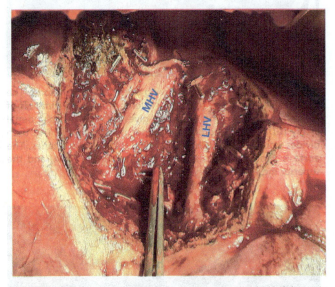

FIGURE 14 • In vivo photograph showing the divided left hepatic vein (*LHV*) as it courses toward the divided middle hepatic vein (*MHV*).

- The obliterated umbilical vein (ligamentum teres) and the obliterated ductus venosus (ligamentum venosum) join it as it enters the left liver.
- The left portal vein most often gives off the dominant portal branch to the caudate lobe and usually does so prior to its segmental arborization.
- The umbilical portion of the left portal vein courses in a vertical orientation in the umbilical fissure. Cephalad it gives branches to segments 4a (medial) and 2 (lateral); caudal it gives branches to segments 4b (medial) and 3 (lateral).[16]

Hepatic Veins

- The hepatic veins divide the liver into its Couinaud sectors.
- The LHV and MHV combine to form a common vein (truncus communis) prior to entering the IVC, although this occurs with some variety (**FIGURES 14** and **15**).
- The caudate lobe has direct venous drainage to the IVC and is not drained by the three major hepatic veins.

Right Hepatic Vein

- The right hepatic vein separates the right posterior and right anterior sections (ie, segments 6 and 7 from segments 5 and 8).
- It drains segments 6 and 7 as well as parts of segment 8.
- There can be accessory right hepatic veins, the most common of which is the inferior right hepatic vein (**FIGURE 16**), which occurs in approximately 10% of patients. The surgeon should be aware of this possible anatomy prior to performing right hepatectomy.[17]

Middle Hepatic Vein

- The MHV follows Cantlie line and is the line of division for right and left hepatectomy.

Chapter 15 SURGICAL ANATOMY OF THE LIVER 117

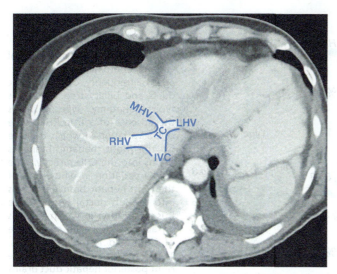

FIGURE 15 • Axial CT scan showing the relationship of the hepatic veins as they converge to the inferior vena cava (*IVC*). The middle (*MHV*) and left (*LHV*) hepatic veins join to form the truncus communis (*TC*), which empties into the *IVC*. The right hepatic vein (*RHV*) is also shown, similarly draining into the *IVC*.

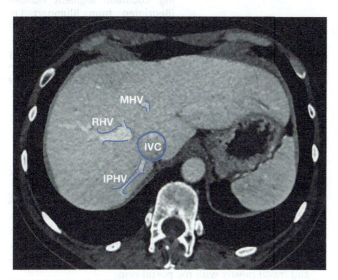

FIGURE 16 • Axial CT showing an accessory hepatic vein. The inferior posterior right hepatic vein (*IPHV*) occurs in approximately 10% of patients. Notice the position of the IPHV, far posterior on the liver. This is of utmost importance to characterize prior to operating on the liver. Also seen are the right hepatic vein (*RHV*), middle hepatic vein (*MHV*), and the inferior vena cava (*IVC*).

- Right hepatectomy is performed just to the *right* of the MHV, preserving its length and ligating its rightward branches.
- Left hepatectomy is conversely performed just the *left* of the MHV, preserving its length and ligating its leftward branches.
- It drains segments 4 and 5 and parts of segment 8.

Left Hepatic Vein

- The LHV drains segments 2 and 3 as well as parts of segment 4.

- Its arborization is variable, and careful identification of both the LHV and MHV is paramount prior to performing LHV ligation for left hepatectomy.

BILIARY SYSTEM

- Bile is made by the hepatocytes and travels via an interlobular network of capillaries and ductules to the minor, then major biliary ductules, and eventually into the hepatic ducts.
- The right and left hepatic ducts come together to form the CHD, which accepts the cystic duct approximately 4 to 6 cm distal to the hepatic duct confluence. This then forms the common bile duct and travels another 4 to 8 cm before joining the pancreatic duct and emptying into the ampulla of Vater.
- There is considerable variation in biliary anatomy. The "typical anatomy" only occurs in 50% to 60% of patients[18,19] (**FIGURE 17**).
- The cystic duct is often tortuous and also often displays variable anatomy leading to misidentification and injury during cholecystectomy.
- The gallbladder sits in the gallbladder fossa between segments 4 and 5 and is attached to the liver surface. It is covered by peritoneum, and its fundus projects beyond the liver anteroinferiorly. Surgical considerations and anatomy of the gallbladder will be discussed further elsewhere in this book.

Right Hepatic Duct

- The right hepatic duct (RHD) is formed from the confluence of the right anterior hepatic duct (RaHD) and the right posterior hepatic duct (RpHD).
  - The RaHD drains the anterosuperior (segment 8) and anteroinferior (segment 5) ducts.
  - The RpHD drains the posterosuperior (segment 7) and posteroinferior (segment 6) ducts.
  - There exists considerable variation in the drainage pattern of the right system. The most common variant is Type C_1, where the RaHD drains directly into the CHD (**FIGURE 18**).
- The RHD is anterior and lateral while in the hilum of the liver; however, intrahepatically, it dives posterior to the portal vein in both RaHD and RpHD branches.

Left Hepatic Duct

- The left hepatic duct is longer than the right and can display similarly variable anatomy.[20]
- It drains the left lateral and medial hepatic ducts.
  - The left lateral hepatic duct drains the laterosuperior (segment 2) and lateroinferior (segment 3) branches.
  - The left medial hepatic duct drains the mediosuperior (segment 4A) and medioinferior (segment 4B) branches.
- Unlike the right side, the left hepatic ductal system remains anterior to the portal vein throughout its intrahepatic and extrahepatic course.

Biliary Drainage of the Caudate Lobe

- The caudate lobe drains directly into the left hepatic duct and RHD, although this is variable.
- There is often a direct branch draining the caudate process into the RHD.

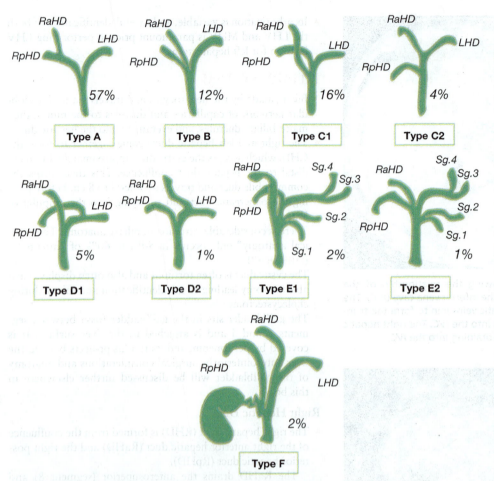

FIGURE 17 • Typical and atypical variant anatomy, with percentages of frequency, of the hepatic ducts and biliary tree. Type A is typical anatomy. Type B shows the absence of a true RHD. Type C is a variation in which the one of the right hepatic branches drains into the CHD directly. Type D is a variation in which one of the right hepatic branches drains into the left ductal system. Type E is a variation in which there is an absence of a true confluence of right and left hepatic ducts. Type F shows a variant where the right posterior hepatic duct drains directly into the cystic duct. *LHD*, left hepatic duct; *RaHD*, right anterior hepatic duct; *RpHD*, right posterior hepatic duct; *Sg*, segmental branch with corresponding Couinaud segment number (Reprinted from Blumgart LH, Schwartz LH, DeMatteo RP. Chapter 2 - Surgical and radiologic anatomy of the liver, biliary tract, and pancreas. In: Jarnagin WR. *Blumgart's Surgery of the Liver, Biliary Tract and Pancreas*. 6th ed. Elsevier; 2017:32-59.e1. Copyright © 2017 Elsevier Inc.)

INNERVATION

- The liver has both sympathetic and parasympathetic innervations.
- The parasympathetic innervation is mostly via the left vagus nerve as it rotates anteriorly upon entering the abdomen. This is the anterior hepatic nerve plexus and travels mostly with the hepatic artery. There are also posterior hepatic fibers, which come from the right (posterior) vagus nerve and travel mostly with the portal vein.
- Sympathetic innervation arrives via the splanchnic divisions of T7-T9, through the celiac ganglion, and runs mostly with the hepatic artery.
- Sensory fibers of the peritoneum of the liver run via the right phrenic nerve, and this leads to referred pain interpreted to be from the subscapular region with hepatic and diaphragmatic irritation from infection, tumor, or insufflation.

LYMPHATICS

- The liver parenchyma drains lymph via empty spaces (space of Disse) between the endothelium and the hepatocytes themselves. This lymph is collected into larger spaces in the portal triad (space of Mall).[21] These are not actual lymphatics but rather nonendothelialized channels through which lymph passes. Lymph is eventually collected in true lymphatics within the portal triad and follows the path of these vessels.
- Lymphatics drain primarily into the lymph nodes of the porta hepatis followed by the celiac nodes. These lymph nodes can

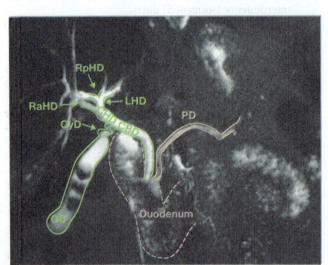

FIGURE 18 • Magnetic resonance imaging (MRI) showing biliary anatomy. The right and left systems draining into the *CHD*. This is joined by the cystic duct (*CyD*), which is notably tortuous as it drains into the biliary tree. This confluence marks the beginning of the common bile duct (*CBD*), which joins the pancreatic duct (*PD*) to drain into the second portion of the duodenum. The gallbladder (*GB*) can also be seen, with three large stones present. This patient's anatomy reveals a common variant (Type C₁), with the right posterior hepatic duct (*RpHD*) joining the left hepatic duct (*LHD*) while the right anterior hepatic duct (*RaHD*) drains directly into the *CHD*.

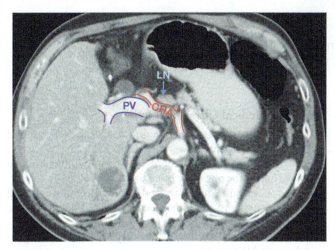

FIGURE 19 • Axial CT showing an enlarged lymph node (*LN*) abutting the celiac bifurcation. A hepatocellular carcinoma can be seen in segment 6. Also labeled are the portal vein (*PV*) and the common hepatic artery (*CHA*).

be evaluated for metastasis prior to resection when indicated (**FIGURE 19**).
- Secondary lymphatics follow the hepatic veins and drain into the phrenic lymph nodes.
- Superficially, beneath Glisson capsule, lymph drainage from the liver follows one of the five avenues[22]:
  - Anterior phrenic lymph nodes: drain anterosuperior surface
  - Lateral phrenic lymph nodes: drain posterosuperior surface
  - Left gastric lymph nodes: drain posterolateral surface
  - Celiac lymph nodes: drain posterior surface
  - Hepatic lymph nodes: drain visceral surface

CONCLUSIONS
- The anatomy of the liver is complex and requires in-depth preoperative study prior to undertaking any liver operation.
- While an improved understanding of segmental anatomy as described by Couinaud has permitted surgeons to perform increasingly specific and parenchymal-sparing resections, the Brisbane classification established consensus terminology for standard liver resections. The inflow and outflow of the caudate lobe are distinct from that of the rest of the liver.
- The liver has many variations of the biliary and vascular anatomy, and preoperative imaging is increasingly important in planning and executing successful liver operations.

REFERENCES
1. Cotran RS, Kumar V, Fausto N, et al. *Robbins and Cotran Pathologic Basis of Disease*. 7th ed. Elsevier Saunders; 2005.
2. Couinaud C. *Le Foie: Études Anatomiques Et Chirurgicales*. Masson; 1957.
3. Couinaud C. *Surgical Anatomy of the Liver Revisited [in French]*. Couinaud; 1989.
4. Goldsmith NA, Woodburne RT. Surgical anatomy pertaining to liver resection. *Surg Gynecol Obstet*. 1957;105:310-318.
5. Bismuth H. Surgical anatomy and anatomical surgery of the liver. *World J Surg*. 1982;6:3-9.
6. Belghiti J, Clavien PA, Gadzijev E, et al. The Brisbane 2000 terminology of liver anatomy and resections terminology committee of the International Hepato-Pancreato-Biliary Association: Chairman, SM Strasberg (USA). *HPB*. 2000;2:333-339.
7. Dodds WJ, Erickson SJ, Taylor AJ, et al. Caudate lobe of the liver: anatomy, embryology, and pathology. *AJR Am J Roentgenol*. 1990;154:87-93.
8. Kumon M. Anatomy of the caudate lobe with special reference to portal vein and bile duct. *Acta Hepatol Jpn*. 1985;26:1193-1199.
9. Abdalla EK, Vauthey JN, Couinaud C. The caudate lobe of the liver: implications of embryology and anatomy for surgery. *Surg Oncol Clin N Am*. 2002;11(4):835-848.
10. Launois B, Jamieson GG. The importance of Glisson's capsule and its sheaths in the intrahepatic approach to resection of the liver. *Surg Gynecol Obstet*. 1992;174(1):7-10.
11. Flint ER. Abnormalities of the right hepatic, cystic, and gastroduodenal arteries, and of the bile-ducts. *Br J Surg*. 1923;10:509-519.
12. Hiatt JR, Gabbay J, Busuttil RW. Surgical anatomy of the hepatic arteries in 1000 cases. *Ann Surg*. 1994;220:50-52.
13. Lin PH, Chaikof EL. Embryology, anatomy, and surgical exposure of the great abdominal vessels. *Surg Clin North Am*. 2000;80:417-433.
14. Healey JE. Vascular anatomy of the liver. *Ann N Y Acad Sci*. 1970;170:8-17.
15. Gumbs AA, Gayet B, Gagner M. Laparoscopic liver resection: when to use the laparoscopic stapler device. *HPB*. 2008;10:296-303.
16. Botero AC, Strasberg SM. Division of the left hemiliver in man—segments, sectors, or sections. *Liver Transplant Surg*. 1998;4:226-231.
17. Makuuchi M, Hasegawa H, Yamazaki S, et al. Four new hepatectomy procedures for resection of the right hepatic vein and preservation of the inferior right hepatic vein. *Surg Gynecol Obstet*. 1987;164(1):68-72.
18. Mortele KJ, Ros PR. Anatomic variants of the biliary tree MR cholangiographic findings and clinical applications. *AJR Am J Roentgenol*. 2001;177(2):389-394.
19. Gazelle GS, Lee MJ, Mueller PR. Cholangiographic segmental anatomy of the liver. *Radiographics*. 1994;14:1005-1013.
20. Janssen BV, van Laarhoven S, Elshaer M, et al. Comprehensive classification of anatomical variants of the main biliary ducts. *Br J Surg*. 2021;108(5):458-462. doi:10.1093/bjs/znaa147
21. Schuppan D, Afdhal NH. Liver cirrhosis. *Lancet*. 2008;371(9615):838-851.
22. Rouviere H. *Anatomy of the Human Lymphatic System*. Tobias MJ, trans. Edwards Brothers; 1938.

Chapter 16: Intraoperative Ultrasound of the Liver

Ankesh Nigam and KMarie King

INTRODUCTION

- Intraoperative ultrasound (IOUS) of the liver involves the use of ultrasound imaging to provide real-time assessment during surgical procedures of the liver.[1-3]
- IOUS is performed directly on the liver, without interference from body wall and other structures, allowing for improved detection, characterization, and localization of liver lesions when compared with percutaneous ultrasound. With the use of high-frequency ultrasound probes, IOUS can detect smaller lesions with higher resolution than either computed tomography (CT) or magnetic resonance imaging (MRI).[4]
- Although the use of IOUS was first reported in the United States in the 1960s, it was not widely adopted because of poor image quality and equipment challenges.[5] With refinement of equipment, Makuuchi et al, in 1981, described the use of IOUS (**FIGURE 1**) of the liver as an adjunct for hepatectomy.[6] Since then, the use of IOUS has expanded to include open ablative techniques and various laparoscopic procedures. IOUS is extremely useful for contemporary hepatic surgery and is a required skill set for hepatic surgeons.
- During laparoscopic surgery, where tactile examination is less feasible, IOUS can be extremely valuable in evaluating the hepatic parenchyma for masses not detected with preoperative imaging and quantifying their relationship to regional structures and hepatic vasculature during the exploratory phase of the operation.
- The following chapter provides a review on the practical aspects of IOUS during hepatic surgery.

Basics of Medical Ultrasonography

- Ultrasound machines generate and receive reflected sound waves at frequencies between 2 and 15 MHz.[7]
- The brightness mode (B mode) gives a two-dimensional image and is the one most often used.
- Sound waves are emitted from the transducer and reflected from the tissue to the transducer creating an image on the screen.
- Fluids transmit more waves than they reflect, producing an echogenic black image.
- Solid material reflects waves, making for a whiter image.
- Stones reflect more waves causing a white image, but they also cause a shadow since the stones do not allow transmittal of waves beyond them.
- Air reflects waves strongly, so it is hard to see beyond it.
- Higher-frequency waves give less penetration but higher resolution.
- Convex transducer spreads waves for a deeper and wider field. Linear transducer makes parallel waves producing a rectangular image; with higher frequency, it creates higher resolution but less penetration.

Applications

- IOUS has numerous applications with the goal of improving surgical decision making, guiding the operation, and thereby improving outcomes. The following are common examples of its use:
  - **Examination of known hepatic lesions** to determine the extent of disease and evaluate the proximity of lesions relative to major structures such as hepatic and portal veins and the vena cava. For primary liver tumors, this can be helpful in staging.
  - **Detection of occult lesions** not detected even with modern preoperative imaging techniques. Subcentimeter metastatic lesions may not be detected by preoperative CT or MRI. Their number and locations may alter the surgical plan. IOUS has a reported sensitivity of 90% for the detection of hepatic lesions with positive and negative predictive values of 90% and 78%, respectively.[2]
  - **Operative planning** as resection planes may not follow anatomic segments and as such, it is important to delineate the mass and relationship to hepatic or biliary pedicles to ensure adequate hepatic vein and biliary drainage. IOUS has been shown to alter the operative plan, when that plan was based on preoperative imaging, in 17% to 44% of cases.[2,8-11]
  - **Targeting** of lesions for biopsy. If an unsuspected lesion is identified during surgery, IOUS-guided biopsy will help to determine the next steps.
  - **Targeting** of lesions for therapeutic ablation, microwave, or cryotherapy. Metastatic disease such as colorectal liver metastases may require a multimodality approach to

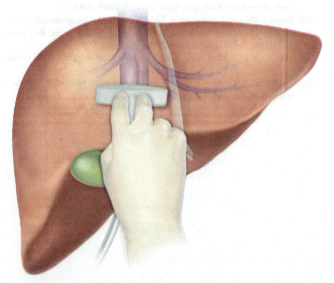

FIGURE 1 • IOUS with T-probe.

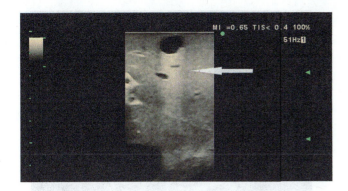

FIGURE 2 • Simple hepatic cyst with posterior acoustic enhancement (arrow).

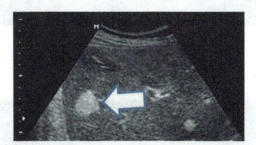

FIGURE 3 • Hemangioma (arrow).

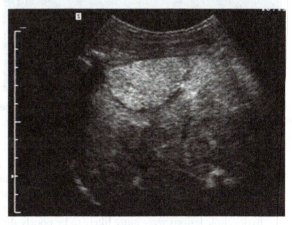

FIGURE 4 • Adenoma.

treatment to achieve optimal control of disease. A combined approach using resection and ablative methods can often allow complete local treatment not otherwise possible.
- **Usefulness of IOUS in the setting of liver-specific MRI and CT** has been questioned. Several studies have found that IOUS improves detection of lesions not seen by modern preoperative imaging.[12,13] With the use of current preoperative chemotherapy, colorectal liver metastases (CRLMs) respond so well they disappear and are not seen with radiologic imaging. In this setting, IOUS has been able to detect these lesions 30% to 58% of the time in centers that perform IOUS regularly, compared with 1% where it is not used routinely.[13] This supports the standard use of IOUS in liver surgery and better outcomes with more regular use.

Liver Parenchyma
- It is important to consider the background liver quality when using the ultrasound to liver tumors.
- Normal liver parenchyma has a homogeneous echo pattern. Steatotic and cirrhotic livers have poor sound transmission and may appear diffusely hyperechoic. This can often make the delineation of pathologic lesions difficult.

Differential Diagnosis of Hepatic Lesions
- If a lesion is encountered, it should be examined in both transverse and longitudinal directions to determine its full extent. Its proximity and extension to neighboring vessels should be determined.
  - Benign lesions
    - Cyst—The ultrasound appearance is a well-defined lesion, with very thin, almost unapparent walls, without circulatory signal on Doppler investigation. The content is transonic suggesting fluid composition (**FIGURE 2**).
    - Hemangioma—Hemangiomas frequently appear as well-circumscribed hyperechoic lesions of varying sizes. Although the lesions are highly vascular, Doppler exploration reveals no circulatory signal, because the blood flow through them is slow (**FIGURE 3**).
    - Adenoma—Adenomas can be exceedingly difficult to distinguish from other benign lesions such as focal nodular hyperplasia. The appearance of adenomas can range from hyper- to hypoechoic; however, they are most frequently hypoechoic (**FIGURE 4**).
  - Neoplastic lesions
    - Hepatocellular carcinoma (HCC)—HCC appearance on 2-D ultrasound is that of an isoechoic or hypoechoic solid tumor, with imprecise delineation, with heterogeneous structure, uni- or multilocular (encephaloid form). HCC may also frequently invade portal and hepatic veins, and so these should be examined even for smaller tumors. Microinvasion seen by IOUS is useful in predicting neoplastic differentiation and prognosis (**FIGURE 5**).[14]
    - Colorectal liver metastases—CRLMs usually appear hypoechoic. They may take on a "target" or "bull's eye" appearance due to alternating layers of hyper- and hypoechoic tissue. This pattern is highly suggestive of malignancy (**FIGURE 6**).

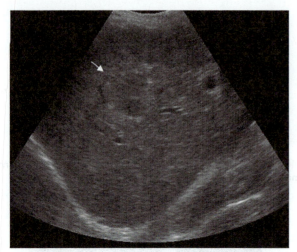

FIGURE 5 • Hepatocellular carcinoma (arrow).

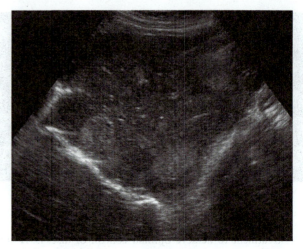

FIGURE 7 • Neuroendocrine tumor.

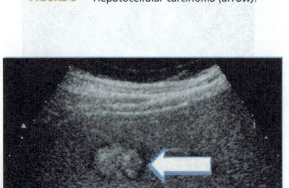

FIGURE 6 • CRLM showing peripheral rim or bull's-eye appearance (arrow).

- Neuroendocrine tumors (NETs)—Because NETs are hypervascular, they often appear as a hyperechoic lesion. However, in one study, 49% appeared hypoechoic, 39% hyperechoic, and 12% isoechoic.[15] Moreover, hypoechoic lesions were more likely to be poorly differentiated and smaller and were associated with shorter disease-free survival (FIGURE 7).

Ultrasound Equipment

- Liver IOUS is best performed using a real-time B-mode scanner system with a 5-MHz or 10-MHz side fire T-shaped linear array probe. Although not always needed, saline or conductive gel can be applied to the liver surface to evaluated surface and liver dome lesions to augment wave transduction. Components for IOUS include the following:
  - Transducer: Transducers help to transmit ultrasound waves through the hepatic parenchyma. There are a variety of probes that are currently available, and selection is based on the goal for the examination, body habitus and quality/character of hepatic parenchyma, and user preference. High-frequency probes allow for more adept superficial imaging, whereas lower-frequency probes allow for deeper evaluation of the parenchyma. The most used probe in open surgery is a T-probe. A flexible laparoscopic probe is useful for laparoscopic procedures, whereas a drop in finger probe is better controlled during robotic operations using a grasper. Probes can either be chemically sterilized or used with a sterile cover. If a cover is used, conductive gel must be placed within the plastic sheath and centered tightly on the probe with a rubber band for the ultrasound waves to transmit. Our group uses chemically sterilized probes (FIGURE 8).

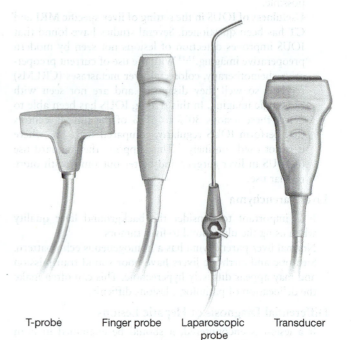

T-probe   Finger probe   Laparoscopic probe   Transducer

FIGURE 8 • Example of some transducer probes available.

  - Processing unit: A variety of processing units are commercially available; most include preset controls to adjust frequency, gain, depth, focus, freeze screens, and calipers to acquire measurements. It is helpful to set the unit for liver imaging to help optimize the picture and to make sure

Chapter 16 INTRAOPERATIVE ULTRASOUND OF THE LIVER

the direction of imaging is correct, inverting the image as need. We find it useful to set the direction of the probe so it is aligned to the CT scan so direct correlations can be made. We recommend familiarizing yourself with the processing unit available in your institution.
- Common controls:
  - Frequency: Determines how much tissue penetration will occur with scanning (higher frequency allows for better resolution but less penetration, the higher the frequency the less the penetrance of ultrasound waves).
  - Gain: Gain amplifies the echography, which manifests as contrast. This determines how the brightness of the image is depicted. To reduce the brightness of an image one would lower the gain.
  - Depth: The depth from which the returning ultrasound signals will be displayed. The scale on the image represents the depth. The maximum amount of depth will depend on the probe frequency. Lower frequencies will allow for improved depth penetration at cost of potentially decreased resolution. Markers on the screen are useful to measure the depth of structures. The depth of imaging can also be appreciated by looking for deep structures through the liver such as the vena cava or the right kidney.
  - Measurements: By freezing the image, calipers can then measure areas of interest.
  - Display: Monitors on the ultrasound unit usually depict black and white images, with color available in Doppler mode. We find it useful to connect the ultrasound unit to external monitors in the room for better positioning of images and larger size. This allows optimal placement of monitors for viewing and teaching purposes and comparison with preoperative images. Images should be saved or printed for the medical record.

Three Modes Commonly Used for Intraoperative Ultrasound of the Liver

- B-mode or 2-D mode: In B-mode (brightness modulation) ultrasound, a linear array of transducers simultaneously scans a plane through the liver that can be viewed as a two-dimensional image on screen (**FIGURE 9**).
- Doppler mode: Information is sampled along a line through the body, and all velocities detected at each time point are presented (on a timeline). When sound is reflected from a moving object, the frequency of the reflected echo changes in proportion to the velocity of the object (**FIGURE 10**).
- Duplex mode: The simultaneous presentation of 2-D (B-mode) and (usually) pulsed wave Doppler information. (Using modern ultrasound machines, color Doppler is always also used; hence the alternative name Triplex.) (**FIGURE 11**).

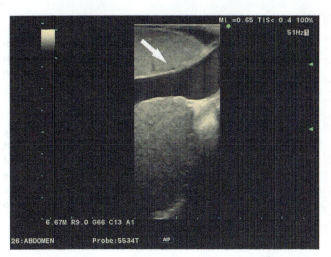

FIGURE 9 • B-mode of the liver with IVC and take off of right hepatic vein *(arrow)*.

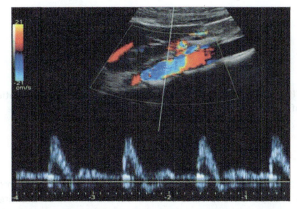

FIGURE 10 • Doppler mode.

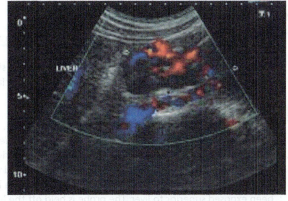

FIGURE 11 • Duplex mode of the liver.

PRESCAN PREPARATION

First Step

- The lights of the operating room should be dimmed to improve visualization of the screen.

Second Step

- No coupling gel unless the transducer is in a sterile bag. If a sterile bag is used, then care should be taken to ensure no air bubbles are present at the contact surface.

Third Step

- Instill saline or water into the abdomen to aid in the transduction of sound waves for surface or liver dome scanning as needed. Most of the liver can be evaluated without fluid in the abdominal cavity.

Fourth Step

- The operator should stand to directly visualize the console monitor. A second monitor placed over the patient's right shoulder or head with the operator standing on the left of the patient provides good in-line visualization. Having the CT or MRI scan on another monitor is useful for direct comparison and localization of lesions and their relationships to vascular structures (FIGURE 12) (Video 1).

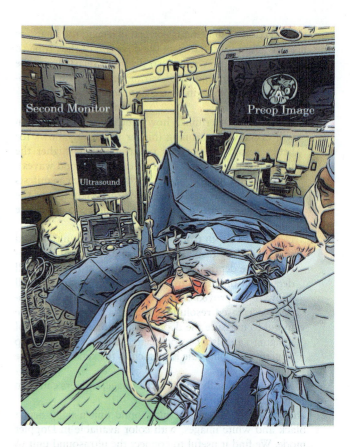

FIGURE 12 • Operating positioning for adequate visualization of the monitor, accessory monitor, and preoperative images.

SCANNING

- Having a systemic technique to hepatic ultrasound is of utmost importance to make sure the liver is evaluated in its entirety and no lesions are overlooked. There are many approaches that have been described. There are two standard methods for ultrasound placement in open and laparoscopic surgeries.

Contact Scanning

- For contact scanning, the probe is in direct contact with the liver surface.
- This technique is used for surveying the liver in most situations, with a systematic approach across the liver surface (FIGURE 13).

Stand-off Scanning

- In stand-off scanning, the surgeon instills water or saline to cover the surface of the liver for coupling to visualize the right posterior segments (segments 6 and 7), the dome around the hepatic veins of the liver is mobilized, and the vena cava has been exposed superior to liver. The probe is held off the liver surface immersed within the water. This technique can also be particularly useful for superficial lesions.

Systematic Approach

- Visually inspect the liver and palpate it looking for masses. Establish whether it is a normal, cirrhotic, or fatty liver. Mobilizing the liver will be helpful for inspection and ultrasonography.

- Identify the confluence of the hepatic veins with the inferior vena cava (IVC). This can be used as a rough indicator of the patient's central venous pressure, or volume status based on IVC distention. Follow the left, middle, and right hepatic veins, respectively.

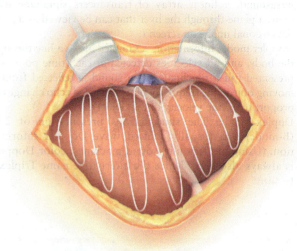

FIGURE 13 • The pattern for scanning with the lawn-mower method.

- Identify the main portal vein and its bifurcation. Follow the left portal vein to identify segment 4 and the bifurcation of segments 2 and 3.
- Again, identify the portal vein bifurcation and follow the right branch to its bifurcation and identify the right anterior and right posterior pedicles.
- Scan over the hilum and identify the bile duct, hepatic artery, and portal vein. Note any lymphadenopathy.
- If there are known lesions, identify these ultrasonographically to determine the echogenic profile that will aid in identifying occult lesions of the same pathology. This is helpful to do early since the image findings will vary depending on the quality of the uninvolved liver.
- Next, survey the entire liver for any additional disease. Repeated scanning is important so as not to miss any unexpected lesions. The two most used survey methods are the lawn-mower method and the pedicle tracking method.

METHODS

Lawn-Mower Method

- The liver is scanned with overlapping fields from the dome to the caudal edge, proceeding from left to right through the entire organ in a sequential manner (FIGURE 13).

Pedicle Tracking Method

- Using this technique, the liver is scanned segment by segment by following the vascular inflow and outflow. The hepatic ultrasonographer should be well versed in hepatic segmental anatomy following Couinaud nomenclature (The Brisbane 2000 terminology of hepatic anatomy and resections).[7]

In-Plane and Out-of-Plane

- It is important to understand the concepts of in-plane and out-of-plane when visualizing structure. In-plane refers to the visualization of structures in their long axis. Out-of-plane refers to visualizing structures at a 90° angle (FIGURE 14).

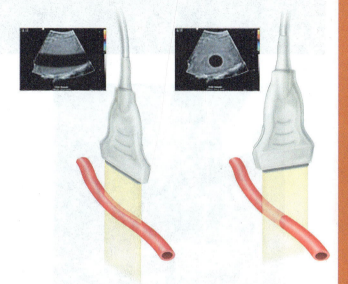

FIGURE 14 • **A,** An ultrasound probe in plane with structure (vessel in this case). **B,** The ultrasound probe at 90° with structure.

IMAGING EXAMPLES

Hepatic Vein Confluence Into Inferior Vena Cava (FIGURE 15)

- The three hepatic veins can be identified entering the IVC near the central diaphragm.
- The middle and left veins can usually be seen forming a common confluence before going into the IVC. It is important to follow the middle hepatic vein as it courses down the liver, since significant bleeding can result when it is encountered during resection. The right hepatic vein is typically posterior and deep.
- The hepatic veins are anechoic vessels, frequently lacking a visible wall structure.

Portal Vein Bifurcation (FIGURES 16 and 17)

- It can be helpful to start at the head of the pancreas and find the portal vein splenic vein junction and travel up toward the liver. This will lead to the hepatic hilum, located at the base of segments 4 and 5. The portal vein can then be identified branching into its main right and left branches.
- The portal veins can be differentiated from the hepatic by their white outline, a result of invested Glisson capsule. The right and left portal veins then ramify into their section branches (anterior and posterior on the right and medial and lateral on the left).
- The arteries and bile ducts run parallel to the portal veins in the liver, branching out into the liver from the hilum. They lie anterior to the portal vein. Duplex color imaging is useful in differentiating the hepatic arteries from the bile ducts.

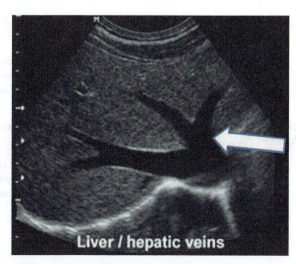

FIGURE 15 • The hepatic vein confluence with the IVC. Note that the left and middle hepatic veins often share a common trunk *(arrow)*.

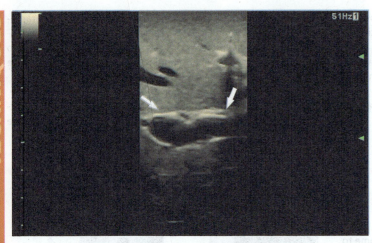

FIGURE 16 • Portal vein bifurcation into its main right and left branches (arrows).

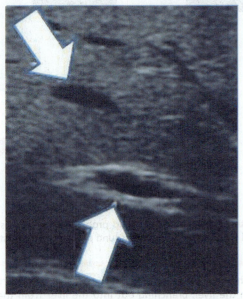

FIGURE 17 • Differentiating portal branches from hepatic vein (top arrow) branches based on the white outline of the portal vein (bottom arrow) branches as they are invested in Glisson capsule.

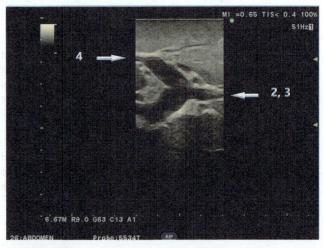

FIGURE 18 • Left portal vein bifurcation into segments 2, 3, and 4 (arrows).

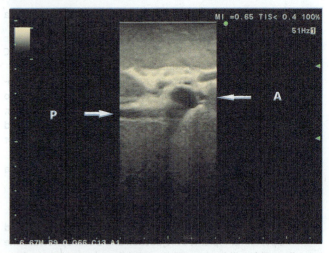

FIGURE 19 • Right portal vein bifurcation into anterior (A) and posterior (P) pedicles (arrows).

Left Portal Vein Bifurcation Into Segments 2, 3, and 4 (FIGURE 18)

- The left portal vein branch is longer than its right counterpart. It turns anteriorly (toward the probe) as it ascends into the umbilical fissure. It then divides into the lateral and medial segments.

Right Portal Vein Bifurcation Into Anterior and Posterior Pedicle (FIGURE 19)

- If one follows the right portal vein from its origin, one can identify the bifurcation into the right anterior (supplying segments 5 and 8) and the right posterior (supplying segments 6 and 7) branches.

Chapter 16 **INTRAOPERATIVE ULTRASOUND OF THE LIVER** 127

TARGETING OF LESIONS FOR ABLATION

- Several different IOUS ablative technologies exist.
- The ablation probe and the ultrasound should be "in plane" so that the approach to the targeting lesion can be visualized. Without doing this it can be difficult to localize the needle of the probe (**FIGURE 20**). The depth of lesion must be appreciated to get the correct angle of insertion into liver, adjusting angle as needed by removing and reinserting probe. Once the probe has reached its intended target, the ultrasound probe can be turned 90° to ensure that it is in the center of the intended target. During ablation, the process can be seen with "whitening" of the ablative area. Following ablation, a significant artifact will be generated, limiting ability to target further lesions in that field. As such, deeper lesions should be targeted first if multiple lesions are being targeted in one area.

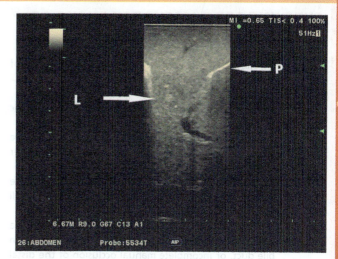

FIGURE 20 • Imaging in-plane targeting of lesion (L) with probe (P) *(arrows)*.

TARGETING OF LESIONS FOR BIOPSY

- Target liver lesions by IOUS for core needle biopsy or aspiration biopsy is similar to ablation.
- Often a spring-loaded biopsy instrument is used. The needle is directed to the lesion by ultrasound held parallel to the needle so that the needle can be seen in its entirety. Since the biopsy instrument typically samples 2 cm in front of the needle tip, care must be taken to position it so that inadvertent biopsy of important vascular or biliary structures is not done and the operator's hand is not in the path of the instrument.
- Sometimes, targeting can be difficult since body wall can interfere with optimal biopsy instrument positioning. In this situation, mobilizing the liver or placing the needle through the abdominal wall may help.

LAPAROSCOPIC ULTRASOUND

- During laparoscopic procedures, the surgeon is not able to palpate the liver to localize lesions. IOUS is needed to identify lesions not seen on the surface and to establish vascular relationships as during open surgery (**FIGURE 21**).
- The goals of laparoscopic IOUS are the same as the ones presented earlier in this chapter in open liver surgery. Using ultrasound probes with varying degrees of freedom, during laparoscopic IOUS evaluation, the special relationships of liver structure can be difficult to comprehend. Changing the direction of the arm of the flexible probes can be helpful in discerning the anatomy.

- If robotic assisted laparoscopic procedures are performed, a drop in probe can be used to scan the liver. Using picture in picture on the console allows for simultaneous visualization of the liver and ultrasound image, making scanning the liver possible. Moreover, with the help of bedside assistance, holding the ultrasound in one arm and guiding a biopsy needle or treatment probe with the other arm, accurate targeting can be done (**FIGURE 22**).

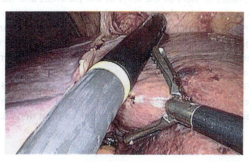

FIGURE 21 • Laparoscopic IOUS. Typically, start high on the patient, to the right of the falciform.

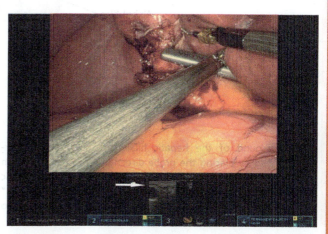

FIGURE 22 • Robotic assisted laparoscopic IOUS with ultrasound image in console showing position of cystic artery crossing over gallbladder neck *(arrow)*. Probe can easily be moved around with grasper.

CHECKING FOR BILIARY LEAK BY USE OF AIR CHOLANGIOGRAM

- This technique has been shown to result in a lower rate of postoperative bile fistula (1.9% vs 10.8%)[16] (FIGURES 23 and 24).
    - A cholangiography catheter is inserted into the cystic duct and secured with a silk tie.
    - A syringe of air is then injected to fill the biliary tree while occluding the distal common bile duct by finger compression.
    - IOUS is then used to look at all liver segments to ensure bile duct patency. If there is an excluded segment, it will have an absence of pneumobilia.
    - Nonvisualization of pneumobilia suggests that there is a bile duct obstruction, a massive air leak via a large open bile duct, or incomplete manual occlusion of the distal common bile duct.

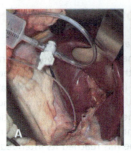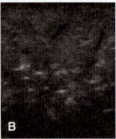

FIGURE 23 • **A,** Injection of air into cystic duct following resection. **B,** Appearance of the liver following injection on air. The appearance is that of "Christmas tree lights" in liver segments that are in continuity.

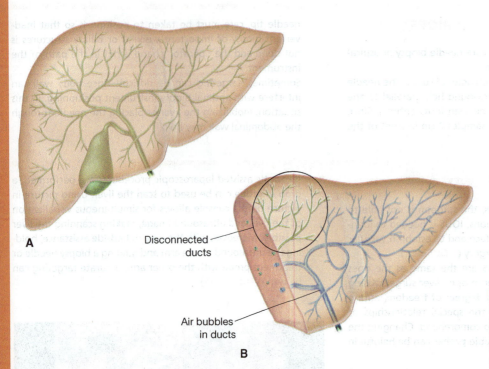

FIGURE 24 • **A,** The liver, prior to resection, showing the biliary system. **B,** The liver, following resection, showing air within segments in continuity and no air in excluded segments.

IDENTIFYING STRUCTURES IN THE HEPATIC HILUM

- Ultrasound of the hepatic hilar structures can be performed by placing the probe directly on the hepatic hilum (FIGURES 25 and 26). The classic appearance of the hepatic hilum on IOUS has been described as "Micky Mouse ears" consisting of the bile duct to the right, the hepatic artery to the left, and the portal vein posteriorly.

- It helps to start at the level of the pancreas and portal vein junction with splenic vein and then go toward liver toward the hilum. Also visualizing the takeoff of the celiac and superior mesenteric arteries helps identify the hepatic artery and any replaced right hepatic coming from the superior mesenteric artery (FIGURE 27).
- The use of IOUS in the hilum can be useful for identifying the level of the hepatic artery bifurcation as well as any other anomalous anatomy such as a replaced right hepatic artery.

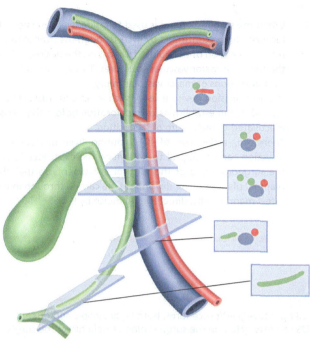

FIGURE 25 • Relationship of structures of the hilum.

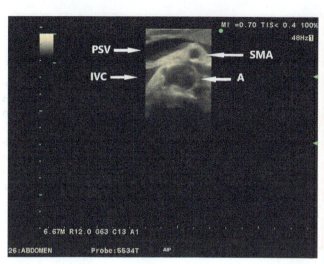

FIGURE 27 • Superior mesenteric artery (SMA), portal–splenic vein (PSV), inferior vena cava (IVC) with left renal vein lying over aorta (A) (arrows).

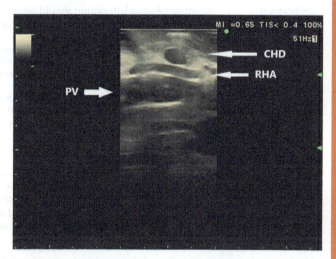

FIGURE 28 • Right hepatic artery (RHA) crossing underneath the common hepatic duct (CHD) with portal vein (PV) posterior (arrows).

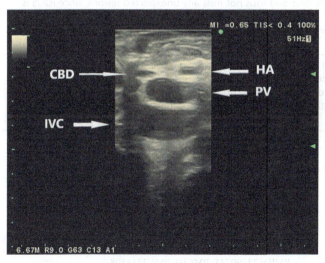

FIGURE 26 • Hepatic artery (HA) to the left, portal vein (PV) posterior, common bile duct (CBD) to the right, and inferior vena cava (IVC) (arrows).

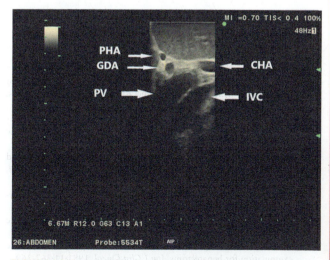

FIGURE 29 • Gastroduodenal artery (GDA) coming off the common hepatic artery (CHA) and traveling down into the neck of pancreas. Note the proper hepatic artery (PHA), portal vein (PV), and the IVC (arrows).

- The location of the right hepatic artery crossing beneath the common hepatic duct is often evident (FIGURE 28).
- The cystic duct can often be seen traveling with the common hepatic duct before it joins the common bile duct.
- The gastroduodenal artery is found by the neck of the pancreas as it comes from the right hepatic artery (FIGURE 29).
- Portal lymph nodes can be appreciated, and tumor presence and invasion into vascular structures can often be seen.

TECHNIQUES

ACTIVE USE OF IOUS DURING LIVER DISSECTION AND RESECTION

- It can often be difficult to know the location of an instrument or line of liver division in relation to the hepatic veins or the portal structures. Mistakes in such areas can result in critical injuries, bleeding, and major complications.
- The location of instruments such as right angle can be visualized during the dissection with liver ultrasound and thus help avoid major vascular injury when trying to encircle portal structures or hepatic veins. Adding fluid to the abdominal cavity can be helpful for this.
- When the surgeon's hand is used to guide liver resection, its location can be confirmed by IOUS through the liver to make sure the location of the guiding hand is on the desired side of the tumor or major vascular structures. This will avoid tumor contaminations or major vascular injury.
- If a liver division devise is used, such as an endovascular stapler, IOUS can establish its correct location before the devise is activated to make sure of its position.
- Therefore, active use of IOUS during liver dissection or resection can be helpful to determine the exact location of the surgeon's hand or the surgical instruments so that the planned planes of liver division can be carried through in the safest manner, with direct live guidance by IOUS.

PEARLS AND PITFALLS

Indications	- Intraoperative ultrasound should be used in all operative liver procedures, both laparoscopic and open. - Even with modern preoperative imaging, IOUS can often change the surgical plan or help direct the surgical technique.
Equipment	- It is important to be familiar with the ultrasound equipment available in the surgeon's hospital. - Using IOUS frequently will help develop expertise in its use and familiarity with the equipment used.
Liver lesions	- Scan a known lesion first to identify the ultrasound imaging characteristics of the pathology of interest in relation to the liver. Lesion imaging can vary with the liver and the pathology. - Use a systematic approach to scan the entire liver and thus not miss any unexpected lesions, since IOUS is more sensitive than preoperative scans. - Mobilizing the liver and placing fluid in the abdomen can be helpful in visualization and thorough scanning.
Targeting	- The targeting needle should be in plane of the ultrasound so that it can be directed to the lesion of concern safely and visualized through its course. - Comparison with preoperative imaging and realizing the location of the surrounding liver structures is helpful when determining the location of the lesion to be targeted by understanding special relationships to these structures.
Active use during liver surgery	- Location of dissecting instruments and the surgeon's hand can be seen in relation to vessels and tumor to help guide the surgery. - This helps determine dissection planes and avoidance of tumor contamination and structural liver injury.

REFERENCES

1. Cervone A, Sardi A, Conaway GL. Intraoperative ultrasound (IOUS) is essential in the management of metastatic colorectal liver lesions. *Am J Surg*. 2000;66(7):611-615.
2. Guimarães C, Correia M, Baldisserotto M, et al. Intraoperative ultrasonography of the liver in patients with abdominal tumors: a new approach. *J Ultrasound Med*. 2004;23:1549-1555.
3. Mazzoni G, Napoli A, Mandetta S, et al. Intra-operative ultrasound for detection of liver metastases from colorectal cancer. *Liver Int*. 2008;28(1):88-94.
4. Xu YW, Fu H. Application of intraoperative ultrasound in liver surgery. *Hepatobiliary Pancreat Dis Int*. 2021;20(5):501-502.
5. Ezaki T, Stansby GP, Hobbs KE. Intraoperative ultrasonographic imaging in liver surgery: a review. *HPB Surg*. 1990;3(1):1-4.
6. Makuuchi M, Hasegawa H, Yamazaki S. Interoperative ultrasonic examination for hepatectomy. *Jpn J Clin Oncol*. 1981;11:367-369.
7. Abu-Zidan FM, Hefny AF, Corr P. Clinical ultrasound physics. *J Emerg Trauma Shock*. 2011;4(4):501-503. doi:10.4103/0974-2700.86646 PMID: 22090745; PMCID: PMC3214508.
8. The Terminology Committee of the International Hepato-Pancreato-Biliary Association. The Brisbane 2000 terminology of hepatic anatomy and resections. *HPB*. 2000;2:333-339.
9. Knowles SA, Bertens KA, Croome KP, Hernandez-Alejandro R. The current role of intraoperative ultrasound during the resection of colorectal liver metastases: a retrospective cohort study. *Int J Surg*. 2015;20:101-106.
10. Joo I. The role of intraoperative ultrasonography in the diagnosis and management of focal hepatic lesions. *Ultrasonography*. 2015;34(4):246-257.
11. Jrearz R, Hart R, Jayaraman S. Intraoperative ultrasonography, and surgical strategy in hepatic resection: what difference does it make? *Can J Surg*. 2015;58(5):318-322.

12. Langella S, Ardito F, Russolillo N, et al. Intraoperative ultrasound staging for colorectal liver metastases in the era of liver-specific magnetic resonance imaging: is it still worthwhile? *J Oncol.* 2019;2019:1369274.
13. Giuliante F, Panettieri E, Ardito F. The impact of intraoperative ultrasonography on the management of disappearing colorectal liver metastases. *Hepat Oncol.* 2015;2(4):325-328.
14. Santambrogio R, Cigala C, Barabino M, et al. Intraoperative ultrasound for prediction of hepatocellular carcinoma biological behaviour: prospective comparison with pathology. *Liver Int.* 2018;38(2):312-320.
15. Dogeas E, Chong CCN, Weiss MJ, et al. Can echogenic appearance of neuroendocrine liver metastases on intraoperative ultrasonography predict tumor biology and prognosis? *HPB (Oxford).* 2018;20(3):237-243.
16. Zimmitti G, Vauthey J, Shindoh J, et al. Use of an intraoperative air leak test at the time of major liver resection reduces the rate of postoperative biliary complications. *J Am Coll Surg.* 2013;217(6):1028-1037.

Chapter 17 | Hepatic Neoplasm Ablation and Related Technology

Ido Nachmany, Niv Pencovich, and Rony Eshkenazy

DEFINITION

- Hepatic ablation represents the use of chemical or physical means to destroy a neoplastic lesion and surrounding normal tissues as an alternative to resection.
- The liver is one of the most common sites for development of malignancy—either primary liver cancer or metastatic disease of an extrahepatic origin.
- As a general concept for primary liver cancers and few of the metastatic diseases, most commonly colorectal cancer, the main curative option is surgical resection by partial hepatectomy or whole liver replacement. A variety of clinical situations preclude this approach; ablation is an attractive and viable option in some of these clinical situations.
- The most common indication for liver resection is colorectal cancer liver metastases (CLM) followed by primary liver cancers (mainly hepatocellular carcinoma [HCC] and cholangiocarcinoma).
- In the case of CLM, about 50% of patients with colorectal cancer will ultimately develop liver metastases. Only about 15% to 20% are resectable at presentation.[1,2]
- Oncologic benefit of liver resection has been shown mainly when complete clearance of metastatic disease is achieved.
- Factors limiting resection include extent of tumor involvement, volume of the postresection liver remnant, anatomic proximity to essential intrahepatic structures, underlying liver disease, and comorbidities.
- HCC is the only universally accepted oncologic indication for orthotopic liver transplantation (OLT). Only a small subset of patients is suitable for OLT, mainly due to stringent criteria influenced by the limited organ availability and inferior long-term survival in patients with locally advanced disease.
- For patients with unresectable liver tumors or those beyond criteria for OLT, life prolongation and control of symptoms are the major goals. This can be achieved by systemic therapy or by different locoregional modalities, grouped under two major categories: tumor ablation and transarterial treatment (chemotherapy infusion, embolization, combination of the two and internal irradiation).
- Ablation can be achieved by direct application of thermal energy (by cooling: cryoablation, heating: radiofrequency ablation [RFA] or microwave ablation [MWA]), chemical ablation: percutaneous acetic acid (PAI) or percutaneous ethanol injection (PEI), or by using electrical field–mediated membrane poration: irreversible electroporation (IRE).
- The most commonly applied modality is thermal ablation using microwave technique (MWA), replacing RFA.
- Based on accumulating data supporting the clinical benefit of ablation techniques, there had been an expansion of the indications. Ablation is now introduced in combination with liver resection and, in limited cases, as a replacement of resection with curative intent.
- Ablation can be performed percutaneously, laparoscopically, or via laparotomy.
- The main advantage of a percutaneous approach is the minimal invasiveness of the procedure.
- The advantages of using ablative modalities in surgery are the ability to reach any territory of the liver, the ability to combine ablation with resection, to protect nearby sensitive structures (like the colon, diaphragm, etc), and the control of inflow and outflow. This may counteract the cooling effect of blood flow in major vessels (referred to as the "heat sink" effect). Laparoscopic ablation may combine the benefits of surgery with those of minimally invasive treatment.
- Studying the long-term effectiveness of ablative modalities has been challenging; in part, this is due to the rapid evolution of ablative tools (probes and energy sources), thus the field is in constant development. Also, the results of most studies are limited by sample size, methodology, and follow-up time.

INDICATIONS

- HCC
  - The vast majority of patients with HCC have background chronic liver disease. The management of these patients takes into account the primary liver disease (synthetic dysfunction and portal hypertension) as well as the extent of the tumor.
  - The most commonly used algorithm outside of the United States for HCC management is the Barcelona Clinic for Liver Cancer (BCLC) staging and treatment strategy.[3] Other criteria (Milan and University of California, San Francisco [UCSF]), as well as others, have also been forwarded.[4]
  - Based on the BCLC algorithm, patients suitable for curative treatment are those with very early and early stages (stages 0 and A).
  - Curative options include resection, liver transplantation, and, in some cases, ablation. The choice between the different options is based on the extent of liver disease, tumor stage, tumor location, and patient comorbidities.[5,6]
  - There are three subsets of patients specifically suitable for ablation:
    - Patients with unresectable HCC beyond transplant criteria. Tumor ablation is usually combined with other treatment modalities, such as transarterial chemoembolization. These patients are not considered curable.
    - Patients with very early stage HCC (stage 0—single, up to 2 cm tumor with Child A cirrhosis, and in good performance status) are usually considered resection candidates. Data suggest that they can also be managed by ablative modalities. The main potential benefit of resection over ablation is the availability of the pathologic specimen. The presence of microvascular invasion or microsatellites in the specimen, which are major risk

factors for recurrence, is considered by some an indication for "salvage OLT."[7,8] Therefore, if the patient is a transplant candidate, resection is preferred over ablation. On the other hand, ablation offers a less invasive procedure and may be attractive alternative to patients.
- Patients with early stage HCC (stage A—up to three lesions, largest ≤3 cm, with Child A–B cirrhosis, and in good performance status) are best treated by OLT unless they have significant comorbidities. In such cases, ablation may be an alternative.
- Colorectal liver metastases
  - The only curative option for patients with CLM is resection, but unfortunately, this is possible in only about 15% to 20% of cases. Some patients may become resectable with neoadjuvant chemotherapy or with anticipated liver remnant volume manipulation such as portal vein embolization, two-stage hepatectomy with portal vein ligation/embolization, associating liver partition and portal vein ligation for staged hepatectomy (ALPPS), and more.[9-12]
  - The advantages of RFA include low complication rates, fast recovery, and good safety profile in patients with marginal liver reserve. The main disadvantages are the higher local recurrence rates and limitations in treating large or multiple lesions.[13]
  - Tumor ablation is a valid option for
    - Patients with limited disease that cannot achieve an R0 resection with surgery
    - Patients who are not surgical candidates due to systemic conditions or because of multiple previous operations on the liver
    - Some authors consider ablation an alternative in patients with resectable metastases. There are currently no prospective studies to support this approach.[13,14] In the future, with improving devices and technique, the equivalence of ablation and resection may eventually be demonstrated.
    - Ablation can also be used in combination with resection of other metastases. This is usually done for relatively small and deeply seated lesions for which resection would dramatically increase the morbidity of the procedure.

CONTRAINDICATIONS

- There are very few contraindications for ablative therapy.
- An absolute contraindication for thermal ablation is abutment of hilar structures, mainly the bile ducts and gallbladder, due to the high risk of thermal injury. This may not apply for IRE.
- Major blood vessels in the immediate vicinity of the target lesion (specifically hepatic veins and large portal branches) are associated with significantly reduced efficacy due to the heat sink effect and it is a risk factor for local recurrence. This can be overcome surgically to some degree by flow manipulation such as the Pringle maneuver or outflow obstruction and thus is not considered an absolute contraindication.

TECHNIQUES

- Chemical ablation with injection (usually percutaneously) of ethanol or acetic acid was used mainly for HCC, because this tumor is soft and accepts the fluid injected well. Currently, use of chemical ablation is not common mainly due to inferior efficacy, as compared to thermal ablation and the need for repeated treatments.[15]
- RFA
  - RFA uses alternating electric field delivered through a needle or multiple needle electrodes. It can be inserted percutaneously, laparoscopically, or at laparotomy (FIGURES 1 and 2).
  - Ions in the tissue follow the direction of the rapidly changing current. This causes frictional energy to produce heat and coagulative necrosis.
  - As temperatures approach 100 °C, changes in the physical properties of the tissue increase impedance and limit the flow of current (tissue desiccation due to evaporation of tissue fluid, charring, and the formation of electrically insulating gas between the electrode and the tissue due to boiling). This limits treatment of larger tumors.
- MWA[16,17]
  - MWA uses electromagnetic radiation, much higher on the spectrum of electromagnetic radiation than RFA (usually in the range of 900-2450 MHz) (FIGURES 3 and 4).
  - Polar molecules in the electromagnetic field (mainly water) try to align in the direction of the current. As the direction changes constantly, continuous realignment causes friction and heating effect. Like RFA, the heat causes cell death by coagulative necrosis.
  - Unlike RFA, MW causes oscillation of water molecules in the entire field, so heat is uniformly distributed in the MW field throughout the activation. This achieves immediate and homogeneous heating and therefore faster tissue destruction.
  - Heat is conducted outside of that field, so the ultimate ablation size is the sum of the microwave field and the conductive heat zone.

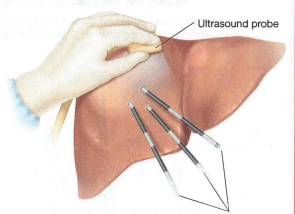

FIGURE 1 • Three RF needles liver insertion.

134 SECTION II SURGERY OF THE LIVER

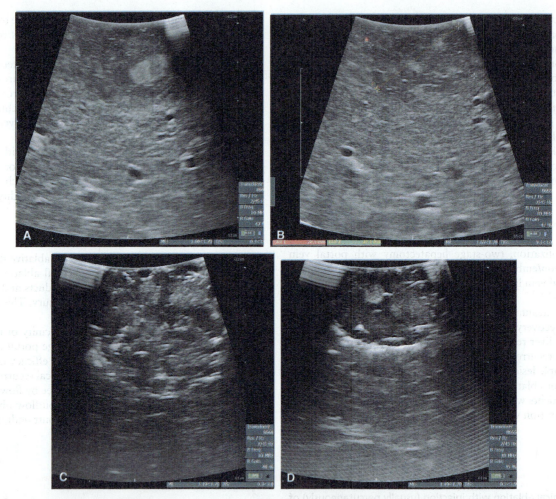

FIGURE 2 • Laparoscopic ultrasound-guided radiofrequency ablation of a peripheral hepatocellular carcinoma. **A**, Before ablation. **B**, Lesion measurements. **C**, During ablation. **D**, Immediate postablation. Note the typical artifacts created by the gas formed by tissue boiling.

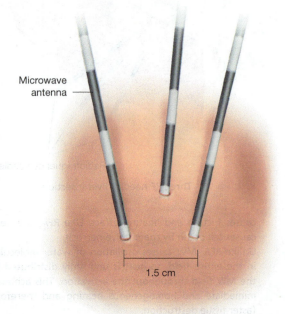

FIGURE 3 • Three microwave antennas arrayed to ablate a large lesion.

- The size of the microwave field is determined by the wavelength and the antenna design.
- Within the microwave field, heat sink and current sink effects are not present. Outside the microwave field (in the conduction zone) there will be a heat sink effect, similar to RFA.[18]
- MWA does not require point-to-point currents.
- No current flows through the patient and no grounding pads are required.
- IRE[19]
  - IRE is based on electric field–mediated nonthermal tissue destruction.
  - IRE is performed by placing electrodes into the tissue and delivering multiple high-voltage electrical pulses to induce pores in the lipid bilayer of cell membrane. This starts a process that leads to cell death.
  - IRE is not influenced by the heat sink effect.
  - Because the location of IRE activity is the cell membrane, acellular structures are preserved. Because hilar structures are wrapped in a fibrous sheet, they are protected. This allows for application of IRE to lesions in the vicinity of intrahepatic vital structures, unlike thermal ablation.[20]

Chapter 17 HEPATIC NEOPLASM ABLATION AND RELATED TECHNOLOGY   135

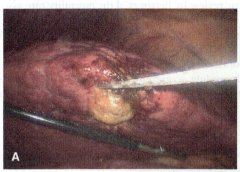
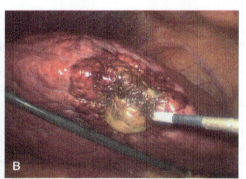
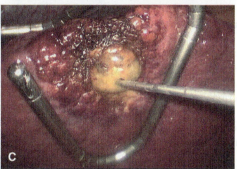

FIGURE 4 • **A–C,** Laparoscopic ablation of a hepatocellular carcinoma using multiple deployments of a microwave probe.

PEARLS AND PITFALLS

Indications	▪ Resection is not an option.
	▪ The lesion is not too big.
	▪ The lesion is not adjacent to a heat sink or vital structure.
	▪ Ultrasound in cirrhotic livers is technically challenging.
Technique	▪ Confirm appropriate probe placement with ultrasound—Record the images.
	▪ Confirm complete destruction of the lesion by ultrasound—Record the images.
	▪ Precoagulation prior to parenchymal transection (**FIGURE 5**).

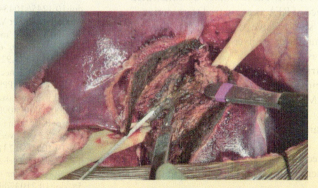

FIGURE 5 • Microwave ablation as a precoagulant strategy prior to parenchymal transection.

OUTCOMES

- Factors influencing outcome include the following:
  - Tumor size: Best results are achieved for the treatment of small tumors less than 3 cm for RFA. MWA achieves effective results in somewhat larger lesions but is also limited by lesion size.
  - Ablation margin: In order to minimize the chance for local recurrence, it is advised to leave a rim of 1 cm of ablated tissue beyond the tumor margin.
  - Vicinity to major vascular structures, mainly large veins, due to the heat sink effect.

- Mode of application: Surgical application usually achieves better outcome than percutaneous.
- Ablation is operator-dependent and therefore experience plays a major role.
- Assessing the isolated effect of ablation is difficult. In most cases, ablation is not considered curative; therefore, it is usually combined with other treatment modalities. Also, there are no high-quality randomized studies, the follow-up is usually short, and the devices used are in constant evolution.[16]
- The most representative benchmark of ablation efficacy is local recurrence at the ablation site. This is widely variable, and in the case of RFA, runs from 2% to 60%.[16]
- HCC
  - A recent updated analysis of the 5- and 10-year therapeutic outcome of percutaneous RFA as first-line therapy for single HCC <3 cm was better than previously reported and demonstrated approximately 83% and 74% overall survival and 20% and 25%, respectively.[21]
  - Randomized control trials comparing hepatic resection vs RFA for small HCC demonstrated comparable results.[5,6,22,23] Complete pathologic response, local recurrence, and overall survival rates for small HCC were similar for RFA, MWA, and cryoablation.[24,25]
  - Combining eight studies and more than 1000 patients, Germani et al.[15] found that RFA was superior to PAI or PEI with regard to survival, complete tumor necrosis, and local recurrence. Other studies corroborated these results.[26]
- CLM
  - During the past decade, RFA has superseded other ablative therapies, due to its low morbidity, mortality, safety, and patient acceptability. However, MWA is gradually becoming the leading modality due to some benefits over RFA including shorter ablation time, higher ablative temperature, more homogenous tissue ablation, less heat sink effect, and probably lower local recurrence rate.[27,28]
  - Multiple studies have compared RFA to liver resection as a radical approach to CLM. These studies demonstrated higher local recurrence of RFA as compared to resection.[29] Nevertheless, recent studies have suggested that thermal ablation may be noninferior to liver resection in certain settings such as in lesions <3 cm.[30,31] A prospective randomized controlled trial aiming to prove noninferiority of thermal ablation compared to hepatic resection in patients with at least one CLM and no extrahepatic disease is currently underway.[32]
  - Liver resection remains the gold standard for the treatment of CLM.[33]
  - In the case of nonresectable CLM, the addition of ablation to systemic chemotherapy increases overall survival.[34]

COMPLICATIONS

- Morbidity and mortality are relatively low. Complications include bleeding, vascular thrombosis, abscess formation, and injury to intrahepatic structures (mainly bile ducts and gallbladder) and extrahepatic organs (colon, duodenum, etc).
- RFA, MWA, and PEI do not show statistically significant difference in mortality or major or minor complications rates.[12,16,35]
- In a systematic review by Bertot et al the mortality rate associated with RFA, MWA, and PEI was 0.15%, 0.23%, and 0.59%, respectively, and the rate of major complications was 4.1%, 2.7%, and 4.6%, respectively.[35] Other studies have corroborated these results.[36,37]
- Needle track seeding is extremely rare. For percutaneous MWA, it was found to be 0.47% per tumor and 0.75% per patient.[38]

REFERENCES

1. Siegel RL, Miller KD, Fuchs HE, Jemal A. Cancer statistics, 2021. *CA Cancer J. Clin.* 2021;71:7-33. doi:10.3322/caac.21654
2. Leporrier J, Maurel J, Chiche L, Bara S, Segol P, Launoy G. A population-based study of the incidence, management and prognosis of hepatic metastases from colorectal cancer. *Br J Surg.* 2006;93:465-474. doi:10.1002/bjs.5278
3. Bruix J, Sherman M, American Association for the Study of Liver Diseases. Management of hepatocellular carcinoma: an update. *Hepatology.* 2011;53:1020-1022. doi:10.1002/hep.24199
4. Yu SJ. A concise review of updated guidelines regarding the management of hepatocellular carcinoma around the world: 2010–2016. *Clin Mol Hepatol.* 2016;22:7-17. doi:10.3350/cmh.2016.22.1.7
5. Feng K, Yan J, Li X, et al. A randomized controlled trial of radiofrequency ablation and surgical resection in the treatment of small hepatocellular carcinoma. *J. Hepatol.* 2012;57:794-802. doi:10.1016/j.jhep.2012.05.007
6. Ng KKC, Chok KSH, Chan ACY, et al. Randomized clinical trial of hepatic resection versus radiofrequency ablation for early-stage hepatocellular carcinoma. *Br J Surg.* 2017;104:1775-1784. doi:10.1002/bjs.10677
7. Ahn KS, Kang KJ. Appropriate treatment modality for solitary small hepatocellular carcinoma: radiofrequency ablation vs. resection vs. transplantation? *Clin Mol Hepatol.* 2019;25:354-359. doi:10.3350/cmh.2018.0096
8. Sala M, Fuster J, Llovet JM, et al. High pathological risk of recurrence after surgical resection for hepatocellular carcinoma: an indication for salvage liver transplantation. *Liver Transpl.* 2004;10:1294-1300. doi:10.1002/lt.20202
9. Lam VWT, Spiro C, Laurence JM, et al. A systematic review of clinical response and survival outcomes of downsizing systemic chemotherapy and rescue liver surgery in patients with initially unresectable colorectal liver metastases. *Ann Surg Oncol.* 2012;19:1292-1301. doi:10.1245/s10434-011-2061-0
10. Adam R, Delvart V, Pascal G, et al. Rescue surgery for unresectable colorectal liver metastases downstaged by chemotherapy. *Ann. Surg.* 2004;240, 644-658; discussion 657-648, doi:10.1097/01.sla.0000141198.92114.f6
11. Petrowsky H, Linecker M, Raptis DA, et al. First long-term oncologic results of the ALPPS procedure in a large cohort of patients with colorectal liver metastases. *Ann. Surg.* 2020;272:793-800. doi:10.1097/SLA.0000000000004330
12. Heinrich S, Lang H. Liver metastases from colorectal cancer: technique of liver resection. *J Surg Oncol.* 2013;107:579-584. doi:10.1002/jso.23138
13. Takahashi H, Berber E. Role of thermal ablation in the management of colorectal liver metastasis. *Hepatobiliary Surg. Nutr.* 2020;9:49-58. doi:10.21037/hbsn.2019.06.08
14. Cirocchi R, Trastulli S, Boselli C, et al. Radiofrequency ablation in the treatment of liver metastases from colorectal cancer. *Cochrane Database Syst Rev.* 2012:CD006317. doi:10.1002/14651858.CD006317.pub3
15. Germani G, Pleguezuelo M, Gurusamy K, Meyer T, Isgrò G, Burroughs AK. Clinical outcomes of radiofrequency ablation, percutaneous alcohol and acetic acid injection for hepatocellular carcinoma: a meta-analysis. *J. Hepatol.* 2010;52:380-388. doi:10.1016/j.jhep.2009.12.004
16. Izzo F, Granata V, Grassi R, et al. Radiofrequency ablation and microwave ablation in liver tumors: an update. *Oncologist.* 2019;24:e990-e1005. doi:10.1634/theoncologist.2018-0337

17. Eisele RM. Advances in local ablation of malignant liver lesions. *World J Gastroenterol.* 2016;22:3885-3891. doi:10.3748/wjg.v22.i15.3885
18. Yu NC, Raman SS, Kim YJ, Lassman C, Chang X, Lu DSK. Microwave liver ablation: influence of hepatic vein size on heat-sink effect in a porcine model. *J Vasc Intervent Radiol.* 2008;19:1087-1092. doi:10.1016/j.jvir.2008.03.023
19. Gupta P, Maralakunte M, Sagar S, et al. Efficacy and safety of irreversible electroporation for malignant liver tumors: a systematic review and meta-analysis. *Eur Radiol.* 2021;31:6511-6521. doi:10.1007/s00330-021-07742-y
20. Charpentier KP, Wolf F, Noble L, Winn B, Resnick M, Dupuy DE. Irreversible electroporation of the liver and liver hilum in swine. *HPB.* 2011;13:168-173. doi:10.1111/j.1477-2574.2010.00261.x
21. Lee MW, Kang D, Lim HK, et al. Updated 10-year outcomes of percutaneous radiofrequency ablation as first-line therapy for single hepatocellular carcinoma <3 cm: emphasis on association of local tumor progression and overall survival. *Eur Radiol.* 2020;30, 2391-2400. doi:10.1007/s00330-019-06575-0
22. Chen M-S, Li J-Q, Zheng Y, et al. A prospective randomized trial comparing percutaneous local ablative therapy and partial hepatectomy for small hepatocellular carcinoma. *Ann. Surg.* 2006;243:321-328. doi:10.1097/01.sla.0000201480.65519.b8
23. Jia Z, Zhang H, Li N. Evaluation of clinical outcomes of radiofrequency ablation and surgical resection for hepatocellular carcinoma conforming to the Milan criteria: a systematic review and meta-analysis of recent randomized controlled trials. *J Gastroenterol Hepatol.* 2021;36:1769-1777. doi:10.1111/jgh.15440
24. Tan W, Deng Q, Lin S, Wang Y, Xu G. Comparison of microwave ablation and radiofrequency ablation for hepatocellular carcinoma: a systematic review and meta-analysis. *Int J Hyperthermia.* 2019;36:263-271. doi:10.1080/02656736.2018.1562571
25. Mulier S, Ni Y, Jamart J, Ruers T, Marchal G, Michel L. Local recurrence after hepatic radiofrequency coagulation. *Ann. Surg.* 2005;242:158-171. doi:10.1097/01.sla.0000171032.99149.fe
26. Dong W, Zhang T, Wang ZG, Liu H. Clinical outcome of small hepatocellular carcinoma after different treatments: a meta-analysis. *World J Gastroenterol.* 2014;20:10174-10182. doi:10.3748/wjg.v20.i29.10174
27. Jabbar F, Syblis C, Sucandy I. The use of thermal ablation in the treatment of colorectal liver metastasis-proper selection and application of technology. *Hepatobiliary Surg Nutr.* 2021;10:279-280. doi:10.21037/hbsn-21-54
28. Takahashi H, Kahramangil B, Kose E, Berber E. A comparison of microwave thermosphere versus radiofrequency thermal ablation in the treatment of colorectal liver metastases. *HPB.* 2018;20:1157-1162. doi:10.1016/j.hpb.2018.05.012
29. Yang G, Wang G, Sun J, et al. The prognosis of radiofrequency ablation versus hepatic resection for patients with colorectal liver metastases: a systematic review and meta-analysis based on 22 studies. *Int J Surg.* 2021;87:105896. doi:10.1016/j.ijsu.2021.105896
30. Tinguely P, Dal G, Bottai M, Nilsson H, Freedman J, Engstrand J. Microwave ablation versus resection for colorectal cancer liver metastases—a propensity score analysis from a population-based nationwide registry. *Eur J Surg Oncol.* 2020;46:476-485. doi:10.1016/j.ejso.2019.12.002
31. Hao W, Binbin J, Wei Y, Kun Y. Can radiofrequency ablation replace liver resection for solitary colorectal liver metastasis? A systemic review and meta-analysis. *Front Oncol.* 2020;10:561669. doi:10.3389/fonc.2020.561669
32. Puijk RS, Ruarus AH, Vroomen LGPH, et al. Colorectal liver metastases: surgery versus thermal ablation (COLLISION)—a phase III single-blind prospective randomized controlled trial. *BMC Cancer.* 2018;18:821. doi:10.1186/s12885-018-4716-8
33. Nieuwenhuizen S, Puijk RS, van den Bemd B, et al. Resectability and ablatability criteria for the treatment of liver only colorectal metastases: multidisciplinary consensus document from the COLLISION trial group. *Cancers.* 2020;12:1779. doi:10.3390/cancers12071779
34. Ruers T, Van Coevorden F, Punt CJA, et al. Local treatment of unresectable colorectal liver metastases: results of a randomized phase II trial. *J Natl Cancer Inst.* 2017;109. doi:10.1093/jnci/djx015
35. Bertot LC, Sato M, Tateishi R, Yoshida H, Koike K. Mortality and complication rates of percutaneous ablative techniques for the treatment of liver tumors: a systematic review. *Eur Radiol.* 2011;21:2584-2596. doi:10.1007/s00330-011-2222-3
36. Lahat E, Eshkenazy R, Zendel A, et al. Complications after percutaneous ablation of liver tumors: a systematic review. *Hepatobiliary Surg. Nutr.* 2014;3:317-23. doi:10.3978/j.issn.2304-3881.2014.09.07
37. Liang P, Wang Y, Yu X, Dong B. Malignant liver tumors: Treatment with percutaneous microwave ablation-complications among cohort of 1136 patients. *Radiology.* 2009;251:933-940. doi:10.1148/radiol.2513081740
38. Yu J, Liang P, Yu X-l, Cheng Z-g, Han Z-y, Dong B-w. Needle track seeding after percutaneous microwave ablation of malignant liver tumors under ultrasound guidance: analysis of 14-year experience with 1462 patients at a single center. *Eur J Radiol.* 2012;81:2495-2499. doi:10.1016/j.ejrad.2011.10.019

Chapter 18 Catheter-Based Treatment of Hepatic Neoplasms

Darren W. Postoak

DEFINITION
- Catheter-based treatment of hepatic neoplasms is a percutaneous, minimally invasive, image-guided therapy in which the anticancer regimen is delivered to the arterial supply of the tumor. The most common therapies are transarterial chemoembolization (TACE) and radioembolization using yttrium-90 (^{90}Y).

DIFFERENTIAL DIAGNOSIS
- Differential diagnosis of the different types of hepatic neoplasms is made by using tissue biopsies, tumor markers, and imaging characteristics. Dynamic computed tomography (CT)/magnetic resonance imaging (MRI) demonstrating intense arterial uptake followed by venous or delayed phase "washout" of contrast is considered to be diagnostic of hepatocellular carcinoma (HCC).[1]
- TACE and radioembolization are usually performed in patients with liver-dominant disease. These tumors may be primary liver malignancies or metastatic disease where the liver is the dominant site of the disease.

PATIENT HISTORY AND PHYSICAL FINDINGS
- A thorough history should be obtained prior to treatment including a past medical history, medications, and allergies. Prior therapy should be evaluated, especially if radioembolization is being considered and the patient has previously had external beam radiation to the liver.
- Performance status (ECOG [Eastern Conference Oncology Group] or Karnofsky) must be evaluated. Patients with poor performance status may not be suitable candidates for intra-arterial therapy.
- Arterial pulse examination is needed for planning of the arterial access site. Typically, the puncture site is the common femoral artery, but this may need to be adjusted if the patient has severe iliofemoral atherosclerotic disease.

IMAGING AND OTHER DIAGNOSTIC STUDIES
- All patients should have a preprocedural multiphase CT or MRI examination. A positron emission tomography/CT may be helpful in some instances.
- Imaging should be evaluated for tumor number, tumor volume, and portal vein invasion/thrombosis. The vascular anatomy should be evaluated for vascular disease and anatomic variants as this may change the treatment plan.
- Laboratory evaluation should include a complete blood count, coagulation profile, creatinine, albumin, and liver function studies.
- Exclusionary criteria include immediate life-threatening extrahepatic disease, tumor volume greater than 50% to 70%, uncorrectable flow to the gastrointestinal (GI) tract, and significant hepatopulmonary shunting.

SURGICAL MANAGEMENT

Preoperative Planning
- Patients need to be well hydrated, typically with 150 to 300 mL per hour of normal saline prior to and during the procedure.
- Preprocedure medications may include antiemetics and steroids.
- Antibiotics are administered as needed. This is important in patients without an intact sphincter of Oddi due to sphincterotomy, biliary stent or catheter placement, and surgical biliary-enteric anastomosis. The regimen is 2 weeks in total, beginning 2 days prior to the embolization procedure.[2,3]
- Radioembolization is a multistep procedure with a need for arterial embolization of vessels leading to the GI tract and a simulation of the procedural injection prior to the actual injection of ^{90}Y particles. This will be discussed in more depth in the "Techniques" section.
- Proton pump inhibitors are started about 2 weeks prior to radioembolization.
- Octreotide pretreatment is indicated in patients with metastatic carcinoid to help prevent a carcinoid crisis. Typically, 250 µg is administered intravenously about 1 hour prior to the procedure.

Positioning
- The patient is placed supine with both groins prepped and draped (FIGURE 1). If there are iliac arterial occlusions or other technical problems, then brachial artery access is the next choice with the left arm being preferred. For brachial access, the arm is extended 45° to 90° away from the body.

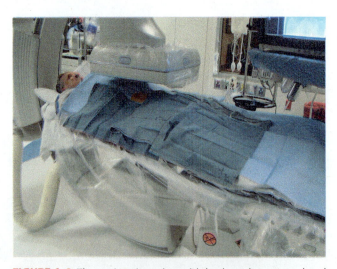

FIGURE 1 • The patient is supine with both groins prepped and draped. The C-arm fluoroscopic unit and monitors are in position to visualize the puncture site in the common femoral artery and the entire abdomen.

TRANSARTERIAL CHEMOEMBOLIZATION

Superior Mesenteric Arteriogram With Venous Phase Imaging

- A 4-Fr or 5-Fr catheter is used to selectively catheterize the superior mesenteric artery (SMA). The arterial phase (FIGURE 2) is inspected for anatomic variants such as a replaced right hepatic artery (FIGURE 3) or other anatomic variants. The potential for "parasitized" blood flow recruited from the SMA to the liver must also be assessed.
- The venous phase (FIGURE 4) is inspected to evaluate patency of the portal vein and to evaluate for hepatofugal flow. TACE can be performed in cirrhotic patients with hepatofugal portal flow, but a smaller volume of liver should be embolized each time.

Celiac and Common Hepatic Arteriograms

- The 4- or 5-Fr catheter is used to selectively catheterize these vessels. The arteriograms (FIGURE 5) are evaluated for anatomic variants such as a replaced or accessory left hepatic artery arising from a gastrohepatic trunk (FIGURE 6) and phrenic arteries, which may arise at the origin of the celiac.
- If the celiac artery is occluded, the occlusion can often be crossed and possibly stented to allow access or the procedure may be performed from the SMA in a retrograde approach via the pancreaticoduodenal arcade (FIGURE 7).
- Evaluate where the arterial supply to the tumors is arising. Try to limit embolization of branches that do not supply the tumors.

Advancement of the Catheter to Point of Embolization

- Commonly, this will be performed using a coaxial microcatheter.
- Advance the catheter as selectively as possible; however, a lobar embolization may be required if the tumors are scattered throughout the liver.

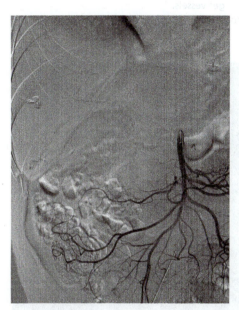

FIGURE 2 • A superior mesenteric arteriogram is obtained to evaluate for anatomic variants. The patient is positioned to visualize the portal vein during the venous phase of the examination.

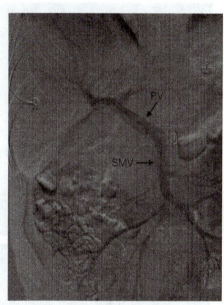

FIGURE 4 • Venous phase following a superior mesenteric arteriogram demonstrates patency of the superior mesenteric and portal veins (same patient as FIGURE 2). PV, portal vein; SMV, superior mesenteric vein.

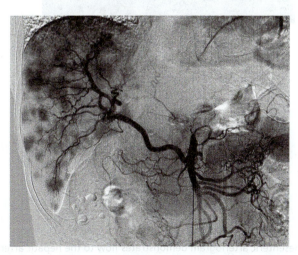

FIGURE 3 • The replaced right hepatic artery is one of the anatomic variants more commonly seen. The replaced right hepatic artery arises as a branch of the superior mesenteric artery.

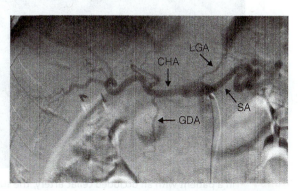

FIGURE 5 • Celiac arteriogram demonstrating typical celiac and hepatic arterial anatomy. CHA, common hepatic artery; GDA, gastroduodenal artery; LGA, left gastric artery; SA, splenic artery.

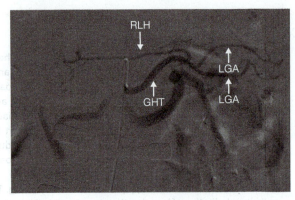

FIGURE 6 • The catheter tip is in a gastrohepatic trunk arising from the celiac artery. The replaced left hepatic artery supplies the left hepatic lobe, whereas the remaining left gastric artery branches supply the fundus of the stomach. When embolizing the replaced left hepatic artery, the catheter must be distal to the left gastric artery branches. GHT, gastrohepatic trunk; LGA, left gastric artery branches; RLH, replaced left hepatic artery.

- In patients with intact gallbladders, evaluate where the cystic artery originates (**FIGURE 8**). Ideally, embolization should be performed distal to the cystic artery. Treatment proximal to the cystic artery can cause a chemical cholecystitis with a more severe postembolization syndrome.
- Arteriogram to evaluate selective cannulation of the feeding vessel(s) and to assess for arteriovenous shunting.

Embolization Using the Embolic Material

- Oily chemoembolization
  - Ethiodol is a poppy seed oil–based contrast. The Ethiodol vehicle is mixed, most commonly with a combination of cisplatin, doxorubicin, and mitomycin-C. The Ethiodol acts as a carrier and the chemotherapy is released slowly from the mixture. The Ethiodol is retained within the tumor and the neovasculature of the tumor (**FIGURE 9**). This is followed by particulate embolization of the target vessels.
- Drug-eluting microspheres

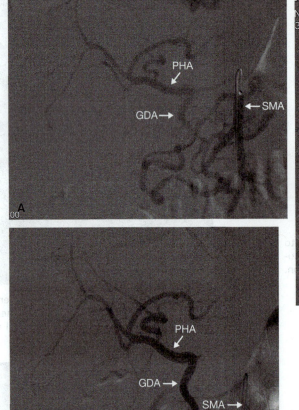

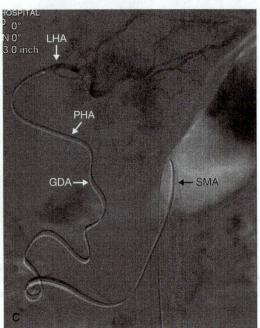

FIGURE 7 • In a patient with an occluded celiac artery, the superior mesenteric arteriogram demonstrates flow to the hepatic arteries via collateral supply (**A**). The pancreaticoduodenal arcade and gastroduodenal arteries are crossed in a retrograde fashion (**B**) with the microcatheter tip eventually placed in the left hepatic artery (**C**) for treatment of left lobar tumor. GDA, gastroduodenal artery; LHA, left hepatic artery; PHA, proper hepatic artery; SMA, superior mesenteric artery.

Chapter 18 **CATHETER-BASED TREATMENT OF HEPATIC NEOPLASMS** 141

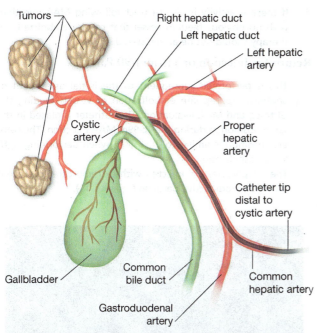

FIGURE 8 • The catheter tip is placed distal to the origin of the cystic artery prior to chemoembolization to prevent a chemical cholecystitis.

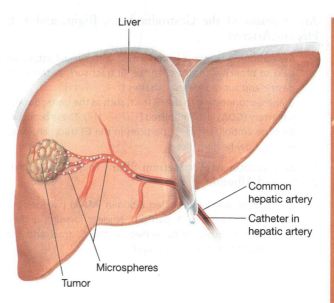

FIGURE 10 • Drug-eluting microspheres block the arterial supply to the tumor and then the chemotherapy drug is slowly released directly to the tumor.

- LC beads are a polyvinyl alcohol–based microsphere and QuadraSpheres are a copolymer microsphere.
- 50 to 75 mg of doxorubicin is loaded into each vial of microspheres with a maximum of two vials being used per procedure. 100 to 300 μm LC beads and 50 to 100 μm QuadraSpheres are commonly used. The particles are then injected (**FIGURE 10**) until there is significant slowing of flow within the target vessels.
- Irinotecan has been used, instead of doxorubicin, in treating patients with colorectal cancer that has metastasized to the liver.
- Transarterial embolization (TAE), also known as bland embolization, has also been performed. TAE uses Ethiodol embolization, particulate embolization, or a combination of both without the addition of any chemotherapeutic agent.

Removal of the Catheters and Sheath

- The puncture site is closed using manual pressure or an arterial closure device.

Follow-up

- Labs in about 4 weeks to evaluate liver function.
- Repeat imaging if needed.
- Repeat embolization, if needed, in about 4 to 6 weeks.

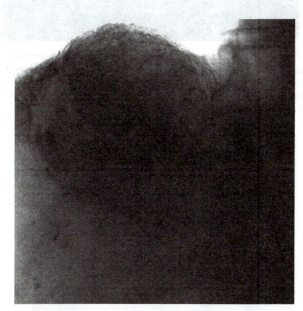

FIGURE 9 • Fluoroscopic image following oily chemoembolization shows the Ethiodol mixture within the tumor.

RADIOEMBOLIZATION

Sir-Spheres or TheraSphere

- ^{90}Y binds to particles that are less than 35 microns in size. Sir-Spheres are resin-based particles, whereas the TheraSphere particles are nonbiodegradable glass microspheres.

Superior Mesenteric, Celiac, and Common Hepatic Arteriograms

- The initial steps are similar to TACE. The arteriograms are evaluated for vessel patency and anatomic variants.

Arteriograms of the Gastroduodenal, Right, and Left Hepatic Arteries

- Evaluation of anatomy is performed with special attention paid to branches that lead to the GI tract such as the right gastric and supraduodenal arteries (**FIGURE 11**).
- Branches connecting to the GI tract, such as the gastroduodenal artery (GDA), are embolized (**FIGURE 12**). These branches must be embolized, as ^{90}Y particles in the GI tract can cause severe, slow-healing ulcers.

Lobar Injection of Technetium-99m (Tc 99m) Macroaggregated Albumin

- The Tc 99m macroaggregated albumin (MAA) particles are used to simulate the ^{90}Y particles. Nuclear imaging is then performed to evaluate for activity in the GI tract and the amount of shunting to the lungs (**FIGURE 13**).

- If there is activity in the GI tract following MAA injection, with no obvious feeding vessel that can be embolized, ^{90}Y therapy should not be administered.

Return for Injection of Yttrium-90 Particles

- This is performed subsequent to the initial assessment of anatomy, appropriate embolization of vessels feeding the GI tract, and MAA evaluation. The catheter is placed in the same position as during the Tc-99m MAA injection. The catheter position is similar to **FIGURE 8** when performing right lobar embolization.
- The ^{90}Y particles are injected with extreme care to prevent spillage of radioactive particles (**FIGURE 14**).

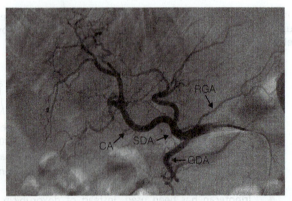

FIGURE 11 • Common hepatic arteriogram demonstrates the anatomy prior to Tc-99m MAA particle injection. Branches leading to the gastrointestinal tract will need to be embolized to prevent ^{90}Y particle reflux to these branches with subsequent injury. CA, cystic artery; GDA, gastroduodenal artery; RGA, right gastric artery; SDA, supraduodenal artery.

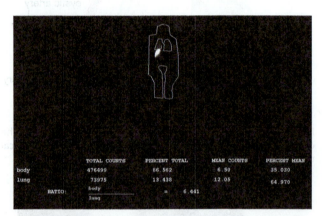

FIGURE 13 • Nuclear imaging following Tc-99m macroaggregated albumin administration demonstrates no activity within the gastrointestinal tract and 13.4% shunting to the lungs. The dose of Sir-Spheres to be given would be reduced by 20% due to the degree of shunting.

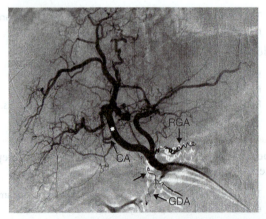

FIGURE 12 • An Amplatzer plug has been used to embolize the gastroduodenal artery (GDA) with microcoils within the right gastric artery (RGA) and supraduodenal arteries. The microcatheter would then be placed distal to the cystic artery (CA) origin for right lobar Tc-99m MAA and ^{90}Y injections (*asterisk*).

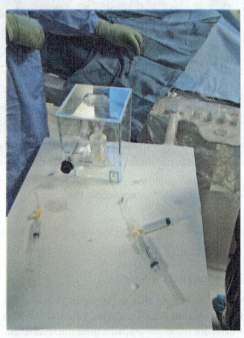

FIGURE 14 • The Sir-Spheres particles are connected to the catheter via a special delivery system to prevent spillage of radioactive material.

- If there is 10% to 15% hepatopulmonary shunting on the MAA study, then the Sir-Spheres dose is decreased by 20%. If the shunting is 15% to 20%, then the dose is decreased by 40%.
- If hepatopulmonary shunting is greater than 20%, then Sir-Spheres are not administered.
- When using TheraSphere, the limitation of what can be administered to the lungs is based on the cumulative dose, irrespective of the lung shunt.

Removal of the Catheters and Sheath

- The puncture site is closed using manual pressure or an arterial closure device.

Follow-Up

- Labs in about 4 weeks to evaluate liver function.
- Repeat imaging if necessary.
- Workup for the second lobar injection is begun about 4 to 6 weeks after the initial side if labs and imaging are adequate. The patient will need an arteriogram and repeat Tc-99m MAA injection as well, prior to radioembolization of the second lobe, if needed.

PEARLS AND PITFALLS

Patient history and physical findings	■ Patients without an intact sphincter of Oddi are at much higher risk of abscess formation and need extended antibiotic prophylaxis. ■ Do not overtreat in patients with borderline hepatic function. The procedure can always be repeated at a later time.
Imaging and other diagnostic studies	■ C-arm CT scan may be helpful to verify that the catheter is in the correct arterial branch as it may be difficult to tell with lesions that are not well visualized (FIGURE 15). ■ Hepatic tumors may be supplied by nonhepatic vessels, especially subcapsular lesions. Parasitized flow from the inferior phrenic, internal mammary, and intercostal arteries may need to be embolized (FIGURE 16). ■ It may be difficult to tell if there is arterial tumor enhancement on a contrasted CT scan with Ethiodol in place. A noncontrast scan (FIGURE 17) is needed for comparison or an MRI can be obtained.

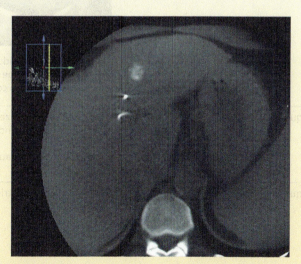

FIGURE 15 • C-arm CT shows tumoral enhancement demonstrating that the microcatheter is within the correct arterial branch prior to chemoembolization. The tumoral enhancement was not appreciated by conventional arteriography.

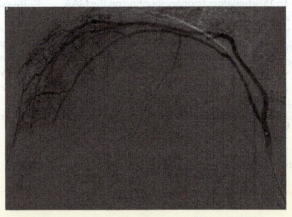

FIGURE 16 • Right inferior phrenic arteriogram demonstrates tumor enhancement in the dome of the liver supplied by the distal phrenic branches. These branches were then embolized.

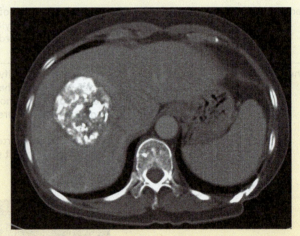

FIGURE 17 • CT scan demonstrates residual Ethiodol within a tumor on a noncontrast examination. A noncontrast examination must be obtained prior to the contrast-enhanced examination to demonstrate the difference between contrast enhancement and residual Ethiodol.

Surgical technique (TACE)	▪ Arterial-portal shunts can be embolized with large particles or coils prior to TACE. ▪ There are more postembolization syndrome symptoms with oily chemoembolization than with drug-eluting microspheres. ▪ Embolization of dome lesions may cause right shoulder pain or hiccups. Steroids (Medrol Dosepak) may be helpful.
Surgical technique (^{90}Y)	▪ Even though the GDA and right gastric arteries are embolized, do not inject ^{90}Y via the common or proper hepatic arteries.

POSTOPERATIVE CARE

- Pain medications
- Antiemetics
- Proton pump inhibitor (radioembolization)
- Steroids (Medrol Dosepak)
- Antibiotics (as indicated)
- Hospitalization for TACE is typically overnight for microsphere embolization and up to several days for oily chemoembolization. Patients that receive radioembolization can typically be discharged the same day.
- Repeat labs and imaging are typically obtained. Protocols are institution-specific and not typically driven by data.
- Further embolization procedures as needed. Imaging after TACE is about 4 to 6 weeks after the completion of embolization. If there is tumor identified on repeat imaging, then embolization is again performed. If no further tumor

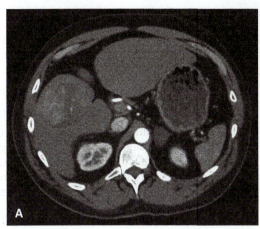
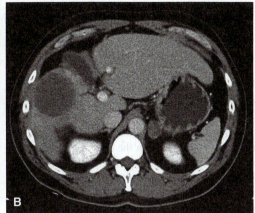

FIGURE 18 • **A,** Initial CT scan demonstrates a large, contrast-enhancing hepatocellular carcinoma in the right lobe of the liver prior to treatment. **B,** A follow-up CT 5 weeks after treatment using doxorubicin-loaded LC beads shows that the tumor is slightly smaller and there is no further contrast enhancement. Repeat imaging would then be performed about 3 months later.

is identified, then imaging is performed every 3 months (**FIGURE 18**).
- Imaging after radioembolization is performed 2 to 3 months after the last lobe is embolized as it can take longer to see the effects.

OUTCOMES

- In 2002, two separate studies demonstrated that TACE for HCC had a statistically significant survival advantage over the best supportive care that was available.[4,5] Since then, other studies have confirmed these findings in patients with well-compensated cirrhosis.
- In patients with limited hepatic reserve or decreased performance status, there have been better outcomes with drug-eluting microspheres as compared to oily chemoembolization.[6] In addition, the treatment was better tolerated by the patients.
- Treatment using drug-eluting microspheres loaded with doxorubicin demonstrated a statistically longer time to progression and fewer recurrences when compared to bland embolization.[7]
- Patients with HCC and Child-Pugh A disease survive significantly longer following ^{90}Y radioembolization than do those patients with Child-Pugh B disease, 17.7 vs 7.7 months, respectively.[8]
- In a study of patients with unresectable, chemoresistant liver metastases treated with ^{90}Y radioembolization, the median survival for patients was 15.2 months for those with colorectal tumors, 25.9 months for those with neuroendocrine tumors, and 6.9 months for those with noncolorectal, nonneuroendocrine tumors.[9]

COMPLICATIONS

- Groin hematoma/pseudoaneurysm
- Liver insufficiency
- Severe postembolization syndrome
- Routine postembolization syndrome is not an unexpected event. Postembolization syndrome includes pain, fever, and nausea/vomiting. Severe postembolization syndrome would necessitate an extended hospital stay or readmission.
- Hepatic abscess
- Cholecystitis
- Nontarget embolization with GI tract ulceration

REFERENCES

1. Bruix J, Sherman M, American Association for the Study of Liver Diseases. Management of hepatocellular carcinoma: an update. *Hepatology.* 2011;53:1020-1022.
2. Geschwind JF, Kaushik S, Ramsey DE, et al. Influence of a new prophylactic antibiotic therapy on the incidence of liver abscesses after chemoembolization treatment of liver tumors. *J Vasc Interv Radiol.* 2002;13:1163-1166.
3. Patel S, Tuite CM, Mondschein JI, et al. Effectiveness of an aggressive antibiotic regimen for chemoembolization in patients with previous biliary intervention. *J Vasc Interv Radiol.* 2006;17:1931-1934.
4. Lo CM, Ngan H, Tso WK, et al. Randomized controlled trial of transarterial lipiodol chemoembolization for unresectable hepatocellular carcinoma. *Hepatology.* 2002;35:1164-1171.
5. Llovet JM, Real MI, Montaña X, et al. Arterial embolisation or chemoembolisation versus symptomatic treatment in patients with unresectable hepatocellular carcinoma: a randomized controlled trial. *Lancet.* 2002;359:1734-1739.
6. Lammer J, Malagari K, Vogl T, et al. Prospective randomized study of doxorubicin-eluting-bead embolization in the treatment of hepatocellular carcinoma: results of the PRECISION V study. *Cardiovasc Intervent Radiol.* 2010;33:41-52.
7. Malagari K, Pomoni M, Kelekis A, et al. Prospective randomized comparison of chemoembolization with doxorubicin-eluting beads and bland embolization with BeadBlock for hepatocellular carcinoma. *Cardiovasc Intervent Radiol.* 2010;33:541-551.
8. Salem R, Lewandowski RJ, Mulcahy MF, et al. Radioembolization for hepatocellular carcinoma using Yttrium-90 microspheres: a comprehensive report of long-term outcomes. *Gastroenterology.* 2010;138:52-64.
9. Sato KT, Lewandowski RJ, Mulcahy MF, et al. Unresectable chemorefractory liver metastases: radioembolization with 90Y microspheres-safety, efficacy, and survival. *Radiology.* 2008;247:507-515.

Chapter 19 Segmental Hepatectomy

June S. Peng, Matthew E. Dixon, and Niraj J. Gusani

DEFINITION

- A segmental hepatectomy consists of surgical resection of one or more functional anatomic segments of the liver, as originally classified by Couinaud (**FIGURE 1**). Nomenclature for liver resections was standardized in the Brisbane conference.[1]
- The most common anatomic segmental resections are (1) right posterior sectionectomy (segments 6 and 7), (2) left lateral sectionectomy (segments 2 and 3), and (3) caudate lobe resection (segment 1).
- Resections of a single segment (with the exception of segment 1, the caudate lobe) or nonanatomic resections without formal inflow or outflow occlusion or delineation of the segmental vascular or biliary anatomy will not be covered in this chapter.
- Segmental resections can be performed using minimally invasive and open approaches.

PATIENT HISTORY AND PHYSICAL FINDINGS

- Patients should be good medical candidates for liver surgery.
- Preoperative planning requires knowledge of previous abdominal surgeries.
- Systemic staging should generally be performed in neoplastic and malignant processes for evaluation of extrahepatic disease. The presence of extrahepatic disease should be considered in conjunction with the tumor type and extent of resection to determine if the patient would benefit from surgery.
- History of jaundice, hepatitis, alcohol, drug abuse, and chemotherapy should be elicited to ascertain the health of the liver.
- Viral hepatitis panel should be obtained if appropriate.
- Liver function should be assessed by the Child-Pugh classification and/or the Model for End-Stage Liver Disease. Neither score has been definitively shown to be superior in determining a patient's ability to tolerate surgery.[2]

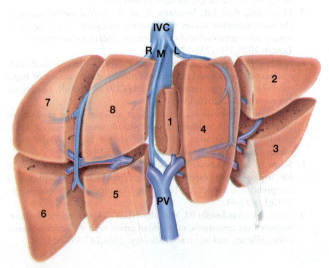

FIGURE 1 • Couinaud segments with vascular anatomy.

IMAGING AND OTHER DIAGNOSTIC STUDIES

- High-quality, multiphase, contrast-enhanced cross-sectional imaging with computed tomography or magnetic resonance imaging should be obtained to evaluate for extent of liver disease and to define anatomy. Both modalities are of similar sensitivity and may be used interchangeably or in combination.
- In a normal liver, a future liver remnant (FLR) composed of at least two contiguous segments with adequate inflow and outflow and measuring 20% of the total liver volume is sufficient to avoid postoperative liver failure. In patients heavily pretreated with systemic chemotherapy (especially >6 months), a higher FLR of at least 30% is desirable. In a cirrhotic liver, a remnant of greater than 40% is recommended, although the FLR may need to be even greater, depending on function of the liver. Segmental hepatic resections rarely induce hepatic insufficiency unless the remnant liver is severely diseased.
- Concern for significant hepatic dysfunction should be investigated with transjugular measurement of the portal pressure gradient (normal, <5 to 8 mm Hg), liver function tests, and biopsy to evaluate for steatosis or cirrhosis. A biopsy of the nontumor liver can also be helpful to assess the degree of liver damage.
- In Asia, indocyanine green clearance testing is often performed to quantify liver health. This is rarely performed in the United States.
- In patients with decompensated cirrhosis (Child B and Child C) and pathologic conditions that benefit from transplantation (hepatocellular cancer, neuroendocrine malignancies, and some hilar cholangiocarcinomas), surgeons should consider a referral for transplantation.

SURGICAL MANAGEMENT

- The indications for hepatectomy include diagnostic uncertainty, symptomatic benign lesions, and malignancy (**TABLE 1**).
- The strongest evidence for hepatic metastasectomy shows that R0 resection prolongs survival and is potentially curative for colorectal carcinomas and neuroendocrine tumors.

Preoperative Planning

- Preoperative cross-sectional imaging should be reviewed with skilled radiologists before surgery and be available throughout the procedure.
- Vascular, particularly hilar, arterial anomalies are common. Inadvertent injury at surgery may be prevented by thorough multiplanar analysis of preoperative imaging.
- 3-D reconstruction is not mandatory, but understanding of all lesions and their relationship to hepatic and portal venous structures is imperative and should be aided with intraoperative ultrasound.

Chapter 19 SEGMENTAL HEPATECTOMY 147

Table 1: Indications for Hepatectomy

Diagnosis
  Focal nodular hyperplasia vs hepatocellular adenoma
Symptoms
  Hemangioma
  Simple cysts
Benign disease
  Refractory abscesses/cholangitis
  Severe hepatolithiasis
Premalignant disease
  Hepatocellular adenoma
  Biliary cystadenoma
Malignancy
  Metastasis
  Hepatocellular carcinoma
  Cholangiocarcinoma

- For postoperative pain control, we employ epidural catheters or single-dose intrathecal morphine with transversus abdominis plane (TAP) blocks for open hepatectomy, and TAP blocks alone for minimally invasive resections with low risk of conversion.
- Low central venous pressure (CVP) anesthesia is a cornerstone in reducing blood loss in hepatic surgeries. To maintain low CVP (5-8 mm Hg), communication with the anesthesia team is critical. We utilize arterial lines for hemodynamic monitoring and rarely use central venous catheters. We typically aim for intravenous crystalloid rate of 1 mL/kg/h prior to specimen removal and utilize stroke volume variation and pulse pressure variation to guide intraoperative fluid management.
- Patients receive prophylactic antibiotics, generally a second- or third-generation cephalosporin for patients without stents, and a broad-spectrum antibiotic such as piperacillin/tazobactam for patients with indwelling stents.
- Most patients undergoing hepatectomy are at high risk for venous thromboembolic (VTE) disease due to age, malignancy, and lengthy major abdominal surgery. Unfractionated heparin is given prior to induction. Patients undergoing hepatectomy for malignant diagnoses are discharged with a 28-day course of low-molecular-weight heparin.

Positioning and Setup

- Open hepatectomy: Patients are generally positioned supine with arms abducted.
- Laparoscopic right posterior sectionectomy or caudate resections are aided by use of a split-leg table or by having the patient in modified lithotomy position with the surgeon between the patient's legs. For a right posterior sectionectomy, we bump up the right side and for extreme lateral right liver lesions, full lateral positioning may be used.
- Open or laparoscopic ultrasound should be routinely performed intraoperatively.
- For laparoscopic cases, we utilize a sealing device, cautery, dissector and scissors, laparoscopic paddle retractor (Medtronic, Minneapolis, MN), stapler with 30-mm curved tip vascular loads, and "quick stitches" (12-cm stitches with two clips on the end). Self-retaining balloon ports can be used to avoid port migration (Applied Medical, Rancho Santa Margarita, CA) and the AirSeal system (CONMED, Largo, FL) to assist with smoke evacuation without losing insufflation pressure.

- See ▶ Video 1.

RIGHT POSTERIOR SECTIONECTOMY (SEGMENTS 6 AND 7)

Exposure and Setup

- For open cases, a right subcostal (with left-sided or midline extension if needed), Makuuchi, or midline incision can be used. A fixed retraction system is employed.
- For laparoscopic cases, a number of different port setups can be used, and our approach is shown (FIGURE 2). The steps of a laparoscopic approach are similar in principle, and a hand-assist port can be placed if needed for hemostasis and retraction, and may be helpful during the learning curve.

Mobilization

- The round ligament is ligated but kept long to allow its use for retraction. The falciform ligament is divided close to the liver, thus minimizing interference from this structure during intraoperative ultrasonography (IOUS).
- Dissection of the apex of the right triangular ligament proceeds from medial to lateral. The peritoneum and areolar tissue surrounding the anterior and lateral aspects of the right hepatic vein (RHV) is cleared. To continue laterally and inferiorly, the liver can be retracted medially and compressed posteriorly.
- If caval compression induces hypotension, temporary release of retraction may be all that is required. Alternatively, raising the inferolateral edge of the right liver will expose the final attachments of the right triangular ligament.
- Complete mobilization of the right liver requires extensive exposure of the lateral and anterior surface of the inferior vena cava (IVC). Medial retraction and cephalad rotation of the inferolateral edge raises the liver off the IVC.
- A variable number of short hepatic vein branches drain the right hepatic lobe directly into the IVC. These should be carefully ligated using 4-0 ties and clips. We avoid use of clips on the hepatic side of these small vessels as they may interfere with parenchymal transection and reserve their use for the branches on the caval side.
- At the proximal and lateral aspects of the IVC, the caval ligament extends from segment 7 to the retroperitoneal tissue behind the IVC. This band can be vascular, and transection should be performed by ligation, stapling, or bipolar energy.

TECHNIQUES

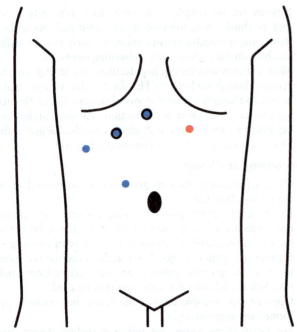

FIGURE 2 • Port setup for laparoscopic right posterior sectionectomy. Rummel tourniquet site indicated by red dot, 5-mm ports shown as solid blue dots, and 12-mm ports shown as blue dots with black outline.

Hilar Dissection and Vascular Control

- Anterior and cranial retraction of the falciform ligament exposes the hilum.
- Antegrade cholecystectomy is performed to expose the right lateral hilar plate.
- IOUS should be used routinely to examine the hepatic parenchyma for known and occult lesions. IOUS confirms vascular anatomy, identifies major vascular branches, and maps the proximity of hepatic and portal vein branches near the lesions.
- The gastrohepatic ligament is opened and an umbilical tape is placed around the porta hepatis and fashioned as a Rummel tourniquet for subsequent Pringle maneuver.
- Dissection begins at the right lateral edge of the hilar plate. Dissection on the contralateral side should be avoided to prevent inadvertent injury and to minimize scarring in case subsequent hepatectomy is required.
- In the right hilum, the right hepatic artery (RHA) is superficial and is dissected first. The RHA typically bifurcates as it enters the right liver. Both the anterior and posterior branches should be identified. A vascular loop facilitates gentle traction, and a bulldog clamp is then placed on the right posterior artery (**FIGURE 3**).
- Perfusion in the right anterior and proper hepatic artery (in the porta hepatis) as well as the left hepatic artery (LHA) should be confirmed by manual palpation, Doppler examination, or IOUS.
- If no deficit is noted, then the clamp may be removed and the posterior branch of the RHA can be divided between 2-0 silk ligatures and 3-0 Prolene suture ligatures. Division will expose the right portal vein (RPV) posteriorly and cephalad to the RHA.

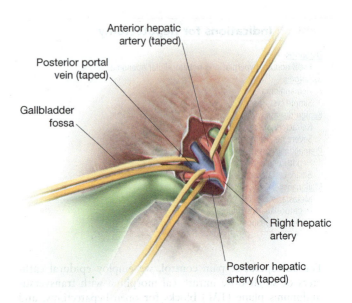

FIGURE 3 • The right portal pedicle is exposed, and the anterior and posterior branches are visualized prior to ligation of the right posterior hepatic artery and portal vein.

- The RPV dissection should identify anterior and posterior branches and left portal vein (LPV). Correct identification of the bifurcation of the RPV and LPV is imperative to avoid ligating or narrowing the main portal trunk or the takeoff of the LPV. During this exposure, posterior branches of the RPV to the caudate can be avulsed. These should be ligated or avoided as the dissection proceeds to avoid unnecessary bleeding. Further dissection along the circumference of the RPV should allow identification and isolation of the right anterior and right posterior branches. In some circumstances, a short segment hepatotomy of segment 6 may be used to access the posterior portal vein. Isolation of the posterior branch may be confirmed by IOUS. The posterior branch of the RPV is encircled with a vessel loop or Penrose drain to allow gentle traction.
- We routinely transect the posterior portal vein with a curved tip vascular stapler. Extreme care is taken during passage of the jaws of the stapler to avoid disruption of nearby vascular branches. If difficulty is encountered, the anvil jaw can be inserted into the opening of the Penrose drain and gentle withdrawal of the Penrose guides the stapler into the appropriate plane.
- We do not routinely perform extrahepatic division of the right posterior hepatic duct. Rather, we prefer to divide it during the parenchymal transection. This technique allows us to safely ligate the duct distal to the bifurcation and avoids unnecessary hilar dissection, which can devascularize or injure the biliary system.
- The posterior section should begin to demarcate. Inflow occlusion is now complete.
- The RHV is not routinely isolated for posterior sectionectomy, but branches are ligated intrahepatically during parenchymal transection.

Parenchymal Transection

- To begin transection, we use cautery to score Glisson capsule and circumferentially mark the line of transection. IOUS may be helpful to identify the extent of the lesion and to mark the medial margin and the locations of the segment 6 and 7 hepatic vein branches.
- The superficial 1 to 2 cm of parenchyma can be transected with an energy source. Bipolar, radiofrequency, or ultrasonic-generated heat energy can be used at the surgeon's preference.
- A Pringle maneuver may be applied to decrease bleeding during parenchymal transection.
- Stapling of the remaining hepatic parenchyma is our preferred means of completing the transection. The thin anvil side of the stapler is tunneled bluntly into the hepatic parenchyma. The stapler should be passed through the parenchyma without resistance. Resistance may indicate that the stapler is encountering the sidewall of a vessel. Forcing the stapler through these branches may cause significant bleeding. Alternatively, a groove for insertion of this end can be created by gentle passage of a closed curved clamp. Closure of the stapler is analogous to crushing the hepatic parenchyma with a metal clamp during the classical crush-clamp hepatic transection.
- Difficulty in closing or firing the stapler may be encountered when (1) too much tissue is between the jaws or (2) the right hepatic duct is ligated and divided.
- The crush-clamp technique can also be used. The energy device can be used to crush parenchyma and control small biliary and vascular branches, with circumferential dissection and stapler for larger branches.
- With the left hand holding the right liver, the line of transection can be controlled. With the fingers in the posterior groove, the IVC is protected and the endpoint of the transection is known at all times.
- For a complete or formal right posterior sectionectomy, the plane of transection should parallel the lateral aspect of the RHV (**FIGURE 4**).

Completion

- After the parenchyma is divided, the specimen is removed from the field. The specimen may be examined with ultrasound while submerged in water or saline to help confirm the adequacy of the surgical margin. We also routinely examine the specimen with the pathologist to orient the specimen, ink the appropriate margins, and assess gross and/or frozen margins intraoperatively.
- Hemostasis is achieved at the cut edge of the liver. We prefer the bipolar, saline-perfused radiofrequency ablation device, which is effective in sealing small vessels and bile ducts. Hemostatic agents and manual pressure can also be utilized.
- Care should be taken to avoid coagulating major biliary branches, as this may lead to subsequent stricture. Any area of bile leak, which might be near a larger bile duct, can also be ligated with absorbable monofilament suture.
- For areas of bleeding near the hilum, where energy devices may risk damage to crucial structures, we employ manual pressure and/or topical hemostatic agents and suturing when necessary.
- We do not routinely place a drain but one can be placed at the surgeon's preference.
- We reapproximate the falciform ligament to prevent rotation of the remnant that may result in kinking and possible occlusion or thrombosis of the hepatic veins.

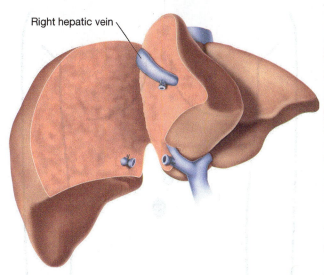

FIGURE 4 • For a complete or formal right posterior sectionectomy, the plane of transection should parallel the lateral aspect of the RHV.

LEFT LATERAL SECTIONECTOMY (SEGMENTS 2 AND 3)

Exposure and Setup

- For open cases, a midline incision is used.
- For laparoscopic cases, many options exist for port placement and our setup is shown (**FIGURE 5**). The steps of a laparoscopic approach are similar in principle to an open resection, and a video demonstrates our approach.

Mobilization

- The round ligament and falciform are divided.
- The left triangular ligament is mobilized. It may be helpful to place a laparotomy pad posterior to the left triangular ligament to help protect the gastroesophageal junction.
- The left hepatic vein (LHV) is cleared, and the surface is visualized extrahepatically.

Hilar Dissection and Vascular Control

- IOUS is used to mark the capsule where the LHV will be encountered. This visual reminder can be useful during parenchymal division.
- The gastrohepatic ligament is divided, including any aberrant LHA. A Rummel tourniquet is fashioned.
- Dissection begins at the left lateral edge of the round ligament, passing into the umbilical fissure.
- The branches of the LHA and LPV supplying the left lateral section can be individually isolated and ligated on the left

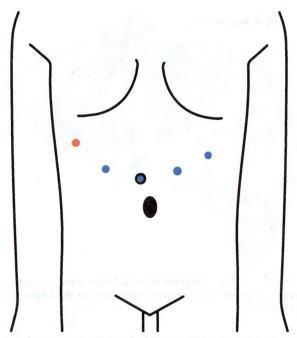

FIGURE 5 • Port setup for laparoscopic left lateral sectionectomy. Rummel tourniquet site indicated by red dot, 5-mm ports shown as solid blue dots, and 12-mm port shown as blue dot with black outline.

side of the round ligament and umbilical portion of the LPV. More proximal dissection on the main LHA and LPV is not necessary. Vascular control can be obtained by a Pringle maneuver, if needed (**FIGURE 6**).
- The LHV is not routinely isolated extrahepatically and is ligated or stapled intrahepatically during transection.

Parenchymal Transection and Completion

- Parenchymal transection can be completed as described in the previous section.
- At the most cranial part of the parenchymal transection, the LHV will be encountered and is best divided with a vascular stapler (**FIGURE 7**).

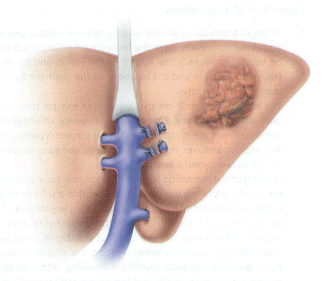

FIGURE 6 • The LPV is shown in the umbilical fissure. The left-sided branches to segments 2 and 3 require ligation or stapling.

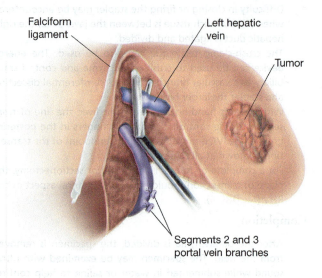

FIGURE 7 • The LHV is divided intraparenchymally with a stapler.

CAUDATE LOBE RESECTION (SEGMENT 1)

Exposure and Setup
- For open cases, a midline incision is used.
- For laparoscopic cases, our port setup is shown (**FIGURE 8**).

Mobilization
- The left triangular ligament is mobilized.
- For larger tumors or tumors that are close to the caudate isthmus, complete mobilization of the right liver is also necessary, including division of the short hepatic branches.
- The peritoneum and areolar tissue surrounding the lateral aspect of the LHV is cleared.
- The gastrohepatic ligament is divided. If an aberrant LHA is present, there should be an attempt to preserve it. However, division of the LHA may be necessary for adequate exposure. After this mobilization is complete, the left liver can be rotated anteromedially to visualize the caudate lobe (**FIGURE 9**).
- IOUS is performed to examine the liver for known and occult lesions.
- The arterial and portal venous inflow arises as smaller posterior branches off the main or left hilar structures.

Chapter 19 SEGMENTAL HEPATECTOMY

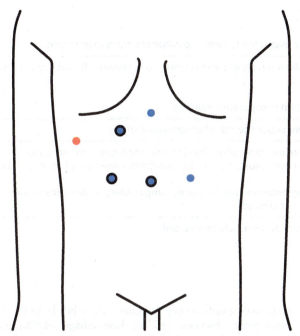

FIGURE 8 • Port setup for laparoscopic caudate resection. Rummel tourniquet site indicated by red dot, 5-mm ports shown as solid blue dots, and 12-mm ports shown as blue dots with black outline.

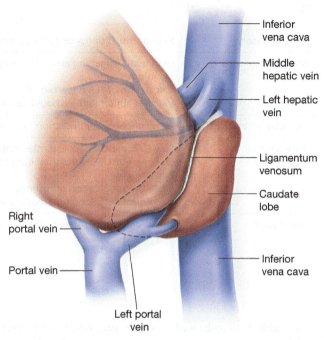

FIGURE 9 • With rotation of the left liver, the caudate lobe is seen in relation to the LHV, ligamentum venosum, the IVC, and a major branch from the LPV.

- The caudate branches to the hilar vessels and bile duct are identified on the anterior surface of the caudate. These can be ligated using energy devices, ligatures, or clips.
- Dissection begins by dividing the caudate isthmus, which crosses anterior to the IVC and fuses with segment 6 at the left lateral edge of the ligamentum teres passing into the umbilical fissure.
- Caudate outflow is via small veins directly into the IVC and the RPV. These should be ligated individually.
- The posterior surface of confluence of the hepatic veins, particularly the middle and left hepatic veins, overlies the cephalad-most aspect of the caudate lobe (FIGURE 10). Safe dissection here requires good mobility of the right and left lobes of the liver.

Parenchymal Transection and Completion

- As described above

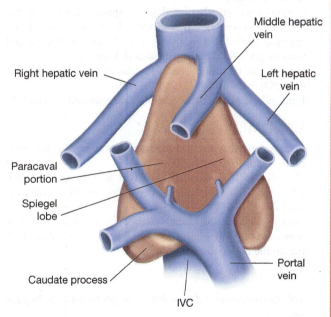

FIGURE 10 • The upper pole of the caudate lobe lies between the IVC and the confluence of the middle and left hepatic veins.

PEARLS AND PITFALLS

Patient history	• Hepatic insufficiency or damage should be evaluated to reduce posthepatectomy liver failure.
Imaging and testing	• High-quality imaging and a thorough understanding of patient anatomy is essential for proper surgical planning. • Calculation of FLR is warranted. • Vascular abnormalities should be detailed on preoperative imaging.
Vascular isolation	• Avoid unnecessary dissection in order to minimize the risk of contralateral injury.
Parenchymal transection	• Low CVP anesthesia is essential to minimize intraoperative blood loss during hepatic transection. • Stapling quickly divides the hepatic parenchyma, vasculature, and bile ducts, minimizing blood loss and bile leaks. • Small venous bleeders encountered during dissection can be simply tamponaded, sealed with an electrosurgical device, or, on occasion, sutured or clipped.
Hemostasis	• Use of energy near major biliary or hilar structures should be avoided.

POSTOPERATIVE CARE

- We utilize an enhanced recovery pathway (ERAS) that defines routine postoperative care.
- VTE prophylaxis is continued, including on the day of surgery as appropriate.
- Prophylactic antibiotics are continued to finish within 24 hours of surgery.
- Patients are routinely placed on phosphorus-containing fluids postoperatively, and electrolyte levels are checked and repleted. Daily brain natriuretic peptide level is checked and used to guide fluid management and diuresis.
- Patients are typically given a low-fat diet by postoperative day (POD) 1.
- Epidurals, if placed preoperatively, are removed on POD 2.

OUTCOMES

- In experienced centers, mortality is less than 3% and morbidity is approximately 20%.[3]
- Overall and disease-specific survival at 5 years can reach 69% and 72%, respectively, depending on the underlying pathology.[4]
- Neoadjuvant or adjuvant systemic treatment, a total of 6 months of perioperative therapy, is recommended depending on the underlying pathology.[5]

COMPLICATIONS

- Volume-outcomes relationships are prominent in hepatic resection.
- Outcomes specific to hepatectomy include bile leaks (5.9%), perihepatic abscesses (3.7%), hemorrhage (0.9%), and hepatic insufficiency (3.1%).[6]
- Bile leaks can be managed by percutaneous drainage or endoscopic retrograde cholangiopancreatography with sphincterotomy to facilitate internal drainage.

REFERENCES

1. Strasberg SM. Terminology of liver anatomy and resections: the Brisbane 2000 terminology. In: Clavien PA, Sarr M, Fong Y, eds. *Atlas of Upper Gastrointestinal and Hepato-Pancreato-Biliary Surgery*. Springer; 2007:313-317.
2. Teh SH, Nagorney DM, Stevens SR, et al. Risk factors for mortality after surgery in patients with cirrhosis. *Gastroenterology*. 2007;132(4):1261-1269.
3. Hamed OH, Bhayani NH, Ortenzi G, et al. Simultaneous colorectal and hepatic procedures for colorectal cancer result in increased morbidity but equivalent mortality compared with colorectal or hepatic procedures alone: outcomes from the National Surgical Quality Improvement Program. *HPB*. 2013;15(9):695-702.
4. Nikfarjam M, Shereef S, Kimchi ET, et al. Survival outcomes of patients with colorectal liver metastases following hepatic resection or ablation in the era of effective chemotherapy. *Ann Surg Oncol*. 2009;16(7):1860-1867.
5. National Comprehensive Cancer Network. *NCCN Clinical Practice Guidelines: Colon Cancer*. National Comprehensive Cancer Network. Accessed September 2, 2013. http://www.nccn.org/professionals/physician_gls/PDF/colon.pdf
6. Zimmitti G, Roses RE, Andreou A, et al. Greater complexity of liver surgery is not associated with an increased incidence of liver-related complications except for bile leak: an experience with 2,628 consecutive resections. *J Gastrointest Surg*. 2013;17(1):57-64. discussion 64-65.

Chapter 20 | Minimally Invasive Segmental Hepatic Resection

Timothy E. Newhook and Hop S. Tran Cao

DEFINITION
- The Tokyo 2020 terminology of liver anatomy and resections update to the Brisbane 2000 system defines anatomical segmentectomy as the complete resection of territory or territories supplied by the third-order portal venous branches of a Couinaud segment.[1]

RATIONALE
- The use of parenchymal-sparing hepatectomy has greatly increased over recent times, and many studies have revealed equivalent outcomes compared with anatomic resection. In view of this, segmental hepatectomy may be preferable as opposed to larger, more complex hepatectomy (ie, right or left hepatectomy) in order to preserve hepatic parenchyma, which is an important concept, particularly in the surgical management of colorectal cancer liver metastases (CLM).
- Parenchymal-sparing approaches are associated with lower postoperative morbidity and liver failure compared with anatomic resection. Moreover, these approaches have been associated with equivalent outcomes compared with anatomic resection even for patients with high-risk biology, such as those with *KRAS*-mutated CLM.[2]

APPROACH
- Minimally invasive hepatectomy can be performed via a laparoscopic approach, hand-assisted laparoscopic surgery approach, and, more recently, using a robotic-assisted laparoscopic approach.

PATIENT HISTORY AND PHYSICAL FINDINGS
- Indications for hepatectomy include primary and secondary malignant tumors in the liver, as well as well-selected benign liver lesions (eg, hepatic adenomas or symptomatic benign tumors).
- A detailed medical and surgical history is imperative with close attention to prior abdominal incisions that may impact minimally invasive access or approaches.

PREOPERATIVE IMAGING
- Liver-specific triple-phase contrast-enhanced computed tomography scans with axial, coronal, and sagittal reformats are critical for operative planning (**FIGURE 1**). Magnetic resonance imaging with Eovist is another complementary imaging modality.
- It is important to delineate intrahepatic structures that will be encountered during hepatic transection, areas of concern for an R0 resection, and vascular anatomic variants.

SURGICAL MANAGEMENT

Preoperative Planning
- Ensure that the patient has sufficient cardiopulmonary reserve to tolerate pneumoperitoneum.
- It is important to recognize prior surgical scars and areas of potential adhesions, as well as limitations to establishing pneumoperitoneum.
- For robotic-assisted laparoscopic hepatectomy, camera port positioning is critical for effective robotic arm use and ports must be placed to minimize exterior collisions.

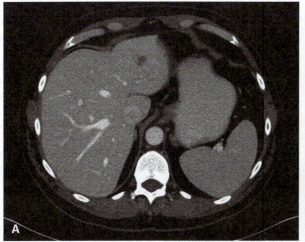 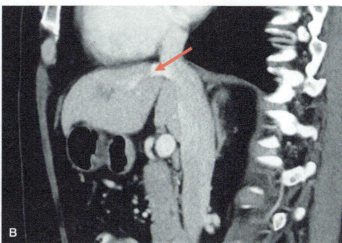

FIGURE 1 • Computed tomography demonstrating a segment II/III colorectal liver metastasis status post preoperative chemotherapy. **A**, axial imaging reveals a 1.0 × 1.3 cm mass and **B**, sagittal reformatted imaging illustrates proximity to the left hepatic vein (*red arrow*).

Positioning

- Patients may be placed supine with arms out for access by the anesthesia team, and patients must be safely strapped to allow for operating table movement.
- Once pneumoperitoneum is established and prior to robot docking, the patient should be placed in reverse Trendelenburg position. For tumors located in the right posterior section, the table is also tilted toward the left side. Alternatively, the patient's right side may be propped up on a bump.

TECHNIQUES

ROBOTIC-ASSISTED BISEGMENTECTOMY 2/3

- Also termed a left lateral sectionectomy, this operation is commonly performed for lesions within segments 2 and 3 that are not amenable to nonanatomic partial hepatectomy.

Port Placement and Instruments

- Port placement is mapped out after pneumoperitoneum has been established to ensure appropriate positioning relative to the target anatomy.
- We avoid placing trocars through the midline, especially through the umbilicus.
- The first robotic port is placed to the right and slightly cephalad to the umbilicus, and additional trocars are introduced under direct visualization across the abdomen (all 8-mm trocars; FIGURE 2).
- The robotic camera is inserted into arm 2, and fenestrated bipolar in arm 1, vessel sealer to be alternated with the monopolar hook in arm 3, and Cadiere forceps in arm 4.
- A 12-mm assistant port with AirSeal is placed in the patient's right lower quadrant or at the anticipated site of extraction at the Pfannenstiel incision.

- Pneumoperitoneum is limited to 12 mm Hg to reduce the risk of gas embolism.
- We routinely plan for inflow control and introduce either an umbilical tape around the porta hepatitis and through a chest tube inserted through the R lower quadrant or a urinary catheter looped onto itself. Compression is applied only if needed, and as in the open setting, would be limited to 15-minute increments with 5-minute breaks in between.

Mobilization of the Left Liver

- The falciform ligament is mobilized from the anterior abdominal wall using the vessel sealer, and the falciform ligament is transected to the hepatocaval confluence.
- The left triangular ligament is dissected from its diaphragmatic attachments (FIGURE 3).

Exposure of the Segment II/III Portal Pedicles

- The liver anterior to the umbilical fissure is transected using vessel sealer, and larger crossing structures are clipped.
- The left side of the umbilical fissure structures is exposed, revealing the segment III then II portal pedicles, which are individually dissected, encircled, and divided with a vascular load of an endoscopic stapler or tied and clipped (FIGURE 4).

Parenchymal Transection and Left Hepatic Vein

- Transection of the hepatic parenchyma continues along the line of demarcation toward the origin of the left hepatic vein.
- Parenchymal transection is performed using the vessel sealer with a crush and clamp technique, followed by bipolar cautery and transection with the same instrument. Moderate-sized structures are clipped on the patient side and transected with the vessel sealer.
- Parenchymal transection continues to the origin of the left hepatic vein, which is encircled, tied, clipped, and divided proximal to its insertion into the inferior vena cava at the hepatocaval confluence (FIGURE 5).
- The remainder of the specimen is transected and placed in a specimen bag.
- The cut surface of the liver is inspected for bleeding and bile leak using a clean gauze, and any hemostasis is ensured using bipolar cautery.
- Bile leaks may be controlled with direct suture ligation.
- The robot is then undocked and abdomen desufflated.
- The specimen is then retrieved via a Pfannenstiel incision, and ports are removed.
- The robotic port sites skin is closed without the need for fascial closure; however, the assistant 12-mm port site fascia is closed either directly with 0-0 Vicryl suture or the abdomen is reinsufflated and a suture passing device is used to close the fascia.

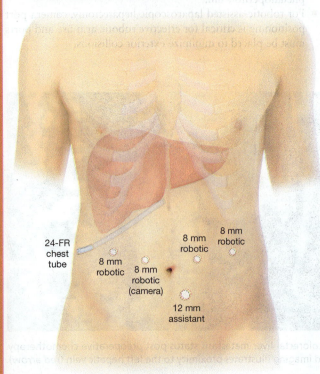

FIGURE 2 • Port placement and setup for robotic-assisted bisegmentectomy 2/3.

Chapter 20 MINIMALLY INVASIVE SEGMENTAL HEPATIC RESECTION 155

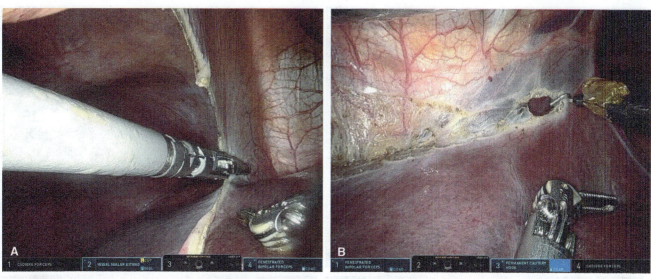

FIGURE 3 • Mobilization of segments II and III. **A,** transection of the falciform ligament and **B,** dissection of the hepatocaval confluence and left triangular ligament.

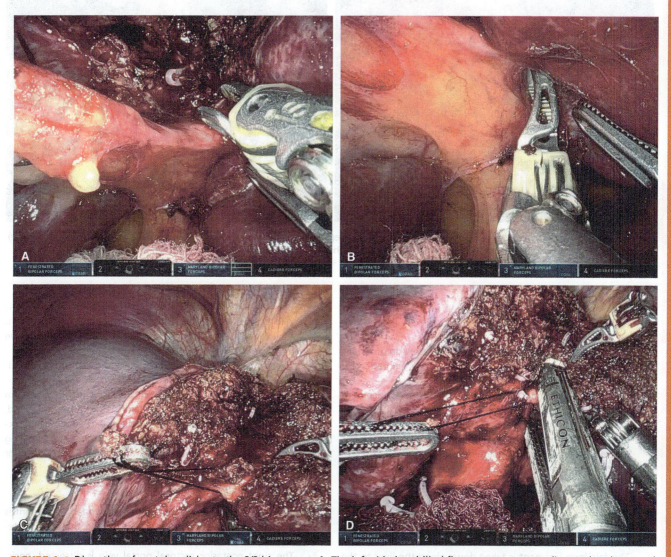

FIGURE 4 • Dissection of portal pedicles to the 2/3 bisegment. **A,** The left-sided umbilical fissure structures are dissected and exposed, hepatic parenchyma is transected adjacent to the segment III pedicle, and **B,** are encircled and **C,** controlled with a suture or vessel loop. **D,** The individual segment II and III pedicles are then transected with a vascular load of either the laparoscopic or robotic stapler.

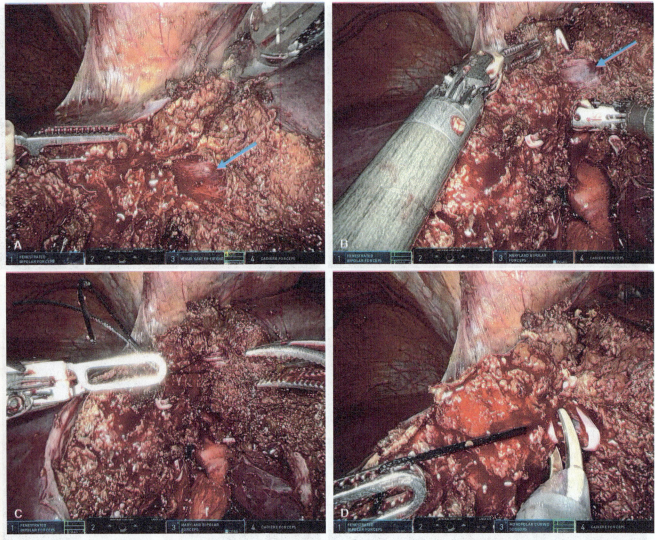

FIGURE 5 • Hepatic transection continues through toward the hepatocaval confluence, **A**, exposing the left hepatic vein (*blue arrow*). **B**, The left hepatic vein is encircled (*blue arrow*), **C**, controlled with a suture tie or vessel loop, **D**, clipped and divided.

ROBOTIC-ASSISTED RIGHT POSTERIOR SECTORECTOMY

- Right posterior sectorectomy involves the resection of lesions in segments 6 and 7 and/or involving the right hepatic vein (**FIGURE 6**).
- Establishing pneumoperitoneum and robotic port placement is similar to prior described bisegmentectomy 2/3 but may bias to the patient's right side.
- Ensuring that the operative table is paired with the robotic platform will ensure adequate positioning with 10 to 12 degrees of reverse Trendelenburg position and slight tilt toward the patient's left.

Mobilization of the Right Liver

- A cholecystectomy is performed initially if a gallbladder remains in situ.
- The falciform ligament is taken down along the liver to the hepatocaval confluence.
- The hepatocaval confluence is dissected and the right hepatic vein is exposed. The dissection is continued anteriorly from the liver and lateral to the right hepatic vein to mobilize the right liver from the diaphragm.
- The right liver is then retracted anteriorly, and the right triangular ligament is taken down.
- The liver is then dissected from the right retroperitoneum using cautery, taking care to avoid the right adrenal gland. With adequate retraction using the fourth arm, the dissection may continue to expose the inferior vena cava, taking care to clip or tie larger short draining veins to the inferior vena cava as needed (**FIGURE 7**).

Dissection of Right Posterior Portal Pedicle

- The right lateral aspect of the hepatoduodenal ligament is dissected toward Rouviere sulcus, exposing the right posterior sectoral portal vein (**FIGURE 8**).
- The right posterior sectoral portal vein is dissected, encircled with a tie for traction, clipped, and divided. The right

Chapter 20 MINIMALLY INVASIVE SEGMENTAL HEPATIC RESECTION 157

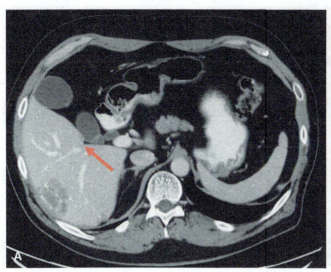 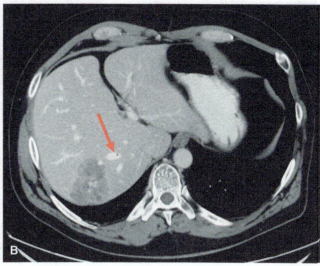

FIGURE 6 • Computed tomography demonstrating a segment VI and VII colorectal liver metastasis status post preoperative chemotherapy. Axial imaging reveals masses in segment VI (red arrow: Rouviere sulcus **(A)** and segment VII with proximity to the distal right hepatic vein (*red arrow*) **(B)**.

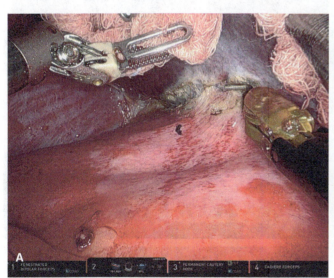 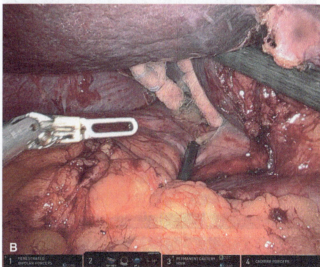

FIGURE 7 • Retroperitoneal dissection and mobilization of the right liver. **A,** The retroperitoneal attachments of the right liver are dissected using cautery and with appropriate retraction **B,** mobilization to the inferior vena cava is achieved.

posterior sectoral hepatic artery is similarly dissected, controlled, and divided.
- Demarcation of the right posterior sector ensues and can be confirmed via indocyanine green injection. The line of demarcation is marked along the hepatic capsule with electrocautery.

Parenchymal Transection and Right Hepatic Vein

- Vessel loops are sutured to either side of the line of demarcation and externalized via stab incisions in the abdominal wall with a suture passer. This facilitates visualization and retraction during parenchymal transection to "open the book" (**FIGURE 9**).

- Parenchymal transection is performed using the vessel sealer with a crush and clamp technique, followed by bipolar cautery and transection with the same instrument. Moderate-sized structures are clipped on the patient side and transected with the vessel sealer.
- Transection of the hepatic parenchyma continues along the line of demarcation toward the right hepatic vein. Once the right hepatic vein is visualized, transection continues toward the hepatocaval confluence keeping the right hepatic vein to the specimen side of dissection.
- The bile ducts to segments 6 and 7 are encountered intrahepatically, dissected, clipped, and divided. Alternatively, these may be stapled or tied and transected.

158 SECTION II SURGERY OF THE LIVER

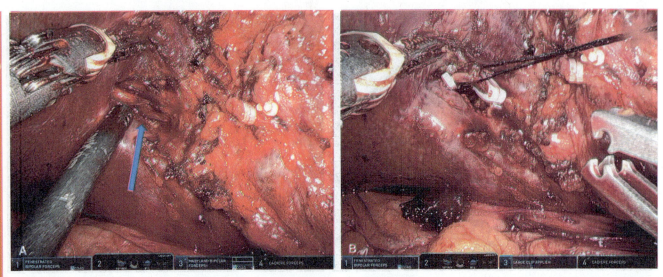

FIGURE 8 • Dissection of the right posterior portal pedicle. **A,** The sulcus of Rouviere is dissected to reveal the right posterior portal pedicle (blue arrow), which is encircled with a silk tie for manipulation/traction. **B,** Using the silk tie for traction, the right posterior portal pedicle is clipped and divided.

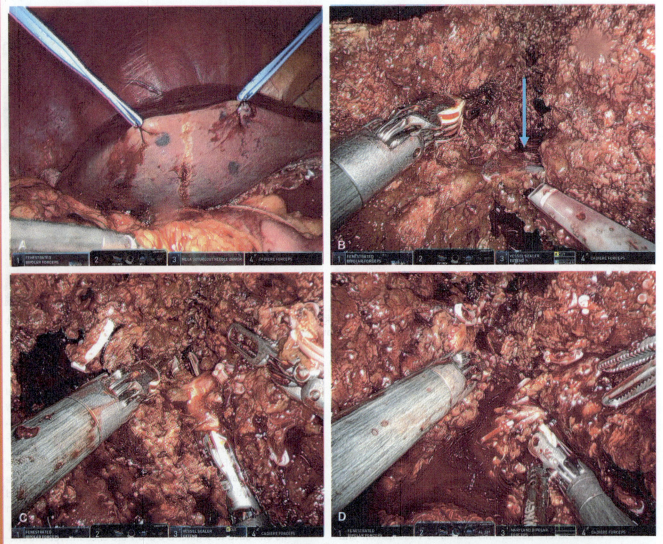

FIGURE 9 • Hepatic transection. **A,** The liver capsule is marked along the line of demarcation, and vessel loops are secured to the liver capsule and drawn transabdominally via suture passer to provide retraction. **B,** Hepatic transection initiates to identify the right hepatic vein (blue arrow) and continues along the left side of the vein. **C,** The right posterior pedicle is encountered intrahepatically, encircled with a silk tie, clipped, and divided. **D,** The distal right hepatic vein is encircled, tied with a silk suture, clipped, and divided.

- Once at the hepatocaval confluence, the right hepatic vein is encircled with a silk tie and ligated, clipped, and divided.
- The right posterior sector is then dissected from the remainder of right hemidiaphragm and placed in a specimen bag.
- The remainder of the specimen is transected and placed in a specimen bag.
- The cut surface of the liver is inspected for bleeding and bile leak using a clean gauze, and any hemostasis is ensured using bipolar cautery.
- Bile leaks may be controlled with direct suture ligation.
- The robot is then undocked and abdomen desufflated.
- The specimen is then retrieved via a Pfannenstiel incision, and ports are removed.
- The robotic port sites skin is closed without the need for fascial closure; however, the assistant 12-mm port site fascia is closed either directly with 0-0 Vicryl suture or the abdomen is reinsufflated and a suture passing device is used to close the fascia.

PEARLS AND PITFALLS

Pitfalls	
	- Port placement in the cephalad-caudad axis is critical so as not to be too close, or too far from your target anatomy.
	- Inflow occlusion via Pringle maneuver, while not absolutely necessary, can be quite helpful if parenchymal bleeding occurs during hepatic transection. Therefore, we advocate for securing inflow occlusion early in the operation so it is ready for use.
	- Misidentification of structures, particularly in the hepatoduodenal ligament can lead to complications. Indocyanine green injection can be helpful for robotic-assisted hepatic segmentectomy for early vasculature and later biliary ductal identification, and may help guide hepatic transection via both positive or negative staining of the target segments. While beyond the scope of this chapter, fluorescence-guided surgery may be helpful.

REFERENCES

1. Wakabayashi G, Cherqui D, Geller DA, et al. The Tokyo 2020 terminology of liver anatomy and resections: updates of the Brisbane 2000 system. *J Hepatobiliary Pancreat Sci*. 2022;29:6-15.
2. Joechle K, Vreeland TJ, Vega EA, et al. Anatomic resection is not required for colorectal liver metastases with RAS mutation. *J Gastrointest Surg*. 2020;24(5):1033-1039.

Chapter 21 | Right Hepatectomy

Rebecca A. Snyder and Alexander A. Parikh

DEFINITION

- A right hepatectomy (or hemihepatectomy) consists of surgical resection of the right hemiliver, consisting of Couinaud segments 5, 6, 7, and 8 (**FIGURE 1**). Nomenclature for liver resections was standardized in the Brisbane conference.[1]

PATIENT HISTORY AND PHYSICAL FINDINGS

- A thorough medical evaluation and assessment of performance status is critical prior to consideration for resection.
- An evaluation of underlying liver disease should include a complete history, including assessment of prior episodes of jaundice, hepatitis exposure, alcohol use, sequelae of cirrhosis and/or portal hypertension, and prior treatment with chemotherapy including type of agents as well as duration of therapy.
- A complete metabolic panel including liver function tests, bilirubin, albumin, as well as complete blood count and a coagulation panel should be obtained in all patients being considered for a major liver resection. A complete viral hepatitis panel may also be considered for potential surgical candidates.
- Thorough assessment of the health of the remnant liver and future liver remnant volume is critical.
- Physical examination findings of chronic liver disease or hepatic insufficiency should prompt further evaluation if the patient remains a surgical candidate.
- If performing a metastasectomy, a thorough evaluation for extrahepatic disease should be performed. Computed tomography (CT) is considered standard of care; a positron emission tomography scan is appropriate in select patients. Findings of extrahepatic disease should prompt multidisciplinary discussion and careful reconsideration of major hepatectomy.
- In appropriate, medically operable patients, resectability is now only limited by the need to preserve adequate hepatic inflow, outflow, and functional hepatic reserve.

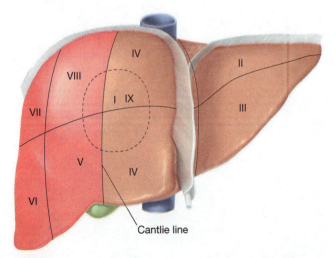

FIGURE 1 • Couinaud segments with right hepatectomy depicted.

- Risk of perioperative morbidity and mortality can be assessed by the Child-Pugh classification or Model for End-Stage Liver Disease (MELD) score, both of which have been correlated with postoperative morbidity and mortality in patients with cirrhosis.[2-5]

IMAGING AND OTHER DIAGNOSTIC STUDIES

- Contrasted cross-sectional imaging is essential in diagnosis and evaluation of suitability for surgery.
- Triple-phase CT (arterial phase, portal venous phase, and hepatic venous phase) is most useful for assessing the relationship of a tumor to vascular structures.
- Magnetic resonance imaging is more sensitive for detection of subcentimeter lesions and is helpful in distinguishing between benign and malignant liver masses.
- In a normal, healthy liver, a future liver remnant (FLR) measuring 20% of the total liver volume constitutes sufficient functional liver volume. In patients with prior chemotherapy exposure, an FLR of 30% is recommended, and in a cirrhotic liver, an FLR greater than 40% is recommended.[6-10]
- When performing a standard right hepatectomy, the remnant left hemiliver is usually of adequate size in a healthy liver. In most cases, this does not require formal volumetric analysis; however, liberal use of volumetry is recommended in patients with underlying liver disease or prior chemotherapy exposure to decrease the risk of postoperative hepatic insufficiency (**FIGURE 2**). In the event of marginal remnant volume, preoperative right portal vein embolization can promote hypertrophy of the FLR.[6]
- Hepatic steatosis can be evaluated by comparison of the densities of liver and spleen on noncontrast images. Significant steatosis can suggest a liver remnant at risk of postoperative failure.
- Patients with a history or laboratory or radiographic findings concerning for significant hepatic injury or dysfunction may be referred for invasive testing of the liver, such as transjugular measurement of the portal pressure gradient (normal <5-8 mm Hg) and/or liver biopsy (to evaluate steatosis or cirrhosis).
- Patients with evidence of decompensated cirrhosis (Child Pugh class B or C) are not candidates for right hepatectomy but may be candidates for liver transplantation in the setting of hepatocellular carcinoma.

SURGICAL MANAGEMENT

- The indications for right hepatectomy include symptomatic benign lesions and malignancy (**TABLE 1**).
- Margin-negative resection of metastatic colorectal cancer has been clearly shown to improve long-term survival, with current 5-year overall survival of approximately 50%.[11,12]
- Parenchymal-sparing or nonanatomic resection is advocated when feasible to preserve normal hepatic parenchyma and

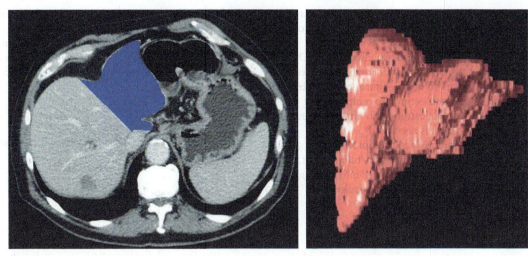

FIGURE 2 • CT volumetry for a right hepatectomy. The calculated future liver remnant (segments I–IV depicted in blue) represents 30% of the total liver volume.

Table 1: Indications for Hepatectomy	
Benign	**Malignant**
Symptomatic hemangioma Hepatic adenoma Biliary cystadenoma Symptomatic focal nodular hyperplasia Traumatic injury	**Primary malignant liver tumors** Intrahepatic cholangiocarcinoma Perihilar cholangiocarcinoma (Klatskin tumor) Hepatocellular carcinoma Biliary cystadenocarcinoma **Secondary malignant tumors** Colorectal liver metastases Neuroendocrine liver metastases Other selected liver metastases (melanoma, breast, renal cell carcinoma etc)

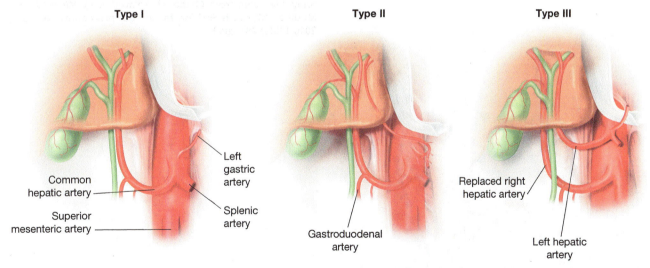

FIGURE 3 • Common variants of hepatic arterial anatomy. Type 1 is considered "standard." Type 2 shows an accessory left hepatic artery (HA) (native left HA present). Type 3 shows an aberrant (replaced) right HA (native right HA absent).

allow for future resection in the setting of recurrent disease. However, formal right hepatectomy is often necessary due to the anatomic relationship of tumor(s) to biliary or vascular structures or the presence of multiple metastatic lesions within the right hemiliver, which would not allow for preservation of sufficient liver parenchyma or a margin-negative resection.

Perioperative Planning

- Preoperative cross-sectional imaging should be carefully reviewed by the surgeon and, if possible, at multidisciplinary tumor board, prior to consideration for resection.
- Hepatic arterial anomalies are common (**FIGURE 3**). Inadvertent injury during an operation can be prevented by thorough preoperative evaluation and multiplanar analysis.

- Three-dimensional (3-D) reconstruction is not mandatory, but an understanding of all the lesions and the relation to hepatic and portal venous structures is imperative. This should be combined with intraoperative ultrasound (IOUS).
- Fluid restriction and maintenance of a low central venous pressure (CVP) is critical to reduce intraoperative blood loss during parenchymal transection. To maintain low CVP (≤5 mm Hg), good communication with the preoperative nursing and anesthesia teams is necessary.
- Patients should receive prophylactic antibiotics with gram negative coverage due to transection of the biliary tract. The authors consider cases with an indwelling biliary device as contaminated and routinely send stents for culture.
- Patients undergoing hepatectomy are at high risk for venous thromboembolic (VTE) events due to age, presence of malignancy, and complex, long major abdominal surgery. Unfractionated heparin or low-molecular-weight heparin can be given subcutaneously prior to induction and redosed every 8 hours as needed.

Positioning

- Supine with arms abducted.
- The sterile field should begin at the nipple line and extend to the pubis.

TECHNIQUES

INCISION AND EXPOSURE

- A right hepatectomy can be performed through a variety of incisions, including a right subcostal, chevron, midline, or modified Makuuchi incision. It is the authors' preference to perform a right hepatectomy using a modified Makuuchi incision for optimal visualization as well as postoperative analgesia (**FIGURE 4**).[13]
- A fixed retractor system is employed with emphasis on the cephalad and lateral retraction of the costal margin to provide adequate exposure (**FIGURE 5**).[13]

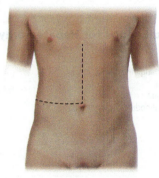

FIGURE 4 • Modified Makuuchi incision for right hepatectomy. (Redrawn from Chang SB, Palavecino M, Wray CJ, et al. Modified Makuuchi incision for foregut procedures. *Arch Surg*. 2010;145(3):281-284.)

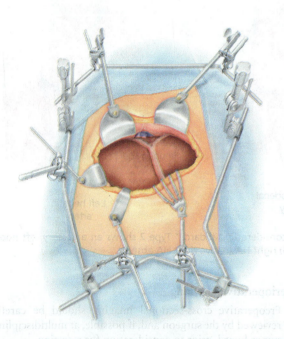

FIGURE 5 • Fixed-retractor setup for right hepatectomy. (Redrawn from Chang SB, Palavecino M, Wray CJ, et al. Modified Makuuchi incision for foregut procedures. *Arch Surg*. 2010;145(3):281-284.)

LIVER MOBILIZATION

- The ligamentum teres and falciform ligament are mobilized from the anterior abdominal wall and maintained as a vascularized flap for future use on the transected liver surface.
- Dissection begins by dividing the coronary ligament followed by the right triangular ligament, working from medial to lateral. The peritoneum and areolar tissue surrounding the anterior and lateral aspects of the right hepatic vein (RHV) is cleared (**FIGURE 6**).
- To continue laterally and inferiorly, the liver can be retracted medially and compressed posteriorly. If caval compression induces hypotension, temporary release of retraction may be all that is required. Alternatively, raising the inferolateral edge of the right liver will expose the final attachments of the triangular ligament.
- Complete mobilization of the right liver requires extensive exposure of the lateral and anterior surface of the inferior vena cava (IVC). Medial retraction and cephalad rotation of the inferolateral edge raises the liver off the retroperitoneum and IVC (**FIGURE 7**).
- Short or lesser hepatic veins from the right liver draining into the IVC will be exposed from distal to proximal IVC. These should be carefully dissected and ligated using ties, suture ligatures, and/or clips. Many patients will also have an accessory right hepatic vein, which can be identified on preoperative imaging and can be divided with a vascular stapler or oversewn with monofilament suture.
- At the proximal and lateral aspect of the IVC, there is a ligamentous band known as Makuuchi ligament or the inferior caval ligament, which extends from segment 7 to the retroperitoneal tissue behind the IVC. Release of this band is critical in the exposure and safe dissection of the RHV. This band can contain a venous tributary; therefore, careful transection with a vascular stapler is an attractive, safe option.
- After mobilization of the liver, IOUS is performed to examine the hepatic parenchyma. This is cross-referenced with preoperative imaging. All known lesions are identified, and the liver is examined for occult lesions. IOUS can confirm vascular anatomy, identify major vascular branches, and map the proximity of hepatic vein and portal vein branches to mass lesions (**FIGURE 8**).

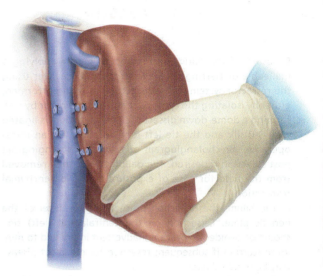

FIGURE 7 • Exposure of the short hepatic veins and IVC. This exposure is obtained by medial rotation and anterior retraction of the right liver. The short hepatic veins from the liver into the IVC are ligated.

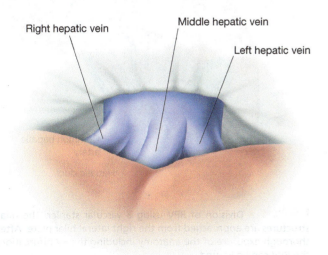

FIGURE 6 • Hepatic veins at the Apex of the falciform ligament. Dissection along the liver surface exposes this confluence. Dissection proceeds from medial to lateral, exposing the RHV without unnecessary dissection of contralateral structures (MHV, LHV).

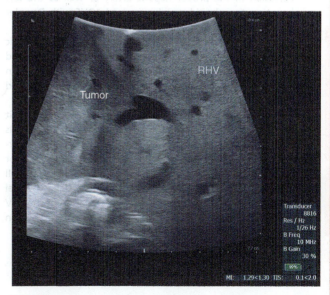

FIGURE 8 • Intraoperative ultrasound image Demonstrating relationship of tumor to the right hepatic vein (RHV).

DISSECTION OF THE RIGHT HEPATIC VEIN

- It is ideal to isolate and ligate the RHV extrahepatically. If this cannot be performed safely due to tumor proximity, the RHV can be divided using a vascular stapler during the parenchymal resection.
- Full exposure and control of the RHV prior to hilar dissection and inflow division is ideal. However, during dissection of the RHV, it is recommended that an umbilical tape and Rummel tourniquet is in place around the porta hepatis to allow for inflow occlusion should venous injury occur.
- The RHV is dissected close to the liver to leave a long cuff of RHV on the IVC in the event of injury. Once fully dissected, the RHV can be isolated with a vessel loop, umbilical tape, or large suture.
- To avoid congestion of the liver, the RHV is not ligated at this time.

HILAR DISSECTION AND VASCULAR CONTROL

- Exposure of the hilum is obtained by gently applying a malleable or Harrington blade to the inferior liver using the retractor system. Cholecystectomy is then performed, either by isolating the cystic duct and artery first or by performing a dome-down dissection. The cystic duct is ligated with 3-0 silk and the tie left long to allow for an intraoperative air cholangiogram or contrast cholangiogram post resection if desired. The gallbladder is then removed from the field for ease of exposure during parenchymal transection.
- In the hilum, the dissection proceeds at the level of the hepatic plate. Dissection on the contralateral (left) side should be avoided to prevent inadvertent injury and to minimize scarring if subsequent resection for recurrent disease may be required later.
- In the right hilum, dissection of the right hepatic artery (RHA) is the first priority. The RHA typically courses posterior to the common bile duct, but awareness of an aberrant course (including the presence of an accessory or replaced RHA) is crucial. The RHA (or its anterior and posterior branches) should be isolated as they enter the right liver. A vascular loop facilitates gentle traction, and a bulldog clamp is used to test clamp the artery to be divided.
- Perfusion in the proper hepatic artery as well as the left hepatic artery should now be assessed. IOUS with Doppler flow can be used for confirmation if needed.
- Once an adequate pulse is confirmed in the proper hepatic artery and left hepatic artery, the RHA can be divided between 2-0 silk ties and 4-0 Prolene suture ligature. Division should expose the right portal vein (RPV) posteriorly and cephalad to the RHA.
- The RPV dissection should establish enough length to permit safe ligation. The first branch of the RPV to the caudate is often divided for adequate length. Dissection must be carried out to identify the bifurcation of the RPV into anterior and posterior branches. Visualization of the left PV as well as the main PV is critical to ensure that the visualized vessel is the RPV and not the main portal vein. Isolation of the RPV may also be confirmed by IOUS. The RPV is circled with an 0-silk tie to allow gentle traction.
- We routinely transect the RPV with a narrow profile vascular stapler (**FIGURE 9**). We typically use an articulating stapler to obtain the optimal angle for transection. Extreme care is taken during passage of the stapler to avoid disruption of nearby tributaries. If the stapler cannot be safely passed, the RPV can simply be ligated with 0-silk until better exposure is achieved during parenchymal transection, at which time it can be safely divided.
- At this point, the right liver should demarcate along Cantlie line (**FIGURE 10**). Lack of inflow can also be confirmed by IOUS if needed.
- Unless an oncologic margin is at risk, the authors do not routinely perform extrahepatic division of the right hepatic duct (RHD). Rather, we prefer to ligate and divide it intraparenchymally with a stapler as described below.
- The previously isolated RHV is divided using an articulating narrow profile vascular stapler (**FIGURE 11**). Vascular occlusion is now complete.

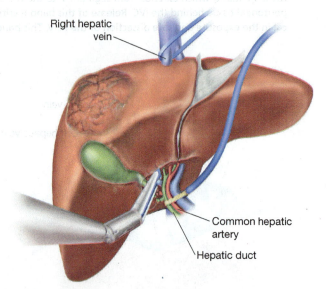

FIGURE 9 • Division of RPV using a vascular stapler. The hilar structures are approached from the right lateral hilar plate. After thorough exposure of the anatomy including the PV bifurcation, the RPV can be ligated.

Chapter 21 **RIGHT HEPATECTOMY** 165

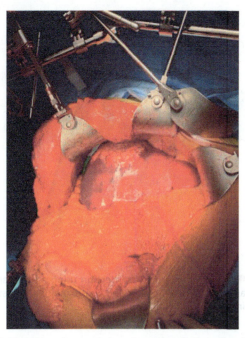

FIGURE 10 • Liver Demarcation along Cantlie line after ligation of RPV and RHA.

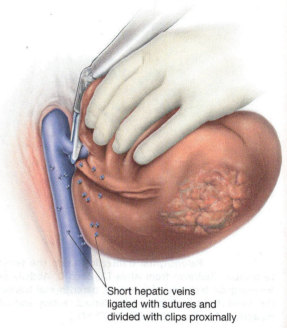

FIGURE 11 • Division of RHV using a vascular stapler. This is the last step of the vascular isolation after completion of inflow ligation (RPV, RHA).

PARENCHYMAL TRANSECTION

- Intraoperative liver ultrasound should be repeated to identify the middle hepatic vein. The transection plane is then marked with cautery on Glisson capsule to the right of the middle hepatic vein and confirmed with cautery to be a safe distance from the vein while allowing adequate distance from the tumor for margins (**FIGURE 12**). It is the authors' practice to put stay sutures on each side of the transection line to provide traction and to elevate the liver off the IVC during transection.
- A Pringle maneuver (inflow occlusion) may be applied to minimize intraoperative blood loss.
- Intraoperative communication with anesthesia is important at this stage in the operation to confirm that the CVP is low (≤5 mm Hg) prior to beginning parenchymal transection to minimize bleeding from intraparenchymal hepatic venous tributaries.
- There are multiple techniques available for transection of the hepatic parenchyma, none of which has shown to be superior to another. Ultimately, surgeon experience and familiarity with a specific technique should guide selection of approach. The authors prefer to utilize a two-surgeon technique in which the liver parenchyma is divided with an ultrasonic dissector in combination with a monopolar dissecting sealer for smaller vessels and clips, ties, or vascular staplers for medium or larger vessels (**FIGURE 13**).
- To begin transection, use sharp dissection with Metzenbaum scissors or cautery to disrupt Glisson capsule. The parenchyma can then be transected with an energy source according to surgeon preference.
- With the left hand holding the right liver, the IVC is protected, and the endpoint of transection is known at all times.
- At any point during the transection, IOUS can be used to confirm the line of resection to ensure adequate margins or reassess the location of the middle hepatic vein.

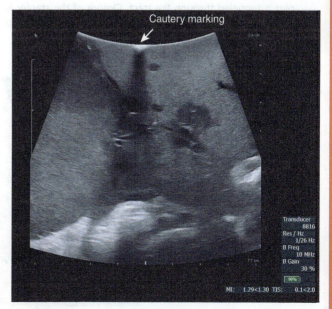

FIGURE 12 • Intraoperative ultrasound showing cautery marking of transection plane and relationship to the tumor.

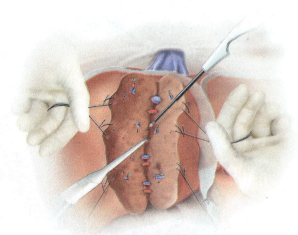

FIGURE 13 • Parenchymal transection using the two-surgeon technique. (Redrawn from Aloia TA, Zorzi D, Abdalla EK, et al. Two-surgeon technique for hepatic parenchymal transection of the noncirrhotic liver using saline-linked cautery and ultrasonic dissection. *Ann Surg*. 2005;242(2):172-177.)

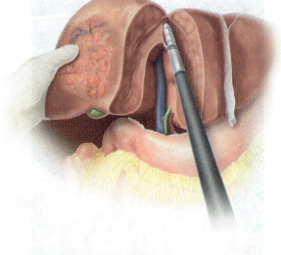

FIGURE 14 • Parenchymal transection using a vascular stapler. The stapler obtains hemostasis and ligates major biliary structures including the right hepatic duct.

- Stapling of the hepatic parenchyma is a commonly employed means of transection, particularly when ligating larger vessels. When stapling is used, the path of the stapler can be guided by creating a parenchymal tunnel with a curved clamp. If resistance is encountered, the clamp should be withdrawn and redirected until no resistance is encountered. Resistance indicates that the stapler is encountering the sidewall of a vessel. Forcing the stapler through these branches will cause significant hemorrhage. Once a tract in the hepatic parenchyma is established, the thin (narrow) arm of the stapler is tunneled through the tract. Closure of the stapler is analogous to crushing the hepatic parenchyma with a clamp (**FIGURE 14**).

- It is the authors' preference to divide the RHD as the last step in the parenchymal transection. This technique allows the safe sealing of the duct at the greatest distance from the left hepatic duct and avoids unnecessary hilar dissection, which can devascularize or injure the common or left hepatic duct.
- After the parenchyma is divided, the specimen is removed from the field (**FIGURE 15**). Immediate gross margin assessment should be performed, either by the surgeon or by pathology.
- Hemostasis is achieved at the cut edge of the liver. Most bleeding is from venules and will cease with gentle compression and patience. It is the authors' preference to apply a hemostatic agent and a lap pad to the cut surface while waiting.

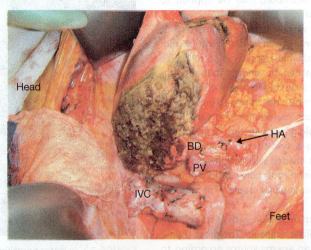

FIGURE 15 • Completed right hepatectomy. BD, bile duct; HA, hepatic artery; IVC, inferior vena cava; PV, portal vein.

- Care should be taken to avoid applying cautery to major bile ducts, as this may lead to subsequent stricture. For areas of bleeding near the hilum, energy devices may risk damage to crucial structures; employ sutures, manual pressure, and/or topical hemostatic agents as needed (such as cellulose matrices or thrombin or fibrin-based sprays or foams).
- The cut surface should be carefully inspected for bile leaks. It is the authors' preference to perform an intraoperative air cholangiogram through the divided cystic duct, which has been shown to decrease the rate of postoperative bile leak.[14] (**FIGURE 16**) Alternatively, a standard contrasted cholangiogram under fluoroscopy can be performed.
- If cholangiography is not feasible (due to prior cholecystectomy, for example), peroxide and/or clean lap pads can be applied to the cut surface to facilitate identification of a bile leak. Any identified bile leak should be controlled with fine monofilament sutures.
- A closed suction drain may be placed adjacent to the transected parenchyma if a persistent bile leak is present despite attempts at repair.
- The falciform ligament should be reapproximated to prevent lateral rotation of the left liver remnant, which could result in occlusion of the middle and left hepatic veins.

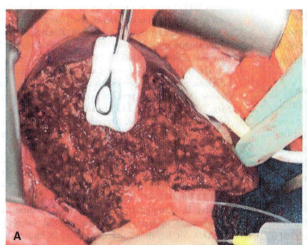 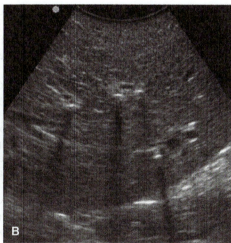

FIGURE 16 • Intraoperative air cholangiogram to assess for bile leak. **A,** Liver ultrasonography during transcystic air injection when the distal common bile duct is occluded by finger compression. **B,** Ultrasonographic visualization of diffuse acoustic shadowing indicates left liver pneumobilia and documents bile duct patency. (Reprinted from Zimmitti G, Vauthey JN, Shindoh J, et al. Systematic use of an intraoperative air leak test at the time of major liver resection reduces the rate of postoperative biliary complications. *J Am Coll Surg*. 2013;217(6):1028-1037. Copyright © 2013 American College of Surgeons. With permission.)

PEARLS AND PITFALLS

Patient history	■ The presence of underlying liver disease should be aggressively evaluated preoperatively to reduce posthepatectomy liver insufficiency.
Imaging and testing	■ Determination of adequate future liver remnant volume with volumetry is critical to avoid posthepatectomy liver insufficiency. ■ Vascular abnormalities and relationships between tumors and major vascular structures should be identified on preoperative contrasted imaging.
Mobilization and vascular isolation	■ Starting the dissection at the right hilar plate minimizes risk of contralateral injury to the remnant vasculature. ■ Dissection of the contralateral liver should be minimized if there is a chance of repeat hepatectomy.

Parenchymal transection	▪ Low CVP anesthesia is key. ▪ Intermittent inflow occlusion (Pringle maneuver) can decrease blood loss. ▪ The transection plan should be evaluated with ultrasound to confirm adequate margins and distance from the middle hepatic vein. ▪ The hepatic parenchyma should be divided efficiently and carefully based on surgeon preference and experience.
Hemostasis and bile leaks	▪ Patient, gentle pressure and use of hemostatic agents are often sufficient to achieve adequate hemostasis post resection. ▪ Use of energy devices near major biliary or hilar structures should be avoided. ▪ Transcystic cholangiogram can be performed to identify postoperative bile leaks. Operative drains should only be placed if a bile leak persists after attempt at repair.

POSTOPERATIVE CARE

- VTE prophylaxis is continued, including doses on the day of surgery as appropriate to the dosing schedule. When resection is performed for malignant indications, 28 days of postoperative prophylaxis with low-molecular-weight heparin should be considered.[15]
- Perioperative antibiotics are discontinued within 24 hours.
- Postoperative phosphate levels are monitored closely and aggressively replaced to aid in liver hypertrophy.
- If an operative drain was placed, daily assessment for bile leak should be performed. If no evidence of ongoing bile leak, the drain should be removed by postoperative day 3. Early drain removal is associated with fewer complications and shorter length of stay and should be prioritized.[16]
- For postoperative pain control, many surgeons utilize either regional anesthetic blocks, such as ultrasound-guided transversus abdominus plane or quadratus lumborum block or epidural analgesia. The authors prefer regional blocks using a long-acting local anesthetic, which appears to be associated with earlier time to ambulation, earlier urinary catheter removal, and fewer hypotensive episodes requiring excess intravenous fluid administration.[17]
- Early ambulation is important for optimal postoperative recovery, including prevention of VTE events. Early involvement of physical and occupational therapy can be beneficial, especially in elderly patients.

OUTCOMES

- In experienced centers, mortality is now less than 2% and morbidity is approximately 30% to 40%.[18,19]

COMPLICATIONS

- Volume-outcomes relationships are well established in hepatic resection.[20,21]
- Overall complication rates range from 30% to 40%. Outcomes specific to hepatectomy include bile leaks (7.8%) and posthepatectomy liver insufficiency (5.3%).[18]
- Persistent bile leaks can be managed by percutaneous drainage or endoscopic retrograde cholangiopancreatography with sphincterotomy to facilitate internal drainage.

REFERENCES

1. Strasberg SM, Belghiti J, Clavien PA, et al. The Brisbane 2000 Terminology of liver anatomy and resections. *HPB*. 2000;2(3):333-339.
2. Farnsworth N, Fagan SP, Berger DH, Awad SS. Child-Turcotte-Pugh versus MELD score as a predictor of outcome after elective and emergent surgery in cirrhotic patients. *Am J Surg*. 2004;188(5):580-583.
3. Schroeder RA, Marroquin CE, Bute BP, Khuri S, Henderson WG, Kuo PC. Predictive indices of morbidity and mortality after liver resection. *Ann Surg*. 2006;243(3):373-379.
4. Teh SH, Christein J, Donohue J, et al. Hepatic resection of hepatocellular carcinoma in patients with cirrhosis: Model of End-Stage Liver Disease (MELD) score predicts perioperative mortality. *J Gastrointest Surg*. 2005;9(9):1207-1215. discussion 1215.
5. Teh SH, Nagorney DM, Stevens SR, et al. Risk factors for mortality after surgery in patients with cirrhosis. *Gastroenterology*. 2007;132(4):1261-1269.
6. Abdalla EK, Barnett CC, Doherty D, Curley SA, Vauthey JN. Extended hepatectomy in patients with hepatobiliary malignancies with and without preoperative portal vein embolization. *Arch Surg*. 2002;137(6):675-680. discussion 671-680.
7. Azoulay D, Castaing D, Krissat J, et al. Percutaneous portal vein embolization increases the feasibility and safety of major liver resection for hepatocellular carcinoma in injured liver. *Ann Surg*. 2000;232(5):665-672.
8. Kubota K, Makuuchi M, Kusaka K, et al. Measurement of liver volume and hepatic functional reserve as a guide to decision-making in resectional surgery for hepatic tumors. *Hepatology*. 1997;26(5):1176-1181.
9. Shindoh J, Tzeng CW, Aloia TA, et al. Optimal future liver remnant in patients treated with extensive preoperative chemotherapy for colorectal liver metastases. *Ann Surg Oncol*. 2013;20(8):2493-2500.
10. Vauthey JN, Chaoui A, Do KA, et al. Standardized measurement of the future liver remnant prior to extended liver resection: methodology and clinical associations. *Surgery*. 2000;127(5):512-519.
11. Kanemitsu Y, Shimizu Y, Mizusawa J, et al. Hepatectomy followed by mFOLFOX6 versus hepatectomy alone for liver-only metastatic colorectal cancer (JCOG0603): a phase II or III randomized controlled trial. *J Clin Oncol*. 2021;39(34):3789-3799.
12. Nordlinger B, Sorbye H, Glimelius B, et al. Perioperative FOLFOX4 chemotherapy and surgery versus surgery alone for resectable liver metastases from colorectal cancer (EORTC 40983): long-term results of a randomised, controlled, phase 3 trial. *Lancet Oncol*. 2013;14(12):1208-1215.
13. Chang SB, Palavecino M, Wray CJ, Kishi Y, Pisters PW, Vauthey JN. Modified Makuuchi incision for foregut procedures. *Arch Surg*. 2010;145(3):281-284.
14. Zimmitti G, Vauthey JN, Shindoh J, et al. Systematic use of an intraoperative air leak test at the time of major liver resection reduces the rate of postoperative biliary complications. *J Am Coll Surg*. 2013;217(6):1028-1037.
15. Key NS, Khorana AA, Kuderer NM, et al. Venous thromboembolism prophylaxis and treatment in patients with cancer: ASCO clinical practice guideline update. *J Clin Oncol*. 2020;38(5):496-520.
16. Fagenson AM, Gleeson EM, Lau KKN, Karachristos A, Pitt HA. Early drain removal after hepatectomy: an underutilized management strategy. *HPB*. 2020;22(10):1463-1470.

17. Qin C, Liu Y, Xiong J, et al. The analgesic efficacy compared ultrasound-guided continuous transverse abdominis plane block with epidural analgesia following abdominal surgery: a systematic review and meta-analysis of randomized controlled trials. *BMC Anesthesiol.* 2020;20(1):52.
18. Bagante F, Ruzzenente A, Beal EW, et al. Complications after liver surgery: a benchmark analysis. *HPB.* 2019;21(9):1139-1149.
19. Pathak P, Tsilimigras DI, Hyer JM, Diaz A, Pawlik TM. Timing and severity of postoperative complications and associated 30-day mortality following hepatic resection: a National Surgical Quality Improvement Project Study. *J Gastrointest Surg.* 2022;26(2):314-322.
20. Glasgow RE, Showstack JA, Katz PP, Corvera CU, Warren RS, Mulvihill SJ. The relationship between hospital volume and outcomes of hepatic resection for hepatocellular carcinoma. *Arch Surg.* 1999;134(1):30-35.
21. Nathan H, Cameron JL, Choti MA, Schulick RD, Pawlik TM. The volume-outcomes effect in hepato-pancreato-biliary surgery: hospital versus surgeon contributions and specificity of the relationship. *J Am Coll Surg.* 2009;208(4):528-538.

Chapter 22 | Minimally Invasive Right Hepatectomy

Iswanto Sucandy, Kaitlyn Crespo, and Allan Tsung

DEFINITION

- Minimally invasive right hepatectomy is defined as resection of segments 5 to 8 using minimally invasive techniques (see Chapter 15, Figure 2). These techniques include the following:
  - Pure laparoscopic.
  - Hand assisted—The surgeon's hand is used to assist during the laparoscopic approach.
  - Hybrid—The liver is mobilized laparoscopically followed by minilaparotomy to divide the liver.
  - Robotic—The liver is resected with robotic technique.

PATIENT HISTORY AND PHYSICAL FINDINGS

- A thorough history and physical examination should be performed for each patient.
- A patient's history is important and should include careful attention to the following:
  - Medical history—Is the liver neoplasm benign or malignant? If the neoplasm is malignant, is it a primary of the liver or a metastasis from another organ? If the lesion is malignant, has the patient had chemotherapy? Does the patient have underlying liver disease such as steatosis or cirrhosis? If steatosis or cirrhosis exists, does the patient have manifestations of advanced liver disease such as esophageal varices, splenomegaly and hypersplenism, ascites, or hepatic encephalopathy? Is the patient's general condition healthy enough to withstand the liver resection?
  - Surgical history—Has the patient had abdominal operation in the past? If so, what type of operation and how many operations? Has the patient had prior liver or biliary tract surgery?
  - Social history—Alcohol use is important for consideration of concurrent liver disease.
  - Functional status should be considered when deciding goals of care and whether surgery is appropriate for an individual patient.
- Physical examination should include evaluation for the presence of advanced liver disease such as jaundice/scleral icterus (can also be present with biliary obstruction), gynecomastia, splenomegaly, ascites, and caput medusa. Findings of advanced malignancy, including supraclavicular lymphadenopathy, should be recognized.

IMAGING AND OTHER DIAGNOSTIC STUDIES

- Abdominal imaging using 1 mm cut computed tomography (CT) or magnetic resonance imaging (MRI) within a short interval of time (within 4-6 weeks) prior to surgery is necessary. Attention should be focused on the number of lesions, the location of the lesions (particularly in relation to the hepatic and portal veins [PVs], bile duct pedicle, as well as the inferior vena cava [IVC]), the character of the background liver (normal, steatosis, cirrhosis), and the proportion of liver that will be left in situ once all hepatic disease is resected (future liver remnant volume).
- For CT scan, a dynamic bolus, contrast-enhanced, multidetector CT using at least a three-phase protocol is ideal. Noncontrast images of the liver are followed by rapid bolus of contrast, and images are immediately obtained during peak arterial enhancement (arterial phase) as well as during PV enhancement (portal venous phase). Hypervascular tumors and tumors that receive their blood supply primarily from the hepatic artery (HA) are best visualized on arterial phase. During the portal venous phase, the liver is maximally enhanced and hypovascular lesions on a background of bright-appearing parenchyma can be well distinguished (**FIGURE 1**).
- Enhanced hepatic MRI is an equivalent alternative. MRI with Eovist intravenous contrast agent is helpful in patients with hepatocellular carcinoma.
- Tissue sampling with core biopsy by ultrasound or percutaneous CT guidance can be useful to make or confirm a diagnosis when necessary.
- Additional diagnostic studies that are necessary prior to operation are basic laboratory tests, including a hepatic function panel and coagulation studies. A complete blood count including a platelet count is important to help detect advanced portal hypertension if the patient has cirrhosis. If disease-specific tumor markers are elevated, they are helpful to confirm a diagnosis as well as to follow patients during a later phase of their treatment.

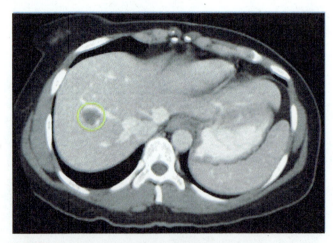

FIGURE 1 • CT image of liver, portal venous phase. Encircled is a metastatic colon lesion to the right liver.

SURGICAL MANAGEMENT AND OPERATIVE TECHNIQUE

- There are several advantages of laparoscopic liver resection when compared with an open technique. These include decreased blood loss, less postoperative pain, quicker return to diet, less blood loss, a shorter length of stay, and decreased postoperative complications.[1] These advantages have been demonstrated in case-controlled studies and prospective randomized study.[2] In addition, oncologic outcomes (margins, survival) are not compromised when laparoscopic technique is used for patients with hepatocellular carcinoma and metastatic colorectal cancer.[3-5]
- During the World Consensus Conference on Laparoscopic Surgery in 2008, the international position on laparoscopic liver surgery was created—this should be used as a guide to determine which patients are eligible for minimally invasive hepatic resection.[6] This statement recommends surgery with minimally invasive technique for patients with a single lesion of 5 cm or less located in segments 2 to 6. It suggests that major liver resection can be performed with minimally invasive technique but only by those experienced both with liver surgery as well as minimally invasive liver resection. Increasing number of surgeons in high-volume centers now operate beyond these criteria as published data describing safety and feasibility of minimally invasive major liver resection emerge. Of importance, the consensus conference suggests that the surgeon should be facile with minimally invasive technique, including the skill of intracorporeal suturing should bleeding become an issue.
- The decision to use hand-assisted vs pure laparoscopic technique is surgeon specific and mostly depends on comfort with either technique. As our own experience in laparoscopic hepatectomy has grown, so has our comfort with performing anatomic hepatic resection in a pure laparoscopic manner. When comparing pure laparoscopic technique with hand-assisted or hybrid technique in 113 patients undergoing anatomic liver resection, we found similar results for estimated blood loss and complications; however, interestingly, shorter operative times were noted in the pure laparoscopic group (188 vs 264 minutes for the pure vs hand-assisted technique, $P < .05$).[7]
- Consideration of the background liver is important to help decide which patients are appropriate for resection—up to 80% of a healthy liver in a relatively healthy patient can be resected without major consequence, more specifically postoperative hepatic insufficiency and hepatic failure. This percentage decreases if the background liver is cirrhotic.
- The technique of minimally invasive right hepatectomy is, as intended, mostly the same as for open surgery except minimally invasive equipment is used.
- Two surgeons who are experienced in hepatobiliary and minimally invasive surgery are appropriate for these cases. An assistant to hold the camera is optimal, thus allowing both hands of both surgeons to be free.

HAND-ASSISTED LAPAROSCOPIC RIGHT HEPATECTOMY

- The patient is positioned supine with the arms tucked. Padded barriers are secured at the patient's feet to prevent sliding with the anticipated use of steep reverse Trendelenburg during the case.
- Access is gained to the abdominal cavity via a 5-mm port ideally in the left upper quadrant (LUQ), and pneumoperitoneum of 15 mm Hg is created. Additional ports are placed using a 5-mm 30° scope for visualization (**FIGURE 2**). These ports include an 8-cm hand access site in the supraumbilical position. Two 12-mm ports are placed in the subxiphoid and right paramedian position, and two 5-mm ports are placed in right subcostal positions. The camera is switched to a 10-mm 30° scope in the right paramedian port.
- The lesion is identified.
- Standing at the patient's left, the surgeon places their nondominant hand through the hand access device.
- The round and falciform ligaments are divided using a sealing device, exposing the anterior surface of the hepatic veins.
- The ligamentous attachments of the right liver are dissected. With the patient in reverse Trendelenburg position and with the right side up, the gallbladder fundus is retracted superiorly via a grasper in the LUQ port. The right lobe of the liver is retracted anteriorly using a closed grasper in the subxiphoid port. With a hand retracting the colon inferiorly, the hepatic flexure is dissected using a cautery device. The colon

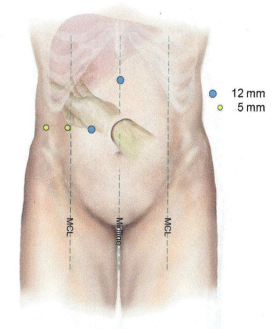

FIGURE 2 • Port placement for minimally invasive right hepatectomy. For the pure laparoscopic method, a 12-mm port is used instead of a hand port in the supraumbilical position. *MCL*, middle clavicular line. (Used with kind permission from Randal S. McKenzie/McKenzie Illustrations.)

is reflected caudally. Attachments to the duodenum are dissected from the liver as necessary. Using hand assistance for ligament exposure, the right triangular and coronary ligaments are dissected up to the origin of right hepatic vein (RHV)/IVC, also using a sealing device (FIGURE 3).

- Laparoscopic ultrasound of the liver is performed via the 12-mm subxiphoid port to confirm intrahepatic anatomy and ensure that the procedure will include the pathology that is anticipated.
- The IVC is dissected (FIGURE 4A and B). For exposure, the gallbladder is retracted superiorly from a grasper in the LUQ port. Hand assistance is used to retract the liver anteriorly, exposing the IVC. The liver is mobilized from the IVC by identifying and ligating short hepatic veins. Ligation is performed using clips, and endoscopic shears or a sealing device is used to cut the veins. This is performed up to the origin of the RHV.
- Cholecystectomy and portal dissection. The hand is removed from the abdominal cavity, and the liver is allowed to rest back in normal position. A 5-mm assist port is placed in the hand access device. The gallbladder is grasped and dissected for cholecystectomy in standard laparoscopic manner. After identifying the critical view, the cystic artery and duct are clipped. The cystic artery and duct are transected. While maintaining superior retraction of the gallbladder, portal tissue is retracted laterally via a grasper in one of the lateral 5-mm ports. The hepatoduodenal ligament is dissected using a combination of an endoscopic dissector and hook cautery via the subxiphoid port. The right HA is identified and defined (FIGURE 5). If space allows, this is stapled using a vascular load roticulating stapler through the 12-mm subxiphoid port. Otherwise, this can be tied laparoscopically, clipped, and then transected. Next, the right PV is identified and defined (FIGURE 6). A silk tie is placed around it (this is not tied), and a grasper in one of the right lateral ports

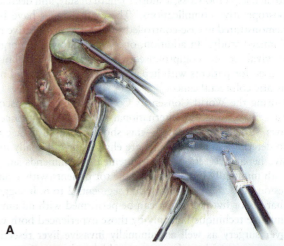

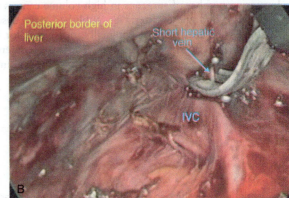

FIGURE 4 • **A,** Dissection of the short hepatic veins from the IVC. Short hepatic veins are defined with a dissector and ligated using a sealing device or clips and shears. **B,** Dissection of the short hepatic veins from the IVC. Short hepatic veins are clipped and divided with shears. (Used with kind permission from Randal S. McKenzie/McKenzie Illustrations.)

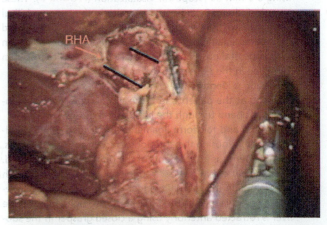

FIGURE 3 • Dissection of the ligamentous attachments of the right liver. (Used with kind permission from Randal S. McKenzie/McKenzie Illustrations.)

FIGURE 5 • Portal dissection. Exposure of the right hepatic artery (RHA).

Chapter 22 MINIMALLY INVASIVE RIGHT HEPATECTOMY   173

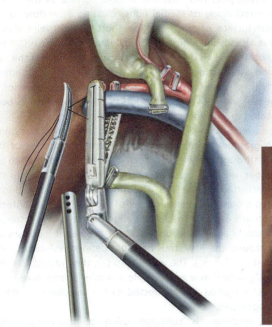

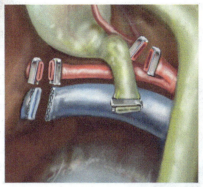

FIGURE 6 • Portal dissection, ligation of the right PV. (Used with kind permission from Randal S. McKenzie/McKenzie Illustrations.)

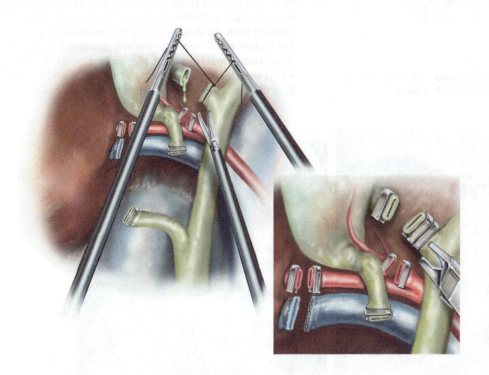

FIGURE 7 • The right HD is identified and defined. It is tied distally, then transected proximally. It is important to identify bile coming from the proximal duct. (Used with kind permission from Randal S. McKenzie/McKenzie Illustrations.)

retracts this tie superolaterally to expose the full length of the vein. A vascular load roticulating stapler is used to ligate and transect the right PV. The right hepatic duct (HD) is identified and defined. It is tied distally, then transected proximally. It is important to identify bile coming from the proximal duct (**FIGURE 7**). Once bile is identified, the proximal duct can be clipped to maintain a clean field. The free, distal end of the right HD is doubly clipped to prevent leak. After the portal dissection is completed, the gallbladder is dissected from the gallbladder fossa.

- The parenchyma is transected. All retracting instruments are removed, allowing the liver to drop. The line of transection is defined using hook cautery, following the line of demarcation on the liver's anterior surface. Ultrasonography is repeated to ensure again that the pathology will be included in the point of transection with desired margins. Figure-of-eight stitches using 0-Polysorb are placed on either side of the line of transection, and these are retracted to either side with graspers (**FIGURE 8**). The parenchyma is coagulated, placing clips when appropriate. Progress is made along the

- line of transection until the RHV is encountered. Using a vascular load roticulating stapler through the 12-mm assist port, the RHV is stapled intraparenchymally, flush to its junction with the IVC. The remaining parenchyma is divided as necessary.
- For tumors that are close to the RHV-IVC junction, the RHV can be isolated and transected in an extrahepatic manner. To accomplish this, first the anterior surface of the RHV is dissected along its medial edge, creating a window to the undersurface of the liver. The short hepatic veins should have already been dissected and ligated along the IVC at this point. The RHV is dissected from the undersurface of the liver using a dissecting instrument while lifting the liver anteriorly (FIGURE 9A). A bending grasper is placed anterior to the RHV and advanced through the window that has been created toward the anterior surface of the liver (FIGURE 9B). The liver is allowed to fall back into place, and the bending grasper is visualized from the anterior surface of the liver through the window created. A vessel loop is fed to the grasper, and the grasper gently pulls back through to the undersurface of the liver. The other end of the vessel loop is fed around the lateral border of the RHV from an anterior approach as well. The lateral edge of the liver is retracted anteriorly again, and both ends of the vessel loops should be around the RHV, thus having a defined isolation of this vein (FIGURE 9C). The vessel loop can then retract the vein gently, acting as a guide while a stapler is introduced. The vessel is ligated and transected with a vascular load roticulating stapler.
- The specimen is collected using a laparoscopic bag. Hemostasis on the resection bed of the liver is ensured.
- Saline and contrast cholangiograms are performed through the cystic duct to confirm no biliary leak. The gallbladder is removed from the abdomen using a laparoscopic bag.
- The abdomen is closed. Laparoscopic equipment is used to remove ports under direct visualization and close fascia using a port site closure device. Fascia at the hand site is closed from the outside in standard manner. The skin is closed.

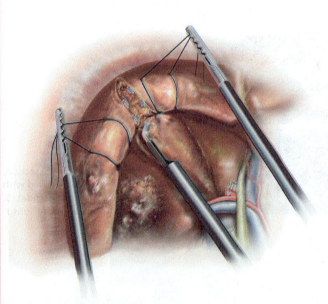

FIGURE 8 • Parenchymal transection. (Used with kind permission from Randal S. McKenzie/McKenzie Illustrations.)

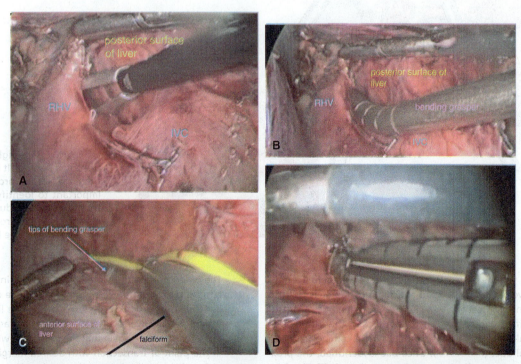

FIGURE 9 • A, Dissection of the RHV extrahepatic ligation. B, Maneuvering around the RHV with a bending grasper. C, Isolating the RHV with a vessel loop. The bending grasper comes anterior to the RHV from the undersurface of the liver. With the liver allowed to fall back into place, a vessel loop is fed to this bending grasper, which then pulls the vessel loop under the liver. D, Division of right hepatic vein with a linear vascular stapler completing outflow control of the right hepatic lobe.

PURE LAPAROSCOPIC RIGHT HEPATECTOMY

- Patient positioning and port placement are similar to that used for the hand-assisted procedure described. Instead of a hand port, however, an additional 12-mm port is used in the supraumbilical position. All steps are the same as described for the hand-assisted procedure except that a laparoscopic instrument is used instead of a hand.
- The round and falciform ligaments are divided using a sealing device, exposing the anterior surface of the hepatic vein (**FIGURE 10A** and **B**).
- The ligamentous attachments of the right liver are dissected. With the patient in reverse Trendelenburg position and with the right side up, the gallbladder fundus is retracted superiorly via a grasper in the LUQ port. The right lobe of the liver is retracted anteriorly using a closed grasper in the subxiphoid port. With a grasper retracting the colon inferiorly, the hepatic flexure is dissected using a cautery device. The colon is reflected inferiorly. Attachments to the duodenum are dissected from the liver as necessary. The right triangular and coronary ligaments are dissected up to the RHV/IVC junction (**FIGURE 11**).
- Laparoscopic ultrasound of the liver is performed via the 12-mm subxiphoid port.
- The IVC is dissected. For exposure, the gallbladder is retracted superiorly from a grasper in the LUQ port. A closed grasper is used via the supraumbilical port to retract the liver anteriorly, exposing the IVC. The liver is mobilized from the IVC by identifying and ligating short hepatic veins (**FIGURE 4B**).
- Cholecystectomy, portal dissection, parenchymal transection. This is similar to what is described in the hand-assisted section.
- The specimen is collected using a laparoscopic bag. Hemostasis on the resection bed of the liver is ensured.
- Saline and contrast cholangiograms are performed through the cystic duct to confirm no biliary leak. The gallbladder is removed from the abdomen using a laparoscopic bag.
- The abdomen is closed. Laparoscopic equipment is used to remove ports under direct visualization and close fascia using a port site closure device. The skin is closed.

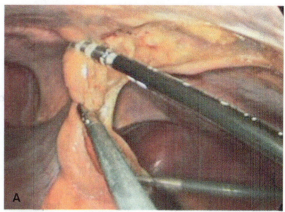
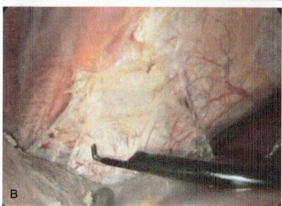

FIGURE 10 • **A,** Laparoscopic dissection of the falciform ligament. **B,** Exposure of the anterior surface of the left/middle hepatic veins after dissection of the falciform ligament.

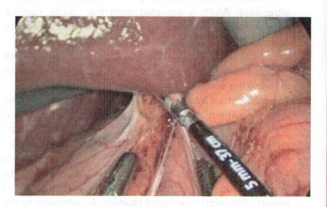

FIGURE 11 • Laparoscopic dissection of ligamentous attachments of the right liver.

ROBOTIC RIGHT HEPATECTOMY

- The patient is positioned supine with the arms extended. Padded barriers are secured at the patient's feet to prevent sliding with the anticipated use of steep reverse Trendelenburg during the case. The operating table is paired with DaVinci Xi robotic surgical system to allow for an intraoperative bed motion. The operating room setup is shown in **FIGURE 12**.
- Access is gained to the abdominal cavity via an 8-mm cutdown incision along the left midclavicular line, and pneumoperitoneum of 15 mm Hg is created. After a diagnostic laparoscopy, three additional 8-mm robotic ports are placed (**FIGURE 13**). A mini Gelpoint is placed via a muscle-splitting incision in the right lower quadrant, slightly caudal to the umbilicus for a bedside surgeon/assistant to work (suction and exposure) and later specimen extraction. The instruments used are as the following:
    - Robotic Arm#1: Bipolar forceps
    - Robotic Arm#2: Camera
    - Robotic Arm#3: Hook/scissors/vessel sealer/Hemolock clips/needle holder/stapler

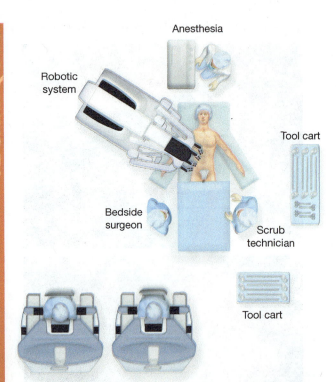

FIGURE 12 • Robotic operating room setup.

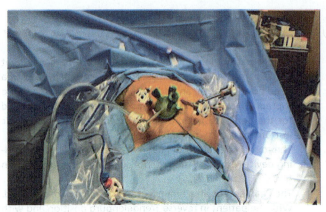

FIGURE 13 • Robotic Port placement.

- Robotic Arm#4: Atraumatic bowel grasper for liver/gallbladder retraction
- Mini Gelpoint: Laparoscopic suction device/robotic ultrasound/specimen extraction

- The lesion is identified using an intraoperative robotic ultrasound, which is operated from the robotic console. Intrahepatic anatomy and its relation to the lesion should be noted.
- The round and falciform ligaments are divided using a hook electrocautery all the way up to the hepatocaval confluence, exposing the anterior surface of the hepatic veins.
- The ligamentous attachments of the right liver are dissected. With the patient in 15° reverse Trendelenburg and with 8° right side up position, the gallbladder fundus and the right lobe of the liver is retracted cephalad toward the patient's left shoulder using a traumatic bowel grasper (Robotic Arm#4). With the assistant retracting the colon inferiorly, the hepatic flexure is dissected using a hook electrocautery or scissors. The colon is reflected caudally. Attachments to the duodenum are dissected from the liver as necessary. With appropriate retraction of the right hepatic lobe, the right triangular and coronary ligaments are exposed and dissected (▶ Video 1). The origin of the RHV/IVC junction is finally cleared using a hook cautery.
- The anterolateral aspect of the IVC is dissected. Adjustment to the atraumatic bowel grasper via robotic arm#4 is periodically made to effectively retract the right liver lobe, exposing the IVC. The liver is mobilized from the IVC by isolating and ligating short hepatic veins, including the Makuuchi ligament. Ligation is performed using either a 3-0 silk tie reinforced by medium-sized Hemolock clips or Hemolock clips (▶ Video 1). This is performed toward the origin of the RHV.

- Cholecystectomy and portal dissection. The gallbladder fundus is grasped retracted cranially using atraumatic bowel grasper. After identifying the critical view, the cystic artery and duct are clipped. The cystic artery and duct are transected. While maintaining superior retraction of the gallbladder and liver using atraumatic bowel grasper, portal tissue is retracted laterally using bipolar forceps. The hepatoduodenal ligament is dissected using a combination of hook electrocautery and Maryland dissector to isolate the right HA (▶ Video 1). After a visual clamping test to ensure preservation of arterial flow in the contralateral HA, the right HA is ligated and clipped. Next, the right PV is identified and isolated (▶ Video 1). A 3-0 silk tie is used to ligate the right PV, reinforced by medium-sized Hemolock clips as well. It is important to make sure the portal vein bifurcation is not narrowed. The right HD can be isolated now if the lesion is close to the bile duct, otherwise we prefer to transect the right HD intraparenchymally.
- The superficial liver parenchyma is then transected using scissors or hook electrocautery following the demarcation line. It is important to allow the liver to drop into its anatomical position to avoid disorientation of the transection plan. Ultrasonography is repeated to ensure again that the pathology will be included in the point of transection with desired margins. Figure-of-eight stitches using 2-0 silks are placed on either side of the line of transection to help open book the liver (▶ Video 1). The deeper liver parenchyma is coagulated using bipolar forceps, and the crossing vascular branches are individually exposed. Vessels that are smaller than 7 mm can be safely divided using the vessel sealer. Larger branches are divided between Hemolock clips. It is important to be aware of the trajectory of the middle hepatic veins at all time. As the parenchymal transection progresses closer toward the right side of the porta hepatis, the right HD is then identified and transected using a robotic stapler (▶ Video 1). Progress is made along the line of transection until the origin of the right HV is encountered. Using a vascular load robotic stapler through arm#3, the right HV is stapled intraparenchymally, flush to its junction with the IVC. The remaining segment 8 parenchyma and attachments to the right hemidiaphragm are divided as necessary (▶ Video 1).
- For tumors that are close to the RHV–IVC junction, the RHV can be isolated and transected in an extrahepatic manner. To accomplish this, first the anterior surface of the RHV is

dissected along its medial edge, creating a window to the undersurface of the liver. The short hepatic veins should have already been dissected and ligated along the IVC at this point. The RHV is dissected from the undersurface of the liver using a Maryland dissector while lifting the liver anteriorly. A vessel loop or 0 silk tie is fed into the space medial to the right HV using the Maryland grasper. The use of a nasogastric tube tied to the vessel loop or silk tie can be useful to facilitate this step. The right HV can then be retracted and stapled using a vascular load reticulating stapler.

- The remaining tissue and ligamentous attachments are divided using a vessel sealer or electrocautery. Sometimes a vein branch is seen entering the phrenic vein or lateral aspect of IVC, which needs to be divided using stapler or Hemolock clips. This is important to recognize in order to avoid bleeding. Finally, the specimen is collected using a laparoscopic specimen retrieval bag. Hemostasis on the resection bed of the liver is ensured (▶ Video 1).
- Saline and contrast cholangiograms through the cystic duct to confirm no biliary leak can be performed prior to closing.
- The abdomen is closed. Robotic system is undocked. Laparoscopic equipment is used to close fascia using a port site closure device. The skin is closed.

Robotic system provides solutions to inherent limitations of straight instruments used in conventional laparoscopy. Robotic system comes with superior three-dimensional visualization, stable platform, improved manual dexterity for the operating surgeon, and better precision during delicate hilar dissection and more importantly facilitates easy suturing for hemostasis and biliostasis. These technical advantages are useful to increase feasibility and reduce unplanned open conversion, especially in major hepatic resection such as right hepatectomy.[8-10]

PEARLS AND PITFALLS

Patient selection	- A careful evaluation of history, examination, and laboratory findings is essential to avoid encountering unexpected liver disease. - High-quality imaging is essential for operative planning to ensure an adequate margin can be obtained.
Operative technique	- Pre- and intraoperative restrictive resuscitation (central venous pressure <5 mm Hg) reduces blood loss. - Attention to hemostasis is essential for minimally invasive liver resection. - Intracorporeal suturing is important to quickly manage bleeding from larger vessels such as hepatic veins, portal vein, and IVC. - Use the shafts of instruments or specifically designed, expanding instruments to retract the liver—puncturing or lacerating the capsule must be avoided. - Be constantly vigilant of potential gas embolism—use reduced insufflation pressure when possible. - Signs of biliary leak must be thoroughly observed on the liver resection surface prior to closing. Placement of suture may be necessary to reduce postoperative complications.
Postoperative care	- Venous thromboembolism remains a risk, even if the international normalized ratio (INR) is elevated. Use chemoprophylaxis.

POSTOPERATIVE CARE

- It is imperative that postoperative care is maintained by a team of individuals familiar with these patients and cases. It is also imperative that care is maintained in a facility equipped to provide care for patients who suffer major postoperative complications, for example, patients who require prolonged intubation or urgent hemodialysis postoperatively. Laboratory tests, including a hepatic function panel and coagulation panel, should be followed and trended.

OUTCOMES

- Laparoscopic and robotic liver resections have been used with increasing frequency. There are several advantages to these techniques, and they include decreased blood loss, less postoperative pain, faster return to diet, and shorter length of stay when compared with open surgery. Oncologic outcomes are not compromised with these techniques, and survival is similar when compared with survival in patients with hepatocellular carcinoma or metastatic colorectal cancer who undergo open surgery. Minimally invasive right hepatectomy is technically demanding and should be performed by surgeons experienced with hepatobiliary surgery.

COMPLICATIONS

- Bleeding
- Infection
- Bile leak
- Liver failure
- Kidney failure in association with liver failure
- Close or positive margins

REFERENCES

1. Nguyen KT, Marsh JW, Tsung A, et al. Comparative benefits of laparoscopic vs open hepatic resection: a critical appraisal. *Arch Surg.* 2011;146(3):348-356.
2. Fretland ÅA, Dagenborg VJ, Bjørnelv GMW, et al. Laparoscopic versus open resection for colorectal liver metastases: the OSLO-COMET randomized controlled trial. *Ann Surg.* 2018;267(2):199-207.
3. Nguyen KT, Gamblin TC, Geller DA. World review of laparoscopic liver resection—2,804 patients. *Ann Surg.* 2009;250(5):831-841.
4. Castaing D, Vibert E, Ricca L, et al. Oncologic results of laparoscopic versus open hepatectomy for colorectal liver metastases in two specialized centers. *Ann Surg.* 2009;250(5):849-855.
5. Zhou YM, Shao WY, Zhao YF, et al. Meta-analysis of laparoscopic versus open resection for hepatocellular carcinoma. *Dig Dis Sci.* 2011;56(7):1937-1943.
6. Buell JF, Cherqui D, Geller DA, et al. The international position on laparoscopic liver surgery: the Louisville Statement, 2008. *Ann Surg.* 2009;250(5):825-830.
7. Cardinal JS, Reddy SK, Tsung A, et al. Laparoscopic major hepatectomy: pure laparoscopic approach versus hand-assisted technique. *J Hepatobiliary Pancreat Sci.* 2013;20(2):114-119.
8. Sucandy I, Giovannetti A, Ross S, et al. Institutional first 100 case experience and outcomes of robotic hepatectomy for liver tumors. *Am Surg.* 2020;86(3):200-207.
9. Sucandy I, Luberice K, Lippert T, et al. Robotic major hepatectomy: an institutional experience and clinical outcomes. *Ann Surg Oncol.* 2020;27(13):4970-4979.
10. Luberice K, Sucandy I, Modasi A, et al. Applying IWATE criteria to robotic hepatectomy: is there a "robotic effect"? *HPB.* 2021;23(6):899-906.

Chapter 23 | Left Hepatectomy

Rebecca Y. Kim and Courtney L. Scaife

DEFINITION

- A left hepatectomy (or hemihepatectomy) consists of surgical resection of the left liver, consisting of Couinaud segments 2 to 4[1] (**FIGURES 1** and **2**). The indications for a left hepatectomy are similar to indications for segmental and major hepatectomy, including diagnostic uncertainty, symptomatic benign lesions, and premalignant and malignant lesions.

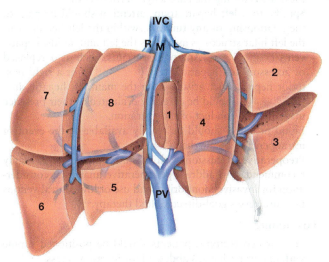

FIGURE 1 • Couinaud segments. The liver is divided into eight anatomic segments with the left and right lobes being separated by Cantlie line (the imaginary line between the gallbladder fossa anteriorly and the IVC posteriorly). The left lobe is made up of segments 2 and 3 (left lateral segments) and segment 4 (left medial segment).

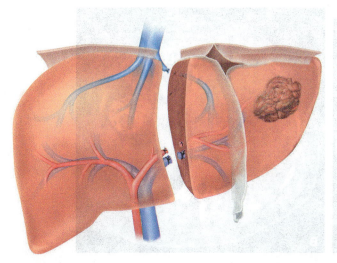

FIGURE 2 • Left hepatectomy involves removal of segments 2 through 4 with division of the left hepatic artery and left portal vein (inflow), left hepatic vein (outflow), and left hepatic duct.

PATIENT HISTORY AND PHYSICAL FINDINGS

Imperative to any major liver resection is an assessment of the patient's overall ability to tolerate a complex abdominal operation. Optimization of preexisting comorbid diseases should occur when feasible.[2-5]

- The patient history should assess for underlying chronic liver disease. Prior episodes of jaundice, gastrointestinal bleeding, ascites, and encephalopathy should be noted. Obesity/metabolic syndrome, chemotherapy exposure, alcohol use, intravenous drug use, participation in high-risk sexual behavior, and receipt of blood transfusions are risk factors for chronic liver disease and warrant further evaluation.
- Physical examination findings concerning for cirrhosis with portal hypertension (**TABLE 1**) are indicative of advanced chronic liver disease, which increases perioperative complication rate.
- For metastatic lesions to the liver, an assessment of tumor biology with demonstrated stability of disease on systemic therapy is critically important. Assessment of durable response to chemotherapy must be weighed against hepatotoxicity of systemic treatment.[6] Multidisciplinary discussions are strongly recommended when considering liver resection for malignant disease.[7-9]

IMAGING AND OTHER DIAGNOSTIC STUDIES

- When the history and/or physical examination findings point to chronic liver disease, additional serologic testing for viral hepatitides, hemochromatosis, Wilson disease, and alpha-1

Table 1: Clinical History and Physical Examination Findings Suggestive of Cirrhosis With Portal Hypertension

History
Jaundice/itchiness
Dark urine
Abdominal pain/bloating
Ascites
Anorexia/cachexia
GI bleeding
Loss of libido or menstrual cycle
Encephalopathy
Fatigue
Weight change
Physical Examination
Jaundice/scleral icterus
Ascites
Caput medusa
Hepatosplenomegaly
Asterixis
Fetor hepaticus
Spider angiomata
Clubbing/palmar erythema
Gynecomastia/testicular atrophy

antitrypsin deficiency may be necessary if the etiology of liver disease is unknown. Liver biopsy may be required to assess for fibrosis/cirrhosis.
- Standard blood work including a complete blood count, complete metabolic panel, and coagulation panel are required prior to proceeding with any major liver surgery.
- In cases of malignancy, appropriate tumor markers, including carcinoembryonic antigen, alpha-fetoprotein, and/or carbohydrate antigen 19-9 levels may provide diagnostic clarity and should be considered as indicated.
- High-quality, cross-sectional imaging is a prerequisite for major liver surgery. Multiphasic computed tomography (CT) and/or magnetic resonance imaging/magnetic resonance cholangiopancreatography should include early hepatic arterial phase and portal venous phase. The number of lesions, the location and relationship of lesions to intrahepatic vascular structures, and the character of the background liver should be noted. Accessory or replaced hepatic arteries are present in roughly half of patients[10]; accessory hepatic veins should also be noted.
- Liver protocol imaging can often obviate the need for invasive biopsy for diagnosis.[11] Simple cysts, hemangioma, focal nodular hyperplasia, and hepatocellular carcinoma have characteristic radiographic findings that can be diagnostic in the appropriate clinical setting.
- Given concern for needle track tumor seeding, hemorrhage, and other biopsy-related complications, percutaneous biopsies have been traditionally discouraged. However, with increased used of neoadjuvant chemotherapy and targeted immunotherapy for primary and secondary liver cancers, the role of percutaneous liver biopsy is evolving, particularly in light of more recent data suggesting the safely of the procedure.[12-15]
- For oncologic resection, appropriate staging should be completed with chest and pelvic imaging. Subcentimeter pulmonary nodules should not preclude hepatic resection.[16-18]
- Nuclear medicine scans, specifically fluorodeoxyglucose–positron emission tomography and somatostatin-receptor analogue studies, have an evolving role in liver resection for metastatic disease. Evaluation of extrahepatic disease is critically important as it portends worse prognosis in metastatic colorectal cancer.[19,20]
- Multidisciplinary discussions are strongly recommended when considering liver resection for malignant disease.[7-9]

SURGICAL MANAGEMENT
Preoperative Planning
- Critical to any major liver operation is thorough understanding of the appropriate preoperative imaging. If necessary, images should be reviewed with a skilled liver radiologist before surgery. Pertinent images should be available throughout the procedure. Understanding the relationship of tumor to major intra- and extrahepatic structures allows the surgeon to anticipate and plan strategies for dealing with these areas during the parenchymal transection.
- Specific to a left hepatectomy, attention should be paid to the relationship of any tumor(s) within the left hemiliver to the left hilar structures as well as the left and middle hepatic veins (**FIGURE 3A**). Anatomic variants, such as a replaced or accessory left hepatic artery (**FIGURE 3B**) or a right posterior hepatic duct arising from the main left hepatic duct (**FIGURE 3C**), should be carefully evaluated as their presence may alter the conduct of the operation.
- Blood products should be readily available in the event of intraoperative hemorrhage.
- Preoperative discussion with the anesthesiologist is highly recommended to address perioperative analgesia, consideration for invasive monitoring, and use of low central venous pressure verses goal-directed fluid therapy.[21-24]

Positioning
- For left hepatectomy, patients should be positioned supine with one or both arms abducted for intra-op access.
- The abdomen is prepped and draped from the nipple line or higher to the symphysis pubis and to the table laterally on both sides.
- A Foley catheter and orogastric tube may be considered.
- Normothermia should be maintained throughout the case.

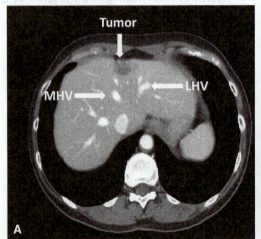 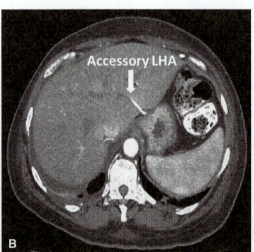

FIGURE 3 • Preoperative imaging and aberrant hepatic anatomy. **A,** CT scan showing the relationship of a metastatic colorectal cancer to the middle hepatic vein (MHV) and left hepatic vein (LHV). **B,** CT scan showing an accessory left hepatic artery (LHA) coming from the left gastric artery. **C,** Schematic demonstrating the right posterior (RP) sectoral duct arising from the left hepatic (LH) duct. When this anatomic variant exists, if the LH duct is transected in plane **A,** the RP segments (6 and 7) will be disconnected from the biliary tree. If the LH duct is transected in plane **B,** the RP ducts will remain connected to the main biliary tree.

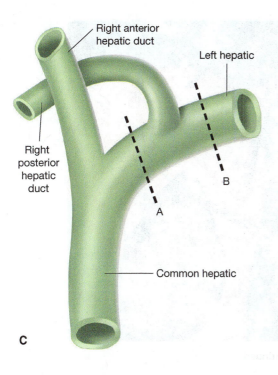

FIGURE 3 • Continued

STEP 1: INCISION AND EXPOSURE

- A left hepatectomy can be performed through a subcostal, chevron, or midline incision. Depending on the location of the lesion, patient factors, and surgeon's comfort, consideration should be given to a minimally invasive approach,[25-28] which is discussed elsewhere. In this chapter, we illustrate a subcostal incision for an open left hepatectomy.

- A right subcostal incision is marked out 2 to 3 fingerbreadths below the costal margin. It is carried out laterally to where the floating 12th rib can be palpated (FIGURE 4A).
- The skin and subcutaneous tissue are opened to expose the anterior fascia. The right anterior rectus sheath is opened to expose the right rectus muscle. The incision is extended medially to the midline. The midline is opened, staying anterior to the preperitoneal fat pad up to the level of the xiphoid

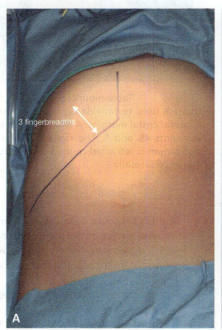
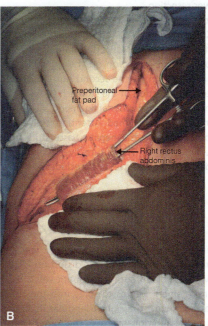

FIGURE 4 • Right subcostal incision with upper midline extension. A, The subcostal portion of the incision should be placed 2 to 3 fingerbreadths below the costal margin. B, The right rectus muscle is divided with cautery. C, The falciform and round ligaments are divided.

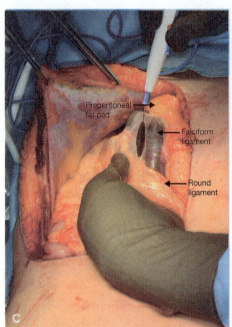
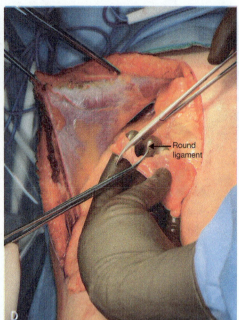

FIGURE 4 • Continued

process. The xiphoid process can be removed to facilitate exposure if necessary.
- The right rectus and lateral abdominal muscles are then divided with cautery (**FIGURE 4B**) and the posterior rectus sheath is exposed. The peritoneal cavity is entered.
- The round ligament is ligated and divided. This can be preserved as a pedicled flap for future use (**FIGURE 4C**).
- The peritoneal surfaces of the abdominal cavity and the future liver remnant are palpated to assess for disease that would preclude liver resection.
- A self-retaining, table-mounted retractor is critical for adequate exposure. Key principles for exposure include cephalad and lateral retraction of the bilateral costal margins. During the hilar dissection, caudad retraction on the right kidney, caudad and medial retraction on the second portion of the duodenum, and lateral retraction of the stomach (**FIGURE 5**) are key to exposing the hepatoduodenal ligament.
- Intraoperative ultrasound is performed. Attention is given to the relationship of tumor(s) to the hepatic vasculature and anticipated transection margin. The future liver remnant is carefully inspected to ensure that no lesions preclude resection.

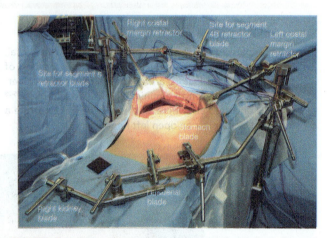

FIGURE 5 • Table-mounted retractor. Abdominal wall retractors are used to provide cephalad and lateral retraction on the bilateral costal margins. A thin, malleable blade is used to retract segments 4B and 6. The right kidney is retracted caudad; the duodenum is retracted caudad and medially; and the stomach is retracted laterally.

STEP 2: MOBILIZATION

- The falciform ligament is divided midway between the anterior abdominal wall and liver capsule. This dissection is carried cephalad toward the diaphragm and hepatic veins.
- Once the falciform ligament begins to splay into the right and left triangular ligaments, the right triangular ligament is released, exposing the anterior surface of the right hepatic vein. Medially, a notch between the right hepatic vein and the common trunk of the middle and left veins can be palpated.
- The left triangular ligament is similarly divided to expose the anterior surface of the common trunk. The left phrenic vein, which drains into the left hepatic vein, serves as a reliable landmark for the identification of the left vein and common trunk.
- Once the anterior surfaces of the hepatic veins are exposed, a lap pad may be placed posterior to the left lateral segments of the liver and anterior to the stomach to protect the stomach from injury. The remainder of the left triangular ligament is divided, exposing the lateral wall of the left hepatic vein.

- If the gallbladder is still present, a standard top-down cholecystectomy is performed. The gallbladder can be left attached to the cystic duct for cholangiogram at the completion of the case.
- The gastrohepatic ligament is opened widely. An accessory or replaced left hepatic artery found in the gastrohepatic ligament is ligated and divided. An umbilical tape or vessel loop may be passed around the hepatoduodenal ligament in preparation for a Pringle maneuver if necessary later in the case (**FIGURE 6**).

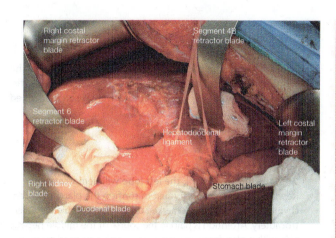

FIGURE 6 • Pringle maneuver. A moistened umbilical tape (or vessel loop) is passed around the hepatoduodenal ligament. As the parenchymal transection is deepened, a Pringle maneuver can be performed by cinching down on the tape or vessel loop to minimize bleeding from inflow vessels.

STEP 3: INFLOW CONTROL

- Any parenchymal bridge between the left lateral and left medial sections are divided, opening up the umbilical fissure.
- The left hilar structures are exposed by scoring the peritoneum at the base of the umbilical fissure. The left hepatic artery is dissected circumferentially. A test clamp is performed by palpating the proper and right hepatic artery or by confirming flow with ultrasound.
- The left portal vein is dissected where it enters the umbilical fissure; it can be divided with a vascular load of a linear cutting stapler (**FIGURE 7**).
- If the caudate lobe is to be preserved, the dissection occurs distal to the caudate branches.

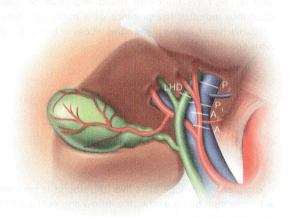

FIGURE 7 • Inflow control. The left hilar structures are exposed. The left hepatic artery is divided proximal to the caudate branch at point A_1 or distal to the caudate branch at point A_2 depending on whether or not the caudate lobe is going to be resected. Similarly, the portal vein is divided proximal to the caudate branch at point P_1 or distal to the caudate branch at point P_2. The left hepatic duct (LHD) can be divided extraparenchymally at this point or intraparenchymally later in the operation.

STEP 4: OUTFLOW CONTROL

- The left lateral section is rotated medially, exposing the caudate lobe and ligamentum venosum (Arantius ligament). The ligamentum venosum is divided caudally, close to its entry into the left hepatic vein.
- Based on the tumor–hepatic vein relationship noted on preoperative imaging and intraoperative ultrasound, a tunnel is carefully developed around the left hepatic vein or the common trunk of the left and middle hepatic veins, anterior to the inferior vena cava. Once isolated, the hepatic vein is divided using a vascular load of a linear cutting stapler.
- If the middle hepatic vein can be preserved based on the location of the lesion, a small hepatotomy can be made between the left and middle hepatic veins, allowing for individual extrahepatic control of the left hepatic vein. Alternatively, the left hepatic vein can be divided intraparenchymally during the parenchymal transection (step 6) if the tumor is located farther away (**FIGURE 8**).

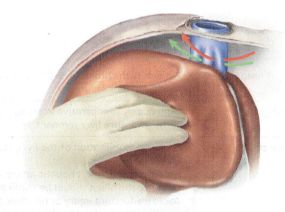

FIGURE 8 • Outflow control. The left lateral segment of the liver is rotated medially to expose the ligamentum venosum. The ligament is divided caudad to the insertion into the left hepatic vein. A tunnel is carefully developed around the left and middle hepatic vein common trunk or around just the left hepatic vein. Care should be taken to stay anterior to the inferior vena cava.

STEP 5: BILE DUCT DIVISION

- The left hepatic bile duct can be identified just above the left portal vein and be divided as it enters the umbilical fissure during step 4 (FIGURE 7). Alternatively, it can be divided intraparenchymally (separately or with the portal triad) during step 6, which minimizes risk to an anomalous right posterior duct arising from the left duct (FIGURE 3C).

STEP 6: PARENCHYMAL TRANSECTION

- With the inflow control, the left lobe will demarcate.
- Repeat ultrasound is performed to confirm the plane of parenchymal transection. This is marked on the liver capsule with electrocautery. Attention is paid to the course of the middle hepatic vein with a plan for preservation or resection depending on the location of the lesion. When possible, the liver should be transected in the ischemic zone to minimize blood loss.
- Electrocautery can be used on the initial 1 to 2 cm of parenchyma, after which any number of methods can be used to divide the parenchyma, including hydrodissection,[29] crush/clamp, and staplers.
- When creating parenchymal tunnels through which staplers can be fired, the clamp should effortlessly be passed. Resistance indicates the presence of a major structure. If resistance is met, a new plane either above or below the previous one should be chosen.
- A Pringle maneuver may be used liberally to minimize blood loss during the transection.
- The line of transection should proceed from caudad to cephalad and anterior to posterior. In addition, the parenchyma is divided anterior to the ligamentum venosum if the caudate lobe is not to be included.
- If not previously divided, the left bile duct and the left hepatic vein can be divided with a linear stapler as encountered during the parenchymal transection.
- Once the parenchymal transection is complete, the cut surface of the liver is inspected for surgical bleeding, which is suture ligated, or bile leaks, which are repaired with fine monofilament suture.
- If a Pringle maneuver was applied, it should be released for assessment of residual bleeding. The cut surface is dried using cautery with care taken to avoid thermal injury to the central biliary structures of the liver remnant.

STEP 7: COMPLETION ULTRASOUND/SALINE AND CONTRAST CHOLANGIOGRAM/ PLACEMENT OF DRAINS AND ABDOMINAL CLOSURE

- A completion intraoperative liver ultrasound is performed with attention being paid to the inflow and outflow of the remnant liver.
- If there is a concern for a biliary leak that cannot be localized, an air or saline cholangiogram can be performed through the cystic duct.[30] The cystic duct is then ligated and divided.
- A closed suction drain may be considered if there is concern for a potential postoperative biliary leak. The incision is closed.

PEARLS AND PITFALLS

Patient history	▪ Patients with chronic liver disease should be aggressively optimized to reduce risk of postoperative liver insufficiency or failure.
Imaging	▪ High-quality preoperative imaging is imperative for operative planning to ensure adequate margin and sufficient future liver remnant.
Inflow control	▪ On initial mobilization of the liver, capsular tears should be avoided as they can cause unnecessary bleeding. ▪ Before taking the left hepatic artery, a test clamp should be performed and maintenance of flow in the right hepatic hilum should be confirmed. ▪ Avoid inadvertent injury or narrowing of the main portal vein by taking the left portal vein high in the umbilical fissure distal to the takeoff of the caudate branch.

Outflow control	▪ Left phrenic vein serves as reliable landmark that can be followed back to the insertion to the left hepatic vein. ▪ Dissection to gain control of the left hepatic vein or the common trunk of the middle and left hepatic veins should be done carefully. Attempts to pass a clamp against resistance can lead to iatrogenic injury to the posterior wall of the hepatic vein or the anterior surface of the vena cava.
Bile duct division	▪ When possible, the bile duct is divided intraparenchymally to avoid injury to an anomalous right posterior duct arising from the left duct.
Parenchymal transection	▪ Several different techniques for parenchymal transection exist. Familiarization and comfort with different techniques is invaluable. ▪ Bile leaks from the cut surface should be identified and repaired immediately when found.

POSTOPERATIVE CARE

- Orogastric tube, if previously placed, can be removed at the end of the case.
- Intensive care unit admission is not necessarily required but depends on patient factors and surgeon preference.
- Adequate analgesia is a key component of the postoperative care. Patient-controlled analgesia and locoregional or incisional blocks should be considered. Nonopiate adjuncts, such as acetaminophen,[31] ketorolac, temperature therapy (ice or heat), and massage therapy, should be used liberally.
- Early ambulation and aggressive respiratory therapy are important to avoid pulmonary complications.
- Laboratory studies including complete metabolic panel and blood counts are obtained as clinically indicated. Particular attention is paid to the serum phosphorus levels with aggressive replacement instituted to assist with liver hypertrophy and regeneration.[32-34]
- If a closed suction drain was placed, the volume and character of the drain output are closely monitored. Bilious drainage is concerning for a bile leak. Should this occur, consider endoscopic retrograde cholangiogram with sphincterotomy and stenting in an attempt to decompress the bile leak to allow spontaneous closure.
- Otherwise, the drain may be removed prior to discharge as long as the output is nonbilious. For high-volume output >200 cc in 24 hours, diuretic therapy may be considered.

OUTCOMES

- A formal left hemihepatectomy is well tolerated by most patients. The length of hospital stay is 7 to 15 days with complication rates 18% to 45%.[35-38] These numbers continue to decrease with advances in minimally invasive techniques.

COMPLICATIONS

- Bile leak
- Liver insufficiency or failure
- Hemorrhage
- Venothromboembolism
- Wound complication
- Disease recurrence

ACKNOWLEDGMENT

We gratefully acknowledge the past contributions by the previous edition author, Jon S. Cardinal, as portions of that chapter were retained in this revision.

REFERENCES

1. Strasberg SM, Belghiti J, Clavien PA, et al. The Brisbane 2000 terminology of liver anatomy and resections. *HPB*. 2000;2(3):333-339. doi:10.1016/S1365-182X(17)30755-4
2. Lambert JE, Hayes LD, Keegan TJ, Subar DA, Gaffney CJ. The impact of prehabilitation on patient outcomes in hepatobiliary, colorectal, and upper gastrointestinal cancer surgery: a PRISMA-accordant meta-analysis. *Ann Surg*. 2021;274(1):70-77. doi:10.1097/SLA.0000000000004527
3. Walcott-Sapp S, Billingsley KG. Preoperative optimization for major hepatic resection. *Langenbeck's Arch Surg* 2017 4031. 2017;403(1):23-35. doi:10.1007/S00423-017-1638-X
4. Fan ST, Lo CM, Lai E, Chu KM, Liu CL, Wong J. Perioperative nutritional support in patients undergoing hepatectomy for hepatocellular carcinoma. *N Engl J Med*. 2010;331(23):1547-1552. doi:10.1056/NEJM199412083312303
5. Barberan-Garcia A, Ubré M, Roca J, et al. Personalised prehabilitation in high-risk patients undergoing elective major abdominal surgery: a randomized blinded controlled trial. *Ann Surg*. 2018;267(1):50-56. doi:10.1097/SLA.0000000000002293
6. Karoui M, Penna C, Amin-Hashem M, et al. Influence of preoperative chemotherapy on the risk of major hepatectomy for colorectal liver metastases. *Ann Surg*. 2006;243(1):1-7. doi:10.1097/01.sla.0000193603.26265.c3
7. Kočo L, Weekenstroo HHA, Lambregts DMJ, et al. The effects of multidisciplinary team meetings on clinical practice for colorectal, lung, prostate and breast cancer: a systematic review. *Cancers (Basel)*. 2021;13(16):4159. doi:10.3390/CANCERS13164159/S1
8. Osterlund P, Salminen T, Soveri LM, et al. Repeated centralized multidisciplinary team assessment of resectability, clinical behavior, and outcomes in 1086 Finnish metastatic colorectal cancer patients (RAXO): a nationwide prospective intervention study. *Lancet Reg Heal Eur*. 2021;3:100049. doi:10.1016/J.LANEPE.2021.100049
9. André T. Centralized multidisciplinary team assessment of metastasis resectability in patients with metastatic colorectal cancer: a fundamental necessity. *Lancet Reg Heal Eur*. 2021;3:100058. doi:10.1016/J.LANEPE.2021.100058
10. Michels NA. Newer anatomy of the liver and its variant blood supply and collateral circulation. *Am J Surg*. 1966;112(3):337-347. doi:10.1016/0002-9610(66)90201-7
11. Chernyak V, Fowler KJ, Kamaya A, et al. Liver imaging reporting and data system (LI-RADS) version 2018: imaging of hepatocellular carcinoma in at-risk patients. *Radiology*. 2018;289(3):816-830. doi:10.1148/RADIOL.2018181494. Accessed November 8, 2021. ASSET/IMAGES/LARGE/RADIOL.2018181494.TBL1.JPEG.
12. Schaffler-Schaden D, Birsak T, Zintl R, Lorber B, Schaffler G. Risk of needle tract seeding after coaxial ultrasound-guided percutaneous biopsy for primary and metastatic tumors of the liver: report of a single institution. *Abdom Radiol (New York)*. 2020;45(10):3301-3306. doi:10.1007/S00261-019-02120-1
13. Chen I, Lorentzen T, Linnemann D, et al. Seeding after ultrasound-guided percutaneous biopsy of liver metastases in patients with

14. Myers RP, Fong A, Shaheen AAM. Utilization rates, complications and costs of percutaneous liver biopsy: a population-based study including 4275 biopsies. *Liver Int.* 2008;28(5):705-712. doi:10.1111/J.1478-3231.2008.01691.X
15. Maturen KE, Nghiem HV, Marrero JA, et al. Lack of tumor seeding of hepatocellular carcinoma after percutaneous needle biopsy using coaxial cutting needle technique. *Am J Roentgenol.* 2006;187(5):1184-1187. doi:10.2214/AJR.05.1347
16. MacMahon H, Naidich DP, Goo JM, et al. Guidelines for management of incidental pulmonary nodules detected on CT images: from the Fleischner Society 2017. *Radiology.* 2017;284(1):228-243. doi:10.1148/RADIOL.2017161659/ASSET/IMAGES/LARGE/RADIOL.2017161659.FIG1 4B.JPEG
17. Schwartz LH, Litière S, De Vries E, et al. Recist 1.1—update and clarification: from the RECIST committee. *Eur J Cancer.* 2016;62:132-137. doi:10.1016/J.EJCA.2016.03.081
18. Loverdos K, Fotiadis A, Kontogianni C, Iliopoulou M, Gaga M. Lung nodules: a comprehensive review on current approach and management. *Ann Thorac Med.* 2019;14(4):226-238. doi:10.4103/ATM.ATM_110_19
19. Adam R, de Haas R, Wicherts D, et al. Is hepatic resection justified after chemotherapy in patients with colorectal liver metastases and lymph node involvement? *J Clin Oncol.* 2008;26(22):3672-3680. doi:10.1200/JCO.2007.15.7297
20. Sawada Y, Sahara K, Endo I, et al. Long-term outcome of liver resection for colorectal metastases in the presence of extrahepatic disease: a multi-institutional Japanese study. *J Hepatobiliary Pancreat Sci.* 2020;27(11):810-818. doi:10.1002/JHBP.810
21. Hughes MJ, Ventham NT, Harrison EM, Wigmore SJ. Central venous pressure and liver resection: a systematic review and meta-analysis. *HPB (Oxford).* 2015;17(10):863-871. doi:10.1111/HPB.12462
22. Mungroop TH, Geerts BF, Veelo DP, et al. Fluid and pain management in liver surgery (MILESTONE): a worldwide study among surgeons and anesthesiologists. *Surgery.* 2019;165(2):337-344. doi:10.1016/J.SURG.2018.08.013
23. Jongerius IM, Mungroop TH, Uz Z, et al. Goal-directed fluid therapy vs. low central venous pressure during major open liver resections (GALILEO): a surgeon- and patient-blinded randomized controlled trial. *HPB (Oxford).* 2021;23(10):1578-1585. doi:10.1016/J.HPB.2021.03.013
24. Wrzosek A, Jakowicka-Wordliczek J, Zajaczkowska R, et al. Perioperative restrictive versus goal-directed fluid therapy for adults undergoing major non-cardiac surgery. *Cochrane Database Syst Rev.* 2019;2019(12):CD012767. doi:10.1002/14651858.CD012767.pub2
25. Fretland AA, Dagenborg VJ, Bjørnelv GMW, et al. Laparoscopic versus open resection for colorectal liver metastases: the OSLO-COMET randomized controlled trial. *Ann Surg.* 2018;267(2):199-207. doi:10.1097/SLA.0000000000002353
26. Wakabayashi G, Cherqui D, Geller DA, et al. Recommendations for laparoscopic liver resection: a report from the second international consensus conference held in Morioka. *Ann Surg.* 2015;261(4):619-629. doi:10.1097/SLA.0000000000001184
27. Robles-Campos R, Lopez-Lopez V, Brusadin R, et al. Open versus minimally invasive liver surgery for colorectal liver metastases (LapOpHuva): a prospective randomized controlled trial. *Surg Endosc.* 2019;33(12):3926-3936. doi:10.1007/S00464-019-06679-0/TABLES/3
28. Ruzzenente A, Bagante F, Ratti F, et al. Minimally invasive versus open liver resection for hepatocellular carcinoma in the setting of portal vein hypertension: results of an international multi-institutional analysis. *Ann Surg Oncol.* 2020;27(9):3360-3371. doi:10.1245/S10434-020-08444-3
29. Aloia TA, Zorzi D, Abdalla EK, Vauthey JN. Two-surgeon technique for hepatic parenchymal transection of the noncirrhotic liver using saline-linked cautery and ultrasonic dissection. *Ann Surg.* 2005;242(2):172-177. doi:10.1097/01.SLA.0000171300.62318.F4
30. Zimmitti G, Vauthey JN, Shindoh J, et al. Systematic use of an intraoperative air leak test at the time of major liver resection reduces the rate of postoperative biliary complications. *J Am Coll Surg.* 2013;217(6):1028-1037. doi:10.1016/J.JAMCOLLSURG.2013.07.392
31. Katayama M, Koizumi S, Kobayashi S. Analgesic safety of periodic intravenous infusion of acetaminophen after hepatectomy: a propensity score matching analysis. *Gastroint Hepatol Dig Dis.* 2019;2(2):1-6.
32. Hallet J, Karanicolas PJ, Zih FSW, et al. Hypophosphatemia and recovery of post-hepatectomy liver insufficiency. *Hepatobiliary Surg Nutr.* 2016;5(3):217. doi:10.21037/HBSN.2015.12.13
33. George R, Shiu MH. Hypophosphatemia after major hepatic resection. *Surgery.* 1992;111(3):281-286. Accessed November 8, 2021. https://pubmed.ncbi.nlm.nih.gov/1311873/
34. Sadot E, Zheng J, Srouji R, et al. Hypophosphatemia as a predictor of organ-specific complications following gastrointestinal surgery: analysis of 8034 patients. *World J Surg.* 2019;43(2):385-394. doi:10.1007/S00268-018-4726-3
35. Valente R, Sutcliffe R, Levesque E, et al. Fully laparoscopic left hepatectomy—a technical reference proposed for standard practice compared to the open approach: a retrospective propensity score model. *HPB (Oxford).* 2018;20(4):347-355. doi:10.1016/J.HPB.2017.10.006
36. Hong SK, Suh KS, Kim KA, et al. Pure laparoscopic versus open left hepatectomy including the middle hepatic vein for living donor liver transplantation. *Liver Transplant.* 2020;26(3):370-378. doi:10.1002/LT.25697
37. Shin YC, Jang JY, Kang MJ, et al. Comparison of laparoscopic versus open left-sided hepatectomy for intrahepatic duct stones. *Surg Endosc.* 2016;30(1):259-265. doi:10.1007/S00464-015-4200-3
38. Chen S, Huang L, nan QF, et al. Total laparoscopic partial hepatectomy versus open partial hepatectomy for primary left-sided hepatolithiasis: a propensity, long-term follow-up analysis at a single center. *Surgery.* 2018;163(4):714-720. doi:10.1016/J.SURG.2017.10.053

Chapter 24 Minimally Invasive Left Hepatic Lobectomy

Epameinondas Dogeas and Amer H. Zureikat

DEFINITION

- A minimally invasive left hepatic lobectomy (also termed left hepatectomy or left hemihepatectomy) is the resection of the liver medial to the midplane of the liver (Cantlie line) using laparoscopic or robotic assistance and is formally defined as the resection of Couinaud segments 2, 3, and 4.[1] A liver resection is termed laparoscopic if it is a pure laparoscopic procedure, a hand-assisted procedure, or a hybrid technique procedure (which begins as a pure laparoscopic or as a hand-assisted procedure with the liver resection done through a mini-laparotomy incision).[2] A left hepatectomy is performed for benign and malignant lesions and for living donor transplantation.

PATIENT HISTORY AND PHYSICAL FINDINGS

- A comprehensive history and physical examination should be performed with attention to signs and symptoms of liver failure, coagulopathy, and cardiac disease.
- The same indications for an open left hepatectomy apply to a minimally invasive left hepatectomy, and the indications for benign lesions should not be relaxed due to the minimally invasive approach.[2] The indications for resection include hepatic adenoma, symptomatic hemangiomas, symptomatic focal nodular hyperplasia, symptomatic giant cysts, hepatocellular carcinoma, and colorectal and neuroendocrine cancer metastases.[3]
- The contraindications for a minimally invasive left hepatectomy include those for an open resection, in addition to decompensated cirrhosis, the inability to tolerate pneumoperitoneum, dense adhesions that are not amenable to minimally invasive adhesiolysis, need for extensive portal lymphadenectomy, concern for gallbladder carcinoma, need for vascular resection, and lesions that are near major vessels.[3,4] Biliary reconstruction is a relative contraindication for robotic assisted surgery depending on the experience of the surgeon.[5]
- Lesion characteristics that are most favorable for laparoscopic resection include solitary lesions, size of 5 cm or less, peripheral location, and those without involvement of the hilum, major hepatic veins, or the inferior vena cava.[2]

IMAGING AND OTHER DIAGNOSTIC STUDIES

- Preoperative imaging is required to evaluate lesion resectability and for surgical planning. Imaging is useful for evaluation of lesion size, proximity to major vessels and bile ducts, aberrant anatomy, and adequacy of anticipated postoperative liver volume and for detection of lung or other abdominal metastases for malignant indications.
- Contrast-enhanced computed tomography (CT) (**FIGURE 1A** and **B**), magnetic resonance imaging (MRI), and positron emission tomography (PET) can be used for preoperative evaluation.[6] A triple-phase CT (arterial, venous, and delayed venous phase) is useful for its spatial resolution and volumetric assessment. MRI is superior for detecting subcentimeter lesions. PET scans may be useful for detecting other sites of metastasis.
- If a quantitative evaluation of liver function is needed, especially for patients who have undergone hepatotoxic chemotherapy, a MEGX (monoethylglycinexylidide) test or indocyanine green clearance test can be used.[6]
- Occasionally, preoperative liver biopsy may be necessary to document the presence or extent of cirrhosis.
- Preoperative laboratory tests include a complete blood count, liver function tests, coagulation profile, and relevant tumor markers in cases of malignant disease.

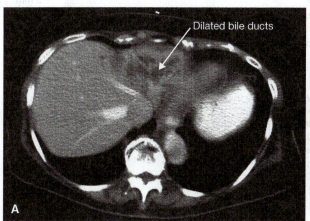 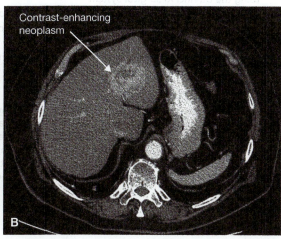

FIGURE 1 • **A,** Female, 84 years, with left hepatic cholangiocarcinoma. **B,** Male, 71 years, with left hepatocellular carcinoma.

SURGICAL MANAGEMENT

Preoperative Planning
- Minimally invasive hepatic surgery should be performed by surgical teams experienced in both advanced minimally invasive techniques and major hepatic surgery.
- All potentially necessary equipment should be readily available, and the patient should be counseled on the possibility for conversion to an open procedure.
- Preoperative portal vein embolization can be considered in order to increase the size of the future remnant liver to a minimum of 25% in the absence of cirrhosis and a minimum of 40% to 50% in well-compensated cirrhosis. PVE is less commonly needed in a left hepatectomy compared with a right.[7]

Positioning
- The operating room is arranged so that the robot can be docked at the head of the table.
- The patient is placed in supine position on a split-leg table in slight reverse-Trendelenburg position. Video monitors are placed to the right and left of the head of the patient.
- A central line and an arterial line are placed for hemodynamic monitoring. Preoperative antibiotic prophylaxis is given and cross-matched blood is made available.
- Judicious administration of intravenous fluid is needed to keep central venous pressure (CVP) less than 5 cm H_2O.
- For a purely laparoscopic resection (no robotic assistance), the operation can be performed with the surgeon standing between the patient's legs or with the surgeon at the patient's left during the hilar dissection and then moving to the right side for the parenchymal transection.[8]
- For the laparoscopic-robotic resection (the focus of this chapter):
  - Laparoscopic portion (liver mobilization): the surgeon stands on the left side, the assistant on the right, and the camera assistant between the legs.
  - For the robotic portion (control of vascular inflow, parenchymal transection, hepatic outflow): the surgeon sits at the console, and the assistant is between the legs (facilitates retraction, suction/irrigation, Ligasure [Covidien, Mansfield, MA] use, suture exchange, exchange of robotic instruments and endovascular stapling).

TECHNIQUES

PORT PLACEMENT (SEE FIGURE 2)
- Pneumoperitoneum is established via a 5-mm OptiView (Ethicon Endo-Surgery, Cincinnati, OH) port in the left mid-abdomen approximately one hands breadth to the left and 2 in above the umbilicus.
- After pneumoperitoneum is established, a 10-mm camera port is placed in the right mid-abdomen approximately one hands breadth to the left and 2 in above the umbilicus. This position is a mirror image of the OptiView port. A smaller 8-mm camera port can be used with the DaVinci Xi Surgical System (Intuitive Surgical, Sunnyvale, CA).
- The abdomen is explored for metastatic disease.
- The full complement of ports is then placed as shown in **FIGURE 2**:
  - three 8-mm robotic ports—R2 on the right, and R1 (OptiView port upsized to robotic) and R3 on the left
  - 12-mm camera port (only 8-mm camera port needed if using the DaVinci Xi Surgical System
  - 12-mm laparoscopic assistant port in right lower quadrant (for stapling, suture access, energy device, suction, clip applier)
  - 5-mm laparoscopic assistant port in left lower quadrant cases (for energy device, suction, clip applier)
- For hepatomegaly or with large tumors, the robotic ports are moved inferiorly toward the level of the umbilicus.[8]
- An intra-abdominal pressure of less than 12 mm Hg is recommended. Although a high intra-abdominal pressure can theoretically improve hemostasis during liver transection, a high intra-abdominal pressure could also potentially increase the risk of gas embolism particularly if injury to the hepatic veins is encountered.[9]

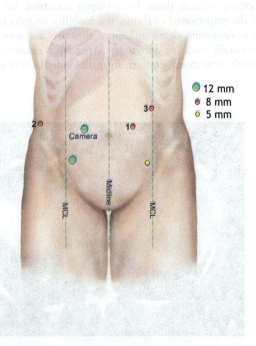

FIGURE 2 • Port sites or left robotic hepatic lobectomy. Red = Robotic arms 1 (usually hook, or grasper), 2 (PK bipolar forceps), 3 (Grasper). Green = Upper (Camera), Lower (Stapler insertion, Passage of Sutures, Gelport specimen extraction). Yellow = laparoscopic assistant port (Suction, Ligasure). Note that a smaller 8-mm camera port can be used with the DaVinci Xi Surgical System.

EXPLORATION AND LESION EVALUATION

- The abdominal cavity and the liver surface are again examined for metastases. All suspicious lesions should be sent for frozen section biopsy.
- Laparoscopic ultrasound of the liver is then performed to confirm resectability of the targeted lesion(s) and the proximity to major vessels as well as to rule out other hepatic metastases.

LIVER EXPOSURE AND MOBILIZATION

- This portion of the operation is performed laparoscopically.
- The falciform ligament and the ligamentum teres are divided with hook electrocautery/Ligasure. These may be divided earlier to help perform the intraoperative ultrasound. The ligamentum teres is left long enough to be used as a handle for the portal dissection.
- The left triangular and left coronary ligaments are also divided using hook electrocautery or the Ligasure device (**FIGURE 3A** and **B**).
- The pars flaccida is opened using the robotic hook/Ligasure staying close to the undersurface of the left lateral section and the caudate lobe. An accessory left hepatic artery may be encountered and is doubly clipped and divided.
- Arantius ligament is then incised using the hook. It runs from the left branch of the portal vein to the left hepatic vein or the common (left and middle) hepatic vein truck. This maneuver can be dangerous since injury to the left hepatic vein can occur. Alternatively, it can be done after the robot is docked to improve visualization.
- The bridge between the left lateral and medial sections (segments III and IVB) is divided with the hook/Ligasure.
- A cholecystectomy is performed to facilitate with exposure of the porta hepatis.

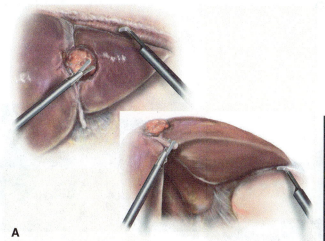
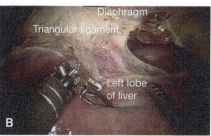

FIGURE 3 • Using the falciform ligament as a handle, the left triangular ligament is divided by a laparoscopic or robotic hook staring from later to medial until the left hepatic vein is visualized before it enters the inferior vena cava (IVC) (**A** and **B**). The pars flaccida is incised, and the ligament of Arantius is divided up to the left hepatic vein.

ROBOT DOCKING

- The robot is docked over the patient's head.
- The R2 (right) arm has the bipolar grasper, R1 (left) arm has the hook, and R3 (left) arm is a Cadiere grasper.

Vascular Inflow Control

- The hepatoduodenal ligament is encircled with tape through the foramen of Winslow to perform the Pringle maneuver intermittently as needed to prevent blood loss.[10]
- The ligamentum teres is retracted anteriorly and cranially to expose the base of the round ligament/umbilical fissure.
- The peritoneum of the left hepatic pedicle is incised, and the left hepatic artery is identified, dissected, and vessel looped. After test clamping and ensuring a good pulse/flow (on ultrasound) in the right porta, the left hepatic artery is transected either between 2-0 silk ties reinforced by clips or by an endovascular stapler (**FIGURE 4A-C**).
- The left portal vein is now identified, dissected using a combination of a hook and Maryland dissector, and vessel looped. Leftward traction on the vessel loop allows the stapler to transect the vein at an ergonomically comfortable angle that does not compromise the bifurcation of the main portal vein (**FIGURE 5A** and **B**).
- The common hepatic duct (**FIGURE 5C**) is followed superiorly just beyond the bifurcation to identify the left hepatic duct. The left hepatic duct is then dissected using the hook along the undersurface of the liver. The left hepatic duct is divided between double clips or ties reinforced with clips.

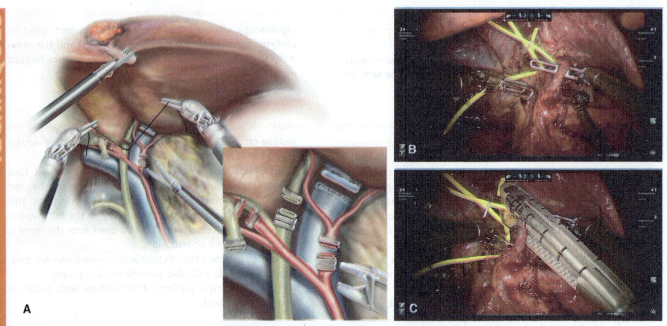

FIGURE 4 • Division of left hepatic inflow. The left hepatic artery is isolated **(A and B)** and taken between 2-0 silk ties reinforce by double clips **(A)** or with a linear vascular stapler **(B and C)**.

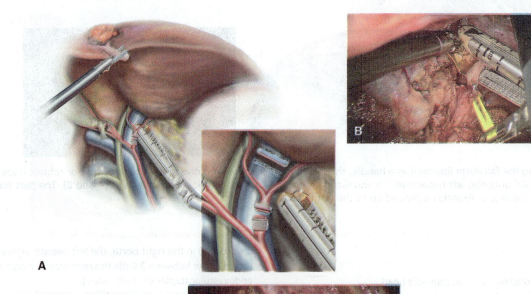

FIGURE 5 • **A,** The left portal vein is transected using a vascular linear stapler. Traction on the bifurcation of the main portal vein using a vessel loop **(B)** prevents inadvertent injury or narrowing of the bifurcation. The left hepatic duct **(C)** is taken between 2-0 ties reinforced by double clips.

PARENCHYMAL TRANSECTION

- A low CVP is maintained during transection to minimize blood loss. Pneumoperitoneum may interfere with CVP readings, and visualization of the vena cava may help determine if the CVP is elevated.
- There is a risk of carbon dioxide venous embolism during parenchymal transection given the combination of pneumoperitoneum during minimally invasive surgery and maintenance of a low CVP.
- Parenchymal transection is then carried out along the line of ischemic demarcation. The plane of transection is marked with electrocautery on the liver slightly to the left of the line of ischemia. The marked line can be assessed by ultrasound as it appears as a hyperechoic line with an acoustic shadow.[8]
- Two large figure-of-eight chromic sutures are placed on either side of the ischemia line and are used as handles to help "open book" the liver (FIGURE 6A).
- Our preferred technique for parenchymal transection proceeds as follows:
  - Transection proceeds from superior to inferior, anterior to posterior direction.
  - The first 1 to 2 cm of the transection is performed with robotic hook electrocautery.
  - The next 1 to 2 cm is performed with the Ligasure device.
  - Deeper dissection utilizes a combination of the bipolar (clamp and crush technique), Ligasure (FIGURE 6B), and clips. This portion of the operation is enhanced by the robotic stereotactic vision and magnification.
- Other transection techniques have been described based on surgeon preference. Instruments that can be used include an ultrasonic scalpel (Harmonic, Ethicon Endo-Surgery, Cincinnati, OH), radiofrequency ablation (Aquamantys, Medtronic, Minneapolis, MN), and ultrasonic aspirator (CUSA, Integra, Plainsboro, NJ) devices. Unlike open resections, argon beam coagulation is not used due to the increase in intra-abdominal pressure (the flow of the argon gas is not pressure regulated) and the potential risk of argon embolism.[11]
- Vessels that are encountered during transection can be clipped and divided with titanium clips (vessels <5 mm) or locking nylon clips (vessels <15 mm) or stapled (larger vessels).

Vascular Outflow Control

- Posteriorly, transection of large tributaries of the left hepatic vein and the left hepatic vein is performed within the liver using vascular load Endo GIA staplers (Covidien, Mansfield, MA). A total of two to three loads is usually necessary (FIGURE 7A and B).

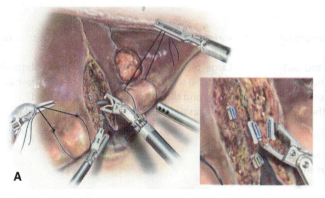
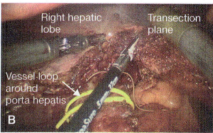

FIGURE 6 • Two figure-of-eight sutures (chromic 2-0 blunt needle) are used as handles to "open book" the liver for parenchymal transection. **A and B,** The robotic hook is used for the first 1 cm depth, followed by the PK robotic bipolar and Ligasure. **C,** Larger sized vessels and bile duct tributaries are clipped as shown.

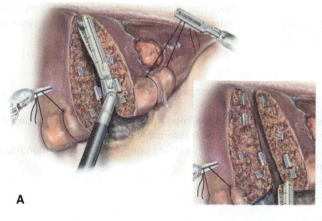
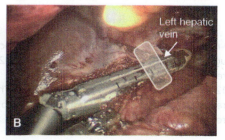

FIGURE 7 • **A and B,** Vascular outflow is taken using an Endo GIA vascular load cartridge. Care must be taken to visualize the tips of the stapler before transection of the left hepatic vein.

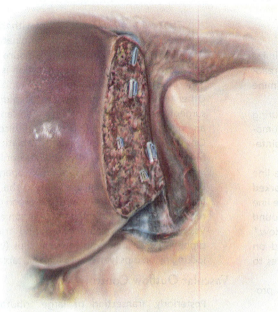
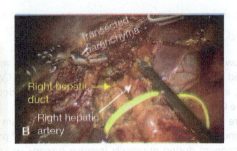

FIGURE 8 • **A,** The cut surface of the liver is examined for bleeding and bile leak. The latter is better visualized after a white sponge/pad is used to compress the liver surface. **B,** Shows the transection surface with the caudate and IVC seen in the left upper quadrant of the picture. Note that a loose vessel loop surrounds the porta hepatis (Pringle); this can be intermittently tightened when bleeding from the cut surface is significant.

- Traction on the middle hepatic vein and vena cava should be avoided.
- Alternatively, a technique where vascular inflow and outflow are controlled before parenchymal dissection has been described.[12] The left hepatic vein is located by identifying the Arantius ligament after lifting the left lobe to the right.

Evaluation of Cut Surface (FIGURE 8A and B)

- The mean arterial pressure and CVP are normalized, and confirmation of hemostasis and absence of bile leak on the cut surface is assessed.[8] A Valsalva maneuver is performed for further evaluation.
- Large bleeders can be suture ligated robotically with ease using 2-0 silk sutures in a figure-of-eight fashion.
- Fibrin and thrombin sealants may be used.
- A cholangiogram is not routinely performed.

SPECIMEN RETRIEVAL

- Intracorporeal sutures are then used to mark the specimen's orientation.
- The specimen is placed in an impermeable plastic bag and removed from the abdominal cavity by enlarging the right lower quadrant incision in order to insert a single site, gas-tight wound protector (Applied Medical, Rancho Santa Margarita, CA) for extraction.
- Note that all robotic instruments should be removed before extracting the specimen to avoid injury when pneumoperitoneum is lost.

DRAIN PLACEMENT AND CLOSURE

- A 19-mm round Blake drain is placed at the resection site through the R3 port and sutured to the skin using 2-0 nylon suture (FIGURE 9).
- The 12-mm camera port site is closed with a Carter-Thomason suture passed in a figure-of-eight fashion using 0 absorbable suture.
- Pneumoperitoneum is then released as the ports are removed.
- The specimen extraction/utility incision is closed using interrupted 0 absorbable suture.
- The skin is closed using 4-0 absorbable monofilament suture.

Chapter 24 MINIMALLY INVASIVE LEFT HEPATIC LOBECTOMY   193

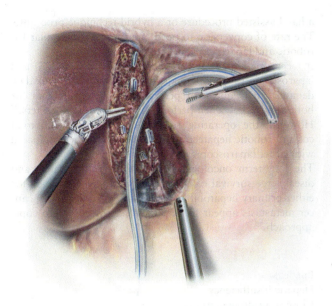

FIGURE 9 • A 19-mm Blake drain is routinely used to drain the resection bed and is usually removed on the 3rd or 4th postoperative day.

CONVERSION

- Conversion should be considered for uncontrolled bleeding and failure to progress. It is recommended to place a mini-laparotomy pad at the bleeding site with the administration of pressure by a laparoscopic grasper while emergent conversion occurs. This will minimize blood loss that can occur while converting to a laparotomy.

PEARLS AND PITFALLS

Port placement	■ Keep a 5-cm distance between ports. Camera port and R1 (dissection arm) should be 5 cm to the right and left of the umbilicus and 2 inches above it. This allows adequate visualization of both the hilar structures anteriorly/inferiorly and the parenchymal transection posteriorly. ■ Robotic arms 2 (bipolar) and 3 (retractor) should be lateral and higher than the camera port and R1. ■ Laparoscopic assistant ports in the right and left lower quadrants must be placed at a slanted angle into the fascia (rather than vertically). This allows minimal collision between the robotic arms and the assistant. It also facilitates easier stapler access to the liver hilum and parenchyma.
Liver mobilization	■ Keeping the round ligament long facilitates its use as a handle for optimal inflow vascular dissection and parenchymal transection. ■ Do not attempt to "overmobilize" the left triangular ligament; this may lead to injury of the left hepatic vein. ■ Use a laparoscopic or robotic bulldog to loosely hold the two ends of the Pringle umbilical tape. In the event of needing a Pringle maneuver, the bulldog can be expeditiously "cinched down" to provide good compression of portal inflow.
Inflow control	■ The robotic Maryland is the most optimal instrument to get around the left portal vein. It is pointed enough to dissect perivascular tissue easily but not sharp enough to readily injure the vessel. ■ Do not grasp vascular structures with the robotic graspers. Use the periadventitial tissue to stabilize the vessel while dissecting it. Lack of tactile feedback can lead to crush injuries to the hepatic artery. ■ A right posterior or anterior duct may insert proximally into the left hepatic duct. This may be injured if the left hepatic duct is not dissected fully.
Parenchymal transection	■ Avoid creating valleys or pits into the liver parenchyma during transection. This makes it difficult to visualize the cut surface and to control bleeding.[8] ■ Have an extra load of the vascular stapler available.
Vascular outflow control	■ This is best approached within the liver. ■ When dividing the middle hepatic vein or left hepatic vein, ensure that the tip of the stapler is seen beyond the vessel.

POSTOPERATIVE CARE

- The orogastric tube is removed at the end of the case.
- ICU admission for major hepatectomy depends on surgeon preference.
- Subcutaneous heparin prophylaxis is started on the evening of surgery.
- Clear liquids are administered on postoperative day 1.
- The Foley catheter is removed on postoperative day 1.
- Diet is advanced as tolerated.

OUTCOMES

- In experienced centers, laparoscopic liver resections are safe and feasible. In a review of 2804 patients, of which 6.8% were left hepatectomies, the overall mortality was 0.3% and overall morbidity was 10.5%.[3] Postoperative morbidity from laparoscopic liver resection is most commonly from liver failure. A conversion rate for laparoscopy to open laparotomy was 4.1% and for laparoscopy to a hand-assisted procedure was 0.7%.
- Compared with open hepatectomies, the advantages of laparoscopic hepatectomies are less blood loss, less time with the Pringle maneuver applied, less postoperative analgesia requirements, a shorter length of stay, and fewer overall complications.[13-15]
- For patients with hepatocellular carcinoma or metastatic disease, margin status, disease-free survival, and overall survival following laparoscopic resection appear comparable with open resection.[16-20]
- Although the operative costs of a minimally invasive hepatectomy are higher than an open approach, this difference may be offset by reduced nonoperative costs due to the shorter length of stay following a minimally invasive resection.[15,21,22]
- A robotic assisted approach with the da Vinci Surgical System (Intuitive Surgical, Sunnyvale, CA) alleviates some of the limitations of laparoscopic surgery such as the fixed pivot point of the instruments, a two-dimensional view, and only 4 degrees of freedom while adding tremor reduction.[5] The advantages of a robotic over a laparoscopic approach could facilitate with the suturing of bleeding parenchyma, performing the hilar dissection, and performing resections that may require intricate biliary-enteric anastomoses.
- Robotic assisted liver resections, including left hepatectomy, are being increasingly performed. Results to date show that it is safe and feasible with a low conversion rate, low estimated blood loss, short length of stay, and limited postoperative morbidity that may be comparable with a laparoscopic approach.[23-27]
- In a matched comparison of robotic vs laparoscopic hepatectomies at the University of Pittsburgh Medical Center, there was no significant difference in estimated blood loss, transfusion rate, R0 negative margin rate, postoperative peak bilirubin, postoperative intensive care admission rate, length of stay, and 90-day mortality. Robotic assisted hepatectomies had a significantly higher overall operating room time (median: 342 vs 261.5 minutes) and operative time (median: 253 vs 199 minutes).[28] However, more robotic assisted hepatectomies were performed in a purely minimally invasive manner, 81%, vs only 7.1% for the laparoscopic approach with the rest of laparoscopic operations involving a hand-assisted procedure or a hybrid technique procedure. The rate of conversion to open laparotomy was similar for robotic and laparoscopic hepatectomy.
- A recent meta-analysis of published robotic (n = 225) and laparoscopic (n = 300) major hepatectomy series to date demonstrated equivalent peri-/postoperative outcomes for both approaches when performed in high-volume centers.[29] However, the operating room, hospitalization, and total costs of robotic hepatectomy appear to be higher compared with either laparoscopic or open surgery.[22]
- The long-term oncologic outcomes, overall survival, and disease-free survival of robotic hepatectomy performed for either primary hepatobiliary malignancies or colorectal cancer metastasis appear to be equivalent to the laparoscopic approach.[30,31]

COMPLICATIONS

- Bile leak
- Hepatic insufficiency
- Close or positive margins
- Hemorrhage
- Wound infection

REFERENCES

1. IHPBA TC of the. Terminology of liver anatomy and resections. *HPB*. 2000;2:333-339.
2. Buell JF, Cherqui D, Geller DA, et al. The international position on laparoscopic liver surgery: the Louisville Statement, 2008. *Ann. Surg.* 2009;250:825-830. doi:10.1097/sla.0b013e3181b3b2d8
3. Nguyen KT, Gamblin TC, Geller DA. World review of laparoscopic liver resection-2,804 patients. *Ann. Surg.* 2009;250(5):831-841. doi:10.1097/sla.0b013e3181b0c4df
4. Vibert E, Perniceni T, Levard H, Denet C, Shahri NK, Gayet B. Laparoscopic liver resection. *Br J Surg*. 2006;93:67-72. doi:10.1002/bjs.5150
5. Idrees K, Bartlett DL. Robotic liver surgery. *Surg Clin*. 2010;90:761-774. doi:10.1016/j.suc.2010.04.020
6. Frankel TL, Gian RK, Jarnagin WR. Preoperative imaging for hepatic resection of colorectal cancer metastasis. *J Gastrointest Oncol*. 2012;3:11-18. doi:10.3978/j.issn.2078-6891.2012.002
7. Vibert E, Kouider A, Gayet B. Laparoscopic anatomic liver resection. *HPB*. 2004;6:222-229. doi:10.1080/13651820410023996
8. Pearce NW, Fabio FD, Hilal MA. Laparoscopic left hepatectomy with extraparenchymal inflow control. *J Am Coll Surg*. 2011;213:e23-7. doi:10.1016/j.jamcollsurg.2011.08.010
9. Otsuka Y, Katagiri T, Ishii J, et al. Gas embolism in laparoscopic hepatectomy: what is the optimal pneumoperitoneal pressure for laparoscopic major hepatectomy? *J Hepatobiliary Pancreatic Sci*. 2013;20:137-140. doi:10.1007/s00534-012-0556-0
10. Rotellar F, Pardo F, Bueno A, Marti-Cruchaga P, Zozaya G. Extracorporeal tourniquet method for intermittent hepatic pedicle clamping during laparoscopic liver surgery: an easy, cheap, and effective technique. *Langenbeck's Arch Surg*. 2012;397:481-485. doi:10.1007/s00423-011-0887-3
11. Figueredo EJ, Yeung RS. Laparoscopic liver resection. *Medscape J Med*. 2008;10:68. http://www.ncbi.nlm.nih.gov/pubmed/18449340
12. Giuro GD, Lainas P, Franco D, Dagher I. Laparoscopic left hepatectomy with prior vascular control. *Surg Endosc*. 2010;24:697-699. doi:10.1007/s00464-009-0613-1
13. Martin RC, Scoggins CR, McMasters KM. Laparoscopic hepatic lobectomy: advantages of a minimally invasive approach. *J Am Coll Surg*. 2010;210:627-634, 634-636. doi:10.1016/j.jamcollsurg.2009.12.022
14. Tsinberg M, Tellioglu G, Simpfendorfer CH, et al. Comparison of laparoscopic versus open liver tumor resection: a case-controlled study. *Surg Endosc*. 2009;23:847-853. doi:10.1007/s00464-008-0262-9

15. Nguyen KT, Marsh JW, Tsung A, Steel JJ, Gamblin TC, Geller DA. Comparative benefits of laparoscopic vs open hepatic resection: a critical appraisal. *Arch Surg.* 2011;146(3):348-356. doi:10.1001/archsurg.2010.248
16. Yin Z, Fan X, Ye H, Yin D, Wang J. Short- and long-term outcomes after laparoscopic and open hepatectomy for hepatocellular carcinoma: a global systematic review and meta-analysis. *Ann Surg Oncol.* 2012;20(4):1203-1215. doi:10.1245/s10434-012-2705-8
17. Kandil E, Noureldine SI, Koffron A, Yao L, Saggi B, Buell JF. Outcomes of laparoscopic and open resection for neuroendocrine liver metastases. *Surgery.* 2012;152:1225-1231. doi:10.1016/j.surg.2012.08.027
18. Cannon RM, Scoggins CR, Callender GG, McMasters KM, Martin RC2nd. Laparoscopic versus open resection of hepatic colorectal metastases. *Surgery.* 2012;152:567-573; discussion 573-574. doi:10.1016/j.surg.2012.07.013
19. Nguyen KT, Laurent A, Dagher I, et al. Minimally invasive liver resection for metastatic colorectal cancer: a multi-institutional, international report of safety, feasibility, and early outcomes. *Ann. Surg.* 2009;250:842-848. doi:10.1097/sla.0b013e3181bc789c
20. Li N, Wu YR, Wu B, Lu MQ. Surgical and oncologic outcomes following laparoscopic versus open liver resection for hepatocellular carcinoma: a meta-analysis. *Hepatol Res.* 2012;42:51-59. doi:10.1111/j.1872-034x.2011.00890.x
21. Koffron AJ, Auffenberg G, Kung R, Abecassis M. Evaluation of 300 minimally invasive liver resections at a single institution: less is more. *Ann. Surg.* 2007;246:385-392; discussion 392-394. doi:10.1097/sla.0b013e318146996c
22. Ziogas IA, Evangeliou AP, Mylonas KS, et al. Economic analysis of open versus laparoscopic versus robotic hepatectomy: a systematic review and meta-analysis. *European J Heal Econ.* 2021;22(4):585-604. doi:10.1007/s10198-021-01277-1
23. Giulianotti PC, Coratti A, Sbrana F, et al. Robotic liver surgery: results for 70 resections. *Surgery.* 2011;149:29-39. doi:10.1016/j.surg.2010.04.002
24. Abood GJ, Tsung A. Robot-assisted surgery: improved tool for major liver resections? *J Hepatobiliary Pancreatic Sci.* 2013;20:151-156. doi:10.1007/s00534-012-0560-4
25. Ho CM, Wakabayashi G, Nitta H, Ito N, Hasegawa Y, Takahara T. Systematic review of robotic liver resection. *Surg Endosc.* 2013;27:732-739. doi:10.1007/s00464-012-2547-2
26. Lee SJ, Lee JH, Lee Y, et al. The feasibility of robotic left-side hepatectomy with comparison of laparoscopic and open approach: consecutive series of single surgeon. *Int J Med Robot Comput Assisted Surg.* 2019;15(2):e1982. doi:10.1002/rcs.1982
27. Cai J-P, Chen W, Chen L-H, Wan X-Y, Lai J-M, Yin X-Y. Comparison between robotic-assisted and laparoscopic left hemi-hepatectomy. *Asian J Surg.* 2022;45(1):265-268. doi:10.1016/j.asjsur.2021.05.017
28. Tsung A, Geller DA, Sukato DC, et al. Robotic versus laparoscopic hepatectomy: a matched comparison. *Ann Surg.* 2013;259(3):549-555. doi:10.1097/sla.0000000000000250
29. Ziogas IA, Giannis D, Esagian SM, Economopoulos KP, Tohme S, Geller DA. Laparoscopic versus robotic major hepatectomy: a systematic review and meta-analysis. *Surg Endosc.* 2021;35(2):524-535. doi:10.1007/s00464-020-08008-2
30. Beard RE, Khan S, Troisi RI, et al. Long-term and oncologic outcomes of robotic versus laparoscopic liver resection for metastatic colorectal cancer: a multicenter, propensity score matching analysis. *World J Surg.* 2020;44(3):887-895. doi:10.1007/s00268-019-05270-x
31. Khan S, Beard RE, Kingham PT, et al. Long-term oncologic outcomes following robotic liver resections for primary hepatobiliary malignancies: a multicenter study. *Ann Surg Oncol.* 2018;25(9):2652-2660. doi:10.1245/s10434-018-6629-9

Chapter 25 Robotic Liver Resection

Cameron Schlegel and David L. Bartlett

DEFINITION

- The use of robotic-assisted surgery for liver resections is mostly dependent on tumor location and the experience of the surgical team. The original indications for the use of robotics have been extrapolated from the Louisville Statement in 2008, which set forth the guidelines for laparoscopic liver resection. Patients with solitary lesions, 5 cm or less, and located in segments 2 to 6 were considered eligible for robotic-assisted surgery.[1]
- These indications have been expanded by most experienced robotic liver surgeons to include more extensive liver resections, including formal anatomic hepatectomies.
- Although absolute contraindications to a minimally invasive approach by an experienced surgeon are few, extra thought should be given to large lesions that may impede mobilization of the liver through a robotic technique. In addition, lesions adjacent to major vascular structures may pose an extra challenge when approaching robotically, particularly in patients with underlying liver disease or high intrahepatic portal venous pressure. Although these patients may still derive benefit from a minimally invasive approach, the surgeon should be prepared to manage additional blood loss and, when necessary, convert to an open procedure.

DIFFERENTIAL DIAGNOSIS

- The differential diagnosis of a liver mass includes both benign and malignant processes. Benign processes are either cystic or solid. Malignant processes are usually solid (**TABLE 1**).

PATIENT HISTORY AND PHYSICAL FINDINGS

- The evaluation of a patient with a liver mass should include a complete history and physical examination.
- History should include questions regarding presence of abdominal pain, weight loss, alcohol use, viral hepatitis, liver disease, tattoos, blood transfusions, and personal or family history of cancer. History should include use of oral contraceptives for women.
- Physical examination should pay particular attention to the presence of abdominal masses, hepatomegaly, splenomegaly, ascites, jaundice, scleral icterus, asterixis, and caput medusa.

IMAGING AND OTHER DIAGNOSTIC STUDIES

- Workup should include blood sent for the following:
  - Complete blood count
  - Blood urea nitrogen
  - Creatinine
  - Electrolytes
  - Liver enzymes
  - Albumin
  - International normalized ratio
  - Viral hepatitis screen
  - Serum ammonia level
  - Tumor markers (carcinoembryonic antigen, α-fetoprotein, cancer antigen 19-9, chromogranin A)
- Imaging studies play a significant role in the diagnoses of liver lesions and in the preoperative planning for liver resection.
- Ultrasound can be useful to differentiate between solid and cystic lesions of the liver, although it is very user dependent and may be limited by interference secondary to presence of bowel gas, obesity, and overlying ribs.
- Contrast-enhanced, triphasic computed tomography (CT) scans are used for diagnosis of liver lesions and preoperative planning for liver resections. These include arterial, portal venous, and delayed phases. Alternatively, a contrasted MRI of the abdomen and pelvis may be used, which offers similar resolution with the avoidance of radiation. Both studies offer excellent ways to assess the characteristic of liver lesions, proximity to major vasculature or biliary structures, and baseline vascular and biliary anatomy and get a sense of the background liver parenchyma.
- Volumetric analysis of a future liver remnant is used to assess feasibility of resection. In general, a functional liver remnant of 20% is desired with a healthy liver and 30% to 50% with a diseased liver. Preoperative portal vein embolization may be considered to hypertrophy the remaining liver prior to resection.
- Other imaging modalities used include positron emission tomography (PET) scan and CT-PET scans. PET imaging is

Table 1: Differential Diagnosis of Liver Mass

Benign	Cystic	Pyogenic abscess Amebic abscess Hydatid cyst Simple cyst
	Solid	Hemangioma Adenoma Focal nodular hyperplasia Biliary hamartoma
Malignant		Hepatocellular carcinoma Cholangiocarcinoma Gallbladder cancer Metastatic colon cancer Metastatic neuroendocrine cancer Metastatic cancer of other etiologies

ideal for many metastatic cancers to the liver, but it is best combined with an intravenous (IV) contrast CT scan so that anatomic relations can be made.

SURGICAL MANAGEMENT

Positioning

- The robot is usually brought from the top or the right side of the operating table.
- The patient is placed in the supine position with the legs split, foot boards placed, and both arms tucked.
- The first surgeon stands on the right side of the table prior to docking the robot, while the second surgeon stands between the legs. An assistant stands on the left side of the table. After docking the assistant surgeon stands between the legs.
- The patient is placed in steep reverse Trendelenburg at all times during the procedure (**FIGURE 1**).

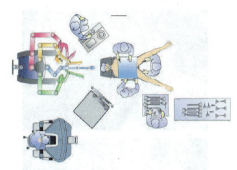

FIGURE 1 • Arrangement of the operating room and placement of the robot. The primary surgeon is positioned between the patient's legs during the laparoscopic portions of the procedure, with the first assistant to the patient's left. The scrub technician is to the patient's right. The anesthesiologist is positioned to the left or the top depending on the robot access. (Reprinted by permission from Springer: Sabbaghian MS, Bartlett DL, Tsung A. Robotic hepatic resections: segmentectomy, lobectomy, parenchymal sparing. In: Kim KC, ed. *Robotics in General Surgery*. Springer; 2014:161-174, with kind permission of Springer Science+Business Media.)

RIGHT HEPATECTOMY

- Port placement
  - Pneumoperitoneum is established through placement of a 5-mm port in the left upper quadrant. This will be exchanged at the end of port placement to become a robotic port.
  - A robotic camera port is placed to the right of the umbilicus.
  - A robotic working port is placed at the level of the right anterior axillary line in the midabdominal region.
  - Another robotic port is placed at the level of the left midclavicular line in the midabdominal region.
  - A fourth robotic port is placed 5 to 7 cm to the left of the above port.
  - A 12-mm laparoscopic assistant port is placed 8 to 10 cm inferior to the robotic ports, usually at the extraction site (lower midline). This port is handled by the bedside surgeon during the robotic part of the procedure for assistance.
  - Another 5-mm assistant laparoscopic port is placed 8 to 10 cm inferior to the robotic ports, straddling the camera (**FIGURE 2**).
- Step 1 (laparoscopic or robotic): The falciform and round ligaments are divided using electrocautery. This exposes the anterior surface of the liver up to the fibroareolar tissue investing the hepatic veins (**FIGURE 3**).
- Step 2 (laparoscopic or robotic): The patient is positioned right side up by rotating the operating table. The hepatic flexure is mobilized to inferiorly reflect the colon. The right lobe of the liver is retracted superiorly. The duodenum is reflected medially. Gerota fascia is retracted inferiorly, and the right triangular and coronary ligaments are divided up to the right hepatic vein (**FIGURE 4**).
- Step 3 (laparoscopic or robotic): Intraoperative ultrasound (IOUS) of the liver is then performed using the 12-mm laparoscopic port. This locates the mass in relation to the segmental

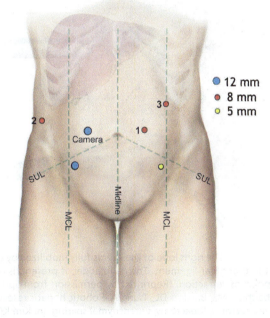

FIGURE 2 • Port placement for right hepatectomy. A 12-mm camera port is placed to the right of the umbilicus. The first robotic port is placed at the level of the right anterior axillary line in the midabdominal region. The second robotic port is placed at the level of the midclavicular line in the midabdominal region. The third robotic is positioned in the left upper quadrant. A 12-mm laparoscopic port is placed 8 to 10 cm inferior and lateral to the camera port. This port is handled by the bedside surgeon during the robotic part of the procedure for assistance. Another 5-mm assistant laparoscopic port is placed 8 to 10 cm inferior and lateral to the second robotic port. MCL, midclavicular line; SUL, spinoumbilical line. (Reprinted by permission from Springer: Sabbaghian MS, Bartlett DL, Tsung A. Robotic hepatic resections: segmentectomy, lobectomy, parenchymal sparing. In: Kim KC, ed. *Robotics in General Surgery*. Springer; 2014:161-174, with kind permission of Springer Science+Business Media.)

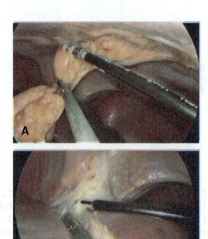

FIGURE 3 • **A,** The round ligament is divided using bipolar electrocautery. **B,** The falciform ligament is divided at the level of the hepatic parenchyma up to the level of the hepatic veins.

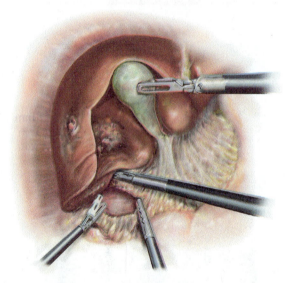

FIGURE 4 • The right lobe of the liver is fully mobilized by dividing the triangular ligament. The gallbladder, if present, is a useful point of retraction. (Reprinted by permission from Springer: Sabbaghian MS, Bartlett DL, Tsung A. Robotic hepatic resections: segmentectomy, lobectomy, parenchymal sparing. In: Kim KC, ed. *Robotics in General Surgery*. Springer; 2014:161-174, with kind permission of Springer Science+Business Media.)

anatomy of the liver and drives the planning of the resection plane.
- Step 4 (laparoscopic or robotic): The short hepatic/caudate veins that insert into the retrohepatic vena cava are divided between clips or with a coagulation device.
- Step 5 (laparoscopic or robotic): The right hepatic vein is encircled with a vessel loop.
- Step 6: Docking of the robot is performed. The camera is aligned with the transection plane of the liver (gallbladder to right hepatic vein origin).

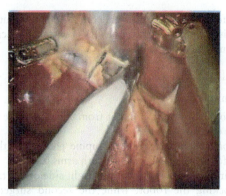

FIGURE 5 • The portal dissection is most safely initiated by identifying the cystic artery and duct (structure being clipped in the figure). These structures are bluntly dissected to their origin as a safe means to identify the right hepatic artery and hepatic duct.

- Step 7: The gallbladder, if present, is retracted cephalad and blunt dissection of triangle of Calot performed so that both cystic artery and duct are identified (**FIGURE 5**). These are ligated after establishing the critical view. The gallbladder is not dissected off the liver bed as it is useful for retraction while dissection is performed at the level of the porta hepatis. The right hepatic artery is identified and ligated between clips and/or ties (**FIGURE 6**). A vascular load for the Endo GIA stapler may be used for the same purpose. The right portal vein is then dissected and identified along its full length. Another load of the vascular stapler is used to transect it (**FIGURE 7**). After transecting the hepatic artery and vein, the right hepatic duct is identified. This is ligated distally then transected (**FIGURE 8**). After completing the dissection at the level of the porta hepatis, the gallbladder is dissected off the gallbladder bed and removed.
- Step 8: The short hepatic veins from the retrohepatic vena cava can be divided with an energy device, clips, and/or ties. The right hepatic vein can be divided extrahepatically if desired, and this is preferable if this region is important for an adequate margin. Alternatively, the vein can also be divided during the parenchymal transection (**FIGURE 9**).
- Step 9: After completing the aforementioned dissection, the parenchyma of the liver is transected. The right lobe of the liver is allowed to drop away, and the falciform is used to retract the left lobe. The line of transaction is based on the demarcated ischemic liver. Hook cautery is used to divide the capsule of the liver. IOUS is performed again to ensure the planned margin. Two figure-of-eight sutures can be placed on each side of the line of demarcation for additional retraction using the robotic arms (**FIGURE 10**). An energy device is used for transecting the parenchyma of the liver. We use a crush technique with the heat sealing device. Clips are applied to larger vessels and the vascular stapler for vessels too large to clip. This is continued until the right hepatic vein is identified. If the right hepatic vein has not been previously divided, a vascular load is applied across the right hepatic vein to complete the resection.
- Step 10: The specimen is retrieved using an EndoCatch bag, then removed through an extension of the inferior 12-mm assistant port (lower midline or Pfannenstiel).
- Step 11: All trocar sites are closed in the regular fashion.

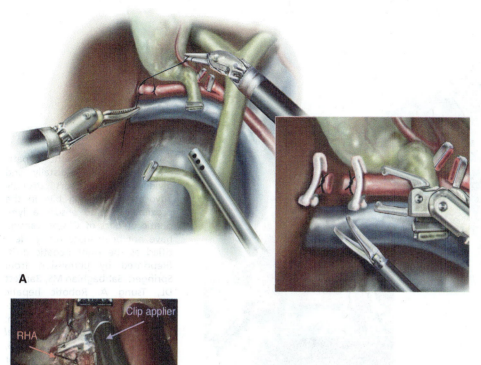

FIGURE 6 • The right hepatic artery is dissected and controlled as it inserts into the liver parenchyma. It is typically posterior to the right hepatic duct and lateral and anterior to the right portal vein. It should be proximally controlled by ligation and a surgical clip. (Reprinted by permission from Springer: Sabbaghian MS, Bartlett DL, Tsung A. Robotic hepatic resections: segmentectomy, lobectomy, parenchymal sparing. In: Kim KC, ed. *Robotics in General Surgery*. Springer; 2014:161-174, with kind permission of Springer Science+Business Media.)

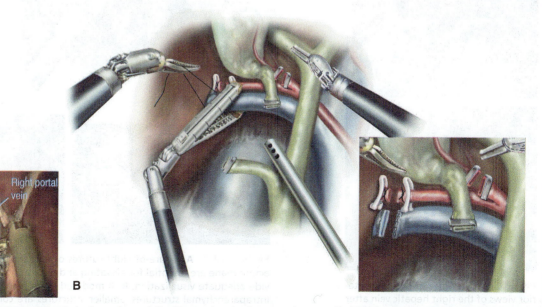

FIGURE 7 • A, The right portal vein is circumferentially dissected and subsequently controlled by a vascular load of the Endo GIA stapler. Use caution during the dissection as a large branch to the caudate lobe is often present. B, Schematic rendition of the dissection and control of the right portal triad. (B, Reprinted by permission from Springer: Sabbaghian MS, Bartlett DL, Tsung A. Robotic hepatic resections: segmentectomy, lobectomy, parenchymal sparing. In: Kim KC, ed. *Robotics in General Surgery*. Springer; 2014:161-174, with kind permission of Springer Science+Business Media.)

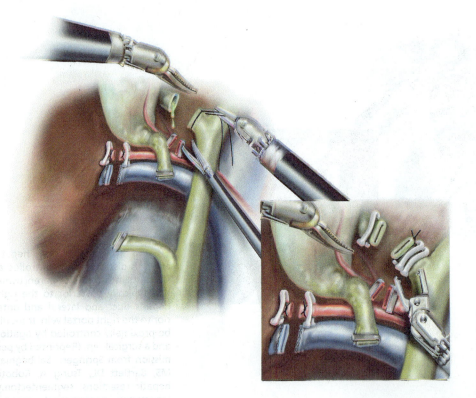

FIGURE 8 • The right hepatic duct is controlled distally and divided. The authors strongly advocate identifying bile in the proximal duct to ensure a lymphatic or part of Glisson capsule have not been inaccurately identified as the right hepatic duct. (Reprinted by permission from Springer: Sabbaghian MS, Bartlett DL, Tsung A. Robotic hepatic resections: segmentectomy, lobectomy, parenchymal sparing. In: Kim KC, ed. *Robotics in General Surgery*. Springer; 2014:161-174, with kind permission of Springer Science+Business Media.)

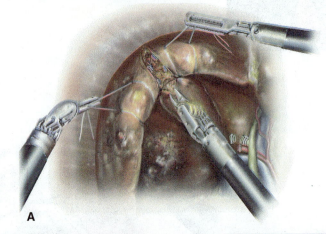

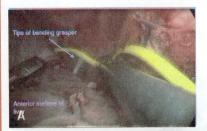

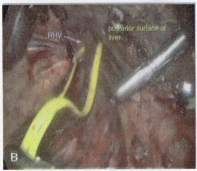

FIGURE 9 • A, Anterior and (B) posterior views of the right hepatic vein after dissection.

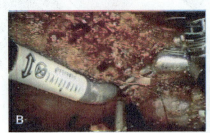
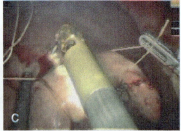

FIGURE 10 • A, Figure-of-eight sutures on either side of the planned transaction plane are essential for elevating and separating the parenchyma to provide adequate visualization. B, A modified crush technique is used to identify intraparenchymal structures. Smaller structures are controlled with clips and/or cautery. C, Larger structures are controlled with stapler firings. (Reprinted by permission from Springer: Sabbaghian MS, Bartlett DL, Tsung A. Robotic hepatic resections: segmentectomy, lobectomy, parenchymal sparing. In: Kim KC, ed. *Robotics in General Surgery*. Springer; 2014:161-174, with kind permission of Springer Science+Business Media.)

LEFT HEPATECTOMY

- Port placement
  - Pneumoperitoneum is established through placement of a 5-mm port in the left upper quadrant. This will be exchanged at the end of port placement to become a robotic port.
  - A robotic camera port is placed to the right of the umbilicus.
  - A robotic working port is placed at the level of the right anterior axillary line in the midabdominal region.
  - Another robotic port is placed at the level of the left midclavicular line in the midabdominal region.
  - A fourth robotic port is placed 5 to 7 cm to the left of the above port.
  - A 12-mm laparoscopic assistant port is placed 8 to 10 cm inferior to the robotic ports, usually at the extraction site (lower midline). This port is handled by the bedside surgeon during the robotic part of the procedure for assistance.
  - Another 5-mm assistant laparoscopic port is placed 8 to 10 cm inferior to the robotic ports, straddling the camera (**FIGURE 11**).
- Step 1 (laparoscopic or robotic): The falciform and round ligaments are divided using electrocautery. This exposes the anterior surface of the liver to the hepatic veins.
- Step 2 (laparoscopic or robotic): With the patient in the left side up position, both left triangular and coronary ligaments are divided until the left hepatic vein is identified. The liver is then retracted cephalad and the gastrohepatic ligament is divided. Care is taken to identify a replaced left hepatic artery and properly control it prior to division, if present.
- Step 3 (laparoscopic or robotic): At this point, the left hepatic vein can be isolated and encircled with a vessel loop if the intention is to divide the vein extrahepatically.
- Step 4 (laparoscopic or robotic): IOUS of the liver is then performed using the 12-mm laparoscopic port. This helps confirm the presence of the mass in the planned resection specimen and its relation to the major structures in the liver. The middle hepatic vein should be preserved, unless this approach will compromise the margin.
- Step 5: Docking of the robot is performed. The camera is aligned with the transection plane of the liver (gallbladder to right hepatic vein origin).

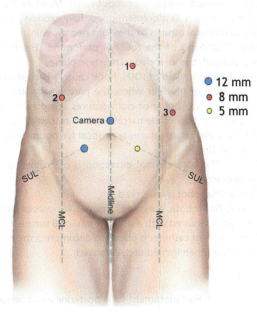

FIGURE 11 • Port placement for a left hepatic lobectomy. MCL, midclavicular line; SUL, spinoumbilical line. (Reprinted by permission from Springer: Sabbaghian MS, Bartlett DL, Tsung A. Robotic hepatic resections: segmentectomy, lobectomy, parenchymal sparing. In: Kim KC, ed. *Robotics in General Surgery*. Springer; 2014:161-174, with kind permission of Springer Science+Business Media.)

- Step 6: Dissection is then carried at the level of the porta hepatis. The ligamentum teres is used to retract the liver anteriorly. The left hepatic artery is identified and ligated between clips. A vascular stapler may be used for the same purpose, if feasible. The left portal vein is then dissected and identified along its full length. A vascular stapler is used to transect it. After transecting the hepatic artery and vein, the left hepatic duct is identified. This is ligated distally and then transected.
- Step 7: At this point, the left hepatic vein can be divided with a vascular stapling device. Note that if done extrahepatically, the middle hepatic vein is also likely being taken.
- Step 8: After completing the aforementioned dissection, the parenchyma of the liver is transected based on the line of demarcation.

LEFT LATERAL SECTIONECTOMY

- Port placement is shown in **FIGURE 11**.
- Mobilization of the liver and control of the left hepatic vein proceeds as described for left hepatic lobectomy.
- The portal structures supplying segments 2 and 3 are controlled with a vascular staple load at the posterior aspect of segment 3 to the patient's right of the falciform ligament.

RIGHT POSTERIOR SECTOR RESECTIONS

- Positioning
  - The patient is positioned in the full right lateral position for posterior-lateral resections.
  - The robot is then brought in toward the left upper corner of the table.
- Port placement
  - In these cases, the ports can be placed laterally on the right side. Rarely, a robotic port through the diaphragm is required.
  - The ports are placed at the costal margin and occasionally between the ribs and through the diaphragm.

- Assistant ports are placed about 10 cm below the robotic ports, straddling the camera (FIGURE 12).
- Step 1 (laparoscopically or robotically): Mobilize the right lobe of the liver as aforementioned, fully exposing the anterior and lateral aspects of the right hepatic vein.
- Step 3: Docking of the robot is performed. The camera is aligned with the intended transection plane.
- Step 4: With the aid of IOUS, hook cautery is used to divide the capsule of the liver where the parenchymal transection will occur. Two figure-of-eight sutures are placed on each side of the line of demarcation and retracted using the robotic arms. These sutures are critical for optimal retraction and visibility.
- Step 5: The parenchymal dissection is performed as previously described.
- Step 6: The robot is undocked.
- Step 7: The robotic ports are removed. If necessary, the diaphragm is repaired with a single figure-of-8 suture.
- Step 8: A chest catheter is placed to decompress the pneumothorax and then immediately removed.

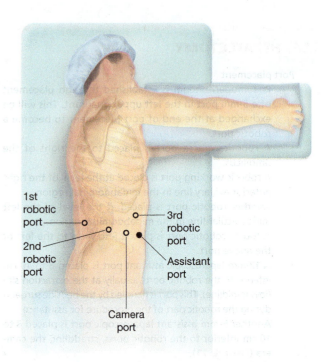

FIGURE 12 • Port placement for a posterior sectionectomy.

PEARLS AND PITFALLS

Preoperative planning	• Cirrhotic or steatotic livers with significantly high intrahepatic portal pressures will be associated with significant blood loss and may be better approached as an open procedure. • Most resections tend to be nonanatomic with the goal to preserve parenchyma and anatomy for future resections. • Flexibility in port placement is important and may vary depending on the location of the lesion, the body habitus, the size of the liver, etc. For example, in some patients, the liver extends well below the costal margin and the ports will need to be placed below the level of the umbilicus.
Operative technique	• A central line should be placed and the central venous pressure monitored and kept low. • Care should be taken to identify major hepatic veins or pedicles by ultrasound in advance of the parenchymal transection so that these are handled carefully. • Although air embolus is a concern, it is rare in practice. Left lateral decubitus positioning and aspiration of air from the right atrium can be performed if necessary. • A Pringle maneuver is recommended to reduce blood loss. • The line of parenchymal transection should be lined up with the camera view and the assistant 12-mm port for stapling. • Obtaining adequate margins can be challenging without the ability to feel the tumor. Ultrasound needs to be used during the parenchymal transection to ensure that the margin is preserved, and the initial marking of the margin by cautery should be generous.

POSTOPERATIVE CARE

- No drain is left next to the resection bed unless a bile leak is identified.
- Orogastric tube is removed in the operating room.
- Patient is transferred to a regular floor monitored bed.
- Daily laboratory tests are ordered including complete blood count, blood urea nitrogen, electrolytes, liver enzymes, bilirubin, and coagulation studies.
- Clear liquids are given on postoperative day 0 or 1 and advanced as tolerated.
- Foley catheter is removed on postoperative day 0 or 1.
- Central venous catheter is removed on postoperative day 0 or 1.

OUTCOMES

- The advantages of minimally invasive surgery are well documented in the literature. These include decreased postoperative pain, early return of activity, decreased postoperative ileus, better cosmesis, and shorter hospital stays.[2]
- The use of robotics offers multiple advantages to the operating surgeon over laparoscopy such as improved

Table 2: Comparison of Robotic and Laparoscopic Groups: Operative and Postoperative Parameters

	Robotic (n = 57)	Laparoscopic (n = 114)	Overall P-value
EBL, median mL	200 (50-337.5)	100 (50-350)	0.097
Transfusion rate (%)	2 (3.8)	7 (7.4)	0.372
Room time, median, min	342 (264-453)	261.5 (199.5-333)	<0.001[a]
OR time, median, min	253 (180-355)	198.5 (137.75-261.5)	0.001[a]
Complication rate (%)	11 (19.3)	29 (26)	0.34
Major complication rate (%)	1 (1.8)	1 (0.9)	0.624
Postoperative peak bilirubin	1.15 (0.7-1.7)	1.2 (0.8-1.6)	0.895
Postoperative ICU (%)	11 (19)	8 (8.5)	0.053
LOS, median, days	4.0 (3.0-5.5)	4.0 (3.0-5.0)	0.10
30-days mortality (%)	0 (0)	1 (0.9)	0.478
90-days mortality (%)	0 (0)	1 (0.9)	0.478
R0 negative margin (%)	40 (95)	98 (92)	0.44

EBL, estimated blood loss; ICU, intensive care unit; LOS, length of stay; OR, operating room.
[a]P < .05.

Table 3: Comparison of Early Robotic vs Later Robotic: Operative and Postoperative Parameters

	Early (n = 13)	Later (n = 44)	Overall P-value
EBL, median, mL	300 (200-600)	100 (50-300)	0.008[a]
Transfusion rate (%)	1 (7.7)	1 (1.9)	0.393
Room time, median, min	466 (349-571.5)	314.5 (257-381)	0.001[a]
OR time, median, min	381 (253-499.5)	232 (175-283)	0.001[a]
Complication rate (%)	3 (23)	9 (20)	0.84
Major complication rate (%)	1 (8)	1 (2)	0.36
Postoperative peak bilirubin	1.30 (1.10-3.65)	1.1 (0.6-1.63)	0.144
Postoperative ICU (%)	3 (23)	8 (18)	0.694
LOS, median, days	5.0 (3.5-10)	4.0 (3.0-5.0)	0.031[a]
30-days mortality (%)	0 (0)	0 (0)	1.00
90-days mortality (%)	0 (0)	0 (0)	1.00
R0 negative margin (%)	10 (77)	29 (66)	0.45

EBL, estimated blood loss; ICU, intensive care unit; LOS, length of stay; OR, operating room.
[a]P < .05.

- three-dimensional imaging, near 360° movement of surgical instruments, along with improved surgeon comfort and precision.[3,4]
- This comes at the cost of prolonged operative times, absence of haptic feedback, higher costs, and a learning curve.[3,4]
- A recent review identified 31 publications that focus on robotic liver resections and provide a description of 1158 resections.[5] These studies capture the growing application of robotic liver resections, with patients ranging in age from 15 to 91 years, of whom 53% had previous abdominal surgeries and 30.4% had cirrhosis.
- Most resections (66.7%) were considered minor, nonanatomic liver resections. These were primarily performed for malignant masses, namely, hepatocellular carcinoma and colorectal metastases. R1 margin resection was reported in 3.6% of patients. Masses ranged in size from 0.2 to 14.5 cm.[5]
- Conversion rates vary in the literature but at higher volume centers have decreased over time and currently range between 3.2% and 4.4%.[6,7] Most common reasons for conversion included confirmation of surgical margin, problems during hilar dissection, long resection planes, and obesity.[8]
- Compared with open procedures, robotic hepatectomies were longer, although patients experience less intraoperative blood loss, lower blood transfusions, decreased length of stay, and lower complication rates.[9]
- For oncologic resections, no significant difference has been reported in rate of R0 resection, overall recurrence, disease-free or overall survival when comparing robotic and open techniques.[10]
- Median operative time is 295.5 min (range 45-1186), with median estimated blood loss 24.5 mL. Median length of stay was 6 days, with 12.2% grade II/III complication rate and a perioperative mortality of 0.3%.[5]
- In a matched series from the University of Pittsburgh comparing patients who received robotic and laparoscopic liver resections, there was no difference in estimated blood loss, hospital length of stay, morbidity, or mortality (TABLE 2). There was an increase in major hepatic resections performed. There was no difference in the conversion rate between the two groups (7% vs 8.8%).[11]
- Upon comparison of early vs late experience with robotic cases, there was a significant difference in estimated blood loss, operative time, and hospital length of stay in favor of the later cases, which reflects the presence of a learning curve (TABLE 3).[11]

COMPLICATIONS

- Bile leak (most common)
- Pulmonary complications
- Wound infections
- Bleeding
- Pleural effusions
- Thromboembolic events
- Ascites
- Hepatic failure

REFERENCES

1. Buell JF, Cherqui D, Geller DA, et al. The international position on laparoscopic liver surgery: the Louisville Statement, 2008. *Ann Surg*. 2009;250(5):825-830.
2. Reddy SK, Tsung A, Geller DA. Laparoscopic liver resection. *World J Surg*. 2011;35:1478-1486.
3. Nguyen KT, Zureikat AH, Chalikonda S, et al. Technical aspect of robotic-assisted pancreaticoduodenectomy (RAPD). *J Gastrointest Surg*. 2011;15(5):870-875.
4. Zeh HJ III, Bartlett DL, Moser AJ. Robotic-assisted major pancreatic resection. *Adv Surg*. 2011;45:323-340.
5. Tsilimigras DI, Moris D, Vagios S, et al. Safety and oncologic outcomes of robotic liver resections: a systematic review. *J Surg Oncol*. 2018;117:1517-1530.

6. King JC, Zeh HJ, Zureikat AH, et al. Safety in Numbers: Progressive Implementation of a Robotics Program in an Academic Surgical Oncology Practice. *Surg Innov*. 2016;23(4):407-414.
7. Wong DJ, Wong MJ, Choi GH, et al. Systematic review and meta-analysis of robotic versus open hepatectomy. *ANZ J Surg*. 2019;89:165-170.
8. Ho CM, Wakabayashi G, Nitta H, et al. Systematic review of robotic liver resection. *Surg Endosc*. 2013;27(3):732-739.
9. Liu R, Wakabayashi G, Kim HJ, et al. International consensus statement on robotic hepatectomy surgery in 2018. *World J Gastroenterol*. 2019;25(12):1432-1444.
10. Wang WH, Kuo KK, Wang SN, Lee KT. Oncological and surgical result of hepatoma after robot surgery. *Surg Endosc*. 2018;32:3918-3924.
11. Tsung A, Geller DA, Sukato DC, et al. Robotic versus laparoscopic hepatectomy: a matched comparison. *Ann Surg*. 2014;259(3):549-555.

Chapter 26 | Vena Cava Resection During Hepatectomy

Aijun Li and Steven J. Hughes

DEFINITION
- Hepatic neoplasms involving the inferior vena cava (IVC) have usually been considered unresectable because of the high surgical risk of massive bleeding and air embolism. However, aggressive surgical approaches for hepatic tumors involving the IVC have recently been reported to have been performed safely and have been shown to alter the natural history of the disease.[1-28]

DIFFERENTIAL DIAGNOSIS
- Intrahepatic cholangiocarcinoma (ICC)[29]
- Hepatocellular carcinoma (HCC)
- Renal cell carcinoma
- Metastatic disease

MEDICAL HISTORY AND PHYSICAL EXAMINATION
- By far, the most frequent indication for IVC resection en bloc with hepatectomy is HCC. As cirrhosis is the major risk for HCC and also the major risk factor for postoperative liver failure, great attention must be paid to history, symptoms, and signs associated with underlying liver disease. In general, hepatectomy that also requires IVC resection is only performed in patients without intrinsic liver disease.
- History
  - Hepatitis
  - Alcohol consumption
- Symptoms
  - Fatigue
  - Encephalopathy
  - Rapid weight gain
- Signs
  - Ascites
  - Asterixis
  - Abdominal or thoracic telangiectasia
  - Cachexia
  - Morbid obesity (steatohepatitis)
  - Extensive pedal edema (IVC compression)
- A thorough evaluation of potential pulmonary and cardiovascular disease must be performed. Patients with significant comorbidities are not candidates for major hepatectomy with en bloc IVC resection.

IMAGING AND OTHER LABORATORY STUDIES
- Ultrasonography (US). US is often the initial diagnostic imaging modality employed but is inadequate to fully evaluate hepatic lesions and IVC involvement.
- Contrast-enhanced computed tomography (CT). In addition to providing information regarding the number, size, and location of lesions, CT is an effective tool to estimate the remnant liver volume.
- Magnetic resonance imaging (MRI) examination. MRI is valuable for characterizing lesions and defining vasculature. It is particularly helpful in diagnosing the extent of tumor thrombus (TT) within the IVC. Magnetic resonance angiography is useful for identifying the major hepatic veins and the IVC and clarifying their relations to any tumor masses.
- Each of these modalities may reveal IVC compression or TT within IVC.
- Patients who are suspected of having malignant invasion of the IVC wall on preoperative radiologic studies should also have echocardiography to assess for extension into the right heart. Such extension is not prohibitive of resection but mandates an operative approach that provides access to the chest, thus increasing morbidity while hope for a surgical cure is fleeting.
- In addition to routine laboratories, all patients must undergo a careful preoperative assessment of liver function and potential underlying disease:
  - Liver function tests
  - Hepatitis serologies
  - Coagulation studies
  - Platelet count

SURGICAL MANAGEMENT
Preoperative Planning
- Preoperative ipsilateral portal vein embolization to create hypertrophy of the planned liver remnant may prevent postoperative hepatic failure after extended major hepatectomy.
- Low-volume resuscitation minimizes blood loss but exaggerates potential hemodynamic instability with clamping of the IVC.
- Venovenous bypass (VVB) with total hepatic vascular exclusion (THVE) facilitates resection of primary and metastatic hepatic neoplasms that invade the vena cava.[21,22] Given the prior pearl, be prepared to use VVB when IVC invasion is suspected (FIGURE 1). Preoperative communication and coordination with perfusion and anesthesia teammates is vital to success in this regard.

Anatomic Considerations
- *Characteristics of the posterior hepatic IVC.* The posterior hepatic IVC extends from the renal veins to the confluence of the right atrium (RA). This is further divided anatomically into the inner segment of the pericardium (intrapericardial IVC), the suprahepatic IVC below the diaphragm, the retrohepatic IVC, and the lower segment of the subhepatic renal vein. The IVC is thick walled, tenacious, elastic, and not particularly susceptible to invasion. The hepatic veins are thin walled but rapidly develop thicker walls as they insert into the IVC. Thus, the proximal portions of the hepatic veins are at greatest risk for injury during the operation. Such injury invariably results in intraoperative hemorrhage and/or air embolism.

- *Characteristics of tumors that involve the IVC.* Most liver cancers near the IVC originate from hepatic segments 1, 4, 5, and/or 8 or in the paracaval portion of the caudate (referred to by some as segment 9).
  - *Caudate tumors*: Anatomically, the hepatic caudate lobe is divided into the left hepatic caudate lobe (Spigelian lobe, caudate lobe proper, segment 1) and right hepatic caudate lobe (dorsal sector). The right hepatic caudate lobe can be further divided into the paracaval portion (segment 9) and the caudate process (segment 10).[23-26] Caudal tumors may either extend anteriorly and thus invade the portal vein and/or the bile duct, resulting in obstructive jaundice, or extend posteriorly and thus invade the IVC. Generally, about one-fourth of caudate tumors involve the IVC.[27,28]
  - *Tumors arising near the root of the hepatic veins*: These tumors typically compress the anterior IVC between the mid and right hepatic veins or between the mid and left hepatic veins. Because the hepatic veins have no valves, are thin walled, and fixed in the hepatic parenchyma, they are unable to retract upon injury and air embolism is liable to occur. To avoid air embolism and massive hemorrhage, the operative strategy should plan to isolate the hepatic veins extrahepatically and occlude them in advance.[17-19] The risk in resecting tumors that are near the confluence of the hepatic veins with the IVC is not rupturing the IVC but injuring the thin wall of the hepatic veins.
  - *Characteristics of inferior vena cava tumor thrombus (IVCTT)*: IVCTT often spreads from the hepatic veins or hepatic short veins.[30-33] IVCTT is clinically classified into three types (FIGURE 2): (1) the posterior liver type (type I), where TT is located in the IVC behind the liver and below the surface of the diaphragm; (2) the superior liver type (type II), where TT extends into the IVC above the surface of the diaphragm but outside the atrium; and (3) the intracardiac type, where TT surpasses the surface of the diaphragm and enters the RA. The operative plan for patients with IVCTT completely depends on this classification of the IVCTT.

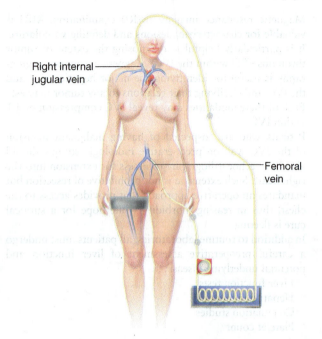

FIGURE 1 • Schematic of a VVB circuit. The left femoral and right internal jugular veins are cannulated percutaneously. The patient is heparinized, and the cannulae are connected to a closed circuit containing a roller pump and a heat exchanger. Blood is drawn from the femoral site and infused into the jugular site.

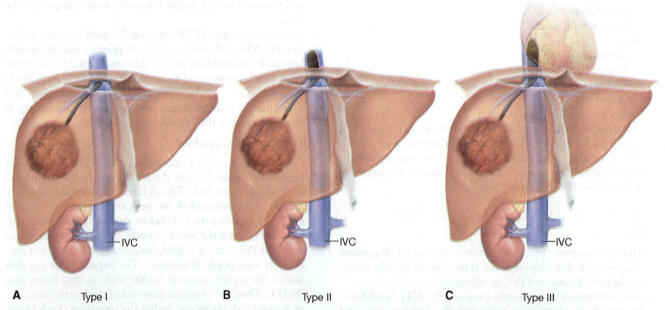

FIGURE 2 • A, The posterior liver type (type I), where thrombus is located in the IVC behind the liver and below the surface of the diaphragm. B, The superior liver type (type II), where thrombus extends into the IVC above the surface of the diaphragm but remains outside the atrium. C, The intracardiac type, where thrombus surpasses the surface of the diaphragm and enters the RA.

Surgical Positioning

- The patient is positioned supine with both arms tucked (access to the chest may be required).
- The patient is prepped from chin to midthigh. The chest should be covered with sterile drapes, if sternotomy is not anticipated, to optimize maintenance of normothermia.
- The authors advocate placement of central lines in the left jugular vein and left femoral vein. These are the access points for VVB should it be required.

Incision

- A right subcostal incision with midline extension to the xiphoid process provides excellent exposure and facilitates extension should a sternotomy prove indicated.
- A fixed retractor is used that is capable of providing adequate exposure. The authors use a Thompson retractor.

HEPATIC NEOPLASM INVASION OF THE INFERIOR VENA CAVA WALL WITHOUT TUMOR THROMBUS

- The liver is fully mobilized.
- An umbilical tape is placed around the hepatoduodenal ligament and vessel loops are placed around the right hepatic vein as well as the confluence of the left and middle hepatic veins. Occasionally, lesion location will preclude this control of both veins. The authors advocate being prepared to perform THVE, and associated VVB if indicated, in this setting.
- Next, assess for IVC invasion vs compression. The underlying pathology will be somewhat predictive of encountering true invasion. HCC most typically will compress but not invade the IVC (FIGURE 3). ICC or metastatic adenocarcinomas are more prone to truly invade the IVC.
- Dissect, control, and divide short hepatic veins working in a caudal to cranial fashion. When the IVC is invaded by a hepatic tumor, the wall becomes pale and stiff. More often than not, there is usually a plane between the tumor and the IVC for separation. Careful identification of this plane may completely avoid injury or need for resection into the IVC.
- Sometimes, after tumors are stripped from the IVC or the IVC outer membranes are compromised by sharp dissection technique, the thinned IVC wall should be repaired with polypropylene 5-0 sutures ideally placed in the transverse axis to prevent narrowing of the lumen.
- If the IVC can be fully dissected, resection proceeds as described in other chapters.
- If the IVC is invaded, the next step is to determine if the segment is short enough to facilitate IVC resection with control using a side-biting vascular clamp such as a Satinsky clamp (FIGURE 4). This clamp is most easily placed after the parenchymal transection when the resection specimen can be retracted to elevate the final area of attachment on the IVC. You may not be able to determine the cranial extent of involvement until the liver has been divided.
- Prior to beginning the parenchymal dissection, get control of the suprahepatic and infrahepatic vena cava by circumferentially dissecting them and placing umbilical tapes (FIGURE 5). Identify and set aside the appropriate vascular clamps you will require should THVE prove indicated. A test clamp of the suprahepatic vena cava should be performed to determine the need for VVB, if THVE is required.
- Hepatic transection proceeds from superficial to deep tissues with the portal trial clamped. The left index finger should be placed up against the lateral wall of the IVC, and the left thumb is put on the medial/anterior aspect of the IVC. This maneuver provides proprioception for the operative surgeon during the transection.
- To facilitate vascular control for subsequent repair, clamp the IVC with a large Satinsky clamp to provide a margin for sharp resection of the involved segment of the IVC (FIGURES 6 and 7).
- If the segment of IVC involvement proves to be more extensive, proceed with THVE to remove the tumor and repair the IVC.
- Sharply excise the lesion with a venous margin that ideally is greater than 0.5 cm.
- Alternatively, the resection can be performed in two steps: to resect and remove the main tumor first, then to clamp the affected part on the IVC wall with Satinsky forceps, cut off the remnant tumor, and finally repair the IVC.
- Assess whether a patch will be required vs primary repair.
    - Simple, longitudinal closure with 5-0 polypropylene is acceptable unless it results in narrowing of the IVC lumen greater than 25%.

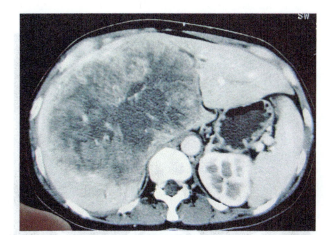

FIGURE 3 • Preoperative CT scan showing a very large liver tumor located at segments 4 to 8 with infiltration into the caudate lobe. The IVC is not clearly identified and invasion of the IVC vs compression cannot be determined. Surgical exploration revealed the IVC was not involved. A right trisegmentectomy was performed.

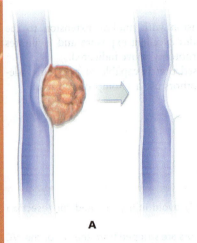
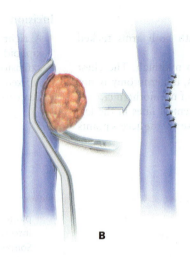
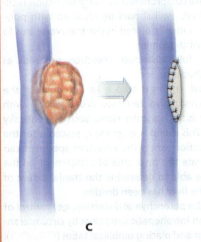
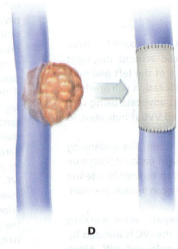

FIGURE 4 • **A,** The IVC is not infiltrated, but the IVC was compressed and flat. The tumor is stripped from the IVC, or the IVC outer membranes are sheared by scissors. **B,** The IVC is partially involved but can be resected under side clamping and then primarily closed with direct longitudinal suturing (result should lead to less than a 25% narrowing of the IVC). **C,** When the IVC is extensively involved (>50% of the diameter), the IVC is resected and reconstructed using a patch (bovine pericardium). **D,** If the defect is large or the IVC is occluded, circumferential excision and primary anastomosis is warranted. An interposition graft should be used only when a long segment of IVC (>3 cm length) is resected.

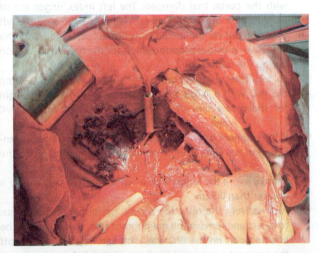

FIGURE 5 • Occlusion of the suprahepatic IVC and infrahepatic IVC using two umbilical tape clamps (total hepatic vascular exclusion). This postresection image (to improve visualization of the placement of the umbilical tapes) was taken after a right trisegmentectomy was performed.

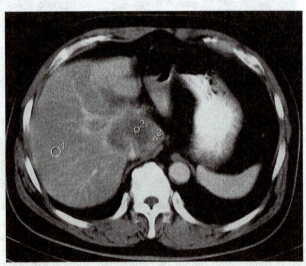

FIGURE 6 • Preoperative CT scan showing a liver tumor located at the caudate lobe with probable invasion of the IVC.

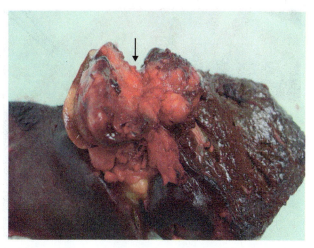

FIGURE 7 • Macroscopic findings of resected specimen. A 4 × 5 × 5 cm IVC infiltrating-type tumor occupied the caudate lobe parenchyma sitting astride the IVC. The *black arrow* indicates the course of the IVC. This lesion was resected using a side-biting vascular clamp. The resultant defect in the IVC required a patch repair.

- Alternatively, if the resection exceeds about half of the circumference, a patch of autologous vein or bovine pericardium can be sewn circumferentially with running 5-0 polypropylene.
- Reported vein grafts for patch repair include saphenous vein, superficial femoral vein, or left renal vein.

■ If the IVC is either extensively infiltrated or completely obstructed, the IVC should be resected and reconstructed using a graft. During segmental resection, vascular clamps should be placed at both proximal and distal sides of the involved part of the IVC. Umbilical tapes will not provide adequate hemostasis.

■ Defects shorter than 3 cm can often be primarily reapproximated with 5-0 polypropylene.

■ If the defect is longer than 3 cm or primary anastomosis is under undue tension, an interposition graft is warranted.

■ Unfortunately, autologous vein grafts are too small to replace the IVC. The favored material for an IVC interposition graft is stented polytetrafluoroethylene (ePTFE).[14,34-46] These conduits are available in varying sizes and are inserted using 5-0 polypropylene running suture.

HEPATIC NEOPLASM WITH INFERIOR VENA CAVA TUMOR THROMBUS

■ Surgery selection depends on the level at which TT enters the IVC (**FIGURE 2**).

■ In surgical manipulation of HCC with TT, it is critical to avoid squeezing the hepatic veins and the IVC in the process of dissecting the tumor, which may result in TT pulmonary embolism. However, "no-touch" technique is almost impossible in the process of dissecting a large tumor mass, and therefore, it is difficult to prevent TT from falling off completely.

- One option to minimize this risk is to implant a device near the IVCTT proximal to the heart before tumor dissection so as to prevent TT fall off. B. Braun's Tempofilter II temporary IVC filter is a device designed for this purpose.[33]
- The filter is implanted under local anesthesia via the right cervical vein 1 day before surgery or in the morning of surgery and fixed in the IVC by means of the delivery rod. It can be withdrawn easily after surgery.
- The device can be fixed securely as long as there is more than 2-cm distance between the TT and the right atrial orifice.

■ For type I tumors
- Explore the location and size of the tumor and location of the IVC first; completely mobilize the liver and expose the IVC above and below the liver.
- The levels for vascular exclusion are at the suprahepatic IVC and infrahepatic IVC (between the adrenal vein and renal vein). Pass umbilical tapes at these levels.
- Use care to minimize manipulation of the involved hepatic vein—tumor embolus is possible.
- Transect the liver parenchyma under Pringle occlusion first, leaving only the affected hepatic vein in continuity with the specimen and the IVC.
- Clamp the IVC.
- Open the hepatic veins and the IVC under direct vision (open the IVC below the liver longitudinally); resect and remove TT under direct vision.
  - As most tumor thrombi are not attached to the wall, they can be removed or dissected from the IVC under direct vision.
  - In some cases where TT is attached to the wall or invades the IVC wall and cannot be removed completely, partial IVC resection plus repair can be performed.
  - In cases where TT has infiltrated the venous wall, adhered with it severely, and obstructed the IVC completely, resect the involved partial IVC together with TT.
  - In cases where complete removal of TT is impossible, IVC replacement can be considered. As the location of type I IVCTT is relatively low, venous TT can be removed surgically by using the standard radical hepatectomy and THVE.
- To restore venous return, control the IVC with a side-biting vascular clamp and release the occluding clamps.
- Irrigate the IVC and suture the luminal wall.

■ In type II tumors, TT has surpassed the level of the diaphragm, thus the TT has to be removed by opening the diaphragm and the pericardium so that the level of vascular isolation of the suprahepatic IVC is above the diaphragm but below the RA (**FIGURES 8** and **9**).
- In type II TT, subdiaphragmatic occlusion of the IVC is not appropriate, as it may cause TT rupture and fall off, resulting in cardiac tamponade, acute pulmonary embolism, and other serious complications.
- Dissect the infrahepatic IVC first and fully mobilize the liver.
- Open the diaphragm anterior to the suprahepatic IVC and enter the mediastinum to expose the right auricle (**FIGURE 10**).

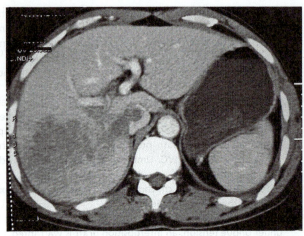

FIGURE 8 • The CT of the case described revealed a large hepatic tumor with TT through the right hepatic vein to the IVC. The patient underwent a combined right hepatic and TT resection.

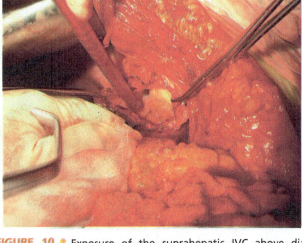

FIGURE 10 • Exposure of the suprahepatic IVC above diaphragm. Note the white pericardium.

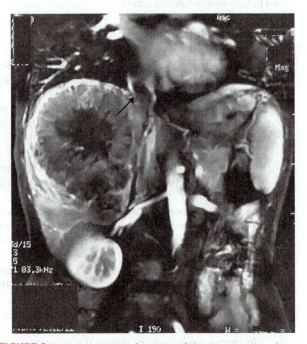

FIGURE 9 • Coronal view of an MRI of the same patient demonstrating TT extending into the suprahepatic IVC (*black arrow*), above the surface of the diaphragm but outside the atrium.

- Control the suprahepatic IVC from within the pericardial space. Place an umbilical tape (**FIGURE 11**).
- Occlude the first portal (Pringle occlusion) and then the infrahepatic IVC.
- Occlude the right auricle with Satinsky forceps (**FIGURE 12**).
- Open the IVC longitudinally and resect the TT together with the tumor under direct vision.
- Before resuming blood flow, the residual TT and clots should be washed out with the help of the blood pressure still existing in the IVC for the sake of avoiding pulmonary embolism caused by air and blood clots.

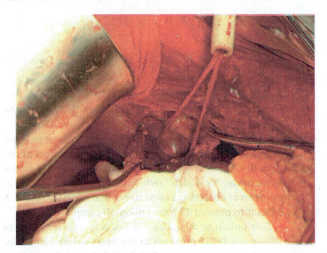

FIGURE 11 • The suprahepatic IVC is circumferentially dissected within the pericardial space, above the diaphragm, and an umbilical tape passed.

- Close the IVC defect with running 5-0 polypropylene (**FIGURE 13**).
- Reversely, release the Satinsky forceps, and then the IVC below the liver, and the first portal occlusion (Pringle occlusion).
- Repair the pericardium and the diaphragm (**FIGURE 14**).
- **FIGURE 15** demonstrates the resected specimen with extension of TT that has been removed.
- Type III TT can extend to the RA (**FIGURE 16**), and therefore, TT removal has to be performed under direct vision using extracorporeal circulation (under cardiopulmonary bypass).[31,32]
- Georgen et al[31] describe an original finger-assisted thoracoabdominal approach for resection of HCC with thrombus extending into the RA, assisted by transesophageal echocardiography, which avoids the need for extracorporal bypass. There are three prerequisites for this procedure:

Chapter 26 **VENA CAVA RESECTION DURING HEPATECTOMY** **211**

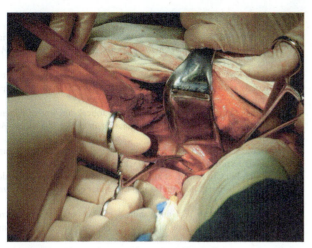

FIGURE 12 • The right atrial appendage was occluded with a Satinsky clamp.

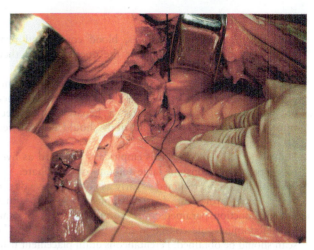

FIGURE 14 • The diaphragm is repaired using interrupted sutures.

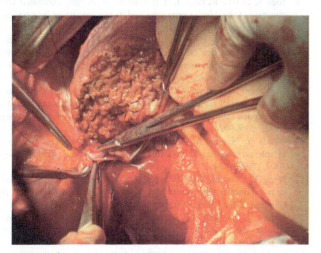

FIGURE 13 • The IVC wall is closed using polypropylene 5-0 suture.

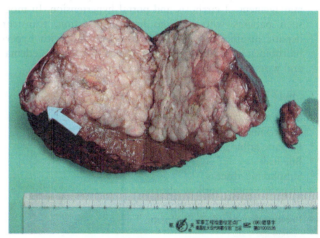

FIGURE 15 • Liver tumor together with thrombus gross pathology. *Arrow* indicated TT in the right hepatic vein; TT of IVC (*right*).

- There are no adhesions to the venous wall of macroscopic thrombus in patients with HCC.
- Complete mobilization of the liver allows caudal retraction of the liver and en bloc retraction of the tumor and the thrombus out of the RA.
- After application of a vascular clamp on the suprahepatic portion of the IVC above the thrombus, a routine hepatic vascular exclusion can be performed to remove the tumor and the thrombus.

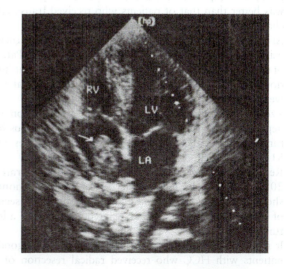

FIGURE 16 • Echocardiography revealing TT (*white arrow*) extending into the RA.

POSTOPERATIVE MANAGEMENT

- Liver function, electrolyte levels, blood count, and prothrombin time are checked after the operation and then daily until discharge.
- Postoperative pain control is best achieved with patient-controlled analgesia. Because of the decreased clearance of liver-metabolized drugs after a hepatectomy, selection and dosing of pain medications should be adjusted accordingly.
- Phosphate supplementation is empirically provided as liver regeneration will consume large amounts of phosphate.
- An oral diet can be resumed as early as postoperative day 3.
- Fever, tachycardia, or hyperbilirubinemia when other hepatic function parameters are normal are signs that an intra-abdominal bile collection may be present, and a CT scan should be obtained. Percutaneous drain placement usually brings about resolution of such collections after a few days; reoperation is rarely necessary.
- The focus of postoperative care in cirrhotic patients is on management of cirrhosis and portal hypertension. In most such patients who undergo hepatic resection, transient hepatic insufficiency develops postoperatively with hyperbilirubinemia, ascites formation, hypoalbuminemia, edema, and worsening of the baseline coagulopathy.

COMPLICATIONS

- Bleeding (hepatic wound surfaces, intraperitoneal, and gastrointestinal bleeding)
- Hepatic failure, renal failure
- Bile leak
- Subphrenic abscess
- Hepatic venous outflow obstruction
- The hepatic wound surfaces infection
- Pneumothorax, pleural effusion

OUTCOMES

- The reported 5-year survival for HCC invading the main trunk of the portal vein and the IVC is 20%,[34] and this was better than that of patients who received transarterial chemoembolization alone.
- Arii et al[35] reported that IVC resection with reconstruction using ePTFE led to a 50% survival at 29 months. Patency of the graft was maintained for the long term without infectious complications. The 1-, 3-, and 5-year survival rates were 63.6%, 38.2%, and 25.5%, respectively.
- Azoulay et al[36] reported their experience with concomitant hepatic and IVC resection in 22 patients with various liver tumors. Actuarial 1-, 3-, and 5-year survival rates were 81.8%, 38.3%, and 38.3%, respectively.
- Recent data[7,31,32,47-50] reported a 5-year survival rate of 20% to 30% and a median survival of 9.8 to 28 months, showing that patients who underwent complete resection of the tumor together with associated TT survived a long time.
- It is now generally accepted that the prognosis is good in patients with HCC who received radical resection of the tumor together with dissection of the IVCTT as long as there is no local or distal metastasis.

REFERENCES

1. Garrean S, Hering J, Helton WS, et al. A primer on transarterial, chemical, and thermal ablative therapies for hepatic tumors. Am J Surg. 2007;194:79-88.
2. Park JH, Koh KC, Choi MS, et al. Analysis of risk factors associated with early multinodular recurrences after hepatic resection for hepatocellular carcinoma. Am J Surg. 2006;192:29-33.
3. Tanaka S, Shimada M, Shirabe K, et al. Surgical outcome of patients with hepatocellular carcinoma originating in the caudate lobe. Am J Surg. 2005;190:451-455.
4. Machado MA, Herman P, Makdissi FF, et al. Anatomic left hepatic trisegmentectomy. Am J Surg. 2005;190:114-117.
5. Chik BH, Liu CL, Fan ST, et al. Tumor size and operative of extended right-sided hepatic resection for hepatocellular carcinoma. Arch Surg. 2007;142:63-69.
6. Ai-jun L, Men-chao W, Guang-shun Y, et al. Management of retrohepatic inferior vena cava injury during hepatectomy for neoplasms. World J Surg. 2004;28:19-22.
7. Sarmiento JM, Bower TC, Cherry KJ, et al. Is combined partial hepatectomy with segmental resection of inferior vena cava justified for malignancy? Arch Surg. 2003;138:624-630.
8. Togo S, Tanaka K, Endo I, et al. Caudate lobectomy combined with resection of the inferior vena cava and its reconstruction by a pericardial autograft Patch. Dig Surg. 2002;19:340-343.
9. Miyazaki M, Ito H, Nakagawa K, et al. An approach to intrapericardial inferior vena cava through the abdominal cavity, without median sternotomy, for total hepatic vascular exclusion. Hepatogastroenterology. 2001;48:1443-1446.
10. Nakagohri T, Konishi M, Jnoue K, et al. Extended right hepatic lobectomy with resection of inferior vena cava and portal vein for intrahepatic cholangiocarcinoma. J Hepatobiliary Pancreat Surg. 2000;7:599-602.
11. Okada Y, Nagino M, Kamiya J, et al. Diagnosis and treatment of inferior vena caval invasion by hepatic cancer. World J Surg. 2003;27:689-694.
12. Wang Y, Chen H, Wu MC, et al. Surgical treatment of hepatocellular carcinoma with tumor thrombus in the inferior vena cava [in Chinese]. Chin J Surg. 2003;41:165-168.
13. Iemura J, Aoshima M, Ishigami N, et al. Surgery for hepatocellular carcinoma with tumor thrombus in the right atrium. Hepatogastroenterology. 1997;44:824-825.
14. Enoki T, Hayashi D, Inokuchi T, et al. Combined right hepatic and retrohepatic caval resection with reconstruction using a polytetrafluoroethylene graft for primary leiomyosarcoma of the liver: report of case. Surg Today. 1999;29:67-70.
15. Smyrniotis V, Arkadopoulos N, Kehagias D, et al. Liver resection with repair of major hepatic veins. Am J Surg. 2002;183:58-61.
16. Kim YI, Chung HJ, Song KE, et al. Evaluation of a protease inhibitor in the prevention of ischemia and reperfusion injury in hepatectomy under intermittent Pringle maneuver. Am J Surg. 2006;191:72-76.
17. Smyrniotis VE, Kostopanagiotou GG, Gamaletsos EL, et al. Total versus selective hepatic vascular exclusion in major liver resection. Am J Surg. 2002;183:173-178.
18. Smyrniotis VE, Kostopanagiotou GG, Contis JC, et al. Selective hepatic vascular exclusion versus Pringle maneuver in major liver resection: prospective study. World J Surg. 2003;27:765-769.
19. Dixon E, Vollmer CM, Bathe OF, et al. Vascular occlusion to decrease blood loss during hepatic resection. Am J Surg. 2005;190:75-86.
20. Gaujoux S, Douard R, Ettorre GM, et al. Liver hanging maneuver an anatomic and clinical review. Am J Surg. 2007;193:488-492.
21. Wakahayashi H, Maeb AT, Okano K, et al. Treatment of recurrent hepatocellular carcinoma by hepatectomy with right and middle hepatic vein reconstruction using total vascular exclusion with extracorporeal bypass and hypothermic hepatic perfusion: report of a case. Surg Today. 1998;28:547-550.
22. Kin T, Nakajima Y, Kanehiro H, et al. Comparison of hemodynamic changes in two vena-venous bypass techniques modified at the portal cannulation site. J Hepatobiliary Pancreat Surg. 1998;5:93-96.

23. Sarmiento JM, Que FG, Nagorney DM. Surgical outcomes of isolated caudate lobe resection: a single series of 19 patients. *Surgery*. 2002;132:697-709.
24. Yamamoto J, Takayama T, Kosuge T, et al. An isolated caudate lobectomy by the transhepatic approach for hepatocellular carcinoma in cirrhotic live. *Surgery*. 1992;111:699-702.
25. Kosuge T, Yamamoto J, Takayama T, et al. An isolated complete resection of the caudate lobe, including the paracaval portion, for hepatocellular carcinoma. *Arch Surg*. 1994;129:280-284.
26. Ortale JR, Borges Keiralla LC. Anatomy of the portal branches and hepatic veins in the caudate lobe of the liver. *Surg Radiol Anat*. 2004;26:384-391.
27. Auh YH, Rosen A, Rubenstein WA, et al. CT of the papillary process of the caudate lobe of the liver. *AJR Am J Roentgenol*. 1984;142:535-538.
28. Donoso L, Martinez-Noguera A, Zidan A, et al. Papillary process of the caudate lobe of the liver: sonographic appearance. *Radiology*. 1989;173:631-633.
29. Ali SM, Clark CJ, Zaydfudim VM, et al. Role of major vascular resection in patients with intrahepatic cholangiocarcinoma. *Ann Surg Oncol*. 2013;20:2023-2028.
30. Malassagne B, Cherqui D, Alon R, et al. Safety of selective vascular clamping for major hepatectomies. *J Am Coll Surg*. 1998;187:482-486.
31. Georgen M, Regimbeau JM, Kianmanesh R, et al. Removal of hepatocellular carcinoma extending in the right atrium without extracorporal bypass. *J Am Coll Surg*. 2002;195(6):892-894.
32. Yamanaka J, Iimuro Y, Kanno H, et al. Liver resection for hepatocellular carcinoma with tumor thrombus in hepatic vein, vena cava, and atrium: long-term prognosis. *Gastroenterology*. 2003;124(4):A695.
33. Stambo GW, Leto J, Van Epps C, et al. Endovascular treatment of intrahepatic inferior vena cava obstruction from malignant hepatocellular tumor thrombus utilizing Luminexx self-expanding nitinol stents. *South Med J*. 2008;14:166-169.
34. Yoshidome H, Takeuchi D, Kimura F, et al. Treatment strategy for hepatocellular carcinoma with major portal vein or inferior vena cava invasion: a single institution experience. *J Am Coll Surg*. 2011;212:796-803.
35. Arii S, Teramoto K, Kawamura T, et al. Significance of hepatic resection combined with inferior vena cava resection and its reconstruction with expanded polytetrafluoroethylene for treatment of liver tumors. *J Am Coll Surg*. 2003;196:243-249.
36. Azoulay D, Andreani P, Maggi U, et al. Combined liver resection and reconstruction of the supra-renal vena cava: the Paul Brousse experience. *Ann Surg*. 2006;244(1):80-88.
37. Iwatsuki S, Todo S, Starzl TE. Right trisegmentectomy with a synthetic vena cava graft. *Arch Surg*. 1988;123:1021-1022.
38. Kumada K, Shimahara Y, Fukui K, et al. Extended right hepatic lobectomy: combined resection of inferior vena cava and its reconstruction by PTFE graft (Gore-Tex). Case report. *Acta Chir Scand*. 1988;254:481-483.
39. Risher WH, Arensman RM, Ochsner JL, et al. Retrohepatic vena cava reconstruction with polytetrafluoroethylene graft. *J Vasc Surg*. 1990;12:367-370.
40. Miller CM, Schwartz ME, Nishizaki T. Combined hepatic and vena caval resection with autogenous caval graft replacement. *Arch Surg*. 1991;126:106-108.
41. Delis SG, Madariaga J, Ciancio G. Combined liver and inferior vena cava resection for hepatic malignancy. *J Surg Oncol*. 2007;96(3):258-264.
42. O'Malley KJ, Stuart RC, McEntee GP. Combined resection of the inferior vena cava and extended right hepatectomy for leiomyosarcoma of the retrohepatic cava. *Br J Surg*. 1994;81:845-846.
43. Ohwada S, Kawashima Y, Ogawa T, et al. Extended hepatectomy with ePTFE graft vena caval replacement and hepatic vein reconstruction: a case report. *Hepatogastroenterology*. 1999;46:1151-1155.
44. Yamamoto Y, Terajima H, Ishikawa Y, et al. In situ pedicle resection in left trisegmentectomy of the liver combined with reconstruction of the right hepatic vein to an inferior vena caval segment transpositioned from the infrahepatic portion. *J Am Coll Surg*. 2001;192:137-141.
45. Lechaux D, Megevand JM, Raoul JL, et al. Ex vivo right trisegmentectomy with reconstruction of inferior vena cava and "flop" reimplantation. *J Am Coll Surg*. 2002;194:842-845.
46. Del Campo C, Konok GP. Use of a pericardial xenograft patch in repair of resected retrohepatic vena cava. *Can J Surg*. 1994;37:59-61.
47. Kuehnl A, Schmidt M, Hornung HM, et al. Resection of malignant tumors invading the vena cava: perioperative complications and long-term follow-up. *J Vasc Surg*. 2007;46(3):533-540.
48. Li AJ, Wu MC, Zhou WP, et al. Surgical treatment of liver cancer involving the inferior vena cava [in Chinese]. *Zhonghua Yixue Zazhi*. 2006;86(24):1671-1674.
49. Hemming AW, Reed AI, Langham MR Jr, et al. Combined resection of the liver and inferior vena cava for hepatic malignancy. *Ann Surg*. 2004;239(5):712-719.
50. Ohwada S, Takahashi T, Tsutsumi H, et al. Hepatocellular carcinoma with a tumor thrombus extending to the tricuspid valve: report of a successful en bloc resection. *Hepatogastroenterology*. 2008;55(84):903-614.

Acknowledgments: *We gratefully acknowledge the previous edition contributions of Dr. Mengchao Wu.*

Chapter 27 Right Hepatic Trisegmentectomy

Jorge Sanchez-Garcia and Ivan R. Zendejas

DEFINITION

- Removal of the liver segments located to the right of the falciform ligament while the left lateral segment with or without the caudate will represent the functional remnant. In other words, this represents the resection of the middle segment (4A and 4B), the right anterior segment (5 and 8), and the right posterior segment (6 and 7, **FIGURE 1**).
- The resection may also include the caudate lobe and all the biliary ducts to the right of the umbilical fissure. This is most frequently indicated in patients diagnosed with hilar cholangiocarcinoma.

DIFFERENTIAL DIAGNOSIS

- Cholangiocarcinoma
- Metastatic carcinoma
- Hepatocellular carcinoma
- Gallbladder cancer
- Liver trauma
- Benign tumors (hemangiomas, adenomas)

PATIENT HISTORY AND PHYSICAL FINDINGS

- Attention must be given to the potential for underlying liver disease and the intended hepatic remnant volume following right trisegmentectomy.

IMAGING AND OTHER DIAGNOSTIC STUDIES

- Triphasic, contrast-enhanced abdominal computed tomography (CT) scan (ideally with coronal, axial, and sagittal fine cuts):
  - Its main value is to identify the vascular structures involved, anatomic variations in the hilar vasculature, and margins to be preserved at the time of surgery (**FIGURE 2**).
  - Examples of CT scans from patients with hepatocellular carcinoma involving the right side and middle segments (**FIGURE 3**) and a right dominant hilar cholangiocarcinoma are shown (**FIGURE 4**).

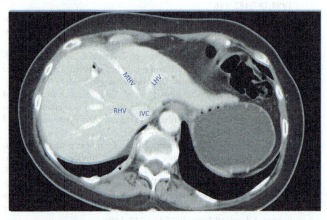

FIGURE 2 • Anatomy of the hepatic veins. The transection plane for a right trisegmentectomy is between the middle hepatic vein (MHV) and left hepatic vein (LHV). IVC, inferior vena cava; RHV, right hepatic vein.

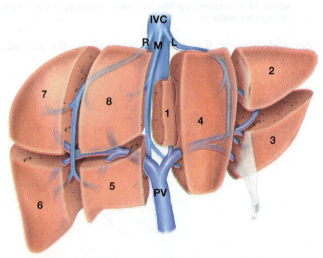

FIGURE 1 • Anatomy of a right trisegmentectomy. Segments 7 and 8 are routinely removed. Segment 1 is selectively included in the resection, depending on the indication and ability to obtain a negative resection margin. IVC, inferior vena cava; PV, pulmonary vein.

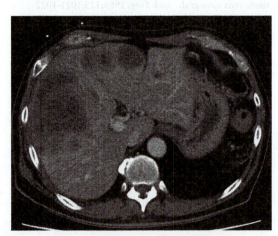

FIGURE 3 • Hepatocellular carcinoma involving the right and middle sectors.

Chapter 27 **RIGHT HEPATIC TRISEGMENTECTOMY** 215

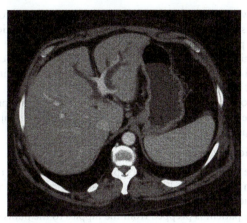

FIGURE 4 • Right dominant hilar cholangiocarcinoma. Note the dilated bile ducts in segment 4, to the right of the falciform ligament, suggesting the obstruction is distal to their confluence with the other ducts draining the left lobe.

- Abdominal magnetic resonance imaging with contrast and delayed liver phase:
  - Equivalent to a contrast CT scan; slightly better at defining parenchyma abnormalities, bile duct anatomy, and in differential diagnosis.
  - The authors favor Gadovist contrast for hepatocellular tumors and Eovist contrast for metastatic tumors.
- Advance imaging with three-dimensional (3D) reconstruction:
  - 3D reconstruction is helpful to estimate the future remnant and understanding the anatomical relationship between the tumor and vessels (**FIGURE 5**).
- Intraoperative ultrasound (IOUS):
  - Essential tool and skill needed during liver surgery. IOUS helps in defining margins, identifying smaller lesions (<1 cm), and visualizing the portal pedicles, hepatic veins, and potential vascular invasion (**FIGURES 6** and **7**).

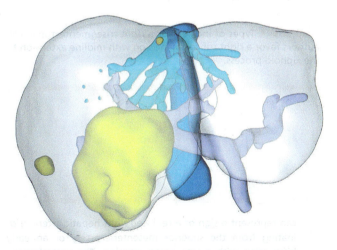

FIGURE 5 • Three-dimensional reconstruction with spatial relationship between the tumor (yellow), the portal vein (purple), and the hepatic veins (blue).

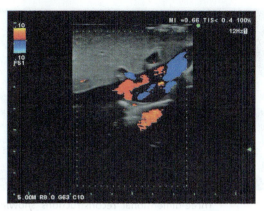

FIGURE 6 • Hepatic vein confluence under intraoperative ultrasound. Fluid-filled structures appear black. Doppler color facilitates identification of cystic lesions from vascular structures. In this image, the left hepatic vein is highlighted by the Doppler signal (blue) and the right hepatic vein is highlighted red as they insert into the inferior vena cava (IVC). The middle hepatic vein in this patient does not fuse with the left hepatic vein prior to IVC insertion and is seen above the IVC without Doppler enhancement.

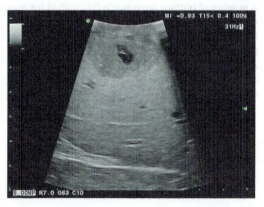

FIGURE 7 • Intraoperative ultrasound of a hepatic neoplasm. The hypoechoic lesion is at the top of the image. The interface with normal parenchyma is readily apparent.

SURGICAL MANAGEMENT

Preoperative Planning

- The volume of the intended remnant liver should to be calculated with preoperative imaging and considered against the patient body weight. Besides the rendition of the remnant volume, the authors favor 3D reconstruction for intraoperative navigation and patient education/orientation (**FIGURE 8**).
- The functional capacity of the remnant liver should be estimated with biological markers (platelets, model for end-stage liver disease score, albumin-bilirubin score, etc) or indocyanine green clearance test.
- Portal vein (PV) embolization of the right lobe (and occasionally segment 4) is often indicated to induce hypertrophy when future liver remnant deems insufficient.
- If PV embolization is performed, CT scan volumetrics are repeated 3 to 4 weeks postembolization to assess adequate hypertrophy of the planned liver remnant.

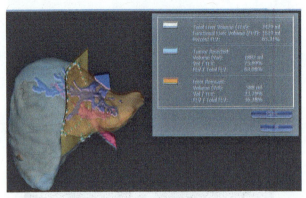

FIGURE 8 • Three-dimensional reconstructions showing the volume of the liver remnant. This particular software package provides the volume and percent of the total volume (table insert).

- Low-volume intraoperative resuscitation reduces blood loss. This approach requires preoperative communication with the preoperative nursing staff and anesthesia.
- Regional anesthesia approaches, such as epidural catheters and transverse abdominis plane block, reduce pain scores and respiratory complications.
- Preoperative steroid (100 mg intravenous methylprednisolone) is associated with reduced peaks of liver injury test values but not improved outcomes.

Positioning

- The patient is placed in a supine position. Tucking the right arm is optional, depending on the retractor to be used on patient's habitus.
- The patient is prepped from the nipples to the pubis on both sides.
- The authors routinely place an arterial line and central venous line for major hepatectomies.

TECHNIQUES

INCISION

- A number of options are possible (FIGURE 9) for appropriate exposure to perform a right trisegmentectomy.
- Bilateral, subcostal incision with upper midline extension (A + B + C).
- A right-sided, hockey stick–type incision (A + C).
- In children, a flat bilateral incision can be used (A + B).
- Removal of the xiphoid process is optional in order to get a better exposure of the suprahepatic abdominal vena cava.

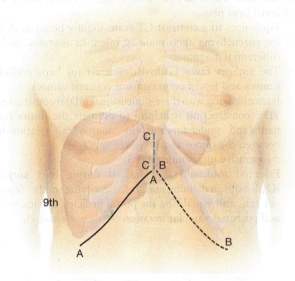

FIGURE 9 • Types of incision for a right trisegmentectomy. The authors favor a right subcostal incision with midline extension to the xiphoid process.

EXPOSURE

- A Thompson retractor facilitates the application of adequate tension of the costal margin to provide exposure to the hepatic veins, suprahepatic vena cava, and porta hepatis.

HILAR PALPATION

- Bimanual palpation of the hilar structures through the foramen of Winslow quickly defines the arterial anatomy (FIGURE 10). A pulse felt inferior posterior to the bile duct can represent a sign of a replaced right hepatic artery originating from the superior mesenteric artery or an early bifurcation with a retroportal position. The gastrohepatic ligament is inspected for the presence of a replaced/accessory left hepatic artery supplying the left lateral segment. The

best place to palpate the left hepatic artery is the umbilical fissure at the base of the liver. The arterial supply of the left lateral segment has to be clearly identified and preserved for a successful outcome.
- Nodal disease can be palpated and fixation of portal structures can estimate tumor extension.

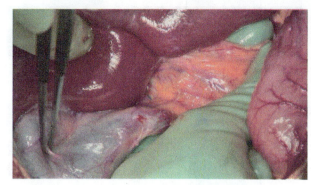

FIGURE 10 • Palpation of the porta hepatis facilitates definition of the arterial anatomy, the presence of involved lymph nodes, and pedicle encasement due to tumor extension.

LIVER MOBILIZATION

- The round ligament is ligated. The falciform ligament is taken down to the level of the hepatic veins. Arantius ligament is taken down to have access to the left hepatic vein. The gastrohepatic ligament is opened with careful attention to preserve the occasional replaced/accessory left hepatic artery. At this point, mobilization of the right lobe is performed (IOUS may be occasionally performed prior to mobilization depending on the tumor size and mobility of the liver) (**FIGURE 11**). The right lobe is mobilized by taking down the right coronary and triangular ligaments and lifting up the right lobe from the bare area with attention to the adrenal gland and the right side of the vena cava. The retrocaval ligament is identified and taken down with a vascular stapler. The short caudate veins are isolated and controlled with ligatures, clips, and/or vascular stapler loads.

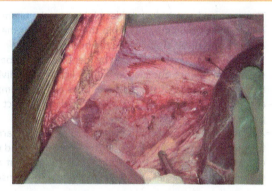

FIGURE 11 • Mobilization of the right lobe. The liver is being manually retracted to the midline, revealing the exposed diaphragm after division of the triangular ligament.

HILAR DISSECTION

- The cystic duct and cystic artery are dissected, ligated, and divided. The right hepatic artery is identified on the right side of the bile duct, ligated, and divided (**FIGURE 12**). There are so many variations in the arterial anatomy that the left hepatic artery flow must be felt and identified with a Doppler probe by doing a test clamp on the right side. The lymphatic and nerve tissue in the porta hepatis will be cleared, and the right PV branches will then be visualized. Alternatively, the right PV can be identified by following the main PV situated laterally and posteriorly in the portal pedicle. Then, the right PV branches are identified and ligated to have access to the main PV, which is encircled with a vessel loop. If the vein is long, then it can be stapled using a vascular load. If it is short, then it will be divided in between clamps and then sutured with continuous 6-0 Prolene sutures. After the inflow is occluded, the area of demarcation will be seen on the right lobe of the liver from the gallbladder fossa to the vena cava area.

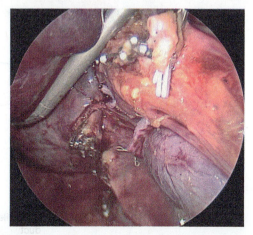

FIGURE 12 • Ligation/stapling of the right-sided structures. The right portal vein has been divided with a linear stapler, and the right hepatic artery and hepatic ducts have been divided between surgical clips.

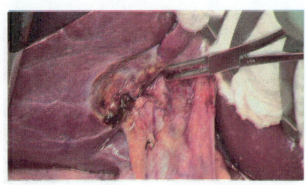

FIGURE 13 • Dissection of the hilar plate. The bifurcation of the hepatic duct can be within the parenchyma of the liver. Glisson capsule has been incised anterior to the hepatic duct in this example (tip of the surgical instrument).

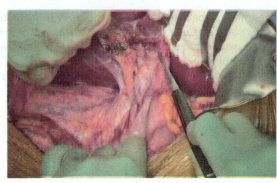

FIGURE 14 • Clear identification of the left bile duct. By elevating the hilar plate, the left hepatic duct is then clearly identified (tip of the forceps).

- The common hepatic duct divides high up on the hilum and, in fact, the division may be within the substance of the liver and only visualized after incising the hilar plate (FIGURE 13). The right branch of the duct will be identified at the base of the liver and, once encircled, it will be ligated and divided. Before the division of the right duct, it is extremely important to demonstrate the integrity of a definite duct that passes into the left side (FIGURE 14).
- At this point, the retractor is adjusted to expose the area of the umbilical fissure (FIGURE 15). The fissure may need to be exposed by transecting the parenchymal bridges that occasionally join the medial and lateral segments. The transverse portion of the umbilical fissure is identified at the base of segment 4B. Except for a few posterior caudate branches, there are no other significant branches in this portion of the PV. If the caudate lobe is to be removed, then these branches are ligated and divided. A replaced or accessory left hepatic artery will be identified at the base of the umbilical fissure. If present, this variant is an advantage as it minimizes the risk of dearterializing the remaining liver. The dissection is then carried out along the right side of the umbilical fissure, ligating all the medial branches to segments 4A and 4B. This can be done via the Glissonian approach (ligating and dividing them individually) or during the parenchymal transection.

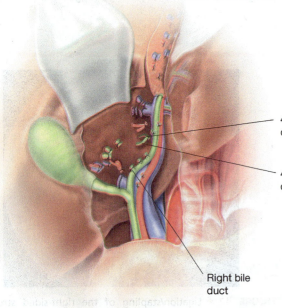

4B bile duct branch

4A bile duct branch

Right bile duct

FIGURE 15 • Dissection of segments 4A and 4B branches. Dissection is carried medial to the left hepatic duct. The dissection plane must be to the right of the falciform ligament to prevent injury to the structures essential to segments 2 and 3.

HEPATIC VEINS DISSECTION

- With the right lobe of the liver fully mobilized to the left side of the vena cava, all the retrohepatic veins are ligated and divided including the right adrenal vein, right caudate vein, and several small posterior hepatic veins. The origin of the right hepatic vein is identified, encircled, and divided with a vascular stapler or between clamps, depending on the vessel length and proximity to the tumor (**FIGURE 16**). After this step, the only patent veins will be the middle and left hepatic veins. The middle vein will be divided during the parenchymal transection as this is typically the safest approach (injury of the left hepatic vein is catastrophic). Alternatively, when an adequate margin is at risk or the anatomy is favorable, the middle vein can be individually encircled by an anterior approach dissecting the tight space between the left and middle vein. A right angle can be used to find this groove, pointing it inferiorly. The left lateral segment is elevated to the right and the ligamentum venosus is divided. The left hepatic vein is identified and the dissection will be carried out on its back wall in a plane just anterior to the vena cava. With careful dissection, the left hepatic vein can be encircled as well as the middle vein. Once again, it is critical to leave the origin of the left hepatic vein intact to secure an adequate venous outflow of the remnant.

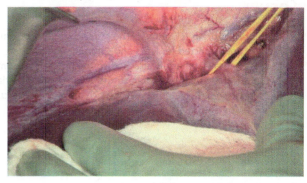

FIGURE 16 • Left/middle hepatic vein isolation. The insertion of the middle hepatic vein into the left hepatic vein is most frequently within the parenchyma of the liver. Thus, it is safest to control and divide the middle vein during the parenchymal transection.

LIVER TRANSECTION

- The transection line for right trisegmentectomy is just to the right of the falciform ligament anteriorly, the umbilical fissure or the round ligament inferiorly, and the anterior surface of the vena cava posteriorly (**FIGURE 17**). A hanging maneuver using a long Penrose drain or an umbilical tape passed behind the substance of the liver can facilitate proprioception of the transection plane. The parenchyma can be divided with a combination of techniques including fragmentation, stapler, or precoagulation. Regardless of the method used, the small portal triads and hepatic vein branches should be clipped or ligated. As the transection continued, the middle hepatic vein will be divided as well. The cut surface of a right trisegmentectomy transection plane is generally small and relatively hemostatic (**FIGURE 18**). Hemostasis on the surface can be achieved with a combination energy devices and chemical products.

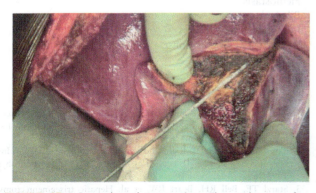

FIGURE 17 • Parenchymal transection. The authors prefer a combination of cautery, clips, and ligatures to perform the transection. The use of a microwave probe is demonstrated in this example.

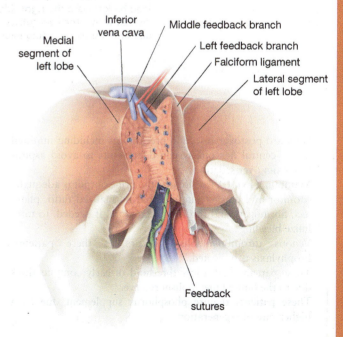

FIGURE 18 • Completion of the parenchymal transection with preservation of the left hepatic vein.

CLOSURE

- The use of a drain is optional. The parenchyma and biliary pedicles are inspected for leaks and sutured as needed.
- The left lateral segment is attached to the anterior abdominal wall with a nonabsorbable suture to prevent potential torsion and the associated catastrophic compromise of vascular inflow or outflow.
- The abdominal wall is then closed in a single- or double-layer fashion with absorbable suture. Skin is then closed with subcuticular sutures or staples.

PEARLS AND PITFALLS

Preoperative planning	- Right trisegmentectomy with caudate lobectomy is indicated for advanced hilar cholangiocarcinoma with involvement of the right-sided bile ducts. Only when the bile duct is divided at the left side of the umbilical fissure a significant negative margin can be achieved. Performance of an R0 resection is essential for a good outcome. - Assessment of the planned liver remnant by volumetrics or other functional assessment is critical for patients requiring trisegmentectomy. - PV embolization should be considered for all potential patients.
Intraoperative monitoring	- Temperature: It is imperative to maintain adequate core temperature to avoid the mortal triad of hypothermia, acidosis, and coagulopathy. The core temperature can be measured with an esophageal probe, or Foley catheter with thermometer of a pulmonary artery catheter, if deemed necessary. - Hemodynamic monitoring includes central line for central venous pressure (CVP) and an arterial line to assure an adequate perfusion in real time.
Operative technique	- The division of the intrahepatic bile duct is critical in the treatment of hilar cholangiocarcinoma because the tumor originates from and extends along the bile duct intramurally or superficially. - The blood supply and duct drainage of segment 4 originate within the umbilical fissure and feed back toward the right side buried in liver substance. These structures should be ligated and divided within the liver substance just to the right of the falciform ligament without entering the umbilical fissure, avoiding injury to the blood supply and drainage of the left lateral segment.

POSTOPERATIVE CARE

- Standard postliver resection precautions including minimal use of central nervous system depressants to avoid aspiration from over sedation.
- Maintain a low CVP as long as the urine output is adequate.
- Monitor and correct international normalized ratio, platelets, fibrinogen, and thromboelastogram, if needed, to minimize bleeding.
- Venous thromboembolism occurs in these patients. Prophylaxis is indicated.
- These patients had a low threshold of early complications due to the limited metabolism reserve.
- These patients require phosphorus supplement due to a higher rate of regeneration.

OUTCOMES

- The 5-year disease-free survival, regardless of underlying histology, is approximately 34.4%.
- The 90-day mortality is 7.6%.

COMPLICATIONS

- Liver failure
- Hemostasis
- Bile leak
- Intra-abdominal abscess
- Respiratory complications
- Wound complications

SUGGESTED READINGS

1. Nagino M, Kamiya J, Nishio H, et al. "Anatomic" right hepatic trisectionectomy (extended right hepatectomy) with caudate lobectomy for hilar cholangiocarcinoma. *Ann Surg*. 2006;243(1):28-32.
2. Shunzaburo I, Starzl T. Right and left hepatic trisegmentectomy. In: Daly J, Cady B, Low D, eds. *Atlas of Surgical Oncology*. Mosby; 1993:369.
3. Starzl TE, Bell RH, Beart RW, et al. Hepatic trisegmentectomy and other liver resections. *Surg Gynecol Obstet*. 1975;141(3):429-437.
4. Yamamoto Y, Yamaoka Y. Right hepatic trisegmentectomy (right trisectionectomy). *Gastroenterol Surg*. 2000;25(7):1101-1109.

Chapter 28 Left Hepatic Trisectionectomy

Jason A. Castellanos and Kamran Idrees

DEFINITION

- First described by Starzl et al[1] in 1982, this procedure entails a standard left hepatic hepatectomy (segments 2, 3, and 4) as well as resection of the right anterior sector (segments 5 and 8) (**FIGURE 1**).
- This operation is performed in a patient with a primary hepatic tumor or metastases involving the left liver invading across the middle hepatic vein toward the right hemiliver and/or portions of segments 5 and 8. In addition, patients with hilar cholangiocarcinoma may require this procedure in order to obtain tumor-free margins.

PATIENT HISTORY AND PHYSICAL FINDINGS

- Careful evaluation of the patient is required to ensure that the future liver remnant provides adequate liver function after resection. This should include assessment of liver function and exclusion of cirrhosis in addition to volumetric evaluation of the expected remnant liver volume on cross-sectional imaging.
- It is imperative to rule out portal hypertension or chronic liver disease, as a majority of the liver will be resected during this procedure.
- Details regarding prior therapy should be obtained.

IMAGING AND OTHER DIAGNOSTIC STUDIES

- Obtain either a liver-devoted magnetic resonance imaging or contrast-enhanced, triphasic computed tomography (CT) scan of the abdomen to identify tumor/s and its relationship to hilar structures and hepatic veins and anatomic variations of hilar vasculature and assess for radiographic signs of cirrhosis (**FIGURE 2**).
- Identify tumor and assess margins for possibility of R0 resection as well as volumetric assessment of future liver remnant.
- For metastatic disease, perform a complete staging evaluation as appropriate for the particular primary neoplasm.
- Intraoperative ultrasound is essential to define margins; exclude presence of disease in the planned liver remnant and visualize hepatic inflow and outflow.

SURGICAL MANAGEMENT

Preoperative Planning

- Assessment of the future liver remnant volume should be calculated with preoperative imaging to ensure adequate liver function after resection—greater than 20% in patients with normal liver function, greater than 30% for patients with evidence of liver disease (nonalcoholic fatty liver disease, chemotherapy-associated steatohepatitis, etc), and greater than 40% in cirrhotic patients.[2,3] If the remnant liver volume is deemed to be too small, then portal vein embolization may be used as an adjunct therapy to hypertrophy the future liver remnant prior to hepatectomy.

Positioning

- The patient should be placed in the supine position with the right arm tucked and prepped from the nipples to the pubis bilaterally.

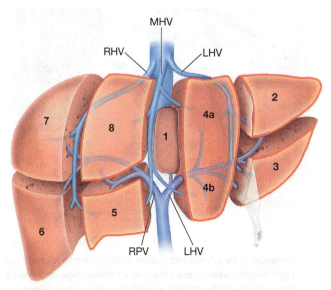

FIGURE 1 • Liver anatomy for left trisectionectomy. Segments outlined in *red* signify the resection margin. LHV, left hepatic vein; MHV, middle hepatic vein; RHV, right hepatic vein; RPV, right portal vein.

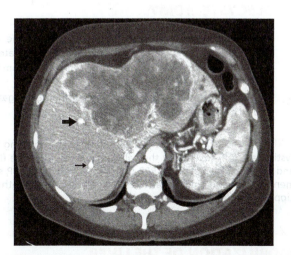

FIGURE 2 • Triple-phase CT scan (portal venous phase) of a cholangiocarcinoma involving segments 1, 2, 3, 4, 5, and 8. The right anterior (*thick arrow*) and posterior (*thin arrow*) pedicles are visible. This patient underwent left trisectionectomy with excision of the caudate lobe, which resulted in R0 excision of the tumor and a favorable outcome.

DIAGNOSTIC LAPAROSCOPY

- Our practice is to perform an initial diagnostic laparoscopy to ensure that there is no evidence of peritoneal disease.
- A supraumbilical incision is made through the skin and subcutaneous tissue using the Hasson technique, and a trocar is introduced into the abdomen, which is then insufflated to a pressure of 15 cm H_2O.
- The abdomen is explored including the hilum of the liver to assess for metastatic disease and periportal adenopathy. If there are no contraindications to operation, we then proceed to incision.

INCISION

- A bilateral subcostal incision is made, with superior extension in the midline to the xiphoid process, and a self-retaining retractor is placed. Another option is a midline incision to just above the umbilicus with a rightward extension (FIGURE 3).
- The xiphoid process may be excised in order to enhance exposure of the confluence of the hepatic veins into the suprahepatic inferior vena cava (IVC).
- The abdomen is inspected again for evidence of distant metastases that would contraindicate proceeding with operation.

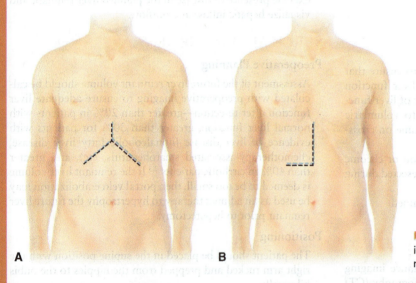

FIGURE 3 • Incisions for left trisectionectomy include **(A)** bilateral subcostal incision and **(B)** long midline incision with rightward extension.

INSPECTION OF THE HILUM, CHOLECYSTECTOMY

- The hilar structures are palpated in order to define any anatomic variations (eg, a posterior pulsation indicates a replaced/accessory right hepatic artery originating from the superior mesenteric artery).
- The cystic duct and cystic artery are identified and ligated, and a cholecystectomy is performed (FIGURE 4).

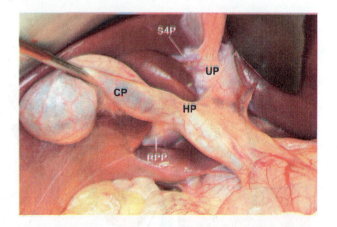

FIGURE 4 • Surface anatomy of the plate system showing the cystic plate (CP) covered by the gallbladder, the hilar plate (HP), and the umbilical plate (UP). RPP, right posterior pedicle; S4P, segment 4 pedicle. (From Fischer JF, ed. *Mastery of Surgery*. 6th ed. Lippincott Williams & Wilkins; 2012.)

MOBILIZATION OF THE LIVER

- The round ligament is ligated and divided, and the falciform, left triangular and coronary ligaments are divided to the level of the hepatic veins. The right coronary and triangular ligaments are transected, exposing the bare area of the liver.
- Intraoperative ultrasound is used at this point to identify the right hepatic vein to plan the line of transection and ensure resectability of the tumor as well as rule out any disease in the future liver remnant.
- After palpation, to identify a potential replaced or accessory left hepatic artery, the gastrohepatic ligament is divided. An

Chapter 28 LEFT HEPATIC TRISECTIONECTOMY 223

- aberrant left hepatic artery may be ligated at this time, as segments 2, 3, and 4 will be resected.
- Mobilization of the right liver is also required in order to facilitate parenchymal dissection along the right hepatic vein. Short hepatic veins are ligated and divided off of IVC. The hepatocaval ligament is then ligated or divided with a vascular stapler.

HILAR DISSECTION

- The hepatoduodenal ligament is opened and the common bile duct, proper hepatic artery, and portal vein are visualized after lymphatic and nerve tissues are cleared (**FIGURE 5**).
- A Rummel tourniquet is placed around the porta hepatis prior to further dissection to facilitate the Pringle maneuver, if needed.
- The left hemiliver is lifted and retracted toward the right to expose the left hilar branches of the portal triad. A vessel loop is placed around the left portal vein, left hepatic artery,

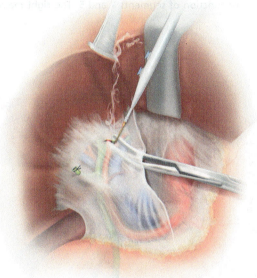

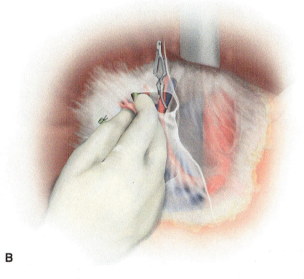

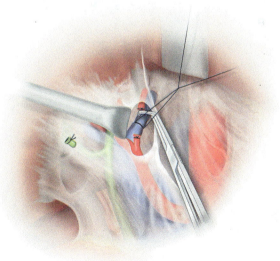

FIGURE 5 • Dissection of the hilum and left pedicle. The hepatoduodenal ligament is opened (**A**), followed by identification of the left hepatic artery (**B**). Clamping of the artery with a bulldog clamp allows for assessment of blood flow to the right liver. The left hepatic artery and vein are ligated (**C**), either with suture ligation or with vascular staplers.

and left hepatic duct to isolate them for ligation. Dissection may be aided by using the caudal stump of Arantius ligament as an anatomic guide toward the left portal vein.
- Ligation of the structures may be performed by an anterior-to-posterior or posterior-to-anterior approach; we prefer to begin ligation with the posterior structures. The left portal vein is ligated and divided first, leaving a distance of at least 5 mm to prevent stenosis of the right portal vein. Next, the left hepatic artery and left hepatic duct are ligated and divided. If the caudate lobe will be resected as well, then the left hilar structures should be ligated as close as possible to their origin.
- Next, the right anterior pedicle is identified with careful dissection in the right portal sheath. Identification of this pedicle can be aided by use of ultrasound, which can determine the location and depth (typically 1-2 cm from the inferior surface) of the pedicles. There are three options that the surgeon may use to approach this structure, depending on the ease of dissection, the extent of tumor involvement of the right portal sheath, and surgeon preference: extrahepatic, intrahepatic, or delayed dissection and ligation. If the anatomy is clear and the tumor does not impair dissection, then the right anterior pedicle may be dissected in the right portal sheath and individual structures of right anterior pedicle selectively ligated (extrahepatic) or right anterior pedicle is transected en bloc with a vascular stapler (intrahepatic pedicle ligation) while the right posterior pedicle is preserved. If the tumor involves the portal sheath, then the pedicle may be ligated during tissue transection instead (delayed) (**FIGURE 6**).
- Machado et al[4] describe an intrahepatic approach to isolating and ligating this structure. A small anterior incision is made in front of the hilum, and the parenchyma is bluntly dissected until the anterior aspect of the pedicle is identified. Another small incision is made perpendicular to the hilum at the junction of segments 1 and 5. The right main sheath is

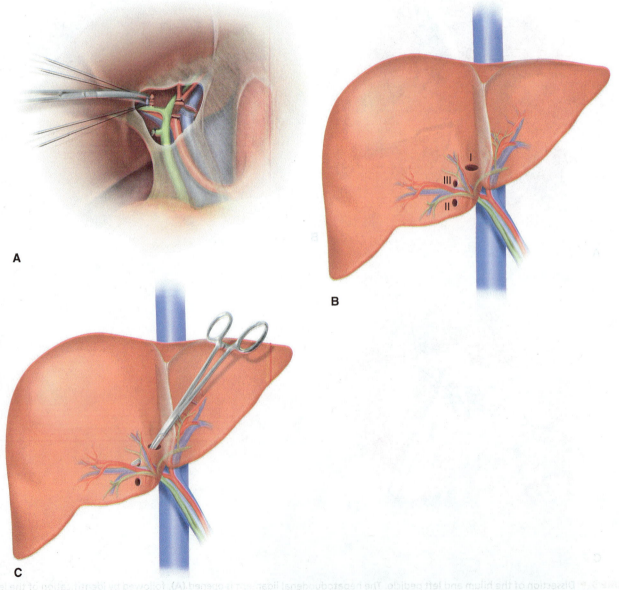

FIGURE 6 • Dissection of the right anterior pedicle. **A,** Extrahepatic selective ligation of the right anterior pedicle using blunt dissection. **B,** Intrahepatic approach to pedicle ligation requires three hepatotomies. An anterior incision is made in front of the hilum (*I*) followed by a vertical incision in segment 5 (*II*), and finally, an incision is made at the right edge of the gallbladder bed (*III*).

then isolated with the use of a large curved clamp inserted between these two incisions, and a vessel loop is placed. A third incision is made on the right side of the gallbladder fossa and a curved clamp used to dissect between this and the first incision, thus isolating the right anterior pedicle.[4]

- It is important to note that the blood supply to segment 7 may come from the right anterior pedicle, and so this must be kept in mind prior to transection in order to ensure adequate blood supply to the remnant liver. Clamping the pedicle prior to transection enables assessment of this relationship if it is not clear on preoperative imaging.

- We ligate these structures using Endo GIA staplers with a vascular load, but if the vessel is too short for this technique, then suture ligation followed by oversewing the distal stump with a continuous 6-0 Prolene may be performed. Our practice is to delay ligation of the right anterior hepatic duct until parenchymal dissection due to the possibility of anatomic variation.

- After ligation of the vessels feeding the left and anterior right liver, the area that will be resected will become demarcated by cyanosis.

DISSECTION OF THE MIDDLE AND LEFT HEPATIC VEINS

- The anterior aspect of the left and middle hepatic veins is exposed by dissection of the falciform left triangular and coronary ligaments as described earlier. The junction of the veins is dissected apart with a blunt right angle, and the left phrenic vein is identified, ligated, and divided at its insertion in the left hepatic vein (**FIGURE 7**).

- With the left lateral section retracted upward, the lesser omentum is divided up to the diaphragm. Arantius ligament (ligamentum venosum), which runs from the left branch of

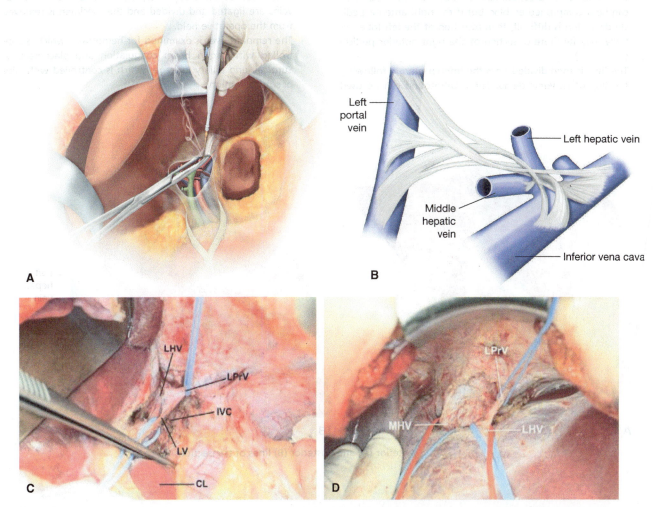

FIGURE 7 • Dissection of the left and middle hepatic veins. **A,** Dissection of Arantius ligament to expose the left and middle hepatic veins. **B,** Arantius ligament inserts onto the left and middle hepatic veins as demonstrated in this schematic. **C,** Isolation of ligamentum venosum (LV) at its junction with the left hepatic vein (LHV). **D,** Operative photo showing extrahepatic isolation of the left and middle hepatic veins together with their common trunk. Division of the left phrenic vein allows an extra length of the left hepatic vein to be isolated. CL, caudate lobe; IVC, inferior vena cava; LHV, left hepatic vein; LPrV, left phrenic vein; MHV, middle hepatic vein.

the portal vein to the left hepatic vein, is then ligated and divided.
- The cephalad stump of Arantius ligament is grasped and used to guide dissection toward the IVC. The ligament will broaden close to the IVC, at which point dissection is stopped and the ligament is retracted cephalad and leftward to create tension that will enable visualization of an avascular plane between the left and middle hepatic veins.[5]
- A vessel loop is then placed around the confluence of the middle and left hepatic veins. The hepatic veins may be ligated at this time if the confluence of the middle and left hepatic vein is already isolated. However, if vascular control cannot be achieved because of tumor proximity, our practice is to first divide the parenchyma and then ligate these vessels. Premature attempts to ligate these vessels may be dangerous as there are posterior tributaries that are difficult to control prior to transection of the parenchyma.
- If the caudate lobe will be resected, then the low hepatic veins that drain the caudate should be ligated and divided prior to transection of the parenchyma.

TRANSECTION OF THE LIVER PARENCHYMA

- 2-0 Chromic stay sutures are placed at the inferior margin of the liver, one on the ischemic left side and one on the normally perfused right side.
- The surgeon should communicate with the anesthesia team at the beginning of the case to ensure a low central venous pressure (CVP) (<3 mm Hg).
- The transection line is scored on the liver capsule following the ischemic demarcation. Resection of the entire specimen can be accomplished en bloc, but if the right anterior pedicle dissection is difficult, then resection of the left lobe initially may facilitate dissection of the right anterior pedicle (FIGURE 8).
- The liver is then divided from the inferior margin following the line of ischemic demarcation. Ultrasound can be used prior to this to ensure that the course of the right hepatic vein is known throughout the liver. Various techniques may be used to transect the liver including stapling, electrosurgery, fragmentation, ultrasonic dissection, radiofrequency energy device dissection, and water-jet dissection (FIGURE 9).
- If the right anterior pedicle cannot be ligated prior to transection of the parenchyma, then the line of transection should be marked 1 cm to the left of the course of the right hepatic vein.
- When transection is complete, the left and middle hepatic veins are ligated and divided and the specimen is removed from the operative field.
- The remnant liver is examined for hemostasis, which is controlled with argon beam coagulation and placement of Surgicel, and biliary leakage, which is controlled with clips or suture ligation.

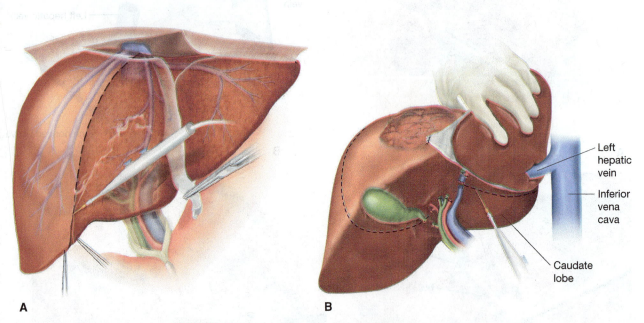

FIGURE 8 • Anterior (**A**) and posterior (**B**) lines of transection.

Chapter 28 LEFT HEPATIC TRISECTIONECTOMY 227

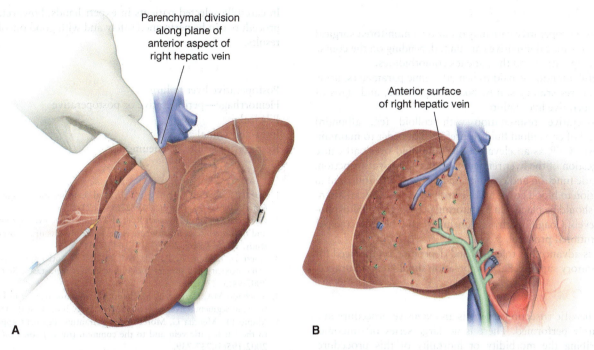

FIGURE 9 • Parenchymal transection and specimen removal. The plane of transection is the anteromedial aspect of the right hepatic vein (**A**). After removal of the specimen (**B**), the right hepatic vein and hilar structures are exposed and careful examination for hemostasis and biliary leakage is performed.

CLOSURE

- Placement of a drain is optional and largely dependent on the clinical scenario. We place drains if there is evidence of biliary leakage or if any biliary reconstruction was performed.

- The incision is then closed in the standard fashion with absorbable suture, and the skin is closed with staples or subcuticular sutures.

PEARLS AND PITFALLS

Operative indications	• Tumor involving the left liver and right anterior section (segments 5 and 8). • No evidence of peritoneal spread or other metastatic disease.
Preoperative assessment	• Ensure normal liver function prior to considering operation. • Assess the volume of future liver remnant preoperatively to decrease the likelihood of postoperative liver failure.
Isolation of the right anterior pedicle	• Ultrasound may be used to help identify structures. • Dissection may be either intrahepatic, extrahepatic, or delayed until transection. • If tumor involves the hilum, then dissection and ligation of the right anterior pedicle should be performed during parenchymal transection. • Ensure that the blood supply to segment 7 is not compromised prior to dividing the right anterior pedicle.

POSTOPERATIVE CARE

- Initial postoperative care may occur on a monitored surgical floor or surgical intensive care unit, depending on the course of the operation and the patient's comorbidities.
- Careful attention is paid to hemodynamic parameters, urine output, respiratory status, body temperature, and signs of postoperative liver failure.
- Postoperative resuscitation with colloid (eg, albumin) instead of crystalloid fluids is preferred in order to maintain a lower CVP, as an elevated CVP and fluid overload cause congestion of the liver remnant and may impair its function.
- Hepatic function and coagulation labs should be followed in addition to blood count and electrolyte panels. Special attention should be placed on monitoring postoperative phosphorus levels. Coagulopathy and anemia should be corrected per institutional protocol.
- Diet is advanced as tolerated and depending on the need for respiratory support. Early ambulation should be encouraged.

OUTCOMES

- Left hepatic trisectionectomy is an extensive procedure and is rarely performed. There is no large series of outcomes describing the morbidity or mortality of this procedure. In carefully selected patients in expert hands, however, this procedure can be performed safely and with good oncologic results.

COMPLICATIONS

- Postoperative liver failure
- Hemorrhage—perioperative or postoperative
- Bile leak
- Intra-abdominal abscess
- Respiratory failure or pneumonia

REFERENCES

1. Starzl TE, Iwatsuki S, Shaw BW Jr, et al. Left hepatic trisegmentectomy. *Surg Gynecol Obstet.* 1982;155(1):21-27.
2. Ferrero A, Vigano L, Polastri R, et al. Postoperative liver dysfunction and future remnant liver: where is the limit? Results of a prospective study. *World J Surg.* 2007;31(8):1643-1651.
3. Zorzi D, Laurent A, Pawlik TM, et al. Chemotherapy-associated hepatotoxicity and surgery for colorectal liver metastases. *Br J Surg.* 2007;94(3):274-286.
4. Machado MA, Herman P, Machado MC. A standardized technique for right segmental liver resections. *Arch Surg.* 2003;138(8):918-920.
5. Majno PE, Mentha G, Morel P, et al. Arantius' ligament approach to the left hepatic vein and to the common trunk. *J Am Coll Surg.* 2002;195(5):737-739.

Chapter 29   Ex Vivo Hepatic Resection

Priyadarshini Manay and Alan William Hemming

DEFINITION

- Ex vivo resection of the liver is a procedure that involves removing the liver from the patient with cold perfusion of the liver with preservation solution on the back table.
- The resection of the tumor and reconstruction of vascular structures can then be performed without time pressure in a bloodless field with subsequent reimplantation of the remnant liver into the patient.

DIFFERENTIAL DIAGNOSIS/INDICATIONS

- Any tumor that cannot be resected with standard techniques can be considered for ex vivo resection. These tumors can be:
  - Primary liver tumors such as hepatocellular carcinoma, cholangiocarcinoma, or hepatoblastoma.
  - Metastatic tumors to the liver such as colorectal metastases, neuroendocrine tumors, GIST.
  - Echinococcal disease that involves inferior vena cava (IVC) and hepatic veins.
  - Tumors that involve the junction of the IVC and the hepatic veins or patients with combined vascular involvement of the hepatic veins and hilar structures are typically considered.

PATIENT HISTORY AND PHYSICAL FINDINGS

- A thorough medical history provides information about the symptoms related to the liver tumor although patients may well be asymptomatic.
- Patients may or may not have signs of liver disease such as jaundice and ascites either of which suggest the patient will not be a candidate for ex vivo resection.
- Patients may have nonspecific symptoms like weight loss, anorexia, or pain.
- With caval obstruction, there may be bilateral pedal edema and the formation of venous collaterals visible on the abdominal wall.
- Associated comorbidities are important to assess with only patients in reasonable physical condition considered for ex vivo resection.
- In patients over 50 years of age or with any cardiac abnormalities, a functional stress test such as dobutamine stress echocardiogram is performed. Any significant cardiac abnormalities would preclude proceeding.
- Renal dysfunction can increase the risk of hepatectomy, and a creatinine >1.3 mg/dL is a relative contraindication to proceeding with this surgery.

IMAGING AND OTHER DIAGNOSTIC STUDIES

- Preoperative imaging has three functions:
  1. To stage the tumor within and outside the liver
  2. To assess position of tumor in relation to hepatic vascular anatomy
  3. To assess the future liver remnant (FLR) volume
- Triphasic computed tomography (CT) (**FIGURE 1**)[1] with 3D reconstruction gives an assessment of liver anatomy and tumor position. CT also allows FLR volume assessment. CT chest and pelvis help assess for distant metastasis.
- MR angiography and venography may be required when all three hepatic veins are involved to the degree that the hepatic venous obstruction prevents adequate flow of contrast into the hepatic veins during CT imaging. MRCP may provide necessary information of biliary anatomy.
- With the technical advances in CT and MR technology, invasive angiography is generally not necessary but can be used if needed in specific cases. Positron emission tomography is generally recommended to rule out the possibility of otherwise undetected extrahepatic disease which would be a contraindication to proceeding.

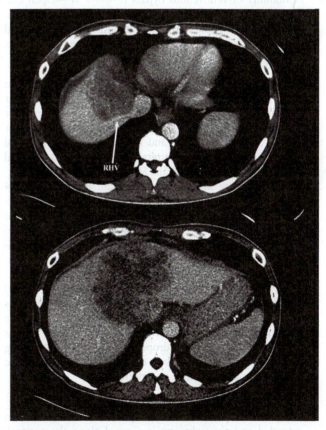

FIGURE 1 • Computed tomography demonstrating a large centrally placed tumor involving all three Hepatic veins. RHV, right hepatic vein. (Reprinted from Hemming AW. Ex vivo and in situ hypothermic hepatic resection. In: Blumgart LH, ed. *Surgery of the Liver, Biliary Tract and Pancreas.* 4th ed. Elsevier; 2006:1472-1483. Copyright © 2007 Elsevier. With permission.)

SURGICAL MANAGEMENT

Preoperative Planning/Considerations

- While an FLR of 25% is acceptable for standard liver resection, cold preservation and reperfusion during ex vivo resection add an additional ischemic injury. In general, a cutoff of >40% for FLR is used for ex vivo liver resections. If FLR is <40%, then preoperative portal vein embolization of the side ipsilateral to the tumor should be considered.[2] Yttrium-90 radiation lobectomy has also been utilized to both reduce tumor size and cause contralateral hypertrophy.
- Three-dimensional imaging is important to plan vascular reconstruction. Such imaging can accurately discover unusual anatomy that may make reconstruction unnecessary. For example, the presence of a large inferior hepatic vein may make main right hepatic vein reconstruction unnecessary. On the other hand, a large segment 6 or segment 8 vein draining into the middle hepatic vein may necessitate additional reconstruction.[3] Consideration of graft material should be undertaken preoperatively with the availability of options such as ringed polytetrafluoroethylene for caval reconstruction or cryopreserved vein graft ensured. Use of autologous vein grafts or falciform/peritoneal grafts should also be planned preoperatively.
- Availability of venovenous bypass (FIGURE 2)[1]—Open cutdown techniques or percutaneous techniques can be utilized for venovenous bypass. Access to femoral vein and internal jugular vein or axillary vein needs to be planned in advance.

Intraoperative Planning/Considerations

- Anesthesia management: This is similar to liver transplant surgery. Maintenance of patient temperature by forced air warming blankets and warming all fluids is required for good outcomes. A Swan-Ganz (SG) catheter is inserted for hemodynamic monitoring and monitoring temperature of blood in the pulmonary artery although transesophageal echo can be substituted for the SG catheter.
- Anhepatic phase management: This can last from 2 to 4 hours. During this period, balancing coagulation is important. Fresh frozen plasma is given as fluid replacement and coagulation products administered with the guidance of thromboelastography. Crystalloid infusion should be minimized. Glucose levels should be monitored closely, and glucose replaced as needed.
- Reperfusion phase management: Pulmonary artery blood temperature can drop to 32 to 33 °C on reperfusion. This can be avoided or managed by warm "blood flushing" the liver as well as temporarily compressing the portal venous inflow when temperature drops below 34.5 °C.[4] Avoiding this extreme temperature drop decreases the risk of cardiac dysfunction abnormalities on reperfusion.

Positioning for Surgery

- The patient is placed in a supine position with the left arm extended and the right arm is secured along the patient's torso.
- The patient is secured to the table at the thighs and the legs.
- Heel pads, sequential compression devices for deep venous thrombosis prophylaxis, and warming devices are also placed.

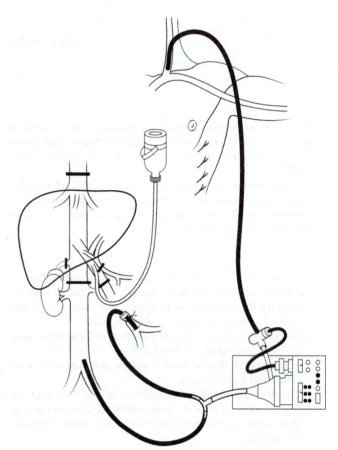

FIGURE 2 • Schematic diagram of venovenous bypass. (Reprinted from Hemming AW. Ex vivo and in situ hypothermic hepatic resection. In: Blumgart LH, ed. *Surgery of the Liver, Biliary Tract and Pancreas*. 4th ed. 2006:1472-1483. Copyright © 2007 Elsevier. With permission.)

- An orogastric tube is inserted to decompress the stomach.
- The patient is prepped and draped from neck to mid-thigh including the left axilla if an axillary vein access is used for venovenous bypass.
- The Thompson or other fixed mechanical retractor is set up as for standard liver surgery.
- The primary surgeon stands at the patient's right and the assistant surgeon at the patient's left.

Incision and Operability

Diagnostic laparoscopy: An initial assessment of operability is undertaken either via laparoscopy or through a limited abdominal incision. Laparoscopy assesses the presence of peritoneal disease that would preclude proceeding with resection.

Limited abdominal incision: A limited incision along the planned final incision is used even after a negative laparoscopy to assess the abdominal cavity. It is not uncommon to have a negative laparoscopy only to find additional small lesions in the liver or elsewhere that would be a contraindication to proceeding. The incision is then lengthened to some variation of a bilateral subcostal incision, with or without a midline extension.

There are three phases to the procedure:
- Assessment of resectability and removal of the liver.
- Liver resection and vascular reconstruction on the back table.
- Reimplantation of the liver autograft.

ASSESSMENT

- Since the indication for *ex vivo* resection is involvement of the hepatic veins with or without caval involvement, the liver may be venous congested, and care must be taken not to injure the liver during mobilization since any small breach of the liver capsule becomes an outflow route for the obstructed venous flow and bleeding can be torrential.
- Venous congestion of the liver is not a contraindication to resection since the planned resection should relieve the venous outflow obstruction.
- Large tumors may restrict the ability to rotate the liver without undue tension, and in these cases, it is prudent to make an early decision regarding *ex vivo* procedure prior to attempting elevation of the liver off the IVC.
- Intraoperative ultrasound is used to assess the level of vascular involvement and to confirm vascular anatomy originally identified on preoperative imaging.
- If a decision is made to proceed with an ex vivo approach, then the following steps are performed:

Preparation of the Hilar Structures

- The arterial anatomy is dissected out and an appropriate site chosen for planned division.
- This will usually be at the level of the common hepatic artery/gastroduodenal artery junction.
- If there is aberrant arterial anatomy, an alternative site may be required depending on the anatomy and portion of the liver that will remain after the resection. The artery is not dissected high into the hilum in most cases in order to preserve small arterial communications to the biliary tree.
- If the tumor involves the hilar structures, the artery must be dissected far enough to determine that there is a usable, tumor-free portion of the respective hepatic artery branch to reconstruct.
- The portal vein is identified, and the common bile duct encircled without skeletonization. A cholecystectomy is performed. The bile duct is reflected off the portal vein taking care to preserve the blood supply, and the neural and lymphatic tissue around the portal vein cleared.
- The infrahepatic IVC is dissected out down to the level of the renal veins and encircled. Planned vascular clamp placement will be immediately above the renal veins although division of the vena cava may be substantially more cephalad. The right adrenal vein should be ligated and divided. Small caudate veins should be divided if accessible. The large size of the tumor may make access to the caudate veins difficult in which case they can be dealt with on the back table.
- The liver is freed from surrounding attachments. If the tumor is infiltrating the diaphragm, the portion of the diaphragm involved is resected *en bloc* with the tumor.
- The suprahepatic IVC is prepared. The phrenic veins are divided, allowing the diaphragm to be dissected away from the IVC, and providing an increased length of intra-abdominal IVC to be available for subsequent clamping and reconstruction. We currently also open the pericardium directly anterior to the IVC and loop the intrapericardial IVC. Control of the intrapericardial IVC allows placement of the clamp on the vena cava within the pericardium either as a primary option for tumors that are very large or as a secondary option in case technical difficulties arise with placement of the original suprahepatic caval clamp. For very large tumors, a median sternotomy can be added to provide excellent exposure to the intrapericardial IVC.
- An assessment of clamp placement and subsequent transection lines is undertaken. The need for vascular conduits for reconstruction is assessed and alternatives for reconstruction contemplated prior to removing the liver. Hepatic venous branches may be reconstructed using hepatic vein or portal vein segments from the side of the liver resected or from autologous vein grafts such as superficial femoral vein, proximal left renal vein, gonadal vein, or saphenous vein panel grafts. Cryopreserved femoral vein grafts can be used for reconstruction of long segments of hepatic veins or IVC; however, the issue of long-term patency is not currently clear. Falciform or peritoneal grafts can be used to form vein patches or constructed into tube grafts. The IVC can alternatively be replaced with 20-mm ringed Gortex tube graft. Planning for these eventualities should take place prior to placement of clamps and removal of the liver.
- Percutaneous access of the internal jugular vein or axillary vein and femoral vein is achieved, the IVC is clamped, and the caval portion of bypass is started. The portal vein is clamped just below the bifurcation and the portal cannula inserted down toward the superior mesenteric vein and secured. The portal vein is completely transected approximately 1.5 to 2 cm below the bifurcation and the portal flow added to the bypass circuit. The liver continues to be perfused by arterial blood at this time.

Liver Removal

- The liver is removed. The bile duct is transected sharply approximately 1 to 1.5 cm below the bifurcation. We do not ligate either end since we may elect to perform a duct-to-duct anastomosis on reimplantation.
- The gastroduodenal artery is ligated and divided. The common hepatic artery is clamped, and the hepatic artery is transected at the takeoff of the gastroduodenal artery such that a branch patch is formed on either side of the arterial transection if possible. The suprahepatic IVC is clamped either below the diaphragm or within the pericardium and the suprahepatic vena cava transected far enough away from tumor to provide an adequate oncologic margin but leaving enough room to perform the suprahepatic caval anastomosis at the time of reimplantation. If the vena cava has been freed of its posterior attachments prior to clamp placement, then the infrahepatic IVC is then divided as cephalad as possible, and the liver is removed and placed in an ice bath. Cold perfusion through the portal vein and hepatic artery is

initiated on the backbench. Cold perfusion can be with either histidine-tryptophan-ketoglutarate (HTK) or University of Wisconsin (UW) solution. If the retrohepatic IVC has not previously been freed up because of the large tumor size and difficulty with access, then the liver can be cold perfused via the portal vein once the suprahepatic IVC is divided. The liver is then rotated forward as in the *ante situm* approach and the retrohepatic IVC freed of attachments. The infrahepatic IVC is then divided, and the liver removed and placed in the ice bath.

- Any bleeding is controlled, and the bypass circuit assessed. Flows of 3 to 6 L/min would be expected on total bypass. The abdomen is loosely packed and covered and attention turned to the back table.

LIVER RESECTION AND VASCULAR RECONSTRUCTION

- Liver resection and vascular reconstruction on the back table (▶ Video 1).

Ex Situ Liver Resection

- Once removed from the patient, the liver is immediately placed in an ice bath and perfused with preservation solution through the portal vein. We use UW solution since it is also the preservation solution we use for cadaveric and live donor liver transplantation; however, HTK solution is also a reasonable choice. After the initial 500 to 1000 mL of solution has been flushed through the liver, the effluent from the IVC should be clear. The hepatic artery and biliary tree are then also flushed with another 200 to 300 mL of preservation solution. The liver is immersed in cold UW and the resection performed.
- Hilar structures are dissected out and divided. Great care must be taken not to divide segmental arteries to portions of the liver that are to remain since their caliber are too small to reconstruct with confidence. Main segmental divisions of the portal vein can usually be repaired and reconstructed. Parenchymal transection can be performed using a variety of techniques including ultrasonic dissection, water jet, or can even be divided sharply with a knife. Small bile ducts and vessels are ligated or oversewn. Large hepatic veins are cut sharply and later assessed for reconstruction.
- Margin should not be compromised in order to minimize the subsequent complexity of vascular reconstruction (FIGURE 3).[5] A key advantage to the ex vivo approach is the ability to extend the resection to obtain negative margins while providing the necessary time and exposure for complex reconstructions.
- At completion of the resection, it is helpful to flush the portal vein, hepatic artery, and bile duct with UW to identify leaks from the cut surface of the liver, which can then be repaired prior to reimplantation. Fibrin glue may be sprayed on the cut surface of the liver to minimize bleeding.

Hepatic Vein Reconstruction

- Hepatic vein reconstruction, with or without IVC reconstruction, is the *raison d'être* for *ex vivo* liver resection. The hepatic veins are relatively thick walled and straightforward to reconstruct within 2 to 3 cm of their merging with the IVC.
- For reconstructions of hepatic veins transected relatively close to the IVC, the liver parenchyma can be trimmed back such that direct reimplantation of the hepatic vein into either the IVC or IVC replacement can be performed.

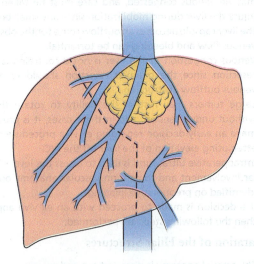

FIGURE 3 • Diagram of resection line for tumor shown in **FIGURE 1**. Note the resection line extends well out the right hepatic vein to obtain negative margins. (Reprinted from McGilvray ID, Hemming AW. Ex vivo and in situ hepatic resection. In: Jarnagin W, ed. *Blumgart's Surgery of the Liver, Biliary Tract and Pancreas*. 6th ed. Elsevier; 2017:1670-1683. Copyright © 2017 Elsevier. With permission.)

- Multiple orifices of hepatic veins can be plastied together or implanted into venous conduits (FIGURES 4-6).[1,5] The farther away from the IVC that the hepatic vein is transected, the thinner the wall of the hepatic vein and the more difficult it is to directly reimplant the vein into the IVC.
- The portal vein bifurcation can be harvested, reversed, and used to reconstruct multiple hepatic vein branches into a single outflow vessel.[6,5]
- Saphenous vein, superficial femoral vein, internal jugular vein, and cryopreserved vein grafts or falciform, peritoneal grafts have all been used to reconstruct hepatic veins.[7-10]
- Segments of uninvolved hepatic vein from the side of the liver resected can be salvaged and used for grafts or patches. Venous grafts should be kept as short as possible and great care must be taken to place the grafts such that they do not kink.
- For extension grafts, the hepatic vein to graft anastomosis is performed first with subsequent reimplantation of the graft into the IVC.

IVC Reconstruction

- If possible, it is preferential to reimplant the hepatic veins into native vena cava. Frequently a large portion of the vena cava that was initially removed with the liver can be salvaged

Chapter 29 EX VIVO HEPATIC RESECTION 233

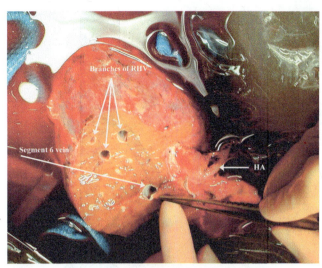

FIGURE 4 • Transection of the liver on the back table yields multiple hepatic vein orifices that will require reconstruction. RHV, right hepatic vein. (Reprinted from Hemming AW. Ex vivo and in situ hypothermic hepatic resection. In: Blumgart LH, ed. *Surgery of the Liver, Biliary Tract and Pancreas*. 4th ed. Elsevier; 2006:1472-1483. Copyright © 2007 Elsevier. With permission.)

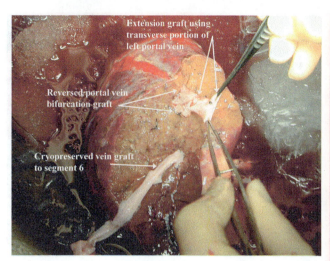

FIGURE 6 • Venous reconstruction on the back table using a reversed portal venous bifurcation graft along with an extension graft to reconstruct the right hepatic vein branches. The segment 6 venous outflow is reconstructed using a cryopreserved venous graft.

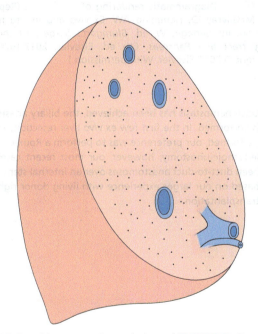

FIGURE 5 • Diagrammatic rendering of **FIGURE 4**. (Reprinted from McGilvray ID, Hemming AW. Ex vivo and in situ hepatic resection. In: Jarnagin W, ed. *Blumgart's Surgery of the Liver, Biliary tract and Pancreas*. 6th ed. Elsevier; 2017:1670-1683. Copyright © 2017 Elsevier. With permission.)

and moved superiorly with the hepatic veins reimplanted into this newly situated portion of IVC.
- Ringed 20-mm Gortex tube graft can then be used to make a composite caval graft with the Gortex graft placed inferiorly.
- Alternatively, a section of the IVC immediately above the renal veins remaining in the patient can be harvested and used as the segment of IVC into which the hepatic veins are reimplanted. A 20-mm ringed Gortex tube graft is then used to replace the segment of IVC immediately above the renal veins.
- In some circumstances it is necessary to reimplant the hepatic veins directly into a relatively stiff Gortex graft that is replacing the IVC. In this situation it is important to make a larger opening in the Gortex than one might expect and to triangulate the anastomosis to prevent the development of an anastomotic stricture.[11]
- At completion of the backbench reconstruction, one has an autograft that is similar to a reduced size or split liver allograft. Total cold ischemic time is between 2 and 6 hours, which is well within acceptable limits when comparing cold ischemic times for split liver or reduced size liver transplantation.

REIMPLANTATION

- Reimplantation is very similar as for reduced size liver transplantation.
- The suprahepatic IVC anastomosis is performed first. If a Gortex graft has been used to reconstruct the IVC, it is shortened such that it will not kink on implantation. Once the back wall of the infrahepatic vena caval anastomosis has been completed, the portal vein is flushed with 500 mL of cold 5% albumin, which is vented through the infrahepatic caval anastomosis.
- The infrahepatic vena caval anastomosis is then completed. The cold rinse washes the UW out of the liver prior to reperfusion. UW contains high levels of potassium and adenosine that can cause dramatic cardiac dysfunction or arrest if allowed into the circulation on reperfusion.

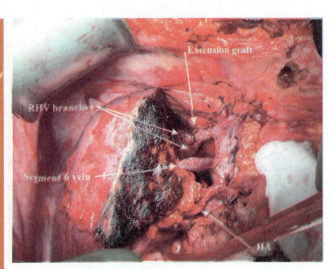

FIGURE 7 • Reimplanted graft with venous and arterial anastomoses completed. RHV, right hepatic vein. (Reprinted from Hemming AW. Ex vivo and in situ hypothermic hepatic resection. In: Blumgart LH, ed. *Surgery of the Liver, Biliary Tract and Pancreas*. 4th ed. Elsevier; 2006:1472-1483. Copyright © 2007 Elsevier. With permission.)

- An alternative to cold flushing the liver prior to reperfusion is to leave the lower caval anastomosis open until after portal reperfusion, venting the initial 300 cc of blood prior to removing the suprahepatic caval clamp.
- There is little evidence to support one technique over the other. We prefer the cold flush technique only because it reduces the number of possible bleeding sites at the time of reperfusion.
- After the infrahepatic caval anastomosis is performed, the portal limb of the bypass circuit is clamped and removed from the portal vein. The portal venous anastomosis is performed.
- The suprahepatic caval clamp is removed and the liver is allowed to perfuse back through the hepatic veins. Any major bleeding is controlled prior to reestablishing the portal flow.
- The portal venous clamp is removed, and the liver is reperfused. Any bleeding from the cut surface of the liver is controlled. The patient is then taken off caval bypass.
- The arterial anastomosis is performed, and the liver is reperfused with arterial blood (**FIGURES 7** and **8**).[1,5] Total warm ischemic time is between 20 and 40 minutes.

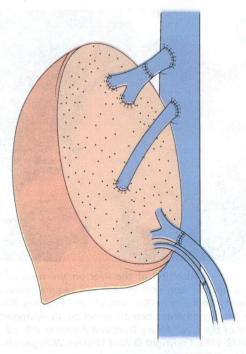

FIGURE 8 • Diagrammatic rendering of **FIGURE 7**. (Reprinted from McGilvray ID, Hemming AW. Ex vivo and in situ hepatic resection. In: Jarnagin W, ed. *Blumgart's Surgery of the liver, Biliary tract and Pancreas*. 6th ed. Elsevier; 2017:1670-1683. Copyright © 2017 Elsevier. With permission.)

- Once hemostasis has been achieved, the biliary anastomosis is performed. In the first few *ex vivo* liver resections that we performed, our preference was to perform a Roux-en-Y choledochojejunostomy; however, our most recent cases have been duct-to-duct anastomoses over an internal stent. This is based on our larger experience with living donor right lobe transplantation.

PEARLS AND PITFALLS

- Almost all liver resections can be performed using standard techniques. One of the advantages of performing ex vivo liver resection is that patients who are felt to be unresectable with standard liver resection techniques are explored with intent to perform ex vivo liver resection and found to be resectable with standard techniques.
- Ligation and division of the phrenic veins as well as right adrenal vein allows extra length of IVC to be obtained and avoids accidental injury at time of clamp placement.

- In bulky tumors, a median sternotomy provides additional excellent exposure to the suprahepatic and intrapericardial IVC. Patient selection is the key to this operation. Patient should be reasonably healthy with no major comorbidities and ideally the FLR should be at least 35% to 40%.

POSTOPERATIVE CARE

- Postoperative care is similar to any major liver resection or liver transplantation.
- Ultrasound with Doppler assessment is performed on postoperative day 1 to assess liver blood flow.
- Transaminases in the 200 to 1000 IU/L are standard but return to near normal by 1 week.
- Hyperbilirubinemia is common and, as one might expect, appears to be worse the smaller the size of the liver remnant. Hyperbilirubinemia of itself is not necessarily concerning if other markers of liver function are improving.
- An early sign that the autograft is functioning is the return of lactate levels to baseline in the first 12 to 24 hours after surgery.
- Maintenance of coagulation parameters, in particular prothrombin time or INR, suggests recovery of liver function. It is, however, frequently necessary to give fresh frozen plasma for the first few days to maintain an INR target less than 2.0.[12]
- Hypophosphatemia can occur between postoperative days 1 and 3 as the liver regenerates. This is an encouraging sign of liver regeneration, but the hypophosphatemia may be profound and need constant intravenous replacement.
- Without much evidence as to its effectiveness, we have used low-dose intravenous heparin (500 units/h) perioperatively and attempt to maintain the hematocrit between 30% and 35%.
- Patients that have Gortex grafts placed are started on low-dose aspirin before discharge and this is maintained for life.

COMPLICATIONS

- Complications are similar to any liver resection with bile leak, bleeding, and infection being the most common. They are managed in standard fashion.
- Complications specific to ex vivo liver resection include liver failure/small-for-size syndrome and vascular thrombosis.
- Liver dysfunction should be assessed with imaging studies of the vascular supply to the liver. Initial ultrasound can document flow in the portal vein, hepatic artery, and hepatic vein outflow. Contrast imaging may be required for confirmation. Any vascular thrombosis requires immediate correction.
- The management of small-for-size syndrome may include pharmacologic management with octreotide, splenic artery embolization or ligation, splenectomy, or temporary partial portosystemic shunting.

REFERENCES

1. Blumgart LH, Belghiti J. *Surgery of the Liver, Biliary Tract, and Pancreas*. Saunders Elsevier; 2007.
2. Hemming AW, Reed AI, Howard RJ, et al. Preoperative portal vein embolization for extended hepatectomy. *Ann Surg*. 2003;237(5):686-693. doi:10.1097/01.sla.0000065265.16728.c0.
3. Lang H, Radtke A, Liu C, Fruhauf NR, Peitgen HO, Broelsch CE. Extended left hepatectomy? Modified operation planning based on three-dimensional visualization of liver anatomy. *Langenbeck's Arch Surg*. 2003;389(4):306-310. doi:10.1007/s00423-003-0441-z
4. Gurusamy KS, Naik P, Abu-Amara M, Fuller B, Davidson BR. Techniques of flushing and reperfusion for liver transplantation. *Cochrane Database Syst Rev*. (3):CD007512. 2012. doi:10.1002/14651858.cd007512.pub2
5. Blumgart L. *Surgery of the Liver, Biliary Tract and Pancreas*. 6th ed. Elsevier; 2017:1670-1683.
6. Hemming AW, Cattral MS. Ex vivo liver resection with replacement of the inferior vena cava and hepatic vein replacement by transposition of the portal vein. *J Am Coll Surg*. 1999;189(5):523-526. doi:10.1016/s1072-7515(99)00192-1
7. Kubota K, Makuuchi M, Sugawara Y, et al. Reconstruction of the hepatic and portal veins using a patch graft from the right ovarian vein. *Am J Surg*. 1998;176(3):295-297. doi:10.1016/s0002-9610(98)00149-4.
8. Kaneoka Y, Yamaguchi A, Isogai M, Hori A. Hepatic vein reconstruction by external iliac vein graft using vascular clips. *World J Surg*. 2000;24(3):377-382. doi:10.1007/s002689910060
9. Kishi Y, Sugawara Y, Akamatsu N, et al. Sharing the middle hepatic vein between donor and recipient: left liver graft procurement preserving a large segment VIII branch in donor. *Liver Transplant*. 2004;10(9):1208-1212. doi:10.1002/lt.20226
10. Dong G. Cadaver iliac vein outflow reconstruction in living donor right lobe liver transplantation1. *J Am Coll Surg*. 2004;199(3):504-507. doi:10.1016/j.jamcollsurg.2004.04.017
11. Lodge JPA, Ammori BJ, Prasad KR, Bellamy MC. Ex vivo and in situ resection of inferior vena cava with hepatectomy for colorectal metastases. *Ann Surg*. 2000;231(4):471-479. doi:10.1097/00000658-200004000-00004
12. Martin RCG, Jarnagin WR, Fong Y, Biernacki P, Blumgart LH, DeMatteo RP. The use of fresh frozen plasma after major hepatic resection for colorectal metastasis: is there a standard for transfusion? *J Am Coll Surg*. 2003;196(3):402-409. doi:10.1016/s1072-7515(02)01752-0

Chapter 30: Surgical Management of Hepatic Trauma

Walter L. Biffl

DEFINITION

- Hepatic trauma is defined as injury to the liver. It may be associated with hemorrhage, bile leak and bile duct injury, or devitalized tissue. There is a spectrum of severity of liver trauma (**TABLE 1**),[1,2] and a broad range of techniques may be employed to manage various injuries.[2-5]

DIFFERENTIAL DIAGNOSIS

- Abdominal trauma can be associated with injuries to any abdominal organ. Major sources of hemorrhage include solid organs (eg, liver, spleen, kidneys) and blood vessels in the retroperitoneum (eg, aorta, inferior vena cava [IVC], renal vessels) or mesentery. Peritonitis may result from any injury to a hollow viscus (eg, bowel, biliary tree, pancreas), including bile leak from a liver injury.

PATIENT HISTORY AND PHYSICAL FINDINGS

- Liver injuries may occur following either blunt (eg, motor vehicle crash, fall) or penetrating (eg, gunshot or stab wound) trauma to the abdomen.
- The liver is one of the most commonly injured organs following blunt trauma, usually following impact to the lower right chest or the abdomen. Any high-energy mechanism should raise concern of intra-abdominal injury.
- The liver, due to its large surface area, is frequently injured in penetrating abdominal or lower thoracic trauma. The path of gunshot wounds to the torso cannot be determined based on physical examination alone.
- Abdominal pain or tenderness on examination raise concern for abdominal injury; however, patients may have significant liver injuries in the absence of pain or tenderness. Vital signs are a critical component of the assessment of trauma patients, and the decision to proceed with surgical (vs nonoperative) management is primarily based on the physiologic condition of the patient. The large majority of liver injuries are managed nonoperatively.

IMAGING AND OTHER DIAGNOSTIC STUDIES

- Ultrasound—in particular, the extended-focused abdominal sonographic examination for trauma (E-FAST)—is commonly used as an initial triage tool in trauma patients. Following blunt trauma, the finding of free fluid in the abdomen in the presence of shock is an indication to proceed to exploratory laparotomy (LAP) without delay. On the other hand, free fluid in a hemodynamically normal patient does not mandate LAP, as many solid organ injuries will stop bleeding spontaneously and do not require any intervention.
- The E-FAST examination is less useful in penetrating trauma victims. Patients with abdominal gunshot wounds should generally undergo immediate LAP. Those with stab wounds should undergo LAP if they exhibit shock, evisceration, or peritonitis. Otherwise, they should be admitted for serial clinical assessments to detect ongoing hemorrhage or hollow viscus injury. The finding of free fluid on FAST does not mandate LAP in stab wound victims.
- Computed tomography (CT) with intravenous contrast is currently the best diagnostic tool for hepatic injury (**FIGURE 1**). CT is indicated in any patient with major abdominal blunt trauma mechanism, abdominal pain or tenderness, hemoperitoneum on E-FAST examination in a stable patient, pelvic fractures, or the potential for abdominal trauma and the inability to clinically assess the abdominal

Table 1: Grading of Liver Injuries

Grade		Injury description
I	Hematoma	Subcapsular, <10% surface area
	Laceration	<1 cm parenchymal depth
II	Hematoma	Subcapsular, 10%-50% surface area; intraparenchymal, <10 cm diameter
	Laceration	1-3 cm parenchymal depth, <10 cm length
III	Hematoma	Subcapsular, >50% surface area or expanding; intraparenchymal, >10 cm diameter or expanding, or ruptured
	Laceration	>3 cm parenchymal depth
IV	Laceration	Parenchymal disruption involving 25%-75% of hepatic lobe or 1-3 Couinaud segments in a single lobe
V	Laceration	Parenchymal disruption involving >75% of hepatic lobe or >3 Couinaud segments in a single lobe
	Vascular	Juxtahepatic venous injuries
VI	Vascular	Hepatic avulsion

Advance one grade for multiple injuries up to grade III.
Reprinted with permission from Moore EE, Cogbill TH, Jurkovich GJ, et al. Organ injury scaling: spleen and liver (1994 Revision). J Trauma. 1995;38(3):323-324.

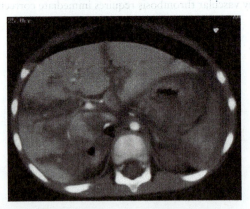

FIGURE 1 • CT scan image of a grade IV liver injury. Despite the extensive injury to the liver, note the relative paucity of blood surrounding the liver. This is a pitfall of FAST ultrasonography, as it detects primarily free fluid. It also speaks to the lack of sensitivity of FAST for individual organ injuries. It detects blood but not the source of the bleeding.

examination (eg, a patient with severe traumatic brain injury following motor vehicle crash).
- The identification of intravenous contrast extravasation on CT warrants consideration of interventional treatment regardless of physiologic condition.
- Arteriography with embolization may be selectively employed as a primary treatment in a stable patient without other indications for LAP. It may also be used as an adjunct to surgical management of liver lacerations with arterial hemorrhage.
- Cholangiography is sometimes useful to determine whether there is biliary injury and ongoing bile leak. This is generally performed later in the postinjury course. The presence of a biliary injury and bile leak generally calls for either surgical or endoscopic intervention.
- Magnetic resonance imaging has little role in the early management of liver trauma.

SURGICAL MANAGEMENT

- Severe abdominal pain or tenderness, peritonitis, evisceration, or shock with a presumed abdominal injury warrant LAP.
- Following stab wounds, the presence of shock, evisceration, or peritonitis is a clear indication for LAP. Gunshot wound to the abdomen, given its high association with significant injury, is an indication for LAP regardless of the initial physical findings. While some centers report reasonable success rates with nonoperative management of isolated penetrating liver injuries, it can be difficult to definitively exclude injuries to the colon, duodenum, gallbladder, or diaphragm without exploration.

Preoperative Planning

- Prior to taking the patient to the OR, the surgeon should communicate with the OR team regarding the suspected diagnoses and planned interventions, anticipated blood loss and transfusion requirements, positioning and incisions, extent of skin preparation, the need for imaging, and any special equipment needs. In a trauma center with a hybrid OR, it may be wise to utilize the room for major abdominal trauma in case angioembolization is necessary. In particular, a patient with abdominal trauma and hemorrhagic shock may prove to be a candidate for adjunctive hepatic artery embolization.

Positioning

- The patient should be positioned supine. It is best to leave both arms out to allow the anesthesiologist's access for venous and arterial catheterization and sampling.

SKIN INCISION

- Exploratory LAP for trauma should be performed through a generous midline abdominal incision. Although it may not initially extend from the xiphoid to pubis, as is classically suggested, once a major liver injury is identified, extension up to the xiphoid process is recommended to afford optimal exposure. Some elective liver surgery is performed through right or bilateral subcostal incisions, with or without cephalad extension in the midline. This may be chosen if the operation is performed later in the patient's clinical course for complications of liver injury, such as hepatic necrosis or bile leak. However, this approach limits access to the lower abdomen. If a midline incision has been made, the surgeon should not hesitate to extend the incision to the right if necessary. Adequate exposure is critical to repairing major hepatic injuries.

ABDOMINAL EXPLORATION

- The initial objective of trauma LAP is to determine if there is exsanguinating hemorrhage and from where it emanates. Blood must be evacuated and the source identified. Primary culprits are solid organs, retroperitoneal blood vessels, and mesentery. The surgeon should be able to rapidly assess the liver for major lacerations, by inspecting it and palpating its surface.

MANUAL COMPRESSION

- The first step in hepatic hemorrhage control is manual compression (**FIGURE 2**). This should be able to control the majority of liver bleeding. The importance of simultaneous aggressive hemostatic resuscitation cannot be overemphasized. Restoration of blood volume and maintenance of tissue perfusion, correction of coagulopathy, and active warming of the patient are critical to avoid the "bloody vicious cycle" that can lead to early mortality.

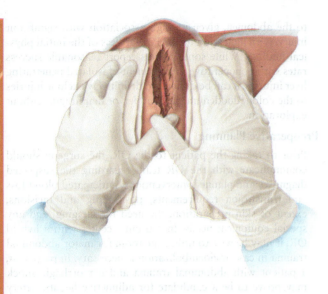

FIGURE 2 • Manual compression of the liver is performed to restore the normal anatomic contour of the liver and tamponade bleeding. This maneuver can control hemorrhage while planning packing or definitive interventions.

PERIHEPATIC PACKING

- Perihepatic packing should be performed in such a manner to maintain hemostatic compression on the liver (FIGURE 3). The supporting ligaments of the liver are left intact at the initial stage, as they may provide tamponade of venous bleeding.

However, should the patient have stellate lacerations or extensive subcapsular injury, one should not hesitate to mobilize the suspensory ligament of the falciform or the right and left triangular ligaments to allow better exposure. Packing should be performed in a systematic fashion, placing packs between the liver and the abdominal wall, diaphragm, and retroperitoneum.

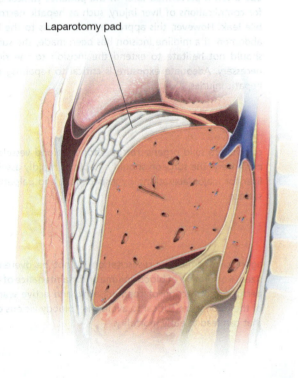

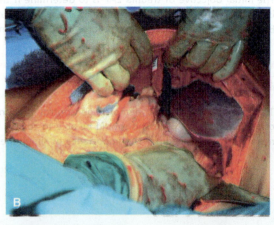

FIGURE 3 • The liver is packed with LAP pads to provide compression against the abdominal wall, diaphragm, and retroperitoneum. **A,** In the sagittal view, packs are present between the liver and the diaphragm and abdominal wall. **B,** In the photograph, the right lobe is compressed by packs.

TOPICAL HEMOSTASIS

- Grade I and II lacerations (see **TABLE 1**) may stop bleeding spontaneously or after a short period of packing (**FIGURE 4**). Ongoing hemorrhage can usually be controlled with electrocautery or argon beam coagulation, with or without application of topical hemostatic agents such as microcrystalline collagen, fibrin glue, or other agents (**FIGURE 5**).

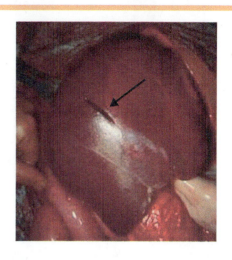

FIGURE 4 • Low-grade lacerations (*arrow*) may often stop bleeding spontaneously or following a brief period of compression or packing.

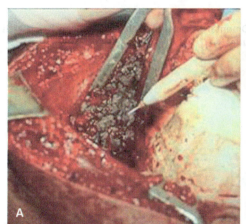
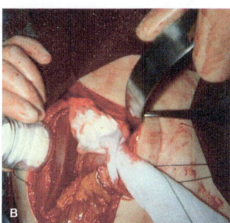

FIGURE 5 • Low-grade injuries with persistent bleeding may be treated by topical hemostatic techniques such as argon beam coagulation **(A)** or microcrystalline collagen application **(B)**.

DAMAGE CONTROL

- In the physiologically compromised patient, the decision to pursue damage control must be made early in order to optimize the patient's chance of survival. Time-consuming efforts to stop relatively minor bleeding should not distract the surgeon from the primary objective. The liver should be packed quickly and other damage control maneuvers completed prior to a temporary abdominal closure. In order to facilitate later pack removal without disrupting clot, a nonadherent plastic drape such as a 3M 1010 Steri-Drape may be spread over the liver surface, with the packs placed on top of the plastic.

DEEP PARENCHYMAL HEMORRHAGE CONTROL

- If the patient's condition allows, the liver should be examined to determine the extent of the injury. Grade II and III lacerations should be inspected to determine whether a discrete vessel may be ligated (**FIGURE 6**). Bleeding can generally be controlled by packing the wound with an omental pedicle or a plug of topical hemostatic agents such as absorbable gelatin sponge wrapped in oxidized regenerated cellulose (**FIGURE 7**). Suture hepatorrhaphy is an option, but one must avoid leaving a large dead space and avoid devitalizing tissue or lacerating vessels or bile ducts. Extensive lacerations may need to be explored to control major vessels. The finger fracture technique allows one to reach major vessels for ligation (**FIGURE 8**). Stapling devices can also be useful in dividing the hepatic parenchyma to reach deep vessels (**FIGURE 9**).

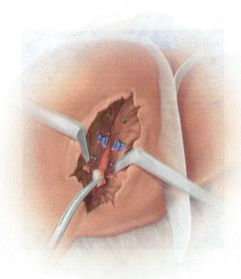

FIGURE 6 • The laceration should be explored to identify discrete vessels to ligate.

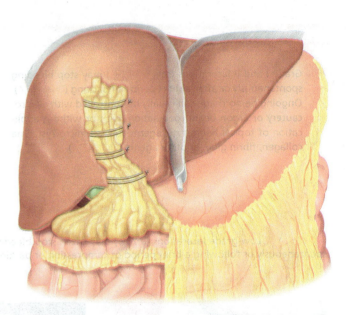

FIGURE 7 • Omental pedicle packing may provide hemostasis for deeper injuries.

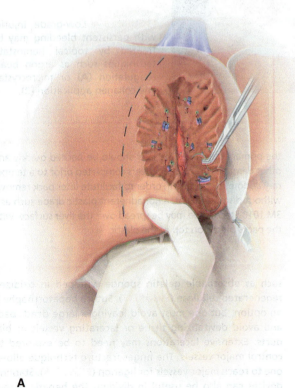

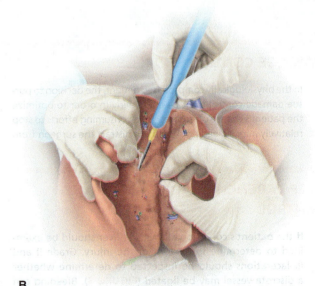

FIGURE 8 • Finger fracture of liver parenchyma **(A)** can provide exposure for clipping or suture ligation of lacerated vessels **(B)**.

Chapter 30 **SURGICAL MANAGEMENT OF HEPATIC TRAUMA** **241**

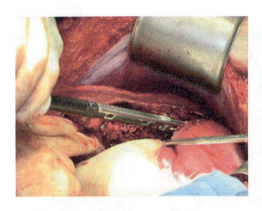

FIGURE 9 • Surgical staplers may be used to divide liver parenchyma to reach bleeding vessels.

BALLOON TAMPONADE

- Transhepatic penetrating wounds may leave a long intracavitary defect that is difficult to access for vascular control. Balloon tamponade may be accomplished by a device originally described by Poggetti and colleagues.[6] This may be fashioned by ligating a 1-in Penrose drain at one end. A red rubber catheter is inserted into the open end and secured with a second ligature. The Penrose drain is pulled through the wound, with the red rubber catheter and drain exiting the abdominal wall. The balloon is inflated with saline to achieve tamponade (**FIGURE 10**).

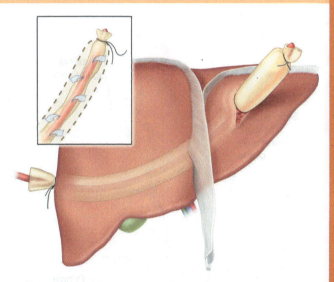

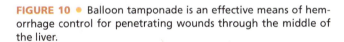

FIGURE 10 • Balloon tamponade is an effective means of hemorrhage control for penetrating wounds through the middle of the liver.

PRINGLE MANEUVER

- Bleeding that persists despite packing may be arterial in origin. The Pringle maneuver—that is, control of the hepatoduodenal ligament with a Rumel tourniquet or vascular clamp—should be employed (**FIGURE 11**). If this controls hemorrhage, it is likely that the bleeding is from either a hepatic arterial branch or major branch of the portal vein. This cannot be left in place for a prolonged period. Intermittent unclamping decreases the degree of ischemia/reperfusion injury. Definitive maneuvers must be undertaken and the clamp should be released within 60 minutes if possible. Ligation of the right or left hepatic artery may control the bleeding. Alternatively, in the appropriate setting, the patient may undergo arterioembolization.

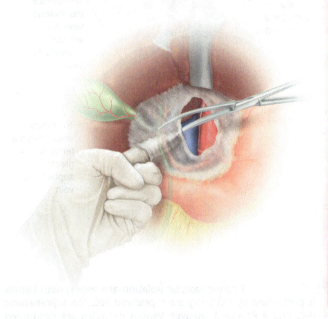

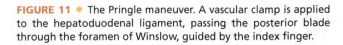

FIGURE 11 • The Pringle maneuver. A vascular clamp is applied to the hepatoduodenal ligament, passing the posterior blade through the foramen of Winslow, guided by the index finger.

HEPATIC RESECTION

- Resection of devitalized tissue may be performed at the initial operation; in the damage control setting, however, this is reserved for subsequent LAP. The extent of devitalized tissue is generally readily apparent (FIGURE 12). Resection may be necessary to control major vascular or biliary structures. Again, in the patient who is severely compromised physiologically, this is best done after resuscitation.

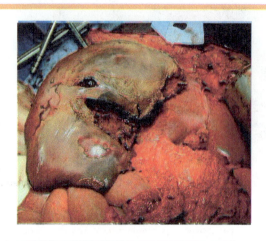

FIGURE 12 • Hepatic necrosis may result from major injury or vascular ligation to control bleeding.

HEPATIC VASCULAR ISOLATION

- Bleeding that persists despite the Pringle maneuver is likely from the hepatic veins. Hepatic vascular isolation with or without venovenous bypass should be considered (FIGURE 13).[7] This entails control of the suprarenal IVC, the suprahepatic IVC, and a Pringle maneuver. If the interruption of venous return results in cardiovascular collapse, the aorta may need to be cross-clamped while venovenous bypass is established. The suprahepatic clamp may be placed below the diaphragm, but this is not ideal. The clamp optimally should be placed within the pericardium. This can be accomplished from within the abdomen, but the exposure is markedly improved by median sternotomy (FIGURE 14).

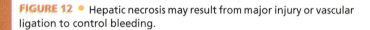

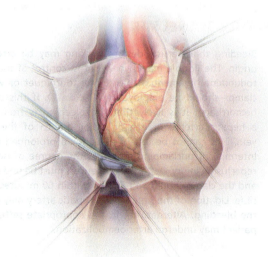

FIGURE 13 • Hepatic vascular isolation and venovenous bypass is performed by clamping the suprarenal IVC, the suprahepatic IVC, and a Pringle maneuver. Venous cannulae are positioned in the femoral vein and superior mesenteric vein, and blood is shunted into the internal jugular vein.

FIGURE 14 • Combining a median sternotomy with a midline LAP incision provides exposure to the hepatic veins and retrohepatic vena cava while avoiding injury to the phrenic nerves. The pericardium and diaphragm can be divided down the center toward the IVC.

CLOSURE

- If the liver is to remain packed, a temporary abdominal closure should be performed. Goals are rapid closure, containment of abdominal viscera, prevent bowel from adhering to fascial edges, allow room for swelling of abdominal viscera, provide a means for egress of ascites, maintain sterility of the abdominal cavity, avoid damage to fascia and skin edges, and minimize cost. The "Vac-Pack" dressing satisfies all of these requirements (FIGURE 15). A plastic sheet is draped over the bowel and extended to the paracolic gutters to keep the bowel from adhering to wound edges. Slits are cut in the sheet to allow egress of ascites. A towel is placed over the sheet to prevent suction drains from adhering to bowel through the slits. Drains are placed on top of the towel. An adhesive drape is placed over the entire wound. Definitive closure may be achieved by simple running fascial suture (eg, no. 2 nylon) and skin staples.

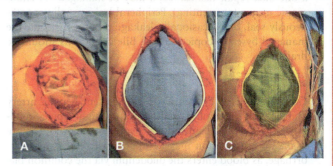

FIGURE 15 • Temporary closure of the abdomen entails covering the bowel with a fenestrated plastic drape (A), placement of closed suction drains and a blue towel (B), followed by an adhesive occlusive dressing (C).

PEARLS AND PITFALLS

Indication for LAP	▪ Unstable patients should go to the OR promptly. Pursuing angioembolization in an unstable patient is not advisable and may prove disastrous.
Incision	▪ A midline incision is the best choice in an unstable trauma patient. The surgeon should not hesitate to extend the incision rightward or into the chest in order to gain exposure and control. Median sternotomy markedly improves exposure for retrohepatic venous repairs.
Damage control	▪ The decision to pack the liver should be made very quickly, as should the decision to adopt a "damage control" strategy.
Resuscitation	▪ Ongoing resuscitation is critical during the operative phase.
Definitive procedures	▪ Avoid major definitive procedures at the first operation, if the patient's condition warrants damage control.

POSTOPERATIVE CARE

- Trauma patients should be monitored for response to resuscitation. Patients who have extensive transfusion may benefit from viscoelastic assays such a thromboelastography (TEG) or rotational thromboelastometry (ROTEM), in order to target coagulation defects and limit unnecessary blood product transfusion. Once resuscitated, postoperative care is routine for abdominal surgery, with provision of diet as tolerated and early ambulation.

OUTCOMES

- Severe liver injuries may be associated with high morbidity and mortality rates. However, patients who survive without significant complications should be expected to have normal life span and functional status vis-à-vis the liver injury.

COMPLICATIONS

Hemorrhage

- Postoperative bleeding is not common outside of the damage control setting. Bleeding may continue despite liver packing.

In this setting, TEG or ROTEM may be helpful in identifying coagulation abnormalities. In this case, depending on the patient's condition, angioembolization may be reasonable to control arterial hemorrhage. On the other hand, if the patient is physiologically compromised, it is prudent to return to the OR to control surgical hemorrhage while resuscitating the patient.

Abdominal Compartment Syndrome

- The abdominal compartment syndrome refers to intra-abdominal hypertension that is associated with organ dysfunction. It is often seen in association with damage control surgery in the presence of liver packing. The accumulation of ascites and retroperitoneal edema, coupled with bowel swelling, lead to a progressive rise in abdominal pressure. Patients may develop abdominal compartment syndrome in spite of an open abdomen, so the intra-abdominal pressure and organ function should be monitored.

Bile Leak

- This is the most common major complication of liver injury. Leaks may come from any biliary repair or anastomosis. They may also originate from peripheral biliary radicals. If a bile duct repair has leaked, it may be managed via endoscopic means (eg, stenting). Peripheral leaks usually spontaneously seal, but occasionally, leakage persists. This may be managed by endoscopic stenting. Bile collections should be drained.

Hemobilia

- Generally caused by injuries to an adjacent hepatic artery and bile duct, hemobilia is heralded by right upper quadrant pain, jaundice, and falling hemoglobin level. A more dramatic presentation may be upper gastrointestinal hemorrhage, as blood enters the duodenum via the common bile duct. Endoscopy can make the diagnosis, as blood is seen exiting from the ampulla of Vater. Angioembolization of the involved artery may be definitive treatment, but occasionally, drainage and/or debridement of a large hematoma/biloma cavity is needed.

Bilhemia

- Bilhemia results from a biliovenous fistula. Bilirubin levels can rise dramatically. Endoscopic biliary stenting may facilitate resolution, but hepatic resection may be required.

Hepatic Necrosis

- Although this may result from the initial injury, ligation or embolization of major vascular branches may also result in hepatic necrosis. This generally requires operative debridement or resection.

REFERENCES

1. Moore EE, Cogbill TH, Jurkovich GJ, et al. Organ injury scaling: spleen and liver (1994 Revision). *J Trauma.* 1995;38:323-324.
2. Coccolini F, Coimbra R, Ordonez C, et al. Liver trauma: WSES 2020 guidelines. *World J Emerg Surg.* 2020;15:24.
3. Kozar RA, Feliciano DV, Moore EE, et al. Western Trauma Association critical decisions in trauma: operative management of adult blunt hepatic trauma. *J Trauma.* 2011;71:1-5.
4. Pachter HL. Prometheus bound: evolution in the management of hepatic trauma—from myth to reality. *J Trauma.* 2012;72:321-329.
5. Peitzman AB, Marsh JW. Advanced operative techniques in the management of complex liver injury. *J Trauma Acute Care Surg.* 2012;73:765-770.
6. Poggetti RS, Moore EE, Moore FA, et al. Balloon tamponade for bilobar transfixing hepatic gunshot wounds. *J Trauma.* 1992;33:694-697.
7. Biffl WL, Moore EE, Franciose RJ. Venovenous bypass and hepatic vascular isolation as adjuncts in the repair of destructive wounds to the retrohepatic inferior vena cava. *J Trauma.* 1998;45:400-403.

SECTION III: Surgery of the Pancreas

Chapter 31 — Pancreaticoduodenectomy: Resection

George Van Buren II and William Edward Fisher

DEFINITION

- Pancreaticoduodenectomy (Whipple procedure) is defined as resection of the pancreatic head, uncinate process, gallbladder, distal bile duct, duodenum, and gastric antrum.
- Pylorus-preserving pancreaticoduodenectomy (pylorus-preserving Whipple procedure) is the same operation with preservation of the gastric antrum, pylorus, and a cuff of proximal duodenum.
- Complete excision of pancreatic head tumors with negative margins maximizes local-regional control and is the standard of care for malignancies of the pancreatic head, ampulla of Vater, duodenum, or distal bile duct.

DIFFERENTIAL DIAGNOSIS

- Pancreatic ductal adenocarcinoma
- Pancreatic neuroendocrine tumor
- Pancreatic cystic neoplasm
- Cancer of the ampulla of Vater
- Distal cholangiocarcinoma
- Duodenal adenocarcinoma
- Biliary stricture
- Chronic pancreatitis

PATIENT HISTORY AND PHYSICAL FINDINGS

- A thorough history and physical examination should be performed prior to treatment.
- Critical history: weight loss greater than 10%, new-onset diabetes, jaundice, vague abdominal pain in mid-epigastrium, pain penetrating to the back (indicates possible celiac involvement), diarrhea (indicating exocrine insufficiency).
- History related to biliary obstruction: jaundice, fever, chills, pruritus, acholic stools, dark urine.
- Risk factors for pancreatic cancer: smoking, chronic pancreatitis, diabetes, age 65 years or older, African American race, obesity, male gender, family history of pancreatic cancer, family history of other malignancy (ie, BRCA2 malignancies).[1]
- Physical examination: scleral icterus, jaundice, signs of malnutrition, cachexia, temporal wasting.
- Ominous signs: A palpable abdominal tumor, ascites, and left supraclavicular lymphadenopathy (Virchow lymph node) may be indicative of unresectable metastatic disease.
- In addition to a history and physical relating to pancreatic cancer, an overall assessment of the patient's functional status should be performed to assure the patient is a candidate for major surgery.
  - If the patient's performance status is poor (Eastern Cooperative Oncology Group score greater than 2 or Karnofsky score of less than 60), they should be considered physiologically borderline resectable.[2]
  - If the patient's carbohydrate antigen 19-9 (CA 19-9) level in the absence of jaundice (total bilirubin <4 mg/dL) is greater than 1000 U/mL, they should be considered biologically borderline resectable.
  - The patient's cardiopulmonary status should also be assessed with an assessment of their exercise tolerance and activity level.
  - Physical examination should look for other sources of chronic disease including carotid bruit, jugular venous distension, rales, wheezing, heart murmur, or clubbing of fingers.

IMAGING AND OTHER DIAGNOSTIC STUDIES

- "Pancreatic protocol" computed tomography (CT) scan of the chest, abdomen, and pelvis is required for all patients. Pancreatic protocol is a triphasic thin (≤5 mm), multislice CT scan with an arterial, venous, and delayed phase in conjunction with sagittal and coronal views. Water is used to opacify the stomach. A properly performed CT scan is perhaps the most critical portion of the preoperative assessment to determine if the patient is a candidate for surgery. The purpose of the CT scan is to detect any metastatic disease and to assess the relationship of the hypoattenuating tumor to the surrounding vasculature. Particular attention is paid to the relationship of the tumor to the portal vein (PV), superior mesenteric vein (SMV), superior mesenteric artery (SMA), hepatic artery, and celiac axis. In addition, a CT scan will aid in identification of aberrant anatomy of the hepatic artery, which is present in 20% of cases and must be noted prior to surgery.
- CT scan of chest is done to evaluate for pulmonary metastasis.
  - Based on imaging, there are well-defined consensus criteria from the Americas Hepato-Pancreato-Biliary Association for resectable, borderline resectable, locally advanced, and metastatic disease. These criteria have been adopted by the National Comprehensive Cancer Network.[3]
  - Resectable tumors demonstrate the following:

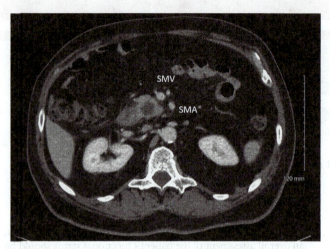

FIGURE 1 • CT scan of a resectable pancreatic cancer. SMA, superior mesenteric artery; SMV, superior mesenteric vein.

- No distant metastases; no radiographic evidence of SMV and PV abutment, distortion, tumor thrombus, or venous encasement; clear fat planes around the celiac axis, hepatic artery, and SMA (FIGURE 1).
- Borderline resectable tumors demonstrate the following:
  - No distant metastases; venous involvement of the SMV/PV demonstrating tumor abutment with or without impingement and narrowing of the lumen, encasement of the SMV/PV but without encasement of the nearby arteries, or short segment venous occlusion resulting from either tumor thrombus or encasement but with suitable vessel proximal and distal to the area of vessel involvement, allowing for safe resection and reconstruction; gastroduodenal artery encasement up to the hepatic artery with either short segment encasement or direct abutment of the hepatic artery, without extension to the celiac axis; tumor abutment of the SMA not to exceed 180° of the circumference of the vessel wall (FIGURE 2).
- Locally advanced tumors demonstrate the following:
  - No distant metastases; unreconstructable SMV/PV occlusion; greater than 180° encasement of SMA, celiac axis, or aortic invasion; metastasis to lymph nodes beyond the field of resection (FIGURE 3).

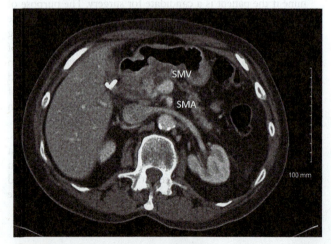

FIGURE 2 • CT scan of a borderline resectable pancreatic cancer. There is a loss of the "fat plane" between the SMV/portal vein confluence. SMA, superior mesenteric artery; SMV, superior mesenteric vein.

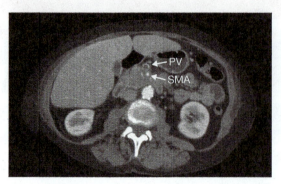

FIGURE 3 • CT scan of an unresectable/locally advanced pancreatic cancer. The lesion has encircled the SMA. PV, portal vein; SMA, superior mesenteric artery.

- Endoscopic ultrasound (EUS): This is an important step in the assessment of many, but not all, pancreatic masses and cystic lesions. EUS is performed to obtain a tissue diagnosis of a solid mass, which will be required if neoadjuvant chemotherapy is planned. Cystic lesions may be characterized by EUS and the fluid may be aspirated and sent for cytology including a mucin stain, carcinoembryonic antigen and amylase concentration, and genetic analysis. Furthermore, EUS may be used as an adjunct to the CT scan to further evaluate venous involvement and can be more sensitive than CT scan in detecting a small mass. If enlarged celiac lymph nodes are seen, they may be biopsied.
- Endoscopic retrograde cholangiopancreatography (ERCP): ERCP may be used to provide biliary decompression. In cholangiocarcinomas, it is necessary to evaluate the entirety of the biliary tree and see the proximal extent of the stricture. This may require a percutaneous transhepatic cholangiogram. In ampullary carcinomas, the mass can be directly visualized and biopsied. A biliary stent should be placed if neoadjuvant therapy is planned, to allow time for referral to a high-volume pancreas surgery center, and in cases where the serum bilirubin is particularly elevated (>10 mg/dL).[4] Although stent placement has been shown to increase infectious complications, prolonged biliary obstruction causing liver insufficiency and coagulopathy adversely affects surgical outcomes.
- Duplex ultrasound of the neck and/or lower extremities is performed selectively in patients who may need to undergo PV resection to evaluate the patency of the internal jugular and deep femoral veins. It may also evaluate the carotids in patients at high risk for atherosclerotic disease.
- Gallium-68 dotatate positron emission tomography (PET)/CT scan: Gallium-68 PET scan is used for localization of primary and metastatic neuroendocrine tumors. Somatostatin analogues are labeled with positron-emitting isotopes including gallium-68 to image somatostatin receptor–expressing tumor cells. It is completed in 2 hours compared to the 2 days for an Octreoscan or metaiodobenzylguanidine scan.
- Tumor markers: Serum CA 19-9 is shown to be predictive of outcomes in pancreatic adenocarcinoma. However, CA 19-9 can be falsely elevated in the setting of obstructive jaundice. If it is more than 1000 U/mL in the absence of jaundice, there should be a high suspicion for metastatic disease.[5] In patients who receive neoadjuvant therapy, CA 19-9 may be used as a marker to assess response. A drop in CA 19-9 of greater than 50% may be predictive of improved survival.[2] A low value is not predictive of favorable biology.

- Liver function test and coagulation profile: Bile salts are required for absorption of vitamins A, D, E, and K. Patients with biliary obstruction may require vitamin K (10 mg administered intramuscularly three times every day) if the prothrombin time/international normalized ratio is prolonged. A serum albumin level of less than 3 may indicate an opportunity for preoperative nutritional prehabilitation.
- Cardiopulmonary clearance and risk assessment by a cardiologist or appropriate internist may aid in perioperative optimization.

SURGICAL MANAGEMENT

Preoperative Planning

- Presentation of the case at a multidisciplinary tumor board with radiology, gastroenterology, medical oncology, radiation oncology, and surgical teams in attendance is optimal in the evaluation of all pancreatic lesions. This allows the case to be reviewed in an objective manner, facilitates enrollment in clinical trials, and allows the development of institutional guidelines of care among all specialties.
- All patients with pancreatic adenocarcinoma, whether resectable, locally advanced, or metastatic, should be offered access to a clinical trial.
- A pancreaticoduodenectomy should be performed at a high-volume center (approximately more than 16 pancreatic resections per year). Resections performed at institutions below that volume have higher perioperative morbidity and mortality rates and worse oncologic outcomes.[6,7]
- Be prepared to alter the sequence of the dissection; anatomic relationships of the tumor drive this up to the point of commitment for resection—unaffected planes should be addressed before embarking on those at risk.

Positioning

- Supine position with both arms out to the side. Tuck the sheet tight under the bed to ensure bed rails are accessible for retractor placement.
- Turn the head to the right with the neck extended to expose the left internal jugular vein.

DIAGNOSTIC LAPAROSCOPY

- Diagnostic laparoscopy: The value of staging laparoscopy has decreased as the accuracy of CT scanning has improved.[3] Laparoscopy should be performed as a prelude to potential surgical resection in selected patients who have pancreatic adenocarcinoma. We advocate selective laparoscopy on the same day as the planned resection in high-risk patients with potentially advanced disease, large (>4 cm) or borderline resectable tumors after neoadjuvant therapy, liver lesions too small to characterize or percutaneously biopsy, any ascites fluid, marked weight loss, hypoalbuminemia, and high (>1000 U/mL) CA 19-9 levels.
- The peritoneum, omentum, and surface of the liver are inspected for evidence of metastasis. A multiport technique with mobilization of the tissues and use of a laparoscopic ultrasound probe is required for a thorough examination.

INCISION

- Pancreaticoduodenectomy can be performed through a midline incision from xiphoid to umbilicus or through a bilateral subcostal incision. A bilateral subcostal incision may be superior in patients with a shorter body habitus or significant obesity. A bilateral subcostal incision can be inferior in patients with a narrow costal angle and may limit exposure to the pelvis in patients with adhesions from previous pelvic surgery.
- The falciform ligament is ligated close to the umbilicus and mobilized to the inferior border of the liver, preserving length and associated adipose and peritoneal surface as a pedicle flap subsequently positioned over the stump of the GDA at the end of the case.
- Placement of wound protector to decrease the risk of surgical site infection especially if a biliary stent is in place.
- Surgical retractor of choice (Bookwalter or Thompson) is placed.

INITIAL ASSESSMENT OF RESECTABILITY

- The initial portion of the procedure is an assessment of resectability.
- The liver and visceral and parietal peritoneal surfaces are thoroughly assessed via a systematic four-quadrant exploration including bimanual palpation of the liver and running the small bowel from the ligament of Treitz to the cecum and palpation of the colon.
- The gastrohepatic omentum is opened, and the region of the celiac axis is examined for enlarged lymph nodes. The base of the transverse mesocolon to the right of the middle colic vessels is examined for tumor involvement.

CATTELL-BRAASCH AND KOCHER MANEUVERS

- The ascending colon and hepatic flexure of the colon are freed of their lateral and superior attachments using an energy device. The colonic mesentery is completely mobilized and reflected medially to expose the second and third portions of the duodenum and the head of the pancreas (FIGURE 4). An avascular plane between these structures will develop over the third portion of the duodenum and extend up to the inferior border of the neck of the pancreas (FIGURE 5). A Kocher maneuver is

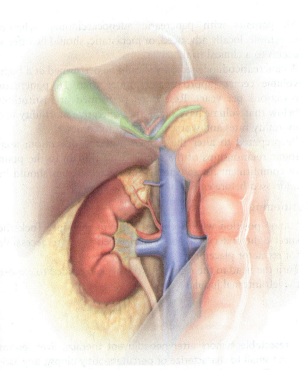

FIGURE 4 • Artist's renditions of the Cattell-Braasch maneuver and subsequent wide Kocher maneuver.

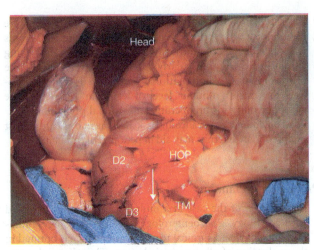

FIGURE 5 • Operative photograph taken during performance of a Cattell-Braasch maneuver exposing the duodenum and pancreatic head. The *white arrow* points to the avascular plane between the transverse mesocolon and the head of the pancreas, which in this view is yet to be dissected from the mesentery and omentum. D2, second portion of duodenum; D3, *third* portion of duodenum; HOP, head of pancreas; TM, transverse mesocolon.

performed by incising the peritoneum along the lateral edge of duodenum. This incision should be extended cephalad into the foramen of Winslow. Incise the avascular ligament that tethers the third portion of the duodenum inferiorly, allowing further dissection behind the head of the pancreas, thus elevating the duodenum and pancreas from the vena cava and aorta. The duodenum is mobilized medially until the left renal vein is seen crossing over aorta.

EXPOSURE OF THE INFRAPANCREATIC SUPERIOR MESENTERIC VEIN

- The gastrocolic omentum is divided, opening the lesser sac and exposing the body and tail of the pancreas. As the gastrocolic ligament is divided, the dissection is kept outside of the gastroepiploic vessels to preserve the gastric vasculature and blood supply to the duodenal cuff. Dissection proceeds from the patient's left to right with the goal of defining the avascular fusion plane between the omentum, the right gastroepiploic vascular pedicle, and the transverse mesocolon. This plane is fully mobilized to expose the pancreatic head. Congenital adhesions of the antrum to the anterior pancreas are then taken along the inferior border of the pancreas working toward the gastroepiploic vein (**FIGURE 6**).
- Dissect the anterior aspect of the middle colic vein(s) and circumferentially dissect the gastroepiploic vein as it inserts into the anterior surface of the SMV at the inferior border of the neck of the pancreas. They may enter as a common trunk (gastrocolic trunk) or separately. There is often a tributary vein inserting into the cephalad (unvisualized) aspect of the gastroepiploic vein. Once isolated, the gastroepiploic vein is ligated and divided (**FIGURE 7**). The middle colic vein may be divided based on anatomy to prevent traction injury or tearing of the vessels later in the dissection.

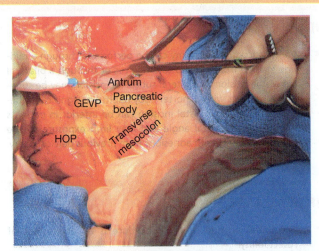

FIGURE 6 • Take down the attachments of the posterior stomach to the anterior aspect of the pancreatic body. After division of the gastrocolic omentum, dissect along the inferior border of the pancreas, up to the gastroepiploic vascular pedicle (GEVP). The head of the pancreas (HOP) is visualized on the left.

- Dissection is continued to further mobilize inferior border of the pancreas to identify and expose the anterior surface of the SMV (**FIGURE 8**).

Chapter 31 PANCREATICODUODENECTOMY: RESECTION 249

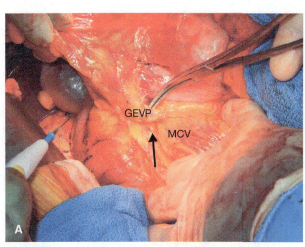 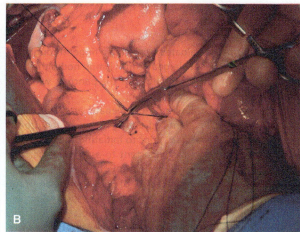

FIGURE 7 • **A,** The gastroepiploic vein is circumferentially dissected (*black arrow* marks the course of the superior mesenteric vein) and **B,** ligated between ligatures and divided. GEVP, gastroepiploic vascular pedicle; MCV, middle colic vein.

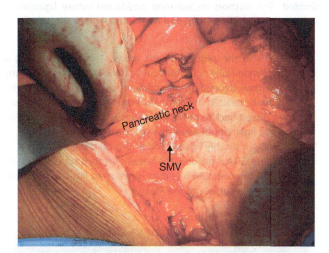

FIGURE 8 • Once the gastroepiploic vein has been divided, the anterior aspect of the superior mesenteric vein (SMV) is exposed. This dissection of the SMV is *continued* inferiorly to the caudad aspect of the third portion of the duodenum.

- At this point, the anterior aspect of the pancreas is fully exposed and the inferior aspect of the neck and body has been dissected, including the anterior aspect of the SMV (**FIGURE 9**).
- The plane anterior to the SMV as it courses behind the pancreatic neck is now initially assessed. Completion of this retropancreatic tunnel should be deferred until the PV is exposed cephalad to the pancreatic neck in subsequent steps. The authors recommend the use of a blunt-tipped instrument such as a Glover clamp to perform this exposure. Care must be taken to carefully assess potential involvement of this plane by tumor or inflammation during this step. Inadvertent injury to the SMV at this point will result in catastrophic hemorrhage that can be very difficult to control given the limited exposure.
- The relation of the tumor to the SMV and artery can now be partially assessed by palpation; however, palpation is not completely reliable, as posterior or lateral extension of the

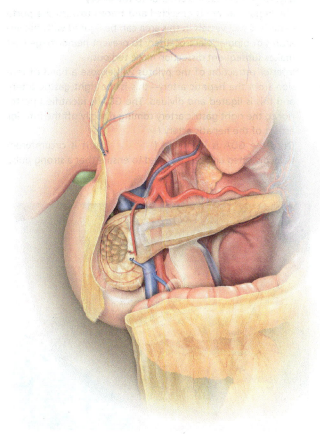

FIGURE 9 • Schematic representation of exposure of the pancreatic head, neck, and body including the anterior aspect of the superior mesenteric vein.

lesion that compromises these margins cannot be completely determined until later in the operation when the neck of the pancreas is divided and the surgeon is committed to resection. The importance of a high-quality preoperative CT scan in predicting this involvement is critical in preventing exploration of unresectable patients.

DISSECTION OF THE PORTA HEPATIS

- The porta hepatis is palpated by placing a finger through the foramen of Winslow. Enlarged or firm lymph nodes that can be swept down toward the head of the pancreas with the specimen do not preclude resection.
- The presence of an aberrant right hepatic artery or other anomalies should be identified during review of the preoperative CT scan. Regardless, prior to initiating the dissection of the porta hepatis, it is important to assess for aberrant hepatic arterial anatomy by palpation of the porta hepatis; it is present in approximately 20% of patients. The aberrant artery commonly arises from the SMA posterior to the pancreas and ascends parallel in a lateral and posterior location to the common bile duct and PV. Possible alterations in this anatomy are reviewed in Chapter 15.
- The proximal hepatic artery is identified usually by removing a lymph node that lies anterior to the artery.
- The hepatic artery is dissected and traced toward the porta hepatis. Small vessels in this area can be ligated with silk ligatures or bipolar electrocautery to prevent hemorrhage that makes subsequent dissection more tedious.
- Inferior retraction of the pylorus will expose a band of tension from the hepatic artery—this is the right gastric artery and this is ligated and divided. The GDA is identified posterior to the right gastric artery coming directly off the inferior aspect of the hepatic artery (**FIGURE 10**).
- Once the GDA is identified (**FIGURE 11**), it is circumferentially dissected and test clamped to ensure that a strong pulse

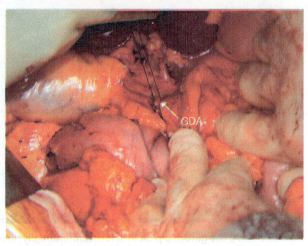

FIGURE 11 • The gastroduodenal artery (GDA) is ligated and divided. The authors recommend additional suture ligation or oversewing the GDA stump and marking it with a surgical clip.

remains in the proper hepatic artery. This test rules out a hemodynamically significant celiac stenosis leading to hepatic blood flow depending on collateral circulation through the pancreatic head. If this clinical scenario is present, the surgeon must dissect back to the celiac axis origin to release the median arcuate ligament or assess the celiac axis origin for stenosis.
- The GDA is doubly ligated and a surgical clip applied.
- Once the GDA is divided, the hepatic artery is retracted medially and the common bile duct is retracted laterally to reveal the anterior surface of the PV (**FIGURE 12**).

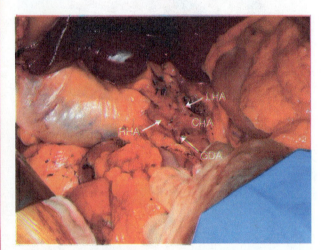

FIGURE 10 • Operative exposure of the common hepatic artery (CHA) and its named branches. The demonstrated anatomy is not classic in that the bifurcation of the right and left hepatic artery (RHA and LHA) occurs prior to the origin of the gastroduodenal artery (GDA). The GDA arises from the RHA. The right gastric artery has been ligated and divided in this photograph.

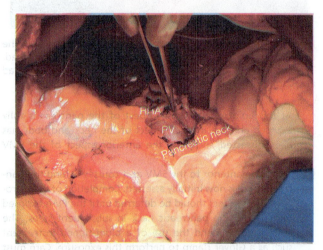

FIGURE 12 • Division of the gastroduodenal artery facilitates medial and cephalad retraction of the hepatic artery and its branches (RHA), exposing the PV cephalad to the pancreatic neck. PV, portal vein; RHA, right hepatic artery.

CREATION OF A TUNNEL BETWEEN THE PANCREATIC NECK AND PORTAL VEIN

- Dissection is performed only on the anterior surface of the vein.
- Dissect the PV superior to the neck of the pancreas. If there is no tumor involvement, the neck of the pancreas will separate from the vein easily. A large, blunt-tipped clamp is a safe instrument to use for this dissection.
- The tunnel under the neck of the pancreas can then be completed mostly under direct vision as one progresses from both the inferior and superior aspects of the pancreas (**FIGURE 13**).
- A vessel loop or umbilical tape is then placed under the neck of the pancreas.
- The common bile duct or hepatic duct (depending on the need for margin) is circumferentially dissected and a vessel loop is placed around the duct (**FIGURE 14**).
- The cystic duct and artery are dissected, ligated, and divided (**FIGURE 15**). A cholecystectomy is performed. Alternatively, it is safer to perform a retrograde dissection of the gallbladder if inflammation is present.
- At this point (**FIGURE 16**), one must commit to resection or abort.

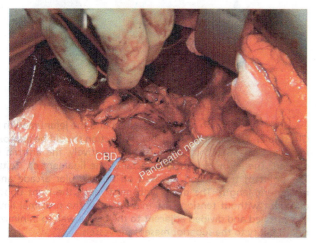

FIGURE 13 • To circumferentially dissect the common bile duct (CBD), continue working anterior to posterior along the lateral margin of the portal vein (PV) establishing a plane between the PV and the CBD. The lateral lymphatic tissues are also dissected so they remain with the specimen. The encircled CBD can be controlled with a vessel loop. If a replaced hepatic artery is present, use care to ensure you establish a plane between the bile duct and the artery.

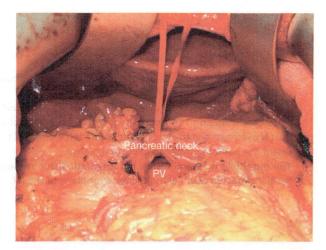

FIGURE 14 • Complete the dissection of the anterior aspect of the portal vein (PV) from the neck of the pancreas. An umbilical tape can be placed to facilitate subsequent parenchymal transection.

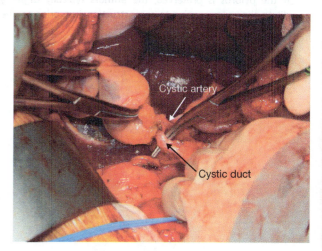

FIGURE 15 • Cholecystectomy is performed. The cystic duct and artery are dissected, controlled with ligatures, and divided.

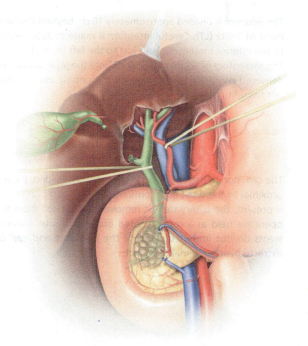

FIGURE 16 • Schematic drawing of the dissection at the point of decision to proceed or abort. The next step commits to resection.

DIVISION OF THE DUODENUM

- If the operative plan is for pyloric preservation, the stomach and proximal duodenum are mobilized off the pancreas, preserving the gastroepiploic vessels down to the pylorus.
- Either the duodenum is divided 1.5 to 2 cm distal to the pylorus-preserving pancreaticoduodenectomy or, alternatively, the antrum is divided (FIGURE 17).
- Antrum division is performed at the branching of the vagus nerves of Latarjet ("crow's feet") usually at the third or fourth transverse vein on the lesser curvature and at the confluence of gastroepiploic veins on the greater curvature.
- If the pylorus is preserved, the authors typically digitally dilate the pylorus prior to reconstruction just prior to the duodenojejunal anastomosis.

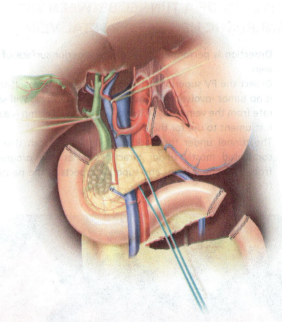

FIGURE 17 • Division of the duodenum and the jejunum with a GIA stapler. The point of duodenal transection should be approximately 2 cm distal to the pylorus. Alternatively, the antrum is divided. The jejunum is divided distal to the ligament of Treitz. The point of transection is based on the vascular arcade and mesenteric length. The distal limb must reach the right upper quadrant without tension. The mesentery of the proximal limb is controlled and divided adjacent to the bowel wall to minimize risk of injury to the superior mesenteric vessels.

TAKEDOWN OF THE LIGAMENT OF TREITZ

- The jejunum is divided approximately 10 cm beyond the ligament of Treitz (LT). Careful attention is made to avoid injury to the inferior mesenteric vein just to the left of the LT.
- The mesentery of jejunum is ligated until the jejunum can be delivered posterior to the superior mesenteric vessels from left to right.
- The mesentery can be taken with ties; however, many surgeons have found that energy devices may speed this portion. Care must be taken as the dissection approaches the mesenteric vessels—the plane of dissection is the bowel wall.

DIVISION OF BILE DUCT

- The common hepatic bile duct is then sharply divided, usually proximal to the cystic duct confluence.
- If present, the biliary stent is removed and passed from the operative field as a contaminated object. Of note, metallic stents do not impact division of the bile duct and can be extracted with minimal resistance.
- Some surgeons obtain cultures of the bile and continue directed, postoperative antibiotic therapy.
- A bulldog clamp is placed on the bile duct to prevent bile from contaminating the field (FIGURE 18). The distal bile duct is oversewn and the ends of the suture left elongated to orient the pathologist to this important margin.
- The distal bile duct and associated lymphatic tissue is then further dissected down along the anterior plane of the PV.

Chapter 31 PANCREATICODUODENECTOMY: RESECTION   253

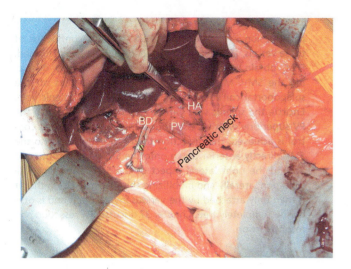

FIGURE 18 • Division of the bile duct. A bulldog clamp is placed proximally to prevent ongoing contamination of the operative field with bile and maintain hemostasis. The bile duct is sharply divided. If present and easily retrievable, the biliary stent is removed and passed off the field. It should be cataloged as removed by the pathologist. The distal bile duct is sutured closed. The ends of this suture are left long to orient the pathologist. BD, bile duct; HA, hepatic artery; PV, portal vein.

DIVISION OF THE PANCREAS

- Hemostatic traction sutures may be placed on the inferior and superior borders of the pancreas around the transverse pancreaticoduodenal vessels prior to division. These sutures should be placed to intentionally ligate the longitudinal arteries within the pancreas; however, care must be taken to ensure they do not entrap the pancreatic duct (**FIGURE 19**).
- The pancreatic neck is divided anterior to the PV (**FIGURE 20**). The authors divide the pancreas with electrocautery on the superior and inferior ends and with the scalpel through the midsection of the pancreas to prevent cautery injury and assist in identification of pancreatic duct. Division is performed just anterior to the PV with a large blunt-tipped clamp being placed behind the pancreas to protect the vein.

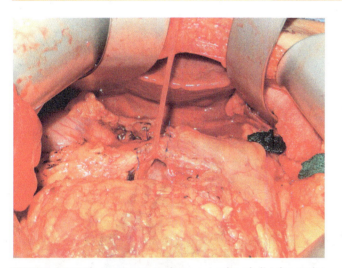

FIGURE 19 • Place sutures at the proximal and distal margins of the pancreatic neck to control the longitudinal arteries and provide retraction.

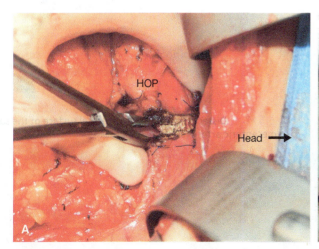
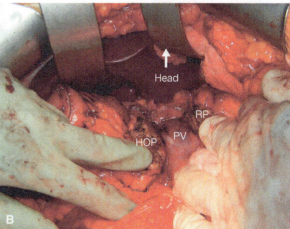

FIGURE 20 • Divide the pancreatic neck. **A,** This is ideally performed sharply with judicious use of cautery to control hemorrhage to facilitate pathologic assessment of the margin. **B,** Once completed, the anterior aspect of the PV is fully exposed. HOP, head of pancreas specimen; PV, portal vein; RP, remnant pancreas.

DISSECTION OF THE LATERAL ASPECT OF THE SUPERIOR MESENTERIC–PORTAL VEIN CONFLUENCE

- The pancreatic head and uncinate process are then dissected off of the right lateral aspect of the SMV, ligating the fragile branches draining the head and uncinate process into the PV (FIGURE 21).
- Superiorly, as the pancreatic head is being retracted inferiorly and laterally, the small venous tributaries from the PV and SMV to the pancreatic head including the superior pancreaticoduodenal vein (vein of Belcher), which inserts at the superior lateral surface of the PV, are ligated.
- Inferiorly, as the pancreatic head is retraced superiorly and laterally, the first jejunal branch will be encountered. If not preserved, the first jejunal branch should be ligated close to the SMV. This will help prevent injury during the dissection and retraction behind the SMA. Efforts to control bleeding once the vessel has retracted may result in injury to the SMA. If the tumor is inferior in location, this ligation is critical. In cases where the tumor is away from the first jejunal branch of the SMV, it can be preserved.
- The SMV is then fully mobilized off the uncinate process to reveal the SMV/PV groove. The vein must be entirely mobilized away from the head of the pancreas to allow for maximal retroperitoneal margin resection (FIGURE 22).
- If the lesion is adhered to the SMV, PV, or confluence of these vessels, an artery-first dissection should be performed. First, obtain vascular control by circumferentially dissecting the SMV. Mobilize the body of the pancreas off the splenoportal confluence and off the proximal splenic vein. Encircle the splenic vein with a vessel loop and encircle the PV superiorly with a vessel loop. Once venous vascular control is achieved, the dissection then proceeds medial to the SMV directly anterior down onto the SMA and is continued around the right lateral aspect of the SMA, retracting the specimen laterally and mobilizing the specimen up so that it is then only attached by the venous involvement and is otherwise completely free. Chapter 37 discusses PV resection and reconstruction.

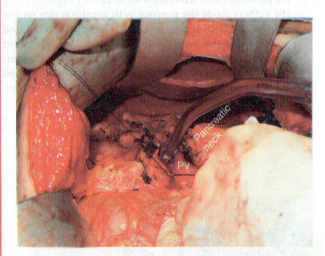

FIGURE 21 • Ligate and divide the lateral venous branches of the pancreas inserting into the superior mesenteric vein (SMV)/PV. Beware the first jejunal branch of the SMV. It inserts into the SMV posteriorly and receives a branch from the uncinate process. PV, portal vein.

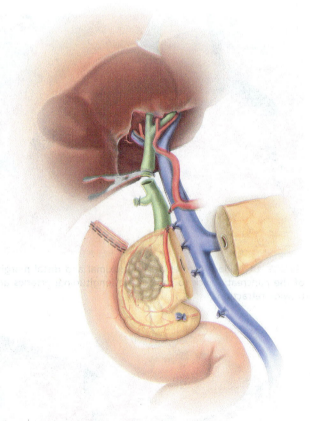

FIGURE 22 • Dissect the anterior and lateral surface of the superior mesenteric artery (SMA).

COMPLETION OF THE RETROPERITONEAL AND SUPERIOR MESENTERIC ARTERY DISSECTION

- In cases without vein involvement, the superior mesenteric-portal vein confluence is retracted medially with a peanut or vein retractor to allow exposure of the retroperitoneal attachments to the SMA.
- The uncinate process is then dissected off of the posterior and right lateral aspect of the SMA, removing all associated autonomic nerve tissue so that the dissection plane is along the adventitia of the SMA. This can be the most tedious portion of the operation, but thoroughly clearing all tissue from the mesenteric vessels minimizes the risk of a margin-positive resection.
- The authors recommend taking the retroperitoneal margin in a controlled fashion with small bites separating out the tissue and division with either suture ties or energy device (FIGURE 23). The authors think that use of a stapler for this portion of the procedure invariably leaves tissue behind on the SMA and will increase the incidence of R1 resections.
- If an energy device is used on this portion, caution must be taken to avoid lateral spread to the SMA, which can result in a postoperative SMA pseudoaneurysm.
- Once the pancreatic specimen is out (FIGURE 24), the remaining pancreatic neck should be fully mobilized approximately 2 cm off of the splenic artery and vein to facilitate the reconstruction.

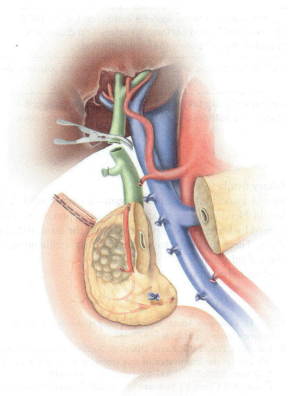

FIGURE 23 • Operative image of the completed dissection. CBD, common bile duct; PV, portal vein; SMV, superior mesenteric vein.

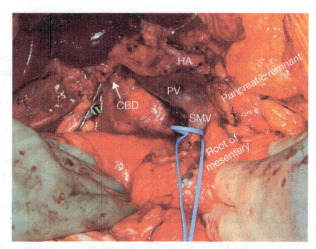

FIGURE 24 • Operative image of the completed dissection. CBD, common bile duct; HA, hepatic artery; PV, portal vein; SMV, superior mesenteric vein.

ORIENTING THE SPECIMEN FOR PATHOLOGIC ANALYSIS

- Before the specimen is sent to pathology, it is critical that the specimen be labeled by the surgeon in a standardized fashion to facilitate communication with the pathologist. We place sutures on the bile duct, pancreatic neck, and retroperitoneal/SMA margin. The SMA margin cannot be marked retrospectively. Furthermore, if any portion of the SMV or PV was resected, the vein should be marked and sent for frozen section.
- Positive resection margins of the pancreatic neck or bile duct may warrant further resection, but recently forwarded data would suggest that this maneuver does not impact outcome.
- If there is concern for a positive margin on the SMA margin on final pathology, no further tissue can be taken and gold fiducial markers can be left in place for postoperative radiation therapy.

PEARLS AND PITFALLS

Preoperative assessment	▪ Failure to identify a replaced hepatic artery on preoperative imaging can result in injury leading to an ischemic injury to the liver and possibly subsequent liver failure.
Opening of the lesser sac	▪ Ligate the gastroepiploic and sometimes middle colic veins early. This provides improved exposure of the SMV and prevents a traction injury to the vein.
Dissection of the SMV/PV confluence	▪ First jejunal branch not being properly ligated can result in injury to the vein with it retracting behind the SMA. Attempts to control this bleeding may result in iatrogenic injury to the SMA.
Retroperitoneal dissection	▪ Complete removal of uncinate process and the mesenteric soft tissue from the SMA decreases the chance of an R1 resection.
Vein involvement	▪ If the tumor is adhered to SMV-PV confluence, we obtain vascular control of the PV, SMV, and splenic vein and dissect medial to the PV/SMV and perform an artery-first dissection. Completing this dissection first decreases clamp time once the vein is divided.
Pancreatic neck	▪ Mobilization of the pancreatic neck off of the splenic artery and vein facilitates a secure pancreaticojejunal anastomosis.
Pylorus preservation	▪ If the pylorus is preserved, the authors typically digitally dilate the pylorus prior to reconstruction once the staple line is removed. The authors think this may reduce postoperative gastroparesis.

POSTOPERATIVE CARE

- Patients should be monitored in the intensive care unit for hemodynamic changes, urine output, or changes in drain characteristics.
- Monitoring of drains: The authors would check postoperative drain amylase on postoperative days 1 and 3. If a pancreatic leak exists, the drain should be left in place. In addition, the drain fluid should be monitored for change in character to bilious or sanguineous. If no pancreatic or biliary leak exists, the drains should be removed on postoperative day 3.
- A low amylase level in the drain does not ensure the absence of a leak. Tachycardia and leukocytosis should drive concern and may warrant CT evaluation.
- Patients should be placed on perioperative antibiotics. If the bile cultures come back positive, the authors continue culture-directed antibiotics for 7 days.

OUTCOMES

- At high-volume institutions, 30-day mortality rates are less than 1.5% and 90-day mortality rates are 4%.
- The overall 1-year survival rate of people with pancreatic cancer is 26%, and the 5-year survival rate is approximately 6%. If the cancer is detected at an early stage when surgical removal of the tumor is possible, the 5-year survival rate is about 22%.

COMPLICATIONS

- Pancreatic fistula
- Delayed gastric emptying
- Biliary fistula
- Fistula-associated pseudoaneurysm—uncommon. Often, a herald bleed presents as an episode of hypotension accompanied by hematemesis and blood from the intra-abdominal drain. These should be treated emergently with angiography
- Wound infection
- Abdominal abscess

REFERENCES

1. Yeo TP, Lowenfels AB. Demographics and epidemiology of pancreatic cancer. *Cancer J*. 2012;18(6):477-484.
2. Katz MH, Pisters PW, Evans DB, et al. Borderline resectable pancreatic cancer: the importance of this emerging stage of disease. *J Am Coll Surg*. 2008;206(5):833-846; discussion 846-848.
3. Callery MP, Chang KJ, Fishman EK, et al. Pretreatment assessment of resectable and borderline resectable pancreatic cancer: expert consensus statement. *Ann Surg Oncol*. 2009;16(7):1727-1733.
4. Kloek JJ, Heger M, van der Gaag NA, et al. Effect of preoperative biliary drainage on coagulation and fibrinolysis in severe obstructive cholestasis. *J Clin Gastroenterol*. 2010;44(9):646-652.
5. Mojtahedi A, Thamake S, Tworowska I, Ranganathan D, Delpassand ES. The value of (68)Ga-DOTATATE PET/CT in diagnosis and management of neuroendocrine tumors compared to current FDA approved imaging modalities: a review of literature. *Am J Nucl Med Mol Imaging*. 2014;4(5):426-434. eCollection 2014. PMID: 25143861.
6. Bressan AK, Aubin JM, Martel G, et al. Efficacy of a dual-ring wound protector for prevention of surgical site infections after pancreaticoduodenectomy in patients with intrabiliary stents: a randomized clinical trial. *Ann Surg*. 2018;268(1):35-40. doi: 10.1097/SLA.0000000000002614. PMID: 29240005.
7. Shah D, Fisher WE, Hodges SE, et al. Preoperative prediction of complete resection in pancreatic cancer. *J Surg Res*. 2008;147(2):216-220.

Chapter 32 Pancreaticoduodenectomy: Minimally Invasive Resection

Song Cheol Kim and Ki Byung Song

DEFINITION

- Pancreaticoduodenectomy (PD) is defined as the resection of the pancreatic head, duodenum, bile duct, and gallbladder, with or without the distal stomach (pylorus preserving), for benign or malignant periampullary diseases.
- Gagner and Pomp first introduced laparoscopic pylorus-preserving PD in an advanced laparoscopic surgical trial in 1994. Subsequently, there has been technical progress in laparoscopic pancreatoduodenectomy (LPD) that includes hand-assisted LPD as well as totally LPD. Robotic surgery is an emerging technology. If robotic system, usually da Vinci, was used to facilitate procedures of resection or reconstruction, it was referred as RPD. LPD and RPD are collectively known as minimally invasive PD (MIPD).

DIFFERENTIAL DIAGNOSIS

- Pancreatic cancer
- Distal bile duct cancer
- Ampullary cancer
- Duodenal cancer
- Pancreatic neuroendocrine neoplasms
- Others

PATIENT HISTORY AND PHYSICAL FINDINGS

- Not all patients are suitable candidates for MIPD. **TABLE 1** shows the currently accepted contraindications for MIPD.
- MIPD with portal vein (PV) resections and reconstructions has been reported. However, locally advanced malignancies may not be technically feasible by minimally invasive approach due to concerns with tumor handling. With increasing experience, MIPD can be attempted for locally advanced malignancies.
- Patient factors, such as body habitus, cardiopulmonary comorbidity, and a history of previous laparotomy, are typical factors that may make MIPD more challenging.
- A history of extensive, previous abdominal surgery or pancreatitis may preclude successful completion of MIPD. Hence, a detailed patient history and medical record review is vital to minimize the rate of conversion.
- A high body mass index (BMI) should be considered a significant factor for morbidity, especially during the learning period. Patients with a high BMI usually have a large amount of parietal and visceral fat, which makes identification of the detailed structures of the inner abdominal organ challenging. Exposure of the third and fourth portions of the duodenum is particularly challenging in the obese patient. Furthermore, the fragile nature of a fatty pancreas leads to difficulties in manipulating or suturing the organ during anastomosis.

IMAGING AND OTHER DIAGNOSTIC STUDIES

- Patients require abdominal or abdominopelvic computed tomography (CT) or magnetic resonance imaging for diagnosis and surgical planning. Multidetector CT (MDCT) is a useful diagnostic tool for detecting the vascular involvement of the tumor, including the PV, the superior mesenteric vein (SMV) or artery, and the celiac axis. MDCT has been reported to have a sensitivity of 85% to 95% and a specificity of 95% for pancreatic cancer.
- The advent of MDCT has eliminated the need for routine magnetic resonance imaging. Heavily weighted T2 imaging sequences in magnetic resonance cholangiopancreatography can depict the pancreatic duct, biliary tree, liver, and vascular structures. Magnetic resonance cholangiopancreatography can replace endoscopic retrograde cholangiopancreatography for imaging of pancreatic and biliary lesions, thereby avoiding endoscopic retrograde cholangiopancreatography-related complications such as bleeding, perforation, and pancreatitis.
- Endoscopic ultrasound (EUS) with a high-frequency probe produces a high-resolution image of the pancreas and its surrounding structures; a small pancreatic mass or cancer can be detected with a sensitivity of 91% to 99% and a specificity of 100%. EUS fine needle aspiration (EUS-FNA) is useful for the diagnosis of an indeterminate pancreatic cystic lesion or when a clinical diagnosis prior to operation is clinically indicated. However, EUS-FNA is not mandatory in operable patients who have been diagnosed with a resectable surgical pancreatic mass by conventional CT and who have clinical signs compatible with a malignant diagnosis. Surgeons should also be mindful of possible risk factors and complications that are associated with an extended surgical time, a possibility that may arise during MIPD. (See the guidelines of the Society of American Gastrointestinal Endoscopic Surgeons.)

SURGICAL MANAGEMENT

Preoperative Planning

- Preoperative palliation of obstructive jaundice may be appropriate for jaundiced patients, but such procedures are associated with an increased risk of operative complications.
- Routine MDCT with arterial reconstruction is useful to evaluate aberrant right hepatic artery in the preoperative planning of MIPD.
- In the case of colon or mesocolon invasion, a bowel prep should be considered before the operation.
- Prophylactic antibiotics and chemical and mechanical venous thromboembolism prophylaxis are warranted.

Table 1: Current Contraindications for Laparoscopic Pancreaticoduodenectomy

Locally advanced malignancies
Obesity (BMI > 35)
Extensive adhesions from previous operations or inflammation
Cardiopulmonary disease that will not tolerate prolonged insufflation of the abdomen
Aberrant anatomy

BMI, body mass index.

LPD TECHNIQUES

- See ▶ Video 1.

Positioning

- The patient is placed in the supine position and an anti-Trendelenburg (10°-30°) is used to expose the surgical field. The surgeon and laparoscopist stood to the right of the patient, with the assistant positioned to the left. Two monitors are placed at the sides of the operator and first assistant. Alternatively, a split-leg positioning can be used for LPD. In this position, the operator stands between the legs of the patient and the assistants stand on either side of the patient.
- A nasogastric tube and Foley catheter are inserted to decompress the stomach and bladder, respectively.
- Intravenous patient-controlled analgesia systems are used to control the pain after the operation.

Trocar Placement

- Open technique is used to establish the pneumoperitoneum through a 12-mm trocar on the umbilicus.
- Thirty-degree angled vision scope is used for visualization. The trocar locations are shown in FIGURE 1.
- An additional three or four trocars are placed under direct vision. Two or three 5-mm trocars (one on the right flank for the left hand of the surgeon and one or two on the left flank for surgical assistance, if necessary) and two 12-mm trocars (one for the laparoscope and one on the umbilicus for the right hand of the surgeon) are employed.
- Abdominal pressure is maintained at 12 mm Hg using carbon dioxide (CO_2) gas insufflation. Keeping the abdominal inflation pressure low, not more than 12 mm Hg, is important to minimize accumulation of CO_2 gas; the LPD procedure can routinely take more than 6 hours.

Division of the Duodenum or Stomach and Identification of the Portal Vein

- The entire abdomen is examined for any abnormalities or metastasis. The entire hepatic and peritoneal surfaces should be inspected. Intraoperative ultrasound may be used for further examination.

- The gastrocolic omentum is dissected to allow entry into the lesser sac (FIGURE 2).
- The gastrohepatic omentum is opened to expose the hepatic artery coursing cephalad to the pancreas. The right gastric artery is ligated using a metal clip and resected using ultrasonic energy device or scissors. After dividing the branches of the right gastroepiploic vessels along the duodenum, the duodenum is divided 2 cm distal to the pylorus using an endoscopic linear stapler (FIGURE 3). Alternatively, resection of the gastric antrum can be performed according to surgeon preference or when there is concern for obtaining an adequate margin. The stomach is placed in the left upper region of the abdominal cavity.

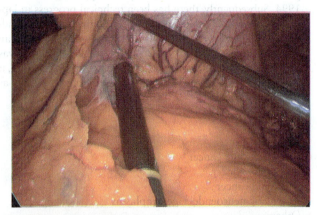

FIGURE 2 • Laparoscopic ultrasound. Laparoscopic intraoperative ultrasound probe is inserted into the 12-mm trocar, and ultrasonography is performed for identifying the location of the lesion.

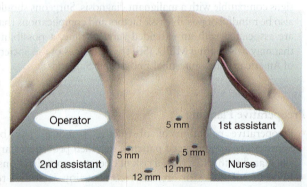

FIGURE 1 • Location of trocar placement for laparoscopic pylorus-preserving PD. Two or three 5-mm trocars (one on the right flank for the left hand of the surgeon and one or two on the left flank for surgical assistance) and two 12-mm trocars (one for the laparoscope and one on the umbilicus for the right hand of the surgeon) are employed.

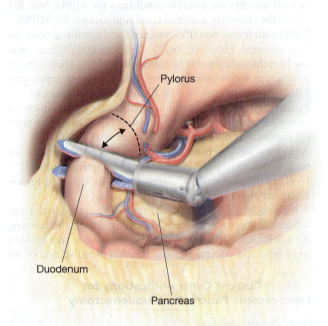

FIGURE 3 • The duodenum is divided approximately 2 cm distal to the pylorus (*dotted line*) using an endoscopic linear stapler. We prefer early division of the duodenum to facilitate the subsequent dissection.

- The PV is identified at the inferior border of the pancreas by distally following the gastroepiploic vein (GEV) to its insertion into the SMV. The GEV is clipped and divided as it inserts into the SMV (**FIGURE 4**). The GEV often drains into the middle colic vein, and in this circumstance, efforts should be made to preserve the middle colic vein.
- The anterior aspect of the retropancreatic segment of the PV/SMV is dissected, creating a tunnel, and potential invasion of tumor into the PV is assessed (**FIGURE 5**).
- The gastrohepatic omentum is opened to expose the hepatic artery coursing cephalad to the pancreas. The right gastric artery is ligated using a metal clip and resected using ultrasonic energy device or scissors.
- The upper border of the pancreas is dissected to establish "Kim triangle," formed by the common hepatic artery, upper border of the pancreas neck, and gastroduodenal artery (GDA) (**FIGURE 6**). The GDA is ligated with Hemo-loc or metal clip and then divided.
- The PV tunnel is completed and gentle upward traction of the isolated pancreas is applied using an umbilical tape in preparation for division of the pancreas.

Mobilization of the Right Colon and Duodenum and Identification of the Superior Mesenteric Vein

- The peritoneum of the hepatic flexure of the right colon is incised. The right colon is mobilized downward and to the left side of the patient to fully expose the second and third portions of the duodenum. The dissection between the mesocolon and the duodenum/pancreatic head proceeds along the avascular surgical plane and is facilitated by the first assistant pulling the mesentery of the right colon toward the patient's left lower quadrant (**FIGURE 7**).
- Mobilization of the third and fourth portions of the duodenum (Kocher maneuver), including division of the ligament of Treitz, is performed (**FIGURE 8**). Careful traction of the duodenum should be applied to prevent perforation. Dissection is continued to the left of the aorta and up to the origin of the superior mesenteric artery (SMA). The ligament of Treitz can be successfully taken down from this exposure in the majority of patients, but occasionally, there are additional peritoneal attachments to the first portion of the duodenum that will need to be divided with exposure beneath the transverse mesocolon. The third and fourth portions of

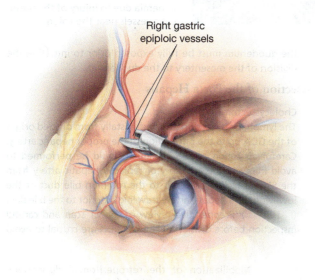

FIGURE 4 • The gastroepiploic vein (GEV) is identified at the inferior border of the pancreas. The GEV is clipped and divided as it inserts into the SMV.

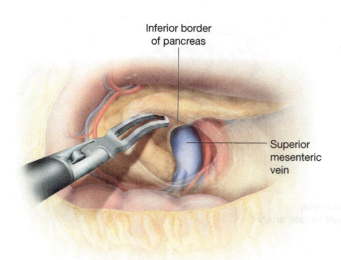

FIGURE 5 • Identification of PV and SMV. The SMV is identified at the inferior border of the pancreas and dissected up to the retropancreatic PV.

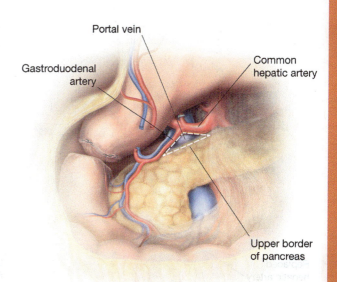

FIGURE 6 • Kim triangle. The outline of common hepatic artery, upper border of the pancreatic neck, and GDA forms a triangle for the tunneling behind the neck of the pancreas. The triangular space is dissected to isolate the pancreas from the PV (tunneling), and gentle upward traction of the isolated pancreas is applied using cotton tape ("lasso technique") in preparation for division of the pancreas.

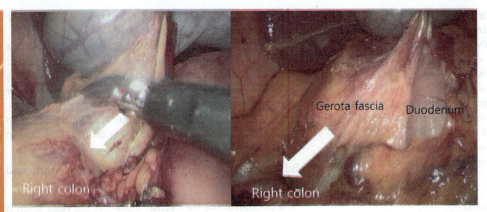

FIGURE 7 • Dissection of coloduodenal avascular plane. The coloduodenal plane is bluntly dissected along the avascular surgical plane. This step is crucial to avoid colonic ischemia due to injury of the mesocolic vessels near the colon.

the duodenum must be fully exposed prior to initiating the division of the mesentery to the duodenum.

Dissection of the Porta Hepatis

- Cholecystectomy is performed.
- The lymphatic dissection proceeds distally from divided origin of the GDA up to the bifurcation of the proper hepatic artery.
- Careful dissection of the bile duct should be performed to avoid injury to the accessory or replaced hepatic artery from the SMA traveling posterior to the common bile duct or the low-lying right hepatic artery traveling anterior to the bile duct (**FIGURE 9**). Preoperative review of the CT scan and careful inspection before division of the bile duct are crucial to avoid

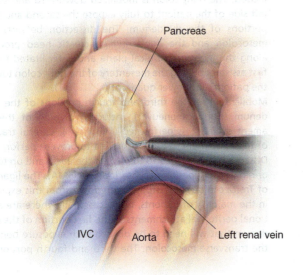

FIGURE 8 • Mobilization of the retroperitoneal duodenum. Kocher maneuver is performed to the left renal vein and aorta. Careful traction of the duodenum should be performed to prevent perforation of the duodenum. A full mobilization of the retroperitoneal duodenum facilitates the separation of duodenum from the root of the mesentery.

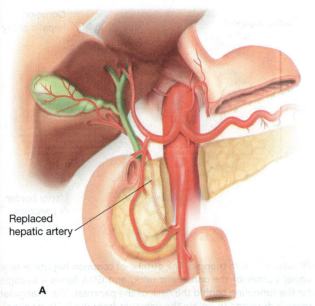
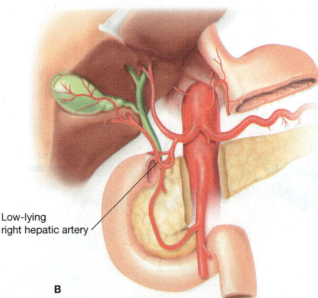

FIGURE 9 • Replaced hepatic artery (**A**) and low-lying right hepatic artery (**B**). Careful dissection of the bile duct should be performed to avoid injury to the accessory or replaced hepatic artery from the SMA traveling posterior to the common bile duct or the low-lying right hepatic artery traveling anterior to the bile duct.

unexpected injury to the hepatic artery because palpation of the porta hepatis is impossible in laparoscopic surgery.
- Mobilize the common bile duct and transect just proximal to the insertion of the cystic duct. However, the resection site of bile duct for extrahepatic cholangiocarcinoma is dependent on the location of the tumor. The proximal duct is controlled with a bulldog clamp. The distal duct is oversewn to prevent contamination and to provide hemostasis. The PV can now be fully exposed by dissecting the soft tissues and lymphatics using ultrasonic shears or bipolar electrocautery.

Division of the Neck of the Pancreas

- Suture ligation of the longitudinal arteries coursing within the parenchyma along the superior and inferior border of the neck of the pancreas can help control bleeding from the cut surface during transection of the pancreas. We prefer to use ultrasonic shears to divide the pancreas to minimize bleeding (**FIGURE 10**).
- Retraction of the pancreas parenchyma using cotton tape to separate the PV/SMV helps prevent injury to the PV. Meticulous control of bleeding from the cut pancreatic surface is necessary to prevent postoperative bleeding and failure of the pancreaticoenteric anastomosis. The pancreatic duct is identified (**FIGURE 11**). A frozen tissue section can be obtained from the margin of the pancreas.

- The SMV and PV are further dissected, identifying, controlling, and dividing the few venous tributaries arising from the head of the pancreas and uncinate process. The authors recommend the use of clips to control these vessels.
- The remaining pancreatic stump is further dissected to provide the 1 to 2 cm of mobility necessary to invaginate the pancreas into the jejunum for the pancreaticojejunostomy (**FIGURE 12**).

Transection of the Proximal Jejunum

- The jejunal mesentery, 10 to 15 cm distal to the ligament of Treitz, is divided between vascular arcades, and the mesenteric vessels are ligated (**FIGURE 13**). The jejunum is transected with an endoscopic linear gastrointestinal stapler. This procedure can be performed to the right side of the base of the mesentery after pulling the jejunum through the retromesenteric space. Alternatively, we perform this procedure in its original position (performing the division of the jejunum and mesentery prior to pulling the jejunum into the right side).
- Although the Harmonic scalpel or bipolar electrocautery is useful for dividing the mesentery of the proximal jejunum, it is prudent to clip the mesenteric (remaining) side.
- The nutrient vessels of the jejunum and duodenum should be taken at the level of the bowel to minimize risk of injury to the cisterna chyle or mesenteric vessels.

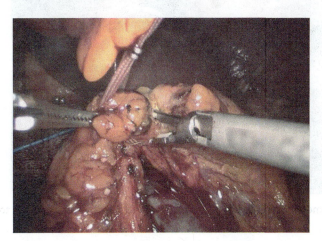

FIGURE 10 • Division of pancreas using ultrasonic shears. Electrocautery can be used depending on the surgeon's preference. We prefer to use ultrasonic shears to divide the pancreas with minimal bleeding.

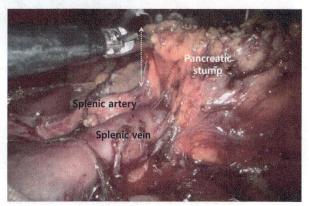

FIGURE 12 • Mobilizing the pancreatic remnant. The remaining pancreatic stump is mobilized by 1 to 2 cm to facilitate invagination of the pancreas into the jejunum for the pancreaticojejunostomy.

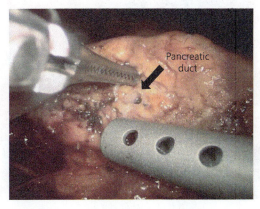

FIGURE 11 • Identification of pancreatic duct.

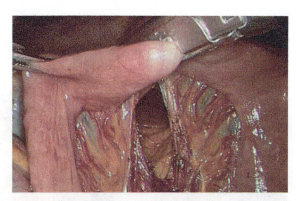

FIGURE 13 • Transection of proximal jejunum. The jejunal mesentery 10 to 15 cm distal from the ligament of Treitz is divided along the mesenteric vascular arch and mesenteric vessels are ligated.

Dissection of the Uncinate Process from the Superior Mesenteric Artery

- This step is the most technically difficult part of the procedure and also the most critical in terms of obtaining tumor-free margins. Elevation of the specimen reveals detailed features of the remaining attachments, including tributaries of the PV or SMV. The first jejunal vein and its tributaries to the uncinate process of the pancreas can also be identified with this lateral anterior traction of the specimen (**FIGURE 14**). Of importance, this maneuver rotates the mesentery facilitating visualization of the SMA; however, this change in the anatomic relationship puts the artery to the right of the PV and at risk for injury.
- To aid in the dissection and to control any unexpected bleeding from the PV or SMV, a surgical vessel loops is applied to the PV and SMV, respectively, just above the splenic vein and the first jejunal vein (**FIGURE 15**). A hooked retractor is useful for traction of the mesenteric root to the left in order to dissect the plane between the uncinate process and the mesenteric veins. Traction with umbilical tape allows the neurolymphatic soft tissues around the SMA to be clearly visualized.
- Two possible methods can be used to dissect between the SMA and the uncinate process: downward (from the common bile duct side to the mesentery of the jejunum) or upward (from the mesentery of the jejunum to the common bile duct side) (**FIGURE 16**). We prefer an upward dissection because this exposes the venous branches more effectively than the downward approach.
- With upward traction of the SMV using vessel loop and caudal traction of the specimen, posterior venous tributaries draining from the uncinate process to the first jejunal vein (two or three veins) can be identified and divided with clips and an ultrasonic energic device. After dividing the tributaries from the first jejunal branch, the soft tissue near the SMA should be dissected to identify one or two inferior pancreaticoduodenal arteries (**FIGURE 17**). An ultrasonic energic device may be used to divide these arteries; however, we prefer to separately clip the remaining pancreaticoduodenal arteries. Occasionally, small branches that cannot be identified may be easily divided using an ultrasonic energic device.
- The remaining dissection of the soft tissue between the SMA and the uncinate process should be performed according to the oncologic status of the disease. For diseases other than

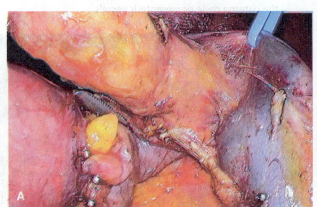
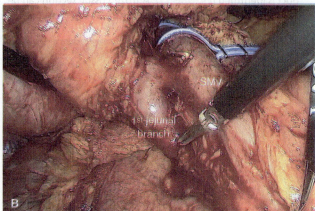

FIGURE 14 • **A** and **B**, Lateral and anterior retraction of the specimen is useful to identify the first jejunal vein and its tributaries to the uncinate process of the pancreas.

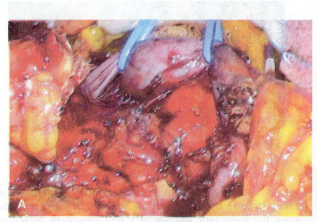
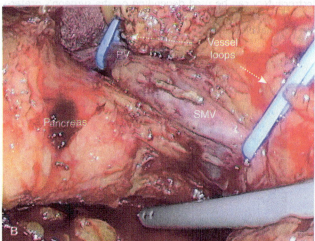

FIGURE 15 • **A** and **B**, Two vessel loops were applied for retraction of portal vein (PV) and superior mesenteric vein (SMV).

Chapter 32 PANCREATICODUODENECTOMY: MINIMALLY INVASIVE RESECTION 263

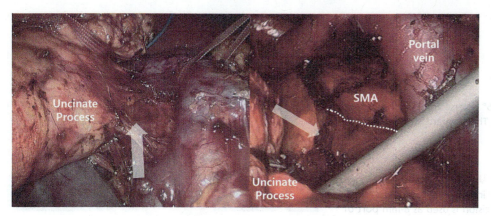

FIGURE 16 • Two possible methods to dissect between the SMA and the uncinate process: upward dissection (from the mesentery of the jejunum to the common bile duct side) or downward (from the common bile duct side to the mesentery of the jejunum). We prefer an upward dissection (arrow) because this exposes the venous branches more effectively than the downward dissection (arrow).

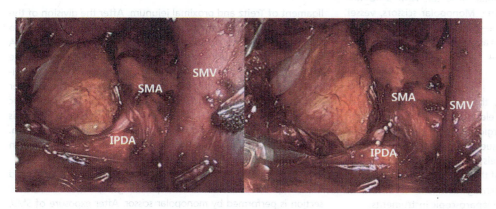

FIGURE 17 • Identification of inferior pancreaticoduodenal arteries (IPDA). After dividing the tributaries from the first jejunal branch, the soft tissue near the SMA should be dissected to identify one or two IPDAs.

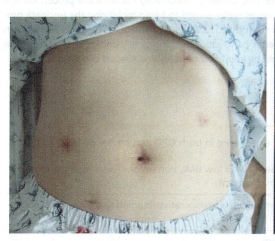
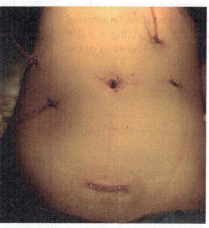

FIGURE 18 • Periumbilical and Pfannenstiel incisions. The specimen is placed in a specimen bag and retrieved at the end of procedure, either through the 2- to 3-cm extension of the umbilical port or a separate Pfannenstiel incision.

pancreatic ductal adenocarcinoma, the dissection can be performed near the uncinate process without risk of injury to the SMA. However, for pancreatic ductal adenocarcinoma, a clear dissection of the neurolymphatic soft tissues of the right side of the SMA is needed to optimize a margin-negative resection.
- Most soft tissues including small mesenteric vessels can be safely sealed with a Harmonic scalpel to transect the pancreas head from the SMA. However, the remaining large superior pancreaticoduodenal vein should be tied or clipped securely.
- The specimen is placed in a specimen bag and retrieved at the end of procedure, either through the 2- to 3-cm extension of the umbilical port or a separate incision (FIGURE 18). The specimen bag containing the gallbladder is removed at the same time.

TECHNIQUES OF RPD

- See ▶ Video 2.

Positioning

The patient is placed in a supine 15° reverse Trendelenburg position with slight right-up position. The assistant stands between the patient's lower limbs.

Trocar Placement

Port placement is described in **FIGURE 19**. Pneumoperitoneum is induced with a Veress needle introduced through a small supraumbilical incision, and this incision is used as 8-mm port of camera. Arm 1—8-mm robotic port—right anterior axillary line. Fenestrated bipolar grasper. Arm 2—8-mm robotic port—right mid-clavicular line. Maryland bipolar dissector. Arm 3—8-mm robotic port—left mid-clavicular line. Monopolar scissors, vessel sealer extend, needle driver. Arm 4—8-mm robotic port—supra-umbilical midline. Camera A 12-mm assistant port is placed on the left area between Arm 3 and Arm 4.

Resection phase of RPD

As energy device for hemostasis, the EndoWrist Vessel Sealer Extend is used. This is a bipolar electrosurgical instrument for use with a compatible da Vinci surgical system. It is intended for grasping and blunt dissection of tissue and for bipolar coagulation and mechanical transection of vessels up to 7 mm in diameter and tissue bundles that fit in the jaws of the instrument. Wristed articulation (fully 60°) is also a big advantage compared with robotic Harmonic scalpel and conventional laparoscopic instruments.

The principle of robotic PD is similar to that of the laparoscopic approach. The operation starts with the opening of the gastrocolic ligament, and the hepatic flexure of the colon is taken down. A Kocher maneuver is performed to completely mobilize to reach the left lateral border of the aorta. For this procedure, Fenestrated grasper of Arm 1 plays an important role in securing a stable view by lifting of the duodenum. The next step is division of the

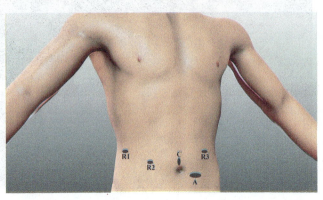

FIGURE 19 • Location of trocar placement for robotic pylorus-preserving PD.

ligament of Treitz and proximal jejunum. After the division of the gastroepiploic vessels, the duodenum is transected using an Endo GIA stapler. The hepatoduodenal ligament is dissected. The CHA lymph node is carefully resected at this point, further exposing the CHA and GDA. By dividing the GDA, the portal vein can be identified lying in a plane deeper than the common bile duct and proper hepatic artery, marking the superior aspect of the retropancreatic tunnel. The gallbladder is taken down. The common bile duct is dissected and isolated, followed by frozen examination of margin. A small bulldog clamp may be introduced to occlude the common hepatic duct to prevent bile spillage in the operative field.

An avascular plane/tunnel is developed between the pancreas and the SMV/portal vein, and after U-tape lifting of pancreas neck, transection is performed by monopolar scissor. After exposure of SMV, gastrocolic trunk is ligated. The head of the pancreas and duodenum are now retracted laterally, toward the right side of the abdomen, and attention is turned to mobilizing the uncinate process off the SMV. The vessel sealer is used to begin mobilizing the uncinate process away from this critical vascular structure. Larger branches such as the inferior pancreaticoduodenal artery and small branches from SMV should be identified carefully and clipped and divided.

PEARLS AND PITFALLS

Indications	• Surgeons wishing to perform MIPD should have sufficient experience in both OPD and advanced MIPD suturing techniques. • The indications for MIPD should be limited initially to patients with low BMI, benign or low-grade malignant disease, or confined malignant disease without vascular involvement.
Preoperative planning	• Palpation cannot be used to identify aberrant arterial anatomy. Review preoperative imaging specifically to this regard.
Technique	• Early division of the duodenum facilitates further dissection. • Proper mobilization of the right colon is crucial to clearly expose the operative field. • Staple and ligate the GDA—Clips will slip off the specimen side during subsequent manipulation of the specimen. Staple lines are at risk for pseudoaneurysm. Ligate above the staple line. • A bulldog clamp on the proximal bile duct prevents contamination and provides hemostasis. • Ligation of longitudinal arteries and division of the pancreatic neck using ultrasonic energy device are essential steps to a hemostatic field. • Anterior and lateral retraction of the specimen is essential for visualization of the attachments of the uncinate process to the SMV and SMA. • Identification and careful division of the first jejunal vein and its tributaries to the uncinate process of the pancreas is critical to prevent unexpected bleeding. • Applying vessel loops around the PV and SMV just above the splenic vein and first jejunal vein can also help control any unexpected bleeding.

POSTOPERATIVE CARE

- In the majority of cases, patients should be transferred to an intensive care unit for monitoring. However, patients may be transferred to a general ward in highly specialized centers.
- Maintenance of nasogastric tube after MIPD does not improve outcomes, and its routine use is not warranted.
- Early and active mobilization and ambulation should be encouraged.
- Early drain removal on postoperative day 3 to 5 following pancreatoduodenectomy is safe and could reduce the incidence of major complications in patients undergoing MIPD.
- Low-molecular-weight heparin or unfragmented heparin reduces the risk of venous thromboembolism with complications and should be continued until postoperative day 3 to 5.
- Intravenous patient-controlled analgesia systems are used to control pain.

OUTCOMES

- When compared with open pancreaticoduodenectomy (OPD), MIPD potentially offers the recognized advantages of minimally invasive surgery, including faster postoperative recovery, improved cosmesis, and fewer wound complications.
- Mortality rates of 3% to 15% for MIPD have been reported. The postoperative major morbidity rate was approximately 4.8% to 24.8%. The operative time is usually longer than that of conventional pylorus-preserving pancreatoduodenectomy. The time between surgery and hospital discharge is the same or less than that of an open procedure. Oncologic outcomes for advanced cancer, such as the number of harvested lymph nodes and the rate of negative margin status, also show results similar to those of open procedures.
- The perioperative outcomes of MIPD in large series are shown in **TABLE 2**.

COMPLICATIONS

- Morbidity rates of between 20% and 40% have been reported. The most common and fatal complications are pancreatic leakage and hemorrhage. The majority of intra-abdominal infections are associated with pancreatic leaks and fistulas.
- Pancreatic fistula
- Hemorrhage
- Delayed gastric emptying

Table 2: Mortality and Morbidity in Large Series of Total Laparoscopic Pancreaticoduodenectomy

Variables	Shyr et al[1]	Zureikat et al[2]	Wang et al[3]	Song et al[4]
Operation type	RPD	RPD	LPD	LPD
Number	304	500	550	500
Conversion (%)	4.8	5.2	2.9	2.3
Mortality (no.)	9	15	5	3
Operative time (median, minutes)	438	415	323.5	402.4
Major complication (%)[b]	12.3	24.8	5.6	4.8
Pancreatic fistula (%)[a]	12.4	7.8	7.5	10.8
Length of hospital stay (median, days)	20	8	13	13.3

NA, not available.
[a]International Study Group on Pancreatic Fistula (ISGPF) grade B or C.[5]
[b]Clavien-Dindo classification ≥ grade 3.[6]

REFERENCES

1. Shyr BU, Shyr BS, Chen SC, Shyr YM, Wang SE. Robotic and open pancreaticoduodenectomy: results from Taipei Veterans general hospital in Taiwan. *Updates Surg*. 2021;73(3):939-946.
2. Zureikat AH, Beane JD, Zenati MS, et al. 500 minimally invasive robotic pancreatoduodenectomies: one decade of optimizing performance. *Ann Surg*. 2021;273(5):966-972.
3. Wang X, Cai Y, Jiang J, Peng B. Laparoscopic pancreaticoduodenectomy: outcomes and experience of 550 patients in a single Institution. *Ann Surg Oncol*. 2020;27(11):4562-4573.
4. Song KB, Kim SC, Lee W, et al. Laparoscopic pancreaticoduodenectomy for periampullary tumors: lessons learned from 500 consecutive patients in a single center. *Surg Endosc*. 2020;34(3):1343-1352.
5. Bassi C, Dervenis C, Butturini G, et al. Postoperative pancreatic fistula: an international study group (ISGPF) definition. *Surgery*. 2005;138(1):8-13.
6. Clavien PA, Barkun J, de Oliveira ML, et al. The Clavien-Dindo classification of surgical complications: five-year experience. *Ann Surg*. 2009;250(2):187-196.

Chapter 33 Pancreaticoduodenectomy: Robotic-Assisted Resection

Brian A. Boone and Herbert J. Zeh III

DEFINITION

- Pancreaticoduodenectomy entails resection of the head of the pancreas and duodenum, which requires mobilization and transection of the pancreas, stomach, common bile duct, and jejunum. This chapter will focus on the resection and extraction of the specimen using a robotic-assisted technique, with subsequent chapters devoted to reconstruction.

DIFFERENTIAL DIAGNOSIS

- Pancreaticoduodenectomy is performed most frequently for premalignant or malignant indications, including duodenal carcinoma, intraductal papillary mucinous neoplasm, mucinous cystic neoplasm, pancreatic neuroendocrine tumor, and cholangio-, ampullary, and pancreatic carcinoma.

PATIENT HISTORY AND PHYSICAL FINDINGS

- The history and physical examination should focus on identifying evidence of metastatic disease, which would preclude resectability.
- The robotic technique is routinely used for both benign, premalignant, and malignant disease.
- Patients are not excluded from the robotic approach based on age, body mass index, or comorbidities.
- Relative contraindications to robotic surgery are the anticipation of vascular resection and reconstruction and extensive prior abdominal surgery.

IMAGING AND OTHER DIAGNOSTIC STUDIES

- The primary goal of imaging modalities for pancreatic cancer is to determine resectability by excluding metastatic disease and involvement of the mesenteric vessels.
- Based on consensus guidelines, resectable tumors are those that have no distant metastasis; have no radiographic evidence of abutment or distortion of the superior mesenteric vein (SMV) and portal vein (PV); and have clear fat planes surrounding the celiac axis, hepatic artery, and superior mesenteric artery (SMA) (**FIGURE 1**). Patients with tumor abutment of the SMV/PV, gastroduodenal artery (GDA) abutment or encasement up to the hepatic artery, or abutment of the SMA less than 180° are considered to be borderline resectable and may benefit from neoadjuvant treatment.
- Computed tomography (CT) scan—A triphasic CT scan of the chest, abdomen, and pelvis with fine cuts through the pancreas is the mainstay of imaging for pancreatic pathology. CT allows for characterization of the pancreatic mass, identifies involvement of the mesenteric vessels, and evaluates for metastatic disease, particularly in the liver or lungs.
- Endoscopic ultrasound (EUS)—This diagnostic modality, although not routinely performed at all institutions, should be considered standard of care in most cases. EUS allows for visualization and biopsy of the mass, particularly if a tissue diagnosis is required for treatment with neoadjuvant or adjuvant chemotherapy. Mesenteric vessel involvement can be evaluated. In addition, suspicious lymph nodes can be identified and biopsied, which helps to accurately stage the patient.
- Staging laparoscopy—The role of stand-alone staging laparoscopy in the management of pancreatic cancer remains controversial and is not routinely performed at most institutions. Robotic pancreaticoduodenectomy begins with a diagnostic laparoscopy and evaluation for liver or peritoneal disease prior to proceeding with surgical resection.

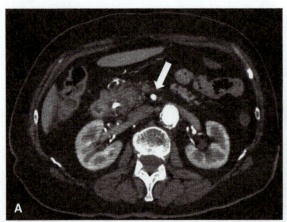
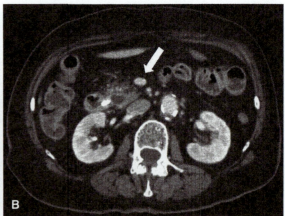

FIGURE 1 • A CT scan demonstrating the tumor relationship to the surrounding vasculature is required to determine resectability during the preoperative planning phase. **A,** CT scan of the abdomen with arterial contrast demonstrating clear fat planes around SMA in resectable pancreatic cancer (*white arrow*). **B,** Venous phase scan demonstrating clear fat planes around SMV (*white arrow*).

Chapter 33 PANCREATICODUODENECTOMY: ROBOTIC-ASSISTED RESECTION

SURGICAL MANAGEMENT

Preoperative Planning

- Determining resectability based on high-quality diagnostic and imaging modalities is the key step in preoperative planning, particularly because the use of the robotic technique precludes the ability of the surgeon to palpate the tumor and readily identify vascular involvement intraoperatively.
- Four units of crossmatched packed red blood cells should be prepared and available.
- Preoperative antibiotics should be administered.

Positioning

- The general setup for the robotic operating room is depicted in **FIGURE 2**. While the Si robot required docking over the patient's head, an advantage of the Xi model is that it can be docked from the right of the table.
- The patient is positioned supine on a split-leg table, which allows space for the assistant surgeon to have access to the abdomen.
- Prior to the start of the procedure, an arterial line is inserted along with large-bore peripheral venous access, a nasogastric tube, and Foley catheter. A convective warming blanket is used on the upper body.

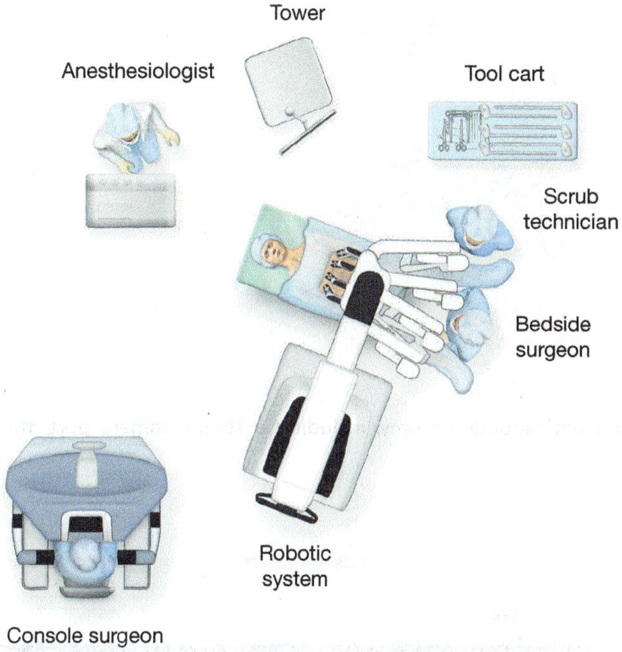

FIGURE 2 • Setup of operating room for robotic pancreaticoduodenectomy for the Si **(A)** and Xi **(B)**. For the Si robot, the robot is placed above the patient's head. The Xi allows for the robot to be docked from the patient's right. A split-leg table is used to allow the assistant access to the abdomen and robotic arms. The robotic console is placed to the side of the room to allow ample space for the circulator and scrub tech.

PORT PLACEMENT

- Seven ports are used for robotic assistance during pancreaticoduodenectomy. Ports include a robotic camera port, three robotic arm ports, two assistant ports, and a 5-mm liver retractor port. Our port location and configuration are displayed in **FIGURE 3**.
- Access to the abdomen is obtained using a 5-mm optical separator port inserted to the left of the umbilicus in the midclavicular line. This port is eventually upsized to 8 mm and serves as a robotic arm.
- Once ports are placed, the bed is placed in reverse Trendelenburg position (15°) with the right side up (7°) slightly and the robot is docked.
- The operating surgeon moves to the robotics console, and the assisting surgeon stands between the legs to exchange instruments, pass needles, and assist with suction and stapling.
- After completion of the resection, a 4- to 5-cm incision to extract the specimen is placed in the left lower quadrant in the left midclavicular line or in the midline utilizing extension of the camera port. After extraction, a laparoscopic wound retractor system is used to maintain pneumoperitoneum and either the assistant port (left lower quadrant extraction) or the camera port (midline) is replaced through the Gelport, depending on the location of the extraction site.

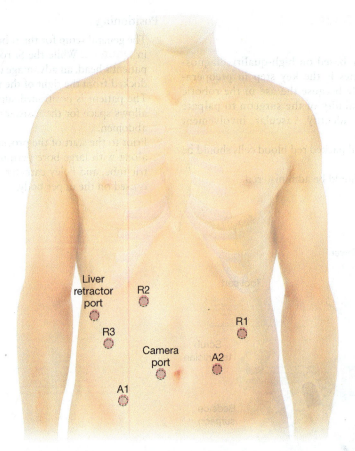

FIGURE 3 • Seven ports are used for robotic assistance during pancreaticoduodenectomy, including a 10-mm camera port, three robotic ports, two assistant ports, and a 5-mm liver retractor port.

MOBILIZATION OF THE RIGHT COLON AND DUODENUM

- The lesser sac is entered by division of the gastrocolic omentum and the right colon is fully mobilized. This step is particularly important if the tumor abuts or involves the portal vein or uncinated process.
- The duodenum is kocherized with mobilization of the third and fourth portions until the jejunum reaches into the right upper quadrant and the SMV is exposed at the root of the small bowel mesentery (FIGURE 4).
- The ligament of Treitz is taken down from the right upper quadrant using hook cautery, and the proximal jejunum is delivered into the right upper quadrant, then divided using a linear stapler (▶ Video 1). The distal jejunum to be used for reconstruction is left in the right upper quadrant.

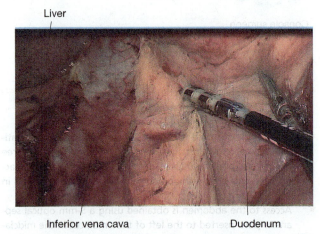

FIGURE 4 • Complete kocherization of the duodenum using laparoscopic instruments brings the duodenum into the left upper quadrant. The inferior vena cava is visualized during mobilization of the duodenum.

MOBILIZATION AND DIVISION OF THE STOMACH

- The posterior stomach is freed from the anterior pancreas.
- The right gastric and right gastroepiploic arteries are ligated close to the stomach with a bipolar electrocautery device (FIGURE 5).
- The stomach is divided with a linear stapler after removal of the nasogastric tube.

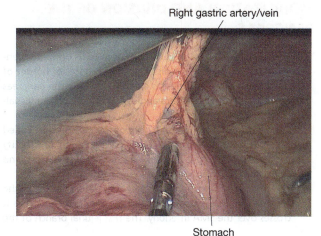

FIGURE 5 • The right gastric artery is identified and ligated close to the stomach using bipolar electrocautery.

DISSECTION OF THE PORTA HEPATIS

- Dissection is continued along the superior border of the pancreas and into the porta hepatis using the robotic hook cautery. The specimen side of the stomach is retracted to the right. The common hepatic artery (CHA) lymph node is identified and removed (FIGURE 6). This allows exposure of the CHA. The CHA is exposed and followed until the right gastric artery and GDA are identified (FIGURE 7). A vessel loop is passed around the GDA, and it is occluded while flow is checked by color flow and 3-D Doppler in the CHA. Once flow is confirmed, the GDA is ligated with a vascular load stapler and reinforced with a 10-mm titanium clip.
- Portal lymph nodes are dissected and removed. The PV and common bile duct are then exposed (FIGURE 8).
- Cholecystectomy may be performed in an antegrade fashion at this point or reserved for after the main specimen is removed.
- The common bile duct is dissected and divided with a vascular load of the endostapler.

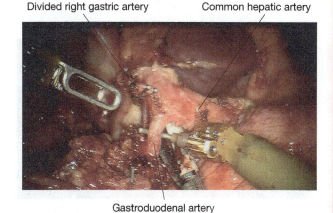

FIGURE 7 • The GDA is identified. Flow in the CHA is confirmed with a vessel loop constricting the GDA. The GDA is then ligated with an endostapler with a vascular load.

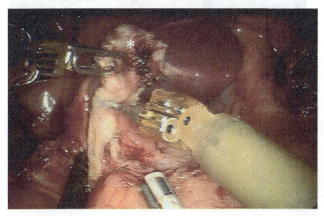

FIGURE 6 • The CHA lymph node is identified (*white asterisk*) and removed using hook cautery. This allows exposure of the CHA.

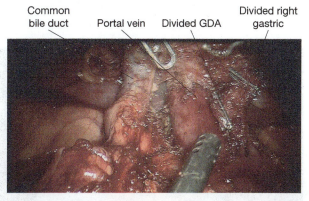

FIGURE 8 • The portal dissection continues until the common bile duct and PV are identified and exposed. Regional lymphadenectomy in the porta hepatis is performed by clearing tissue from the hepatic artery beginning proximal to the station 8A lymph node to distal to the takeoff of the right gastric, the anterior and lateral surface of the portal vein, and around the bile duct above the planned site of transection. The bile duct is then stapled.

MOBILIZATION AND DIVISION OF THE PANCREAS

- The right gastroepiploic vein is followed to its origin to identify the SMV. The SMV is dissected off the inferior border of the pancreas, and a tunnel is created between the pancreas and PV. The robotic camera angles allow for excellent visualization of the tunnel (**FIGURE 9**).
- Once a tunnel is formed, the neck of the pancreas is divided with electrocautery (**FIGURE 10**). Care is taken to identify the pancreatic duct, divide the duct sharply with scissors, and leave small extension on it.
- The pancreas is then mobilized, first at the lateral border of the SMV/PV. The first jejunal branch of the SMV is identified as it crosses over the SMA inferiorly. The first jejunal branch of the SMV is preserved by taking several small recurrent branches to the uncinate process using the bipolar energy device.
- The SMV/PV is brought medially, exposing the SMA, which is then dissected along the plane of Leriche (**FIGURE 11**).
- The superior and inferior pancreaticoduodenal artery are individually identified and secured with clips, silk ligatures, or LigaSure, depending on size and location (**FIGURE 12**).
- The superior uncinate branch of the PV is identified and ligated with the bipolar vessel sealer, vascular load stapler, clips, or silk ligature.
- The specimen is removed in an EndoCatch bag through a 4- to 5-cm extraction incision in the left midclavicular line or in the abdominal midline through the camera port site. Following removal of the specimen, the resection field is prepared for reconstruction (**FIGURE 13**).

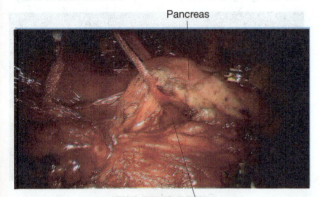

FIGURE 9 • Dissection at the inferior border of the pancreas allows the tunnel underneath the pancreas and over top of the mesenteric vessels.

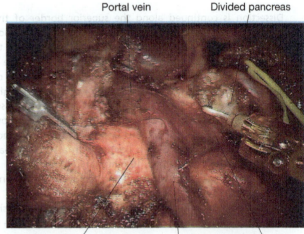

FIGURE 11 • The uncinate process is dissected using a combination of hook cautery and fine scissors.

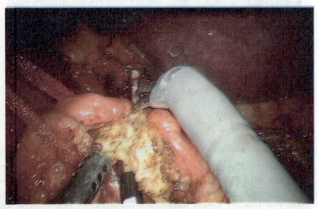

FIGURE 10 • The pancreas is divided using cauterized scissors. The enhanced camera angles on the robotic system allow for excellent visualization during the tunnel and subsequent division of the pancreas.

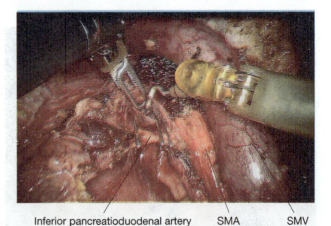

FIGURE 12 • Retraction of the SMV medially exposes the SMA to allow for dissection along the plane of Leriche. The inferior pancreaticoduodenal artery is identified and ligated.

Chapter 33 PANCREATICODUODENECTOMY: ROBOTIC-ASSISTED RESECTION

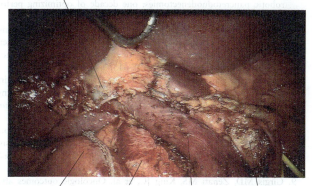

FIGURE 13 • The resection bed following removal of the specimen. The field is now prepared for reconstruction.

PEARLS AND PITFALLS

Preoperative planning—determination of resectability	■ Invasion of the tumor into the mesenteric vessels cannot be fully assessed by palpation until after the pancreatic neck is divided and the surgeon is committed to resection; therefore, a high-quality preoperative CT and planning are required to determine resectability.
Port placement	■ If the ports are placed too close together, the robot arms will hit each other.
Dissection of the porta hepatis	■ Assess for aberrant vascular anatomy such as a right hepatic artery from the SMA, which occurs in up to 20% of patients.
Hanging technique for uncinate	■ The third robotic arm must rotate the specimen laterally and superiorly to allow for adequate exposure of the SMA.

POSTOPERATIVE CARE

- Following completion of the operation, the patient is extubated and transferred to a monitored floor bed. Based on our enhanced recovery protocol, the nasogastric tube is removed prior to completing the operation.
- A drain is left in the pancreatic bed, and a drain amylase is checked on postoperative days 1 and 3. Drains with normal amylase are removed prior to discharge.

OUTCOMES

- Although no randomized trials have been completed comparing robotic and open pancreaticoduodenectomy, the preliminary experience of several groups suggests that outcomes of robotic pancreaticoduodenectomy are comparable with those of open surgery.[1-4] Several series have consistently demonstrated a reduction in estimated blood loss and potential for lower rates of pancreatic leak with the robotic approach.
- The largest series of robotic pancreaticoduodenectomy from a single institution was recently reported,[5] with outcomes for 500 pancreaticoduodenectomies listed below:
  - Thirty-day and 90-day perioperative mortality was 1.4% and 3.1%, respectively.
  - Clinically significant morbidity (grade 3 or 4 Clavien Dindo) affected 24% of patients.
  - Median operative time was 391 minutes with significant improvement noted over the experience.
  - The median estimated blood loss was around 250 mL for the series.
  - Conversion to open was required in 5.2% of cases.
- Although early series demonstrated a significant learning curve associated with optimization of robotic pancreaticoduodenectomy, the experience of surgeons who underwent comprehensive robotic pancreatic surgery training suggests a dramatic reduction in the learning curve.[6-9]

COMPLICATIONS

- The types of complications following robotic pancreaticoduodenectomy are identical to those of open surgery. The incidence and severity appear to be similar to that of open surgery in series detailing outcomes of robotic pancreaticoduodenectomy:[3-7]
  - Pancreatic leak
  - Pseudoaneurysm
  - Delayed gastric emptying
  - Infection (wound, intra-abdominal abscess)
  - Biliary leak
  - Gastric leak
  - Gastric outlet obstruction
  - Bowel obstruction

REFERENCES

1. Liu Q, Zhao Z, Zhang X, et al. Perioperative and Oncological outcomes of robotic versus open pancreaticoduodenectomy in low-risk surgical candidates: a Multicenter Propensity score-matched study. *Ann Surg.* Published online August 19, 2021. doi:10.1097/SLA.0000000000005160
2. Zureikat AH, Postelwait LM, Liu Y, et al. A Multi-Institutional comparison of perioperative outcomes of robotic and open pancreaticoduodenectomy. *Ann Surg.* 2016;264(4):640-649.
3. van Oosten AF, Ding D, Habib JR, et al. Perioperative outcomes of robotic pancreaticoduodenectomy: a propensity-matched analysis to open and laparoscopic pancreaticoduodenectomy. *J Gastrointest Surg.* 2021;25(7):1795-1804.
4. Cai J, Ramanatha R, Zenati MS, et al. Robotic pancreaticoduodenectomy is associated with decreased clinically relevant pancreatic fistulas: a propensity-matched analysis. *J Gastrointest Surg.* 2020;24(5):1111-1118.
5. Zureikat AH, Beane JD, Zenati MS, et al. 500 minimally invasive robotic pancretoduodenectomies: one decade of optimizing performance. *Ann Surg.* 2021;273(5):966-972.
6. Rice MK, Hodges JC, Bellon J, et al. Association of mentorship and a formal robotic proficiency skills curriculum with subsequent generations' learning curve and safety for robotic pancreaticoduodenectomy. *JAMA Surg.* 2020;155(7):607-615.
7. Schmidt CR, Harris BR, Musgrove KA, et al. Formal robotic training diminishes the learning curve for robotic pancreatoduodenectomy: implications for new programs in complex robotic surgery. *J Surg Oncol.* 2021;123(2):375-380.
8. Ryoo DY, Eskander MF, Hamad A, et al. Mitigation of the robotic pancreaticoduodenectomy learning curve through comprehensive training. *HPB (Oxford).* 2021;23(10):1550-1556. doi:10.1016/j.hpb.2021.03.010
9. Girgis MD, Zenati MS, King JC, et al. Oncologic outcomes after robotic pancreatic resections are not inferior to open surgery. *Ann Surg.* 2021;274(3):e262-e268.

Chapter 34

Pancreaticoduodenectomy: Pancreaticojejunostomy

Charles M. Vollmer Jr.

DEFINITION

- Pancreaticojejunostomy is defined as the anastomosis of a remnant pancreas to the jejunum—requisite for reestablishing intestinal tract continuity following pancreaticoduodenectomy (PD).
- Although there are numerous options available to restore continuity of the pancreas to the enteric tract following PD, central pancreatectomy, or distal pancreatectomy (rarely), pancreaticojejunostomy is the most frequently applied approach worldwide (≈90%).[1] Furthermore, there are a number of technical variations available for this procedure including "dunking" and "invagination" approaches. This chapter depicts construction of the widely prevalent double-layered, duct-to-mucosa, end-to-side pancreaticojejunostomy—chosen for 76% of PDs constructed worldwide.[1]
- This chapter's importance lies in the following: Although the first half of PD hinges on the optimal resection of diseased tissue, which determines long-term (usually oncologic) outcomes, the reconstruction phase sets the tone for the immediate postoperative recovery period through the prevention of complications. Chief among these is pancreatic anastomotic failure, which occurs roughly 15% of the time.

PATIENT HISTORY AND PHYSICAL FINDINGS

- The updated, international consensus definition of this complication has been enthusiastically adopted by most pancreatic surgeons (International Study Group on Pancreatic Surgery [ISGPS]).[2] Subsequently, patient-specific risk factors for clinically relevant leaks have been identified as (1) soft gland texture, (2) small pancreatic duct diameter, (3) pathology exclusive of pancreatic cancer or pancreatitis, and (4) elevated blood loss.[3] These variables forming the components of the Fistula Risk Score (FRS) are best elucidated at the time of the operation and should factor into decision-making as understanding them can influence intraoperative and postoperative management techniques.[4,5] Contemporary "Master" pancreatic surgeons place considerable emphasis on the operative technique aspects of anastomotic reconstruction.[5]

SURGICAL MANAGEMENT

Pancreatic Transection

- A successful anastomosis begins well before the reconstruction phase of the procedure. Limiting blood loss and careful handling of the pancreas during the resection stage should be regular goals.[6]
- Once an appropriate site of transection over the portal vein canal is chosen, it is helpful to place hemostatic transfixion sutures on each side of the proposed plane. There are two reproducible horizontal arterial arcades coursing a few millimeters within the superior and inferior borders of the pancreas. A 2-0 silk, figure-of-eight suture is deeply placed into each border and on each side of the transection plane (total of four). Care must be taken to not place these too deeply into the parenchyma on the left (stay) side, such that the pancreatic duct is inadvertently occluded. This is not a concern on the right side where the pancreatic head specimen will ultimately be removed. Once tied down, these sutures are not cut but rather maintained long on a snap to aid in leverage of the distal gland during the reconstruction phase (FIGURE 1).
- Transection can occur via a number of techniques including scalpel or staplers. However, Bovie cautery is preferred for its ability to limit blood loss. A needle-tipped cautery provides good precision with focused coagulation. The "cut" mode is used to transect the capsule and most of the parenchyma, whereas focal use of the coagulation mode is valuable to control distinct blood vessels when encountered. This approach proceeds through the majority of the gland until the area of the duct is anticipated. Sharp transection of this area is preferred to prevent thermal damage to the duct. While doing this, one can "bow" the transection plane away from the parenchymal face to try to provide a cuff of duct that does not retract back within the parenchyma.

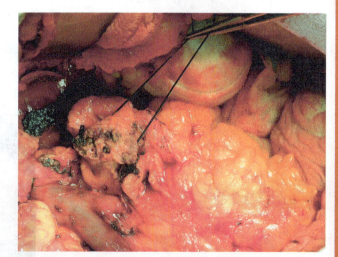

FIGURE 1 • En face picture of the transection plane of the pancreatic neck. Two sutures are placed into the parenchyma to control the superior and inferior vascular arcades. These also provide leverage in "lifting" the pancreatic remnant out of the retroperitoneum for the anastomotic construction.

- Cautery is then focally applied to dry up any oozing from the cut edge of the pancreas. There is quite often a reproducible, pesky arterial vessel on the posterior edge of the gland just beneath where the duct lies.
- The distal pancreatic remnant should be elevated off of the splenic vein beneath it for a distance of at least 2 to 3 cm. This, along with traction on the transfixion sutures, will expose the back side of the gland so that the posterior row of the outer anastomotic layer can eventually be created. This is generally an avascular plane until the point where the splenic vein (and/or artery) becomes incorporated by pancreatic parenchyma.

The Setup

- Once hemostasis of the pancreatic transection planes is achieved, the pancreaticobiliary drainage limb is introduced to the right upper quadrant (RUQ). Although many achieve this by placing it through the transverse mesentery in a retrocolic position, the author prefers to lay the limb in a completely retromesenteric fashion. The limb is introduced from the infracolic compartment (left side of midline) through the previous ligament of Treitz canal to the RUQ. Once placed in apposition with the remnant pancreas and the transected bile duct, this, in essence, becomes a "neoduodenum" (FIGURE 2). However, this may also be achieved in the more traditional fashion mentioned earlier, particularly in the cases where the patient has significant central obesity.
- Remember the hallmark surgical dictum that the success of an anastomosis is predicated on the following factors: (1) healthy tissue with a good blood supply, (2) lack of tension, and (3) freedom of distal obstruction. You can assure that the pancreaticobiliary drainage limb has a good pulse by palpating the vascular arcade within the mesentery after it has been placed in the desired position. Meticulous technique during the jejunal resection should assure that there is not a mesenteric hematoma, which might compromise the health of the limb. Do not shortchange the length of proximal jejunum, which is originally resected, as this will shorten the mesenteric "leash" and therefore place tension on the limb as it reaches to the RUQ.
- Hemostasis of the transection plane of the neck of the pancreas is achieved by judicious use of the needle-tipped Bovie cautery on a low power (15-20). Energy near the pancreatic duct is avoided.
- The pancreatic duct diameter is examined and measured with a flexible ruler. An absorptive "Weck-Cel" arrowhead spear is useful in keeping the duct dry both now and later, when precision is needed during suture placement in the duct (FIGURE 3).
- The duct can be actively dilated by placing the tips of a fine instrument (Gemini or pediatric right angle) within the duct and gently spreading and holding them open, being careful to not disrupt the duct tissue. Finally, the patency of the course of the pancreatic duct should be assured by advancing a 5-Fr or 8-Fr pediatric feeding tube within the duct in a retrograde manner. These are flexible and safer than a rigid probe, which might be advanced inadvertently through the duct wall and even the parenchyma. This is particularly important in cases of chronic pancreatitis, where distal strictures may lurk.
- The operative field is then prepared by covering the retraction devices with an arrangement of white towels which, in effect, excludes the retractor from the field and provides a neutral background to better visualize fine, colored monofilament sutures (FIGURE 4).

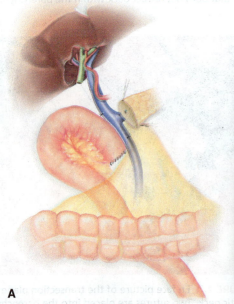
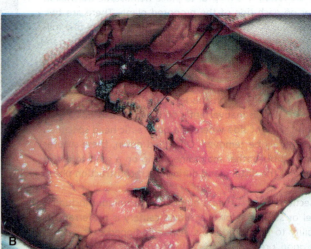

FIGURE 2 • **A,** The pancreaticobiliary limb is positioned in the right upper quadrant by bringing it behind the mesenteric stalk through the ligament of Treitz canal. **B,** In effect, this becomes a neoduodenum, as it lays comfortably in apposition with the pancreas and bile duct. Undue tension on this limb can be avoided by resecting at least 20 cm of proximal jejunum initially.

Chapter 34 PANCREATICODUODENECTOMY: PANCREATICOJEJUNOSTOMY

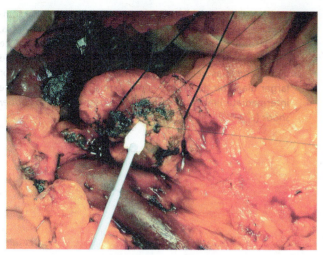

FIGURE 3 • An *arrowhead* Weck-Cel facilitates precise visualization of the pancreatic duct.

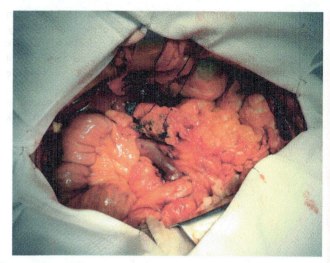

FIGURE 4 • Placement of four white surgical towels around the periphery of the incision enhances visualization of fine suture and prevents it from tangling on the retractors.

TECHNICAL CONSIDERATIONS

- The inner (duct-to-mucosa) anastomosis is constructed with monofilament absorbable suture. A 6-0 caliber is favored for normal to small ducts, but a 5-0 caliber can be used on larger, dilated ducts (≥8 mm). In select circumstances in *extremely* small diameter ducts (1-2 mm), a 7-0 caliber may be necessary. Remember that smaller grade suture has smaller needles and thus creates smaller puncture holes in the tissue. Double-armed sutures provide the most flexibility for needle placement, as some sutures are best applied from in to out, whereas others are optimally placed from out to in. This should be determined on a suture-for-suture basis, depending on how the arc of the needle is applied the most effortlessly *and precisely* through the duct.

- Due to the precision required for this step, a Castro Viejo needle driver commanded through the finger tips is recommended rather than a bulky, longer driver controlled in the palm. Finer sized ducts (<3 mm) may benefit from the use of Loupe glasses for magnification.
- The author routinely *avoids* placing *internal* pancreaticoenteric stent across the anastomosis, in light of its inefficiency in preventing pancreatic fistula, particularly in presumably vulnerable high-risk patients.[7] However, to increase precision of the needle placement in precarious ducts, some surgeons do find value in creating the anastomosis with a small pediatric feeding tube temporarily in place during the anastomotic construction.
- On the other hand, externalized stents *do provide certain value* in "high" FRS situations (FRS 7-10).[8]

THE INNER LAYER—FRONT ROW

- The objective of this step is to "open" the duct orifice and further elevate the face of the transection plane into the field. The appearance of the transected duct can be compared to the face of a clock (**FIGURE 5**).
- Start by placing the 12 o'clock suture. These needles are curved considerably, and thus, the hand motion should allow for perpendicular placement of the needle tip into the parenchyma about 2 mm behind the duct. A curving motion will deliver it about a millimeter into the duct lumen, where it should be retrieved using a smooth "roll out" motion rather than a "tugging" technique. Efficiency and precision of movements are tantamount at this stage.
- The two limbs of the suture are gathered, and the needle from the parenchymal side is removed while the needle attached to the limb emanating from the duct is maintained. A *straight snap* is used to identify that this is an ordinal point (3-, 6-, 9-,

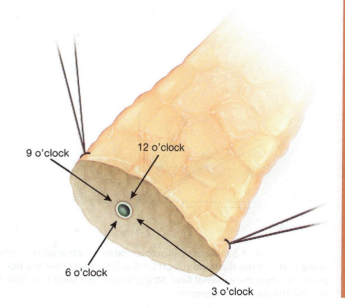

FIGURE 5 • Clock-face orientation of the pancreatic duct at the transection plane.

and 12-o'clock positions; FIGURE 5) and is placed off the field in a manner that elevates the pancreas out of the incision slightly.
- The next moves consist of placing the 9 o'clock and 3 o'clock (horizontal plane) sutures which, when under tension, will fully "open up" the lumen of the duct (FIGURE 6). These are also gathered with *straight* snaps.
- Next, the two limbs can be completed from the horizon to the zenith (3- to 12-o'clock positions and 9- to 12-o'clock positions, respectively). A 3-mm duct will usually accommodate two evenly placed sutures in each of these limbs, for a total of seven sutures placed during this sequence (FIGURE 7A). However, there is room for flexibility to add more sutures as necessary (three to four per quadrant) for larger diameter ducts. To keep a semblance of order, these intermediate limb sutures should be gathered with *rubber shods* (FIGURE 7B).

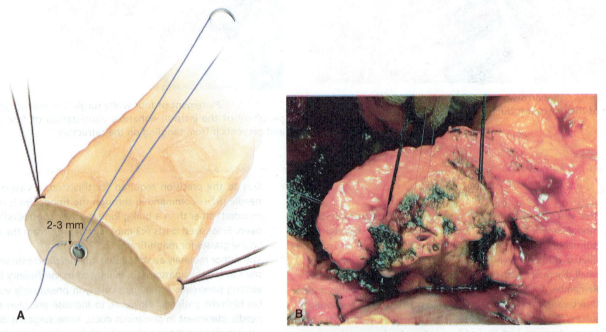

FIGURE 6 • **A,** Placement of the 9 o'clock stitch from in to out on the pancreatic duct, incorporating a few millimeters of parenchyma around the duct. **B,** Placement of these initial stitches in the front row provides better exposure for subsequent stitch placement.

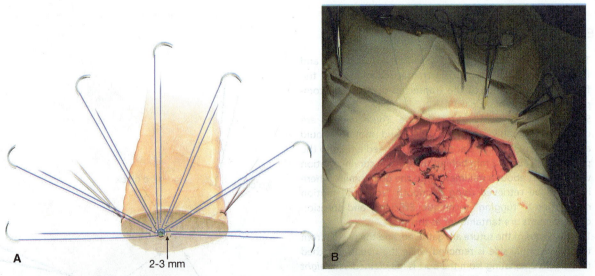

FIGURE 7 • **A,** A 3-mm duct will accommodate seven double-armed sutures on the anterior row. Needles should be maintained on the limbs that exit the duct and cut off on the sides that enter the duct. **B,** To maintain consistency, sutures should be carefully laid out in an array across the external field. Straight snaps are used to gather the corner sutures, whereas rubber shods delineate other positions around the duct circumference.

PREPARATION OF THE ENTEROTOMY

- An appropriate-sized enterotomy is created on the antimesenteric side of the pancreaticobiliary drainage limb, about 5 cm upstream from the oversewn staple line. Care should be taken to match the diameter of this to correspond to the size of the pancreatic duct lumen. Do not make the enterotomy too big; in fact, undersize it if anything, as the opening tends to expand as you are working on it.
- A needle-tipped Bovie cautery works nicely here (**FIGURE 8**). Use the "cut" mode to precisely open the serosal level. Then, create a pinpoint opening of the mucosa in an atraumatic fashion. Avoid manipulating this fragile tissue with unnecessary instrumentation to minimize bleeding, hematomas, and edema.
- To optimize orientation and control of the mucosal outpouching, place four 6-0 absorbable sutures at the ordinal positions (3, 6, 9, and 12 o'clock) (**FIGURE 9A**). In doing so, the clock faces of the duct and the enterotomy should now mirror themselves (**FIGURE 9B**). These sutures should be very small bites, which tack the mucosa to the serosa in the four corners (**FIGURE 9B**, *inset*). Again, the precision of a Castro Viejo instrument is preferred to minimize tissue trauma.

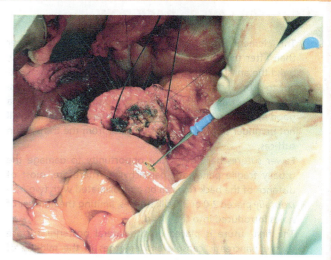

FIGURE 8 • The enterotomy is created with excellent precision using a needle-tipped Bovie cautery. The serosal layer is opened about 2 mm for a corresponding 3-mm wide pancreatic duct. Create a pinpoint opening in the mucosa at first.

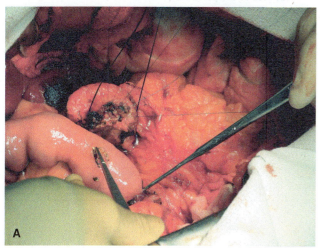

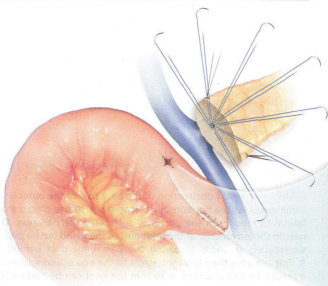

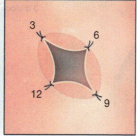

FIGURE 9 • **A**, In order to "tidy up" the enterotomy, 6-0 absorbable sutures are applied to each corner by tacking the mucosa to a small (1 mm) bite of serosa. Use care to prevent undue manipulation of the mucosa. **B**, These sutures prevent puckering of the mucosa (*inset*) and again indicate a clock-face configuration, which now forms a mirror image of that of the duct.

THE OUTER LAYER—BACK ROW

- This element is best achieved earlier in the process rather than after the inner layer has been completed. In essence, build the anastomosis from the ground upward. It is important to properly size up where the sutures will be placed vis-à-vis the duct and enterotomy. In doing so, you can assure a good apposition of the duct and the enterotomy, which will not be under tension. About 2 cm back from the transection suffices.
- Fewer sutures here mean less opportunity to damage the usually fragile pancreatic parenchyma. Therefore, most of distance of the back row can be approximated with two *horizontally* placed 2-0 or 3-0 silk sutures, limiting the number of holes introduced into the gland.
- The first suture is placed on the lateral posterior surface of the pancreatic capsule and emerges in the midline of the pancreas about 1 cm behind the transection edge (**FIGURE 10A**). Care is taken to keep this bite rather superficial so as not to incorporate the pancreatic duct beneath—yet deep enough to "grip" enough parenchyma so that it does not rip through when being tied down.
- This is then brought across to the bowel, where the direction of the needle travel is now from medial to lateral on a line about 2 to 2.5 cm peripheral from the enterotomy (**FIGURE 10B**). Assuming the enterotomy is situated at the true antimesenteric edge of the bowel circumference, this essentially equates to about a quarter of the way from the interface of the bowel and its mesentery.
- A second posterior suture is placed in an analogous fashion. This time, however, the first move is from lateral to medial on the bowel—meeting at the site of the prior suture (**FIGURE 11A**), and then across to the gland where it is placed in a medial to lateral trajectory (**FIGURE 11B**). Thus, the knots of each of these sutures are both tied down laterally.
- Extra security of the periphery of this row can be achieved by one to two additional silk sutures on each side, tied again on the outside. The bowel now lies in direct apposition with the cut face of the pancreas (**FIGURE 11C**).

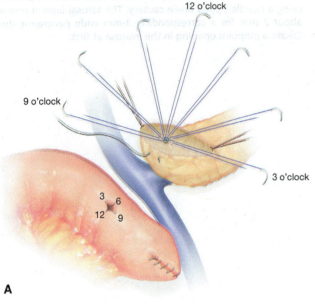

FIGURE 10 • **A,** Construction of the back row of the outer layer commences with a horizontally oriented silk suture placed from lateral to medial on the posterior surface of the pancreas. The needle should emerge at the midpoint of the gland but be placed superficially to avoid involving the pancreatic duct behind it. **B,** This suture is then brought across to the bowel and applied in a medial to lateral direction so that the knot can be tied on the periphery of the pancreas.

Chapter 34 PANCREATICODUODENECTOMY: PANCREATICOJEJUNOSTOMY

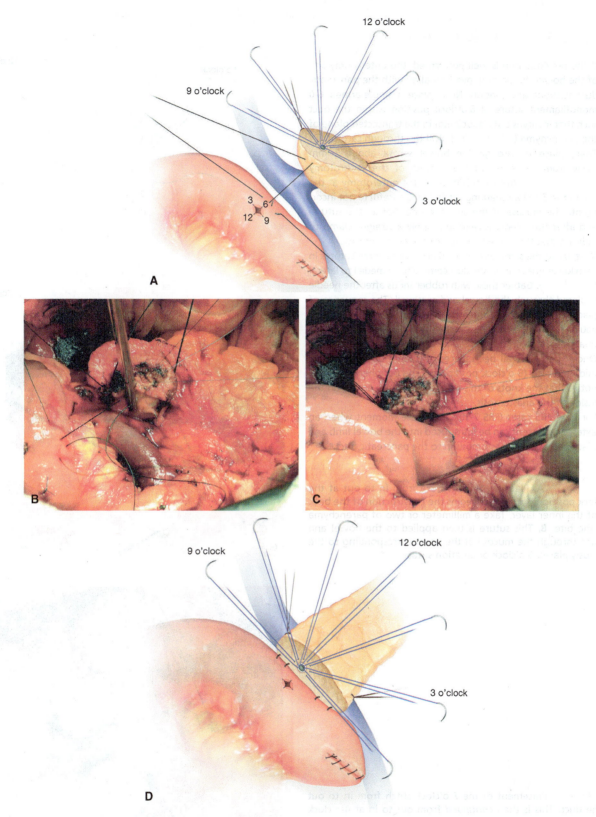

FIGURE 11 • **A,** The back row is *continued* in an analogous fashion. First, a silk suture is placed from lateral to medial in the horizontal plane on the bowel to meet the prior stitch. **B,** Then, the suture is applied from the midpoint of the pancreatic parenchyma laterally to the inferior border of the posterior pancreas. **C,** Demonstration of the relative distance of suture placement. Sutures on the posterior pancreatic parenchymal surface should be about 1 to 2 cm behind the transection margin, whereas the position on the bowel usually corresponds to about one-fourth around the circumference from the enterotomy site. **D,** Once the back wall is completed with a few additional sutures on the periphery, the enterotomy will be appropriately positioned across from the orifice of the pancreatic duct.

THE INNER LAYER—BACK ROW

- If the previous step is well performed, the enterotomy site of the bowel should "roll over" to align with the pancreatic duct without any tension. Now, place a single-armed 6-0 monofilament suture at 6-o'clock position within the duct such that it curves out about 2 mm in the transected plane of the parenchyma (**FIGURE 12A**). Roll this through carefully.
- Then, place it through the bowel serosa about 2 mm away from the edge of the mucosa of the enterotomy (**FIGURE 12B**). Advance this through the enterotomy at the site of the 6 o'clock marking stitch, being careful to not incorporate the mucosa of the opposite side. Gather the suture, and after the needle is removed, apply a *straight clamp* to indicate that this is the midpoint of the posterior row.
- Next, using the same technique, place two to three sutures in each lower quadrant of the duct coming from medial to lateral (**FIGURE 13**). Gather these with rubber shods after the needle is placed through the bowel and removed. The sequence of placement of this row is demonstrated in **FIGURE 14**. Again, you can be flexible with how many sutures are needed on each quadrant based on the actual duct diameter.
- Once these have all been placed, tie them down from the middle suture (6-o'clock position) to the periphery. You will notice that the knots of this absorbable suture are all on the inside of the anastomosis.
- For high FRS cases (FRS 7-10), this is the moment when an externalized stent can be introduced into the bowel limb and placed across the anastomosis in to the pancreatic duct.[8]

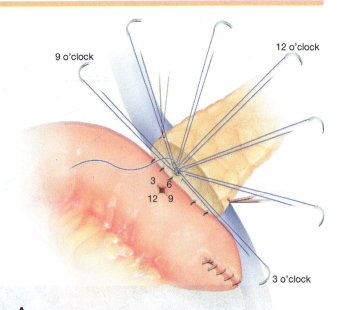

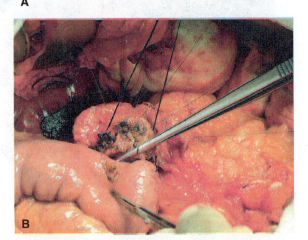

FIGURE 12 • **A,** Placement of a suture from in to out at the 6-o'clock position of the duct begins the construction of the back row of the inner layer. Take a millimeter or two of parenchyma with the bite. **B,** This suture is then applied to the bowel and brought through the mucosa at the point corresponding to the previously placed 6 o'clock orientation suture.

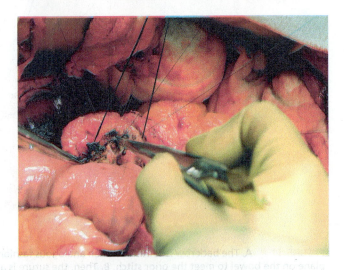

FIGURE 13 • Placement of the 7 o'clock stitch from in to out on the duct. This is then *continued* from out to in at 4-o'clock position on the bowel.

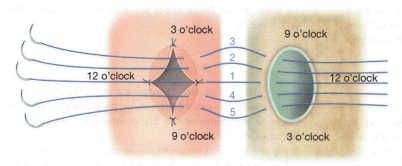

FIGURE 14 • Sequence of placement of sutures for the back row of the inner layer. The general theme is to work from medial to lateral for optimal exposure of needle placement.

COMPLETION OF THE INNER LAYER—FRONT ROW

- Now it's time to revisit the originally placed sutures from the front row of the inner layer. These are placed serially across to the enterotomy—this time working from the lateral (3- and 9-o'clock) positions up to the zenith (12-o'clock position) (FIGURE 15A). The sequence of placement is depicted in FIGURE 15B.
- Ensure that the suture limbs are unwound completely before placing across to the enterotomy, as twisted sutures across the anastomosis will lead to a leak. Again,

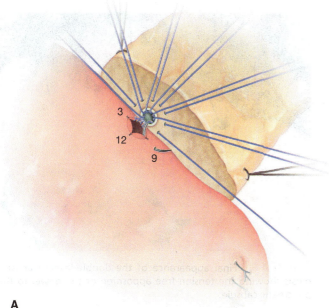

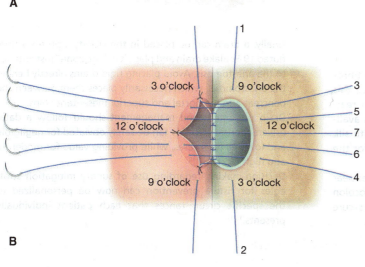

FIGURE 15 • A, Completion of the front row of the inner layer starts by placement of the previously placed corner sutures (either 3-o'clock or 9-o'clock position) from in to out on the enterotomy. B, The optimal sequence of this placement is depicted, reflecting a general movement from the horizon (3- and 9-o'clock positions) up to the zenith (12-o'clock position). Place all sutures across to the bowel before any one of them is tied.

be careful not to incorporate the mucosa of the back wall of the enterotomy. Only once, all the sutures from both limbs are placed across to the bowel should you tie them down. These knots will now be external to the anastomosis.

THE OUTER LAYER—FRONT ROW

- The pancreaticojejunal reconstruction is completed by securing the front row of the outer layer. The 2-0 silks are placed carefully into the pancreas about half a centimeter behind the cut edge of the parenchymal transection edge (FIGURE 16). Although these need to be substantial—particularly in softer glands—take care to stay superficial to the inner anastomosis, particularly as you get closer to the center of the gland, where the parenchyma becomes more shallow.
- Bring these sutures across to the serosa of the bowel limb. Allow for some distance (5-10 mm) between the inner anastomosis and the needle placement into the bowel. This allows for enough redundancy such that the bowel will roll over to the face of the transection without placing undue tension to the pancreatic capsule (FIGURE 17).
- The greatest of care is needed when tying these sutures down to avoid "sawing" through the parenchyma. Avoid "bobbing" movements as you are tying these knots, as this will lift the suture out of the field and thus cause a linear tear through the parenchyma. Tie down to the pancreas!

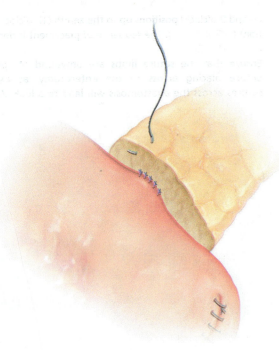

FIGURE 16 • The front aspect of the outer layer is completed by placing silk sutures into the pancreatic parenchyma. Once placed across to the bowel, tie these down with the greatest of care because the pancreas capsule is vulnerable to tearing. Again, work from the lateral aspects of the gland sequentially to the midpoint (directly over the inner anastomosis).

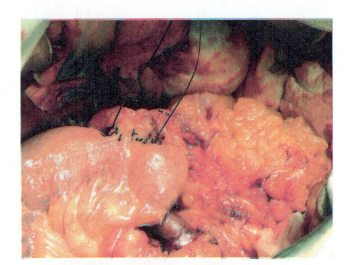

FIGURE 17 • Final appearance of the double-layered anastomosis showing the tension-free apposition of the bowel to the pancreatic capsule.

FINAL STEPS

- In select circumstances, some pancreas will have a fibrofatty layer on their anterior surface. Try to preserve this when initially dissecting and transecting the pancreas, and keep it attached to the pancreatic body. If it is available, it can be applied across to the bowel wall with silk sutures to essentially provide a third layer (hood) for the anterior row.
- You may also be able to attach the redundant bowel near the distal staple line to elements of the transverse mesocolon inferior to the pancreatic anastomosis in order to help secure or "hitch" the limb to prevent an outright dehiscence.
- Finally, a drain can be placed in the vicinity. I prefer a thin, fluted 19-Fr Blake drain and place it in "the zone" just anterior to the anastomosis. Avoid placing rigid drains directly behind the anastomosis, which necessarily places them between the pancreas and the portal and superior mesenteric veins.
- Drain placement and management should follow a data-driven approach. Drains can be safely obviated for negligible and low FRS (0-2) cases, while providing value for moderate and high FRS risk.[3-10]
- Decision-making regarding use of sundry mitigation strategies for fistula prevention can now be personalized to the specific circumstances that each patient individually presents.[10-12]

Chapter 34 PANCREATICODUODENECTOMY: PANCREATICOJEJUNOSTOMY

PEARLS AND PITFALLS

Prelude	- A good pancreaticojejunostomy begins during the resection phase with attention to detail. Minimize unnecessary blood loss and avoid undue tissue trauma to the pancreatic parenchyma. - Although finesse is required for the first half (resection phase) of PD, the tone of the reconstruction phase is markedly different, with concentration on a more deliberate pace focusing on detail, and the surgeon should reorient their mindset accordingly at this point of the case.
Setup	- Assure that the pancreaticobiliary drainage limb is viable, nonedematous, and healthy with good blood flow, with adequate laxity to the RUQ structures. - To minimize technical mishaps with fine-caliber sutures, cover the retractor system with a field of white towels. - Castro Viejo needle drivers provide the precision necessary for the delicate suturing required. Loupe magnification is also valuable.
The inner layer	- Control the operative field by consistently applying straight clamps to gather ordinal (3-, 6-, 9-, and 12-o'clock positions) sutures. Employ rubber shods for the intervening positions. - Use a deliberate, rolling motion in placing the suture through the duct and parenchyma, taking advantage of the natural arc of the needle. Avoid tugging motions when controlling and removing the needle.
The outer layer	- Take care to keep the bites shallow, yet substantial, so as to avoid the inner layer of the anastomosis or pancreatic duct distal to it. - Careless suture tying at this point can lead to tissue fractures of the pancreatic capsule, even in firm glands. - "Roll" the jejunum over to the pancreas, providing a hood effect anteriorly.

POSTOPERATIVE CARE

- Expected outcomes can now be forecast on a case-by-case basis based on the FRS catalog.[12]
- Drain management is predicated on drain amylase values in the recovery period.[9,13] Early drain removal (POD 3-4) is now established as the best approach. The drain can be removed if the patient appears clinically well, the drain amylase level is low (generally under 300 International Unit [IU]), the volume is reasonable, and the fluid does not appear sinister.[2] Drain amylase kinetics are also useful in decision-making.[13]
- Initial (POD 1) drain amylase values over 5000 IU, as well as those that remain static or escalate over the first 3 days, are highly suggestive of a leak in evolution and warrant the continuation of external drainage and possibly, more intervention (radiology assessment, percutaneous or operative procedures, etc).[13]
- External stents, when applied for high FRS cases, can be capped prior to discharge and removed at 1 month.
- If a postoperative leak is clinically apparent, general guidelines for management are provided in a review by Malleo et al.[14]

OUTCOMES

- This described pancreatic anastomotic technique has resulted in a 3.5% clinically relevant fistula rate in the author's last 250 cases in patients with an average FRS of 3.4.[15] Further advice from contemporary "Master" pancreatic surgeons is available, and an audio overview of these concepts can also be found here: https://soundcloud.com/cjs-podcast/e82-charles-vollmer-on-pancreatic-fistulas.[5,16]

REFERENCES

1. McMillan MT, Malleo G, Bassi C, et al. Defining the practice of pancreatoduodenectomy around the world. *HPB*. 2015;17(12):1145-1154.
2. Bassi C, Marchegiani G, Dervenis C, et al. The 2016 update of the international study group (ISGPS) definition and grading of postoperative pancreatic fistula: 11 years after. *Surgery*. 2017;161(3):584-591.
3. Pratt W, Callery MP, Vollmer Jr CM. Risk prediction for development of pancreatic fistula utilizing the ISGPF classification Scheme. *World J Surg*. 2008;32(3):419-428.
4. Callery MP, Pratt WB, Sanchez N, et al. A prospectively validated risk score model for pancreatic fistula after pancreaticoduodenectomy. *J Am Coll Surg*. 2013;216(1):1-14.
5. Casciani F, Bassi C, Vollmer CM. Decision points in pancreatoduodenectomy: insights from the contemporary experts on prevention, mitigation, and management of postoperative pancreatic fistula. *Surgery*. 2021;170(3):889-909. E-pub April 20, 2021.
6. Trudeau MT, Casciani F, Seykora TF, et al. The influence of intraoperative blood loss on fistula development following pancreatoduodenectomy. *Ann Surg*. 2020. Epub Nov 12, 2020.
7. Sachs TE, Kent TS, Pratt WB, et al. The pancreaticojejunal anastomotic stent: friend or foe? *Surgery*. 2013;153:651-662.
8. McMillan MT, Ecker BL, Behrman SW, et al. External stents for pancreatoduodenectomy provide value only in high risk scenarios. *J Gastrointest Surg*. 2016;20(12); 2052-2062.
9. Trudeau MT, Maggino L, Chen B, et al. Extended experience with a dynamic, data-driven selective drain management protocol in pancreatoduodenectomy: progressive risk stratification for better practice. *J Am Coll Surg*. 2020;230(5):809-817.
10. Casciani F, Trudeau MT, Vollmer CM. Of fistula and football. *Ann Surg*. 2021;273(4):e142-e145.
11. Puri P, Vollmer CM. Strategies for prevention and treatment of pancreatic fistula. In Shen P, Rocha F eds. *Optimizing Outcomes for Liver and Pancreas Surgery*. 1st ed. Springer; 2017.
12. Trudeau MT, Casciani F, Ecker BL, et al. The fistula risk score catalogue: toward precision medicine for pancreatic fistula following pancreatoduodenectomy. *Ann Surg*. 2022;275(2):e463-e472.
13. Zureikat AH, Casciani F, Ahmad SB, et al. Kinetics of postoperative drain fluid amylase values following pancreatoduodenectomy: new insights to dynamic, data-driven drain management. *Surgery*. 2021;170(2):639-641.
14. Malleo G, Vollmer CM. Post-pancreatectomy complications and their management. *Surg Clin*. 2016;96:1313-1336.
15. Ecker BL, McMillan MT, Maggino L, Vollmer CM. Taking theory to practice: quality improvement for pancreatoduodenectomy through the development and integration of the fistula risk score. *J Am Coll Surg*. 2018;227(4):430-438.
16. Vollmer CM (Invited Guest). *Masterclass on Pancreatic Fistula. Cold Steel Podcast—Sponsored by the Canadian Journal of Surgery*. 2021. https://soundcloud.com/cjs-podcast/e82-charles-vollmer-on-pancreatic-fistulas

Chapter 35 | Pancreaticoduodenectomy: Pancreaticogastrostomy

Sarah Meade, Jennifer F. Tseng, and David McAneny

DEFINITION

- Pancreaticogastrostomy (PG) is defined as an anastomosis of the pancreas remnant to the stomach following pancreaticoduodenectomy or central pancreatectomy. This technique was originally described in 1946 by Waugh and Claggett.[1]

DIFFERENTIAL DIAGNOSIS

PG is an option for restoration of pancreaticoenteric continuity regardless of the indication for pancreatic resection. The following features provide rationale for this technique:

- PG is facilitated by the natural anatomic proximity of the overlying stomach to the pancreatic transection margin.
- A terminal end of small bowel may be prone to vascular compromise, such as impaired venous outflow, and that could adversely affect a pancreaticojejunostomy (PJ). In contrast, the stomach receives blood from—and drains blood through—several vessels, presumably enhancing the perfusion of the PG.
- From a technical perspective, the stomach has more substance than the jejunum, making it more favorable for the purchase of sutures.
- The proximal jejunum produces enterokinase and possesses a relatively neutral pH, and both of those factors promote activation of the pancreas proenzymes.[2] Activated enzymes leaking from the pancreas anastomosis may destroy retroperitoneal and peripancreatic tissues, resulting in hemorrhage and sepsis. Conversely, the stomach lacks enterokinase and typically presents an acidic milieu, hostile conditions for enzyme activation. As a result, an anastomotic PG leak may be less likely than a PJ to autodigest the retroperitoneal tissues and cause sepsis and major hemorrhage from pseudoaneurysm formation. Interestingly, the lack of activated pancreas enzymes reaching the gut after PG does not seem to confer an increased likelihood of postoperative pancreatic exocrine sufficiency or a diminished quality of life, compared to patients with a PJ.[2]
- The PG provides an opportunity to evacuate pancreatic fluid from the gastric lumen via a nasogastric tube early after resection. Even if there were a small disruption of the PG suture line, suctioning prevents—or at least minimizes—leakage of gastric and pancreas fluid from the gut into the abdominal cavity. Furthermore, nasogastric suctioning obviates the need for intraperitoneal drains that may increase the chances of surgical site infection.
- Notably, patients requiring extensive gastric resections (eg, to obtain sufficient tumor-free margins) may not be candidates for a PG if the gastric pouch is too far from the pancreas remnant. Another limitation may be the potential for an ischemic section of gastric wall between the PG and the gastrojejunostomy.

PATIENT HISTORY AND PHYSICAL FINDINGS

- Acute leakage from a pancreatic anastomosis may cause sepsis, hemorrhage, and death; controlled leaks may become a chronic fistula. (Postoperative pancreatic fistula [POPF] occurs with a frequency of 5%-30%.[3,4]) Risk factors for anastomotic leak include a soft gland, a small pancreatic duct, underlying condition (eg, absence of chronic pancreatitis), reduced regional blood supply, and surgeon experience.[5] A recent meta-analysis of randomized control trials comparing PG to PJ[6] reports postoperative rates of 4.9% mortality, 15.3% delayed gastric emptying, and 10.3% hemorrhage. In one study,[7] 82.3% of postoperative deaths after pancreaticoduodenectomy were due to intra-abdominal complications such as hemorrhage, sepsis, and POPF; of those deaths, 70.5% were attributable to POPF alone. PG is a technical alternative to PJ that conceivably reduces the likelihood of an anastomotic leakage and the associated morbidity.

SURGICAL MANAGEMENT

Preoperative Planning

- No special preparation is necessary in advance of a PG when compared to PJ.
- Techniques for creation of PG vary among surgeons, but this anastomosis may have a shorter learning curve than PJ, as several authors believe that it is technically easier to achieve secure invagination of the pancreatic remnant with PG.[2,8,9]

TECHNIQUES

TELESCOPIC INVAGINATION

- The typical PG involves invagination of the right edge of the pancreas remnant into the gastric lumen with a handsewn anastomosis, in either two layers[4] or one layer.[10] The authors prefer to perform this anastomosis first during reconstruction of gastrointestinal (GI) continuity.
- The surgeon mobilizes about 4 cm of the right aspect of the pancreas remnant (closest to the resection margin), while preserving the perfusion to the remainder of the gland (FIGURE 1).
- The external suture line of the anastomosis comprises interrupted sutures that incorporate both the seromusculature of the posterior gastric wall (just proximal to the level of the anticipated gastrostomy) and a reasonable depth of the periphery of the anterior aspect of the pancreas remnant so that about 2 cm of pancreas parenchyma will ultimately protrude into the gastric lumen

Chapter 35 PANCREATICODUODENECTOMY: PANCREATICOGASTROSTOMY 285

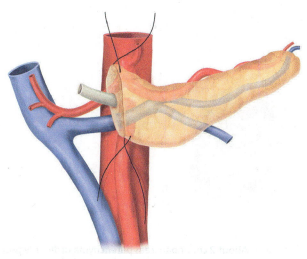

FIGURE 1 • The pancreatic remnant is mobilized approximately 4 cm from the resection margin while maintaining perfusion to the remainder of the gland.

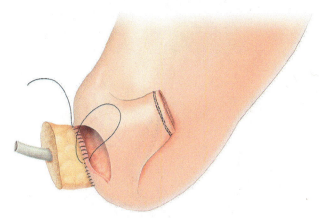

FIGURE 3 • After creation of the gastrotomy, the internal anastomotic layer is circumferentially fashioned using the full thickness of the gastric wall and the periphery of the anterior aspect of the pancreas remnant, with running absorbable sutures.

(FIGURE 2). A plastic stent, ordinarily a #5 pediatric feeding tube, is positioned in the pancreatic duct so that about 5 cm of the stent resides within the duct and 3 cm of the stent will be in the gastric lumen. The stent can be secured with a 4-0 polydioxanone (PDS) suture capturing both the stent and the edge of the pancreatic duct. This stent helps the surgeon avoid incorporation of the pancreatic duct in the suture lines. It is important to advise the patient and family about the presence of the stent so that they are not startled when it is eventually expelled.

- A gastrotomy is performed on the posterior wall of the stomach, transverse to the axis of the stomach and at the junction of body and antrum. The length of the gastrotomy is typically about 3 cm but may be adjusted depending upon the diameter of the pancreas.
- The internal layer of the anastomosis includes the full thickness of the gastric wall (adjacent to the initial silk suture line on the proximal side of the gastrotomy) and the periphery of the anterior aspect of the pancreas remnant. We place 3-0 Vicryl sutures, starting next to the center of the silk suture line and proceeding toward the superior and inferior poles of the gland with separate running sutures (FIGURE 3).
- The pancreas is manipulated to deliver the mobilized portion of the gland into the gastric lumen.
- The inner anastomosis is completed with the same running 3-0 Vicryl sutures, incorporating the full thickness of the gastric wall on the distal side of the gastrotomy and the periphery of the posterior side of the pancreas.
- The outer layer of the anastomosis is completed with interrupted 2-0 silk sutures, including the seromusculature of the stomach and the periphery of the posterior side of the pancreas (FIGURE 4).
- About 2 cm of pancreas parenchyma ordinarily projects into the gastric lumen upon completion of the PG, and this area may be inspected for integrity and hemostasis during the creation of the gastrojejunostomy (FIGURE 5). That also provides an opportunity to position the tip of the nasogastric tube slightly proximal to the PG so that the foreign body does not disturb the PG.

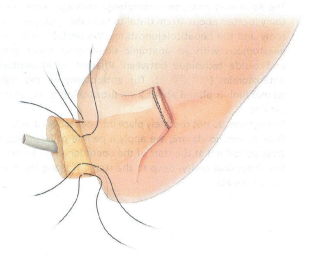

FIGURE 2 • The external suture line of the pancreaticogastrostomy anastomosis comprises interrupted nonabsorbable sutures incorporating both the seromusculature of the posterior gastric wall and a reasonable depth of the anterior aspect of the remnant pancreas.

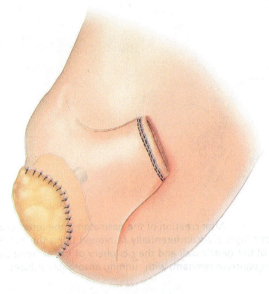

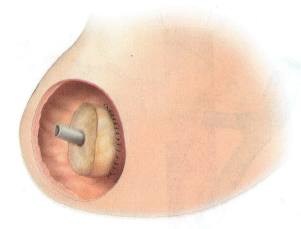

FIGURE 4 • After manipulating the mobilized portion of the gland into the gastric lumen and completing the inner anastomosis, the outer layer of the anastomosis is completed with interrupted nonabsorbable sutures that incorporate the seromusculature of the stomach and the periphery of the posterior surface of the pancreas remnant.

FIGURE 5 • About 2 cm of pancreas parenchyma ordinarily projects into the gastric lumen upon completion of the pancreaticogastrostomy, and this area may be inspected for integrity and hemostasis through the distal stomach during the creation of the gastrojejunostomy.

- We restore continuity of the upper GI tract with a Roux-en-Y configuration (**FIGURE 6**). The hepaticojejunostomy is constructed with an anatomic end-to-side, functional end-to-end technique, between the cut edge of the hepatic duct and an antimesenteric enterotomy located a few centimeters distal to the proximal staple line of the right jejunal limb, depending upon the laxity of the small bowel. We generally use interrupted 3-0 PDS, although the suture size may be adjusted depending upon the diameter of the hepatic duct and the thickness of its wall.
- The gastrojejunostomy is performed next. We do not preserve the pylorus. Instead, we amputate a short length of the prepyloric antrum, the pylorus, and the duodenal cuff (that resulted from the division of the first portion of the duodenum during the pancreatoduodenectomy). This provides a suitable diameter of the gastrotomy, hopefully limiting the prospects of delayed gastric emptying due to anastomotic edema. The gastrojejunostomy is also performed with an anatomic end-to-side, functional end-to-end technique, between the cut edge of the distal antrum and an antimesenteric enterotomy located about 2-3 cm from the proximal staple line of the left jejunal limb.
- The Roux-en-Y anatomy is completed with a jejunojejunostomy located about 40 cm distal to both the gastrojejunostomy and the hepaticojejunostomy. We perform this final anastomosis with an anatomic side-to-side, functioning end-to-side technique between adjacent antimesenteric enterotomies (**FIGURE 6**). The enterotomy on the right jejunal limb is placed about 2 cm proximal to its distal staple line.
- The authors do not routinely place intraperitoneal drains.
- Prior to wound closure, we apply a pedicle of ligamentum teres (mobilized at the start of the operation upon entering the abdominal cavity) deep to the stomach along the right side of the PG.

Chapter 35 PANCREATICODUODENECTOMY: PANCREATICOGASTROSTOMY

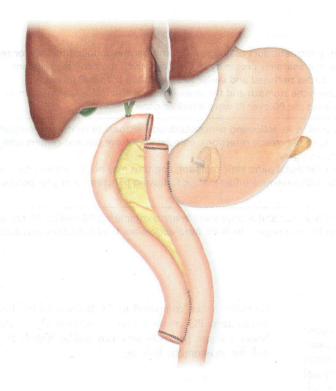

FIGURE 6 • Completed gastrointestinal reconstruction with a Roux-en-Y configuration.

DUCT TO MUCOSA

- In hopes of improving durable patency of the PG, Telford and Mason[11] described an alternative technique that involves direct mucosa-to-mucosa apposition of the pancreatic duct and a small gastrostomy (FIGURE 7).
- The first layer of this two-layer anastomosis includes the periphery of the posterior semicircumference of the cut edge of the pancreas remnant and the seromusculature of the adjacent posterior gastric wall, using interrupted silk sutures. A small gastrotomy is performed opposite the pancreatic duct, and interrupted absorbable monofilament sutures are placed between the deep half of the pancreatic duct mucosa and the corresponding full thickness of the gastric wall. The suture knots reside in the lumen.
- The original report by Telford and Mason proposed that a silastic stent be placed at this time.
- The anterior suture line of the inner row (between anterior pancreatic duct and gastrotomy) is created with the interrupted absorbable monofilament suture knots lying outside the lumen.
- The anastomosis is completed with interrupted silk sutures to appose the anterior semicircumference of the pancreas edge to the adjacent seromusculature of the gastric wall.

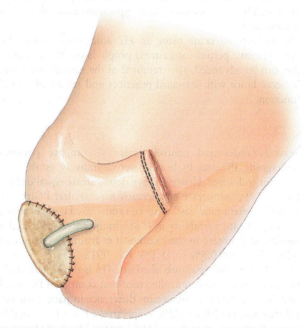

FIGURE 7 • Duct-to-mucosa anastomosis as described by Telford and Mason. A direct duct-to-mucosa apposition is created between the pancreatic duct and a small gastrotomy.

PEARLS AND PITFALLS

History and physical examination	• PG is an attractive option for pancreatic duct drainage following pancreatoduodenectomy or central pancreatectomy, considering the anatomic proximity of the stomach to the pancreas remnant. Furthermore, the stomach is better perfused and easier to suture than the small intestine. • Physiologic differences between the stomach and the small intestine also influence the activation of pancreatic proenzymes, favoring the PG over PJ were a leak to occur.
Surgical management	• The advantages of PG compared to PJ, following pancreatoduodenectomy or central pancreatectomy, could attenuate the morbidity of pancreatic resections, especially for surgeons and centers with relatively low volumes of pancreas surgery. • PG mandates mobilization of the distal pancreatic remnant, and thus may not be technically feasible in all cases, particularly those with extensive inflammation following pancreatitis or preoperative radiation therapy.
Outcomes	• In several randomized controlled trials and a large meta-analysis comparing PG and PJ, PG has equivalent or better outcomes than PJ, with respect to POPF, intra-abdominal fluid collection, and quality of life measures.[7,8]

POSTOPERATIVE CARE

- A nasogastric tube is left in place about 3-4 days and should be diligently maintained so that it consistently sumps, evacuates pancreatic fluid from the gastric lumen, and prevents a gastric dilatation that could disturb the PG. A typical configuration of a PJ results in bile passing—and possibly refluxing across—the gastrojejunostomy. However, a PG with a Roux-en-Y reconstruction diverts bile from the stomach so that gastric output via the nasogastric tube is modest. This also promotes decompression and collapse of the stomach.
- The authors advocate using an H2 antagonist during the postoperative period for gastritis prophylaxis. The patient's diet can be advanced, after removal of the nasogastric tube, in accordance with standard practices and return of bowel function.

OUTCOMES

- Several randomized control trials[2,5,6,9] compare patients undergoing PG and PJ but do not definitively establish a superior technique. However, they demonstrate equal or better rates of postoperative pancreatic fistulas after PG rather than PJ. A meta-analysis[11] of seven randomized control trials, with significant variability in PG technique, demonstrated a significant decrease in the likelihood of fistula development with PG vs PJ (10.5% vs 18.1%, $P < .001$).
- The RECOPANC trial published in 2015 is the largest, multicenter randomized controlled trial that compared PG to PJ and demonstrated no significant difference in pancreatic fistula formation (20% vs 22%, respectively, $P = .617$).[13] In this series, there was an increased incidence of bleeding events in the PG group vs the PJ series (21% vs 11%, $P = .023$). In terms of quality of life metrics, fewer PG patients reported steatorrhea (13% at 12 months) than did PJ patients (22% at 12 months). Emotional and social functioning scores were also significantly better after PG than PJ, while insulin requirements were similar.
- PG is an attractive option for pancreatic duct drainage that does not adversely affect postoperative morbidity and mortality when compared to PJ. Because of its theoretical advantages, PG creation may be particularly desirable for lower volume pancreas surgeons and/or glands at greater risk for anastomotic leakage.

COMPLICATIONS

- Pancreatic fistula
- Intra-abdominal sepsis
- Postoperative intra-abdominal fluid collections
- Postoperative hemorrhage
- Delayed gastric emptying

REFERENCES

1. Waugh JM, Clagett OT. Resection of the duodenum and head of the pancreas for carcinoma. *Surgery*. 1946;20:224-232.
2. Yeo CJ, Cameron JL, Maher MM, et al. A prospective randomized trial of pancreatogastrostomy or pancreatojejunostomy after pancreaticoduodenectomy. *Ann Surg*. 1995;222:580-588.
3. Büchler MW, Friess H, Wagner M, et al. Pancreatic fistula after pancreatic head resection. *Br J Surg*. 2000;87:883-889.
4. Delcore R, Thomas JH, Pierce GE, et al. Pancreatogastrostomy: a safe drainage procedure after pancreatoduodenectomy. *Surgery*. 1990;108:641-645.
5. Kawai M, Tani M, Hirono S, et al. How do we predict the clinically relevant pancreatic fistula after pancreaticoduodenectomy? An analysis in 244 consecutive patients. *World J Surg*. 2009;33:2670-2678.
6. Ma S, Li Q, Dai W, Pan F. Pancreaticogastrostomy versus pancreaticojejunostomy. *J Surg Res*. 2014;192:68-75.
7. Duffas JP, Suc B, Msika S, et al. A controlled randomized multicenter trial of pancreatogastrostomy or pancreatojejunostomy after pancreaticoduodenectomy. *Am J Surg*. 2005;189:720-729.
8. Keck T, Wellner UF, Bahra M, et al. Pancreatograstrostomy versus pancreaticojejunostomy for RECOnstruction after PANCreatoduodenectomy (RECOPANC, DRKS 00000767) perioperative and long-term results of a multicenter randomized controlled trial. *Ann Surg*. 2016;263(3):440-449.
9. Bassi C, Falconi M, Molinari E, et al. Reconstruction by pancreaticojejunostomy versus pancreaticogastrostomy following pancreatectomy: results of a comparative study. *Ann Surg*. 2005;242:767-771.
10. Aranha GV. A technique for pancreaticogastrostomy. *Am J Surg*. 1998;175:328-329.
11. Telford GL, Mason GR. Pancreaticogastrostomy: clinical experience with a direct pancreatic-duct-to-gastric-mucosa anastomoses. *Am J Surg*. 1984;147:832-837.

Chapter 36 | Laparoscopic and Robotic Pancreaticojejunostomy

Ibrahim Nassour and Steven J. Hughes

DEFINITION

- Laparoscopy indicates the use of a camera combined with minimal access techniques to perform surgical procedures.
- Robotic surgery is another form of minimally invasive technique where the DaVinci platform is used to perform the operations. The use of the robot in pancreatic surgery has been steadily increasing over the last decade.[1]
- Pancreaticojejunostomy (PJ) is the operative anastomosis of a remnant pancreas (distal pancreas) to a limb of jejunum to restore continuity of pancreatic secretions into the intestinal tract. This procedure is necessary following pancreaticoduodenectomy.

PATIENT HISTORY AND PHYSICAL FINDINGS

- Pancreatic texture will vary depending on the underlying indication for pancreaticoduodenectomy as well as associated patient factors. The pancreatic duct may also vary in size, depending on whether the duct has been previously obstructed, has been involved in intraductal papillary mucinous neoplastic changes, or is of normal caliber.
- The major risk of PJ is leakage of pancreatic secretions leading to abscess or fistula. A classification scheme for the severity of this complication has been characterized by the International Study Group of Pancreatic Fistula.[2]
- This complication is less frequent when the pancreas is firm in texture, thus providing a substrate that firmly anchors sutures and is not prone to laceration.

SURGICAL MANAGEMENT

Laparoscopic Positioning

- The patient is positioned supine; tucking of the arms is not necessary (**FIGURE 1A**). Some surgeons prefer a "split-table" approach, where the surgeon is positioned between the patient's legs.
- Reverse Trendelenburg position facilitates the exposure. Thus, a footboard should be used.

Robotic Positioning

- The patient is positioned on the split-leg table. The legs are abducted so that the assistant can stand between the legs (**FIGURE 1B**).
- The left arm is extended and placed on an arm board, while the right arm is tucked.
- The table is placed in steep Trendelenburg position and rotated 45° away from anesthesia so as to allow the DaVinci Si robot to be docked at the head of the table. The robot is docked from the right side of the patient if the Xi system is used.

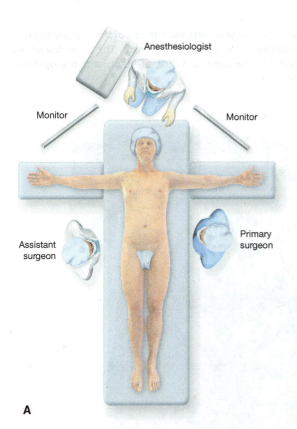

FIGURE 1 • Positioning for laparoscopic (**A**) and robotic approaches (**B**).

290　SECTION III　SURGERY OF THE PANCREAS

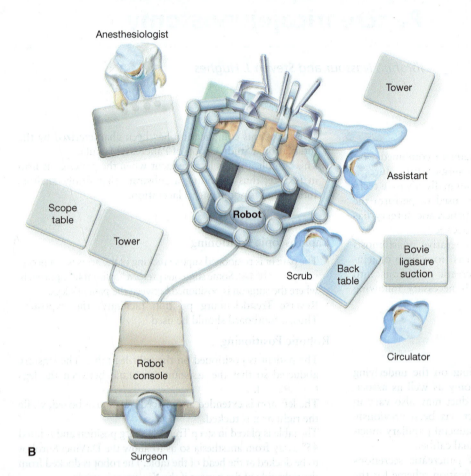

FIGURE 1 • (Continued)

LAPAROSCOPIC TROCAR PLACEMENT

- Trocar placement is depicted in FIGURE 2A.
- Five access points are the minimum required to perform the technique laparoscopically. A fixed retractor is placed in the far-right port to elevate the left lobe of the liver and improve exposure to the pancreatic remnant. The other trocars are used for the camera, a first assistant, and the operative surgeon.

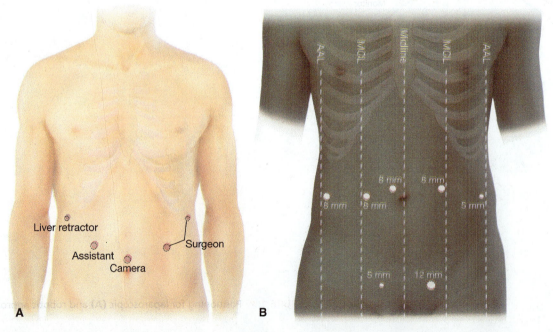

FIGURE 2 • Trocar placement for laparoscopic (A) and robotic (B) approaches. AAL, anterior axillary line; MCL, midclavicular line.

ROBOTIC TROCAR PLACEMENT

- Trocar placement is depicted in **FIGURE 2B**.
- The 12-mm camera port for the Si or the 8-mm port for the Xi is placed 3 cm above and to the right of the umbilicus.
- Two 8-mm robotic trocars are placed in the right anterior axillary (P3) and mid-clavicular (P2) line at the same level as the camera and another 8-mm trocar (P1) is placed in the left mid-clavicular line.
- A 12-mm assistant port is placed in the left lower quadrant a handbreadth below and between the camera and P3. A 5-mm assistant port is placed in the right lower quadrant a handbreadth below and between the camera and P2. The Mediflex liver retractor is introduced through a 5-mm trocar, which is placed laterally inferior to the left costal margin.

MOBILIZATION OF THE REMNANT PANCREAS

- To complete the posterior suture row of the anastomosis, a minimum of 1 cm and ideally 2 cm of the remnant pancreas must be mobilized (**FIGURE 3**). Increased mobilization of the remnant pancreas facilitates elevation of the gland during the anastomosis and results in improved visualization.
- The reconstructive limb should be fashioned focusing on adequate mesenteric length and preservation of the arterial and venous blood supply. Several options regarding reconstructive anatomy are available. The authors favor positioning the reconstructive limb posterior to the mesenteric vessels as a "neoduodenum."[3] Given the natural orientation of the mesentery of the proximal jejunum, this reconstructive approach minimizes the length of the mesentery necessary to perform the PJ in a tension-free environment. This approach also reduces the potential for internal hernia or other technical errors associated with creating a window in the transverse mesocolon. Importantly, this approach avoids excessive rotation of the jejunal limb behind the mesenteric vasculature.

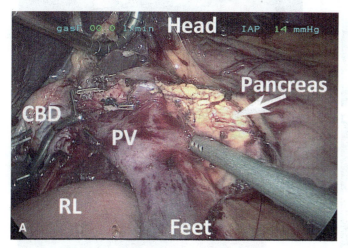
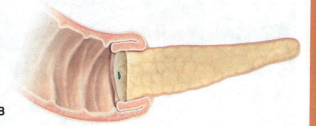

FIGURE 3 • **A,** The surgical field prior to initiation of the pancreaticojejunostomy. After completion of the dissection, the pancreatic neck is circumferentially mobilized for at least 1 to 2 cm. CBD, common bile duct; PV, portal vein; RL, reconstructive limb of jejunum. **B,** Schematic drawing of the completed anastomosis with the pancreas intussuscepted approximately 1 cm into the end of the reconstructive limb of jejunum.

LAPAROSCOPIC END-TO-END INTUSSUSCEPTING ANASTOMOSIS
(▶ VIDEO 1)

- The anastomosis is constructed with a running 4-0 polydioxanone suture on a vascular RB-1 needle. A double-armed suture measuring 40 cm in length (20 cm for each arm) is fashioned by tying two sutures together. The suture is placed through a 12-mm trocar and one arm is positioned out of the surgical field in the left upper quadrant. This arm will be used later for the anterior suture line. The staple line on the reconstructive limb of jejunum is removed using electrocautery.
- The anastomosis is initiated by placing the first suture in the reconstructive limb as shown in **FIGURE 4**. This will facilitate forehand suturing for the entire anastomosis and place the tension of posterior suture line on the serosa of the bowel rather than the soft parenchyma of the pancreas. This suture should be placed at the antimesenteric border of the reconstructive limb.
- The first bite of the pancreatic parenchyma is placed backhand at the cephalad aspect of the remnant pancreas as depicted in **FIGURE 5**. This suture is typically oriented transverse to the longitudinal plane of the pancreatic remnant. Subsequent sutures in the pancreas will be oriented longitudinally.

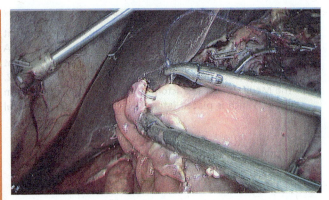

FIGURE 4 • The initial bite of tissue is taken in the jejunum in a longitudinal, distal-to-proximal orientation. This suture should be placed at the antimesenteric border to facilitate the orientation of the reconstructive limb to the base of the mesentery. By starting the posterior row on the side of the jejunum, this row and the anterior row of the anastomosis are placed forehand.

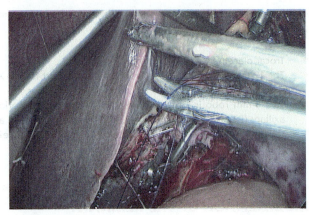

FIGURE 6 • To place the second bit of the posterior row in the jejunum without locking the suture, the needle is passed posterior to the strand that now bridges the jejunum and pancreas. The second bite of jejunum is then taken, advancing 3 to 4 mm along the posterior row.

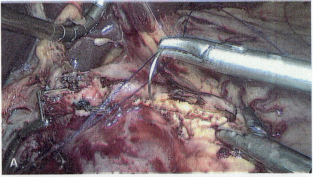

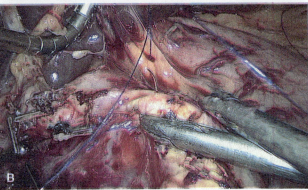

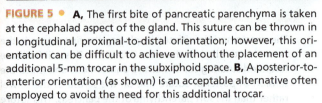

FIGURE 5 • **A,** The first bite of pancreatic parenchyma is taken at the cephalad aspect of the gland. This suture can be thrown in a longitudinal, proximal-to-distal orientation; however, this orientation can be difficult to achieve without the placement of an additional 5-mm trocar in the subxiphoid space. **B,** A posterior-to-anterior orientation (as shown) is an acceptable alternative often employed to avoid the need for this additional trocar.

- The suture is then passed posterior to the suture that now bridges the bowel and the pancreas as shown in **FIGURE 6**. This maneuver is essential to prevent locking of the suture as the posterior suture line of the anastomosis is initiated.
- An additional purchase of the reconstructive limb is taken and then the suture is "parachuted" down to appose the reconstructive limb to the remnant pancreas (**FIGURE 7**). Care

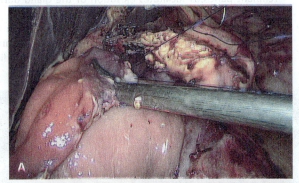

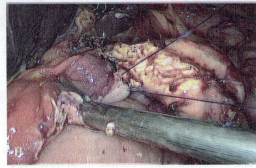

FIGURE 7 • The suture is parachuted, bringing the pancreas and jejunum into apposition. **A,** The knot that was fashioned to create the double-armed suture (cannot be visualized in this photograph) is brought into apposition with the serosa of the jejunum and then the suture is tightened while the jejunum is grasped and moved into position adjacent to the pancreas. **B,** The serosa of the jejunum is now in apposition with the posterior capsule of the pancreas.

should be taken to ensure that the knot securing the two arms of the suture is in good apposition to the serosa of the bowel. Failure to do so will subsequently impact the ability to obtain adequate tissue apposition at the cephalad aspect of the anastomosis with the first tissue bites of the anterior suture line.
- The first assistant provides exposure and maintains tension on the suture line by grasping the suture with an atraumatic grasper approximately 1.5 to 2 cm above suture line

Chapter 36 LAPAROSCOPIC AND ROBOTIC PANCREATICOJEJUNOSTOMY 293

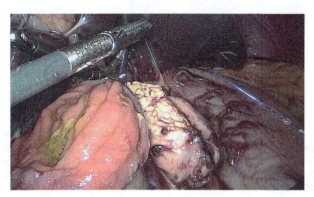

FIGURE 8 • The first assistant provides anterior tension to the suture line. This tension also facilitates exposure to the posterior surface of the pancreas.

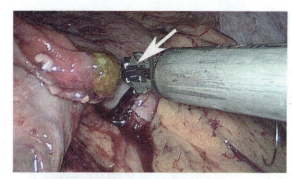

FIGURE 10 • At the caudad aspect of the posterior suture line, a Lapra-Ty is placed to maintain tension.

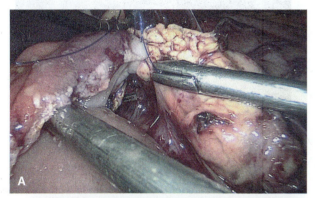

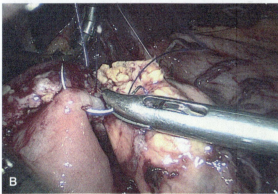

FIGURE 9 • **A,** Formation of the posterior row is *continued* with a forehand bite of the pancreas, followed by **(B)** a seromuscular bite of the adjacent jejunum. The surgeon then applies tension to the stitch and passes it back to the assistant who again maintains tension and exposure. This process is repeated every 3 to 4 mm until the caudad aspect of the suture line is reached.

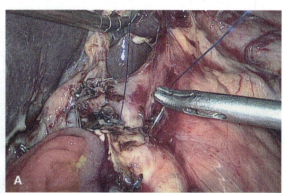

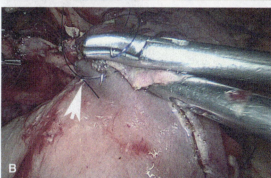

FIGURE 11 • **A,** The first bite of the anterior suture line is taken in the cephalad aspect of the pancreas. **B,** Placement of the initial bite of jejunum. The *arrow* marks the suture knot that holds the two arms of the suture together and is now located at the cephalad aspect of the posterior suture line.

- as shown in **FIGURE 8**. The posterior suture line is then run continuously (**FIGURE 9**). The operating surgeon sets the tension of the suture on the tissue after each bite of jejunum, and then passes the suture on tension to the first assistant. At the caudad aspect of the pancreas, the suture is held by the placement of a Lapra-Ty (**FIGURE 10**).
- The anterior suture line is performed next. The first bite of tissue is taken on the cephalad aspect of the pancreas immediately adjacent to the initial suture of the posterior row (**FIGURE 11**). The first bite of the reconstructive limb is similarly positioned

in close proximity to the knot that holds the two arms of the suture together and also serves to provide tension on the cephalad aspect of the posterior suture line (**FIGURE 12**).
- The assistant applies tension to the suture line after each subsequent bite of jejunum as the primary surgeon inverts the mucosa of the bowel. Applying this tension to the left side of the patient facilitates the drawing of the jejunum up over the anterior aspect of the pancreas, thus inducing the intussusception.
- As this suture line is continued caudally, the intussusception progresses, and typically, the tension on the jejunum will lead to completion of the intussusception prior to the placement of the last few bites of tissue (**FIGURE 13**).
- At the completion of this suture line, a second Lapra-Ty is placed to maintain tension. The suture is then tied (**FIGURE 14**).

SECTION III SURGERY OF THE PANCREAS

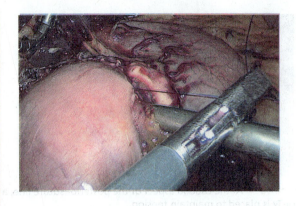

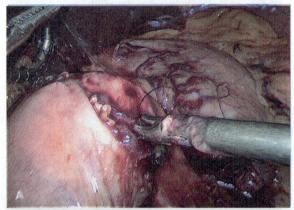

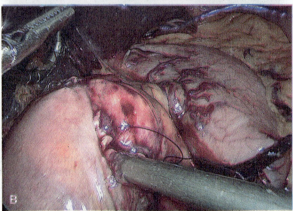

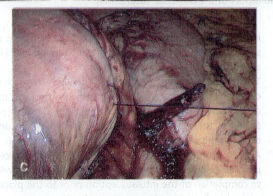

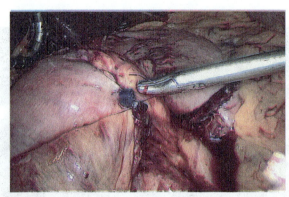

FIGURE 12 • The surgeon inverts the jejunal mucosa as the first assistant applies tension to the suture. This tension should be applied to the patient's left to facilitate rolling of the jejunal wall over the anterior aspect of the pancreas, resulting in the pancreas intussuscepting into the lumen of the jejunum.

FIGURE 14 • The anterior suture is secured with a second Lapra-Ty and the anterior and posterior sutures are tied.

FIGURE 13 • **A–C,** As the anterior suture line nears completion, a final tuft of jejunal mucosa is typically present and subsequently inverted with each additional suture until the intussusception of the pancreas into the lumen of the jejunum is complete.

Chapter 36 LAPAROSCOPIC AND ROBOTIC PANCREATICOJEJUNOSTOMY

END-TO-SIDE, DUCT-TO-MUCOSA (BLUMGART) ANASTOMOSIS

- There are two technical challenges to laparoscopically performing this proven approach to PJ.[4]
  - The surgeon must maintain an organization system for the multiple, interrupted sutures that are placed and not immediately tied.
  - Orienting the course of the needle during the placement of the duct-to-mucosa sutures with the standard trocar placement can prove difficult. The strategic placement of an additional 5-mm trocar(s) (often best positioned in the midline, below the xiphoid) can overcome this challenge.
- The anastomosis is initiated by the placement of a series of 3-0 polyglactin sutures on an SH-1 needle. These interrupted sutures are placed full thickness as depicted in FIGURE 15. The suture passes anterior to posterior through the full thickness of the pancreas. A longitudinal, seromuscular bite of jejunum is taken posterior to the intended duct-to-mucosa anastomosis at the antimesenteric border, and the suture is brought back through the full thickness of the pancreas. Care is taken not to traverse the pancreatic duct with these sutures. Typically, five to six sutures are required. To maintain organization of the suture pairs, clips should be applied across the paired strands. This approach will also maintain proximity of the bowel to the pancreas as the duct-to-mucosa sutures are placed. Varying the length of each suture can also be helpful in maintaining organization.
  - Two 4-0 polyglactin sutures on an RB-1 needle are then placed in a duct-to-mucosa fashion as shown in FIGURE 16. Once both are placed, these sutures are tied down, bringing the bowel and pancreatic duct into apposition. Care must be taken to prevent any tension to the anastomosis at this point, as these sutures will easily tear through the soft pancreatic duct.
  - The anterior row of duct-to-mucosa anastomosis is then fashioned with additional interrupted 4-0 polyglactin sutures (FIGURE 17). Some surgeons favor the placement of a silastic stent prior to this step to prevent accidentally incorporating the back wall of the

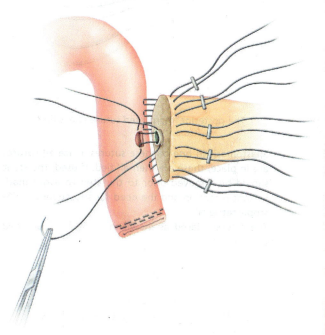

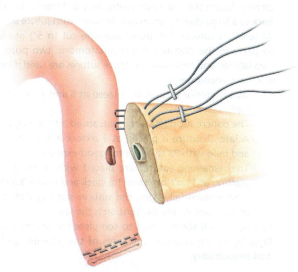

FIGURE 15 • An end-to-side, duct-to-mucosa pancreaticojejunostomy is initiated by placing a posterior row of sutures. This row opposes the posterior aspect of the pancreas to the reconstructive jejunal limb. The sutures are placed through the full thickness of the pancreas to allow all of the sutures to be thrown prior to tying the sutures. This provides additional exposure during subsequent steps but does mandate that an organizational system is employed to prevent confusion regarding the paired strands.

FIGURE 16 • Typically, two sutures are placed to initiate the posterior aspect of the duct-to-mucosa anastomosis. As shown, the knots are positioned outside of the lumen. Some surgeons place these sutures so that the knots are within the lumen.

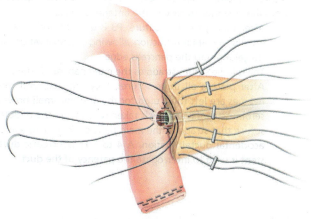

FIGURE 17 • The anterior duct-to-mucosa sutures are placed. An optional silastic stent can be placed to prevent inadvertently incorporating the posterior wall of the anastomosis. This may be particularly useful when the pancreatic duct is of small caliber. The stent should be removed prior to completion of the anastomosis.

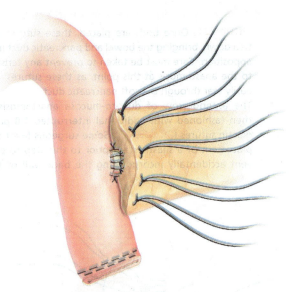

FIGURE 18 • The posterior interrupted suture line is tied.

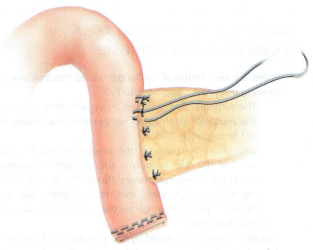

FIGURE 19 • Construction of the anterior suture line to approximate the anterior aspect of the pancreas to the jejunum. Note the incorporation of the tied suture placed as shown in FIGURES 15 and 18.

anastomosis in one of these sutures. Once all sutures are in place, these are then all tied. If used, the stent should be removed prior to this step to avoid inadvertent retention and the need for subsequent endoscopic retrieval.
- The sutures placed as shown in FIGURE 15 are tied (FIGURE 18).

- The anterior row of sutures is oriented longitudinally in the pancreatic parenchyma and then a seromuscular bite of the jejunum is taken. The pioneer of this anastomotic technique advocates incorporating the tied suture from the posterior sutures to minimize laceration of the often-soft pancreas tissues (FIGURE 19).

ROBOTIC END-TO-SIDE, DUCT-T-MUCOSA (MODIFIED BLUMGART) ANASTOMOSIS
(▶ VIDEO 2)

- Three horizontal mattress sutures are placed using 2-0 v-20 silk sutures cut to 8″. The sutures are placed full thickness on the pancreas first, from the anterior surface to the posterior surface. Then, a horizontal seromuscular bite of the jejunum is taken. Finally, a full-thickness bite is taken on the pancreas from the posterior surface to the anterior surface.
  - After taking the first suture, P3 is used to grab it and provide a cranial retraction allowing approximation of the jejunum to the pancreas edge.
  - The middle suture straddles the main pancreatic duct.
  - After placing all three sutures, they are tied, and the needles are left to be used for the anterior small bowel seromuscular layer. Care is taken when tying the middle suture that straddles the main pancreatic duct to avoid accidental ductal ligation. A 4 to 5 Fr pancreatic duct stent is used to interrogate the patency of the duct.
- P1 is switched to a monopolar scissors and used to perform an enterotomy on the antimesenteric border of the jejunum directly facing the main pancreatic duct and then is switched back to a large dual function needle driver with suture scissors.
- At least six sutures (5-0 polydioxanone cut to 5″) are used to perform the duct-to-mucosa anastomosis: two posterior, two lateral, and two anterior. More sutures are used if larger ducts are encountered.
  - Two posterior sutures are placed at 5 and 7 o'clock and tied.
  - The pancreatic duct stent is advanced into the jejunum.
  - A lateral suture is placed at 9 o'clock and kept untied and held with P3 to allow for good exposure.
  - The remaining sutures are placed without tying them starting at 11 o'clock then 1 o'clock and finally 3 o'clock.
  - Start sequentially tying the sutures starting with the 9 o'clock one where the tension is the least.
- Finally, the 2-0 silk are used to complete the anterior outer layer by taking seromuscular bites of the jejunum and are tied sequentially.

PEARLS AND PITFALLS

Patient history and physical findings	• Anticipate a soft-textured pancreas in the clinical setting of neuroendocrine, intrapancreatic bile duct, and duodenal neoplasms. A soft-textured gland is associated with higher complication rates.
Surgical management	• Adequate mobilization of the pancreatic remnant is essential for placement of posterior sutures. • Place additional 5-mm trocar(s) in the subxiphoid space or elsewhere if the orientation of the stitch cannot be optimized with the standard trocar placement during laparoscopic surgery. • If using the interrupted suturing technique, keep the sutures as short as possible and strictly adhere to an organization method, ie, clip paired strands together. • Robotic surgery provides increased range of motion and magnification, which facilitates performing a duct-to-mucosa anastomosis.
Postoperative care	• Bleeding (either intraluminal or via operatively placed drains) that occurs after 5-7 days in the setting of a pancreatic fistula is due to a life-threatening pseudoaneurysm until proven otherwise. • Delayed gastric emptying should be assumed to be due to an evolving pancreatic fistula.

POSTOPERATIVE CARE

- Patients typically require admission postoperatively to a closely monitored setting.
- Drain amylases are obtained on postoperative days 1 and 3.
- Drains can be removed, provided the amylase content is less than 5000 IUD on postoperative day 1 and has decreased significantly on postoperative day 3.
- Drains rich in amylase content should be left in place until the content returns to that of serum, or the drain output is less than 10 mL/d.
- Sandostatin therapy does not reduce rates of pancreatic fistula but may shorten the time required for a fistula to close.
- Delayed gastric emptying often accompanies evolving pancreatic fistula. If a surgical feeding system was not placed at the time of the operation, a nasojejunal feeding tube can be placed, understanding that this is associated with increased risk given the recent enteric anastomosis. Alternatively, total parental nutrition may be necessary. Nutritional support should be in place by postoperative day 7.

COMPLICATIONS

- Fistula[2]
- Delayed gastric emptying[5]
- Hemorrhage (pseudoaneurysm)[6]
- Sepsis
- Death

OUTCOMES

- The overall fistula rate should be approximately 25% (range of 15%-40%) over a large series and typically correlate with the percentage of soft glands in the series.[7-10]

REFERENCES

1. Hoehn RS, Nassour I, Adam MA, Winters S, Paniccia A, Zureikat AH. National trends in robotic pancreas surgery. *J Gastrointest Surg*. 2021;25(4):983-990. doi:10.1007/s11605-020-04591-w
2. Bassi C, Marchegiani G, Dervenis C, et al. The 2016 update of the International Study Group (ISGPS) definition and grading of postoperative pancreatic fistula: 11 Years after. *Surgery*. 2017;161(3):584-591. doi:10.1016/j.surg.2016.11.014
3. Hughes SJ, Neichoy B, Behrns KE. Laparoscopic intussuscepting pancreaticojejunostomy. *J Gastrointest Surg*. 2014;18(1):208-212. doi:10.1007/s11605-013-2308-0
4. Grobmyer SR, Kooby D, Blumgart LH, Hochwald SN. Novel pancreaticojejunostomy with a low rate of anastomotic failure-related complications. *J Am Coll Surg*. 2010;210(1):54-59. doi:10.1016/j.jamcollsurg.2009.09.020
5. Wente MN, Bassi C, Dervenis C, et al. Delayed gastric emptying (DGE) after pancreatic surgery: a suggested definition by the International Study Group of Pancreatic Surgery (ISGPS). *Surgery*. 2007;142(5):761-768. doi:10.1016/j.surg.2007.05.005
6. Wente MN, Veit JA, Bassi C, et al. Postpancreatectomy hemorrhage (PPH)–An International Study Group of Pancreatic Surgery (ISGPS) definition. *Surgery*. 2007;142(1):20-25. doi:10.1016/j.surg.2007.02.001
7. Berger AC, Howard TJ, Kennedy EP, et al. Does type of pancreaticoduodenostomy after pancreaticoduodenectomy decrease rate of pancreatic fistula? A randomized, prospective, dual-institution trial. *J Am Coll Surgeons*. 2009;208(5):738-747. doi:10.1016/j.jamcollsurg.2008.12.031
8. Kennedy EP, Yeo CJ. Dunking pancreaticojejunostomy versus duct-to-mucosa anastomosis. *J Hepato-bil-pan Sci*. 2011;18(6):769. doi:10.1007/s00534-011-0429-y
9. Nassour I, Wang SC, Christie A, et al. Minimally invasive versus open pancreaticoduodenectomy: a propensity-matched Study from a National Cohort of patients. *Ann Surg*. 2017;268(1):1. doi:10.1097/sla.0000000000002259
10. Nassour I, Wang SC, Porembka MR, et al. Robotic versus laparoscopic pancreaticoduodenectomy: a NSQIP analysis. *J Gastrointest Surg*. 2017;244(4):10-19. doi:10.1007/s11605-017-3543-6

Chapter 37 Portal Vein Resection and Reconstruction

Ibrahim Nassour, Alessandro Paniccia, and Steven J. Hughes

DEFINITION

- Borderline resectable pancreatic cancer is anatomically defined by tumor contact with the superior mesenteric vein (SMV)/portal vein (PV) of >180° or contact of ≤180° with contour irregularity of the vein or thrombosis of the vein but with suitable vessel proximal and distal to the site of involvement allowing for vein reconstruction.
- En bloc SMV/PV resection with immediate reconstruction with the goal of achieving R0 is accepted as a standard of care and is safely performed by high-volume pancreatic surgery centers.
- Benchmark outcomes for pancreatoduodenectomy with portomesenteric venous resection have been established and could be used as reference in clinical practice.[1]

PATIENT HISTORY AND PHYSICAL FINDINGS

- Neoadjuvant chemotherapy is recommended in borderline resectable pancreatic cancer. FOLFIRNOX and Gemcitabine-Abraxane are the two regimens used.
- There is variability among institutions in the use of neoadjuvant radiation following chemotherapy. Placement of fiducial markers may be useful for targeting purposes.
- History of hypercoagulopathy, thromboembolic events, lower extremity edema, and previous central lines are the important considerations for surgical planning.

IMAGING AND OTHER DIAGNOSTIC STUDIES

- The preferred modality of imaging is thin-slice, multidetector computed tomography (CT) with angiography using a dual-phase pancreatic protocol. The images are obtained in the pancreatic and portal venous phase of contrast enhancement (**FIGURE 1**)
- Imaging should be performed at least at presentation and within 4 weeks of surgery following neoadjuvant therapy. Decisions about management should involve a multidisciplinary team at a high-volume center.

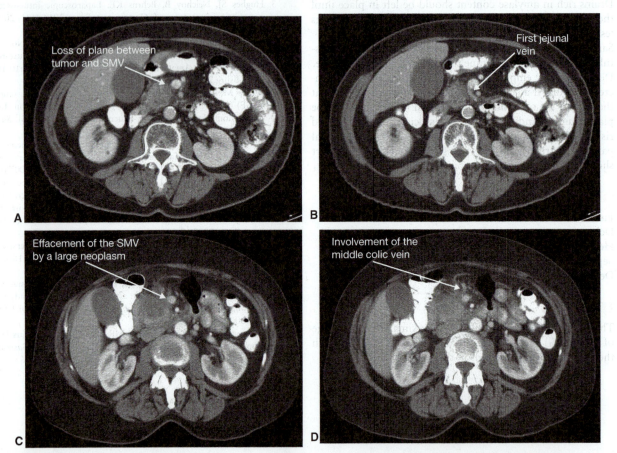

FIGURE 1 • **A,** Computed tomography (CT) of a patient with pancreatic cancer demonstrating superior mesenteric vein (SMV) involvement. **B,** The insertion of the first jejunal branch proved to be involved. The resulting lateral wall defect was repaired with a bovine pericardial patch. **C,** CT of a patient with large pancreatic cancer demonstrating 180° effacement of the SMV and **(D)** middle colic vein involvement. An interposition graft was planned and ultimately required to obtain an R0 resection and perform the subsequent reconstruction.

- Loss of fat plane, tumor abutment, and focal narrowing of the mesentericoportal complex are predictive of SMV/PV involvement. Imaging may fail to detect venous invasion in up to 40% of the cases, ultimately requiring vein resection.[2]
- A baseline CA19-9 level should be measured at the time of diagnosis or after biliary decompression once bilirubin is within normal limits. Subsequent decrease of CA19-9 levels—especially normalization following neoadjuvant therapy—is a good prognostic factor.

PREOPERATIVE PLANNING

- An accurate preoperative assessment of vessel invasion is paramount to allow for appropriate operative planning and selection of adequate conduit if needed.
- When anticipated preoperatively, en bloc vascular resection results in lower rates of positive margins in comparison to unplanned resections.
- Ensure availability of other hepatopancreaticobiliary surgeons or vascular surgeons, depending on the surgeon expertise. One of the theoretical advantages of using expert assistance includes a decreased ischemia time that ultimately leads to less bowel edema, postoperative ileus, and anastomotic leak.
- Based on the CT scan, estimate the length of the PV involved and the resulting defect requiring reconstruction (**FIGURE 2**).
  - A defect measuring less than 2 cm can usually be repaired primarily.
  - A defect up to 4 to 5 cm can also be repaired primarily in an end-to-end fashion. This may need mobilizing of the

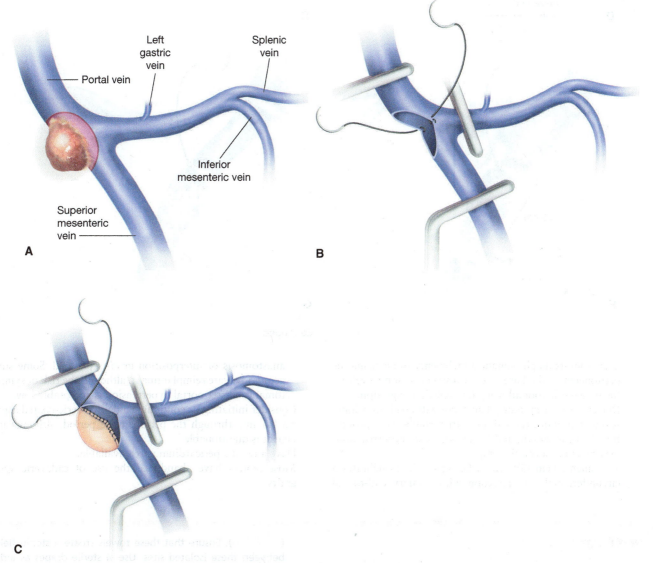

FIGURE 2 • Potential resection options and the associated reconstruction approaches in ascending level of complexity. **A,** A common location for a lesion that involves the lateral aspect of the portal vein (PV) but where the medial wall (involving the splenic vein [SV]/PV confluence) can be preserved. The *red line* indicates the planned vein resection margin. **B,** Transverse closure of a longitudinal lateral wall defect. **C,** Use of a patch to repair a large lateral wall defect. **D,** A lesion resulting in significant narrowing of the superior mesenteric vein (SMV) requiring excision of the vein. The *red areas* represent the planned resection margin. **E,** Primary end-to-end venous anastomosis for reconstruction. This approach is appropriate when the vein defect is less than a 4 to 5-cm gap or with mesenteric mobilization; the ends can be approximated without tension. **F,** Reconstruction using an autologous vein graft (gap in excess of 4 to 5 cm or under tension). **G,** If the SV confluence with the SMV is involved, reconstruction of SV inflow is optional.

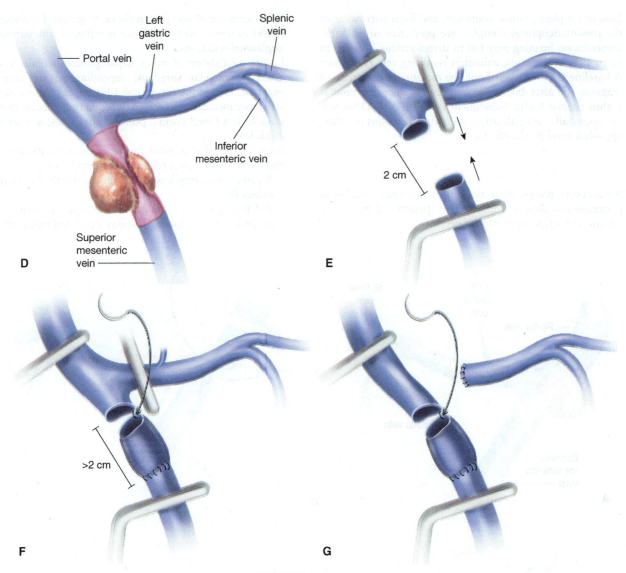

FIGURE 2 • Continued

liver from its diaphragmatic attachments and incising the peritoneum at the base of the transverse colon to release the mesenteric root allowing for cephalad migration.
- Defects measuring more than 5 cm will result in a long-segment conduit; the risk of graft thrombosis is proportional to the length, and longer segment reconstructions may preclude surgical therapy.
- The splenic vein (SV) could be ligated if it facilitates a circumferential vein resection with primary end-to-end anastomosis or interposition graft is planned. Some surgeons advocate reimplanting it, although the risk of symptomatic sinister portal hypertension is acceptably low.
- Consider initiating or continuing a daily enteric-coated aspirin (81 mg) through the perioperative period, although its benefit is questionable.[3]
- Have a bovine pericardium patch available.
- Most centers have abandoned the use of cadaveric vein grafts.

POSITIONING

- The patient is placed in a supine position with the left arm tucked allowing access to the left neck in case the jugular vein is needed as a graft (FIGURE 3).
- An upper or lower body active warming device is placed depending on the planned source of conduit.
- Prepare the patient's skin. Then, isolate the left neck or left thigh and abdominal operative fields with sterile towels (FIGURE 4). Ensure that these towels create a sterile field between these isolated sites. Use ¾ sterile drapes as indicated to achieve this objective. The authors support the use of iodine-containing, self-adhesive barriers to secure these fields under the additional overlying draping and reduce the risk of surgical site infections.
- To minimize the risk of hypothermia, drape the patient such that only the abdominal operative field is exposed. This drape will be cut to expose the graft harvest site when indicated.

Chapter 37 PORTAL VEIN RESECTION AND RECONSTRUCTION

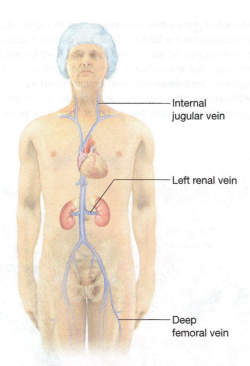

FIGURE 3 • Autologous sources of interposition vein grafts include the jugular, left renal, and deep femoral veins.

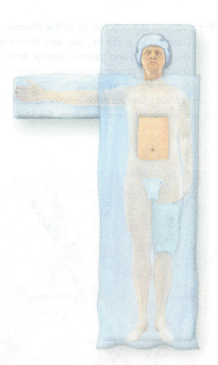

FIGURE 4 • The patient is positioned supine with the left arm tucked. The left leg is prepared and draped with towels, then the abdomen is prepped and draped in a way that should access need to be obtained for the left leg, the draping can be removed or exposed by cutting through the overlying drape without compromising either aseptic operative field.

INCISION AND EXPOSURE

- A midline incision from the xiphoid to just below the umbilicus is preferred to allow for adequate exposure of the upper and mid-abdomen and to allow for complete mobilization of the right colon and retroperitoneal attachments of the small bowel mesentery.

DISSECTION

- The dissection proceeds for the most part as presented in detail in Chapter 31, but may include limiting particular portions of the dissection; *most importantly, the uncinate process/superior mesenteric artery (SMA) dissection is performed prior to dissection of the SMV/PV.*
    - Perform a complete Cattell-Braasch maneuver, fully mobilizing the retroperitoneal attachments of the cecum, right colon, and small bowel mesentery to the left of the aorta and up to the third portion of the duodenum.
    - As part of the Kocher maneuver, establish a plane between the third portion of the duodenum and the aorta and extend this dissection cephalad to the origin of the SMA (**FIGURE 5**).
    - Mobilize the ligament of Treitz and derotate the small bowel such that the cecum is in the left upper quadrant.
    - These maneuvers will provide excellent exposure and mobility of the mesentery to facilitate primary reconstruction without undue tension following mesentericoportal resections up to 3 to 5 cm in length.
- This mobilization will also expose the anterior aspect of the left renal vein—a potential source of reconstruction conduit.
- Open the lesser sac (omental bursa) and expose the pancreatic head. Assess the root of the transverse mesocolon and bimanually palpate the lesion. Also, palpate the course of the SMA with respect to the palpable lesion.
- Proceed with the dissection of the inferior and superior borders of the pancreas, identifying the anterior borders of the SMV and PV proximal and distal to the area of tumor involvement, respectively.
- By palpation and visualization, identify the relationship of the tumor with respect to the SV/SMV confluence.
- Establish the plane between the root of the mesentery and the third and fourth portions of the duodenum and uncinate process.
- Determine resectability with respect to involvement of the SMV/PV and the extent of resection required.
    - Unless a plane can be readily established anterior to the SMV/PV confluence (ie, only the lateral wall of the vein is involved), save the division of the pancreatic neck for later.

- Proceed with the other steps of the dissection.
    - Dissect the porta hepatis and divide and control the bile duct and gastroduodenal artery.
    - Divide the proximal gastrointestinal tract (duodenum or stomach).
- Approaching from the posterior–inferior, dissect the uncinate process and duodenal mesentery from the SMA, hugging the adventitial plane while working caudad to cephalad until the lateral aspect of the SMA has been fully dissected up to its origin from the aorta. An energy device can be used for much of this dissection, but the authors recommend ligation or suturing of any identified inferior pancreaticoduodenal artery (**FIGURE 6**).
- Alternatively, the SMA dissection can be facilitated by approaching it from the anterior aspect, inferior to the

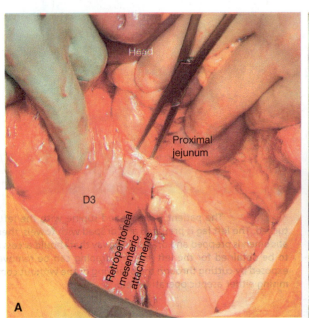
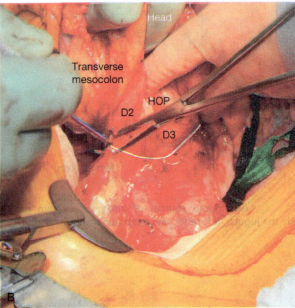

FIGURE 5 • **A,** Completely mobilize the right colon and the retroperitoneal attachments of the small bowel. **B,** Extend the dissection by mobilizing the retroperitoneal attachments of the duodenum and pancreatic head to the origin of the superior mesenteric artery (*white line* represents plane of dissection). D2, second portion of the duodenum; D3, third portion of the duodenum; HOP, head of the pancreas.

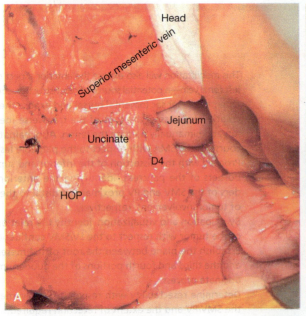
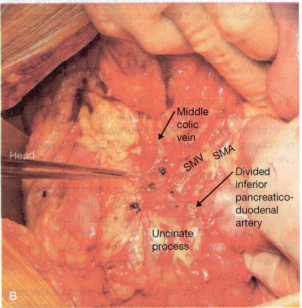

FIGURE 6 • Establish the plane between the root of the mesentery and the third and fourth portions of the duodenum and uncinate process. **A,** Mobilize the uncinate process along the adventitia of the superior mesenteric artery (SMA) (*white line* represents plane of dissection). **B,** Control the inferior pancreaticoduodenal arteries with ligatures. HOP, head of the pancreas; SMV, superior mesenteric vein. D4, fourth portion of the duodenum.

takeoff of the middle colic artery but superior to the arborization of the artery. First, isolate and encircle with a vessel loop the SMV well inferior to the tumor (FIGURE 7). Dissect down to the adventitia and then continue dissecting along the right lateral border until you break through to the posterior dissection plane. Once this maneuver has been performed, continuing the dissection cephalad is straightforward from the posterior–inferior approach described earlier.
- Confirm the resection plan and required reconstruction. Particularly, determine if an interposition graft will be required. Harvesting of this graft *should be performed first* to minimize vascular clamp time and the resultant bowel edema that impacts reconstruction of intestinal continuity.

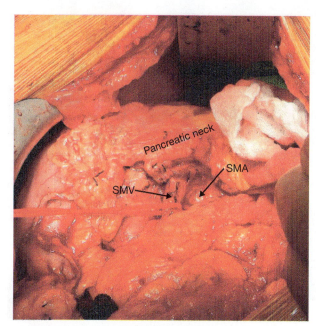

FIGURE 7 • Circumferentially dissect the superior mesenteric vein (SMV) and control it with a vessel loop. This also provides an anterior approach to the distal superior mesenteric artery (SMA). This approach also provides safe access to the adventitial plane of the SMA.

PROCURE THE RECONSTRUCTION CONDUIT

- Intravenously administer unfractionated heparin sulfate (50 IU/kg) and allow time for the drug to circulate. This step can be skipped if the anticipated reconstruction time will be short.
- Have a basin with heparinized normal saline (100 IU/mL) available to store the conduit.

Left Renal Vein

- When of adequate length, the left renal vein is an ideal source of conduit as it can be procured without establishing another surgical field, is typically of appropriate caliber, and has a relatively thick wall that holds sutures well.
- Assess the left renal vein for caliber and length (from the insertion of the left gonadal vein to the inferior vena cava) and determine if it is suitable as the conduit for reconstruction. If the interposition graft is of an anticipated length of 5 cm, the length of conduit should be slightly longer.
- Circumferentially dissect the vein and control it with vessel loops. Using vascular clamps, control the vein proximally and distally and sharply excise the conduit. Place it in heparinized saline (100 IU/mL).

- Use a running 5-0 Prolene to control the proximal renal vein and vena cava.

Femoral Vein or Saphenous Vein

- The deep femoral vein is also an excellent source of conduit as it is relatively thick walled, of good caliber, and never inadequate in length, and complications associated with the procurement site are rare.[4] Alternatively, the saphenous vein instead can be used with similar outcomes.
- Prepare the surgical field for conduit procurement by cutting the overlying draping. Use additional towels as indicated.
- Use a clean set of instruments and keep them separate from those used for the abdominal surgical field.
- The left thigh is more readily available.
- See Lee et al. for details of the exposure and other details of the technique.[5]

Jugular Vein

- The left jugular vein is the preferred conduit for PV reconstructions at some centers.

VASCULAR CONTROL AND RESECTION

- If the pancreatic neck has not been divided, establish a plane posterior to the pancreas at the level of planned transection (this is often at the level of the pancreatic body to the left of the SMV/PV confluence). Divide the pancreas and obtain hemostasis on the cut surface.
- Isolate and control the SV with a vessel loop (FIGURE 8). During this dissection, be mindful of the left gastric vein. It typically inserts into the cephalad aspect of the SV approximately 1 cm proximal to the SMV/PV confluence. It is at risk for injury during isolation of the SV or inserting distal to the point of control; this will lead to a lack of hemostasis after clamping during the vein resection. The authors typically ligate and divide this vein.
- The insertion of the inferior mesenteric vein into the SV is quite variable. It may need to be independently isolated if it inserts in close proximity to the SMV/PV confluence.

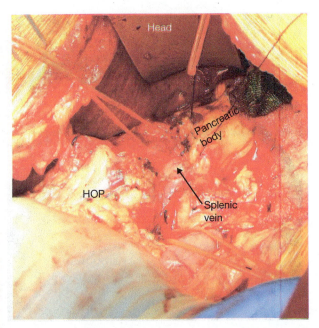 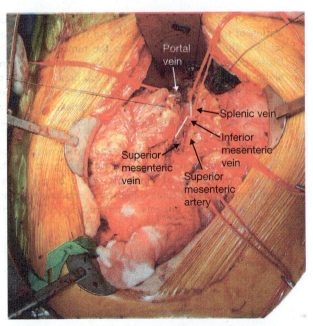

FIGURE 8 • If indicated, isolate and control the splenic vein (SV). In this circumstance, the tumor is attached to the lateral aspect of the superior mesenteric vein (SMV)/portal vein (PV) confluence. The pancreas has been divided to the left of the pancreatic neck to provide an adequate margin and expose the anterior surface of the SV. During this dissection, be mindful of the left gastric vein. It typically inserts into the cephalad aspect of the SV approximately 1 cm proximal to the SMV/PV confluence. It is at risk for injury during isolation of the SV or inserting distal to the point of control; this will lead to a lack of hemostasis after clamping during the vein resection.

- Circumferentially dissect the SMV proximal to the area of venous involvement. Control it with a vessel loop. Be mindful of the first jejunal branch of the SMV. This vessel usually receives a larger tributary vein from the uncinate process and injury or loss of control can be quite challenging. Furthermore, obtaining control proximal to the vessel will not lead to a hemostatic field.
- Get control of the PV above the planned level of vein resection. Identify the posterosuperior pancreaticoduodenal vein (PSPDV or vein of Belcher) and isolate, ligate, and divide it.
- At this point, proximal and distal control has been achieved (**FIGURE 9**).

FIGURE 9 • Proximal and distal control with complete mobilization of the uncinate process off of the superior mesenteric artery. The *white lines* represent the planned venous resection lines. This plan includes a tangential proximal anastomosis that incorporates and aberrant inferior mesenteric vein insertion into the superior mesenteric vein (SMV) and ligation of the splenic vein.

- If a conduit was not procured, intravenously administer unfractionated heparin sulfate (50 IU/kg); allow at least 1 minute for the drug to circulate prior to placing clamps. The authors prefer to have the clamps relatively remote from the planned resection planes; this length provides better exposure and mobility of the vessels during the reconstruction.
- Mark the anterior surface of the vessels using a marking pen. This will facilitate maintenance of the vessels' orientation. Alternatively, consider marking the anterior aspect of the vein with a fine monofilament suture. Loss of this orientation is surprisingly easy and can result in torsion and narrowing of the reconstruction. Sharply divide the vein(s) along the planned resection plane.
- Orient the pathologist to the specimen using sutures. One or more of these sutures should identify the venous margins.

RECONSTRUCTION

- The vascular reconstruction proceeds immediately.
- Place moistened white towels around the field and over the fixed retractor blades/arms to better see the fine reconstructive suture and avoid tangling it on the retractor.
- Use 6-0 Prolene on a fine vascular needle for the repair.
- The authors do not reverse the systemic anticoagulation effects of the heparin unless necessary to control nonsurgical bleeding at the completion of the procedure.

Primary Transverse Closure

- Place single-armed 6-0 Prolene sutures at the (1) anterior and (2) posterior longitudinal midpoints of the venotomy

(**FIGURE 10**). The two stitches are placed longitudinally, 1 mm from the cut edge from outside in and then immediately back inside out so that they can be tied and result with the knot outside the lumen.

- Begin with the posterior suture, advancing 1 mm cephalad from outside the lumen into the lumen.
- Run the posterior suture visualizing the placement of the sutures from inside the lumen until the anterior suture can be used to complete the anastomosis with visualization from outside the vessel lumen.
- Release the PV clamp to allow retrograde blood flow. Allow the vessel to fill, thus degassing the anastomosis. Hold minimal tension on the sutures to allow the suture line to maximally expand before tying the two sutures together to

Chapter 37 PORTAL VEIN RESECTION AND RECONSTRUCTION 305

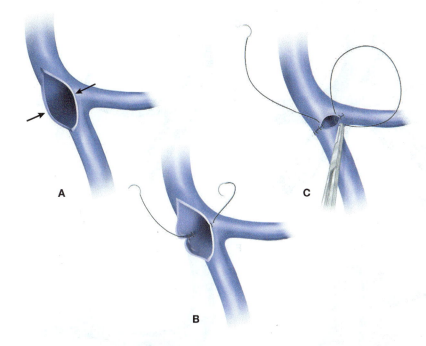

FIGURE 10 • A transverse closure of a longitudinal defect. **A,** The suture line is initiated at the anterior and posterior midpoints of the longitudinal venotomy (*arrows*). **B,** The posterior suture is run first, visualizing the repair from inside the lumen of the vessel. **C,** The anterior suture completes the anastomosis.

complete the anastomosis. Alternatively, an air knot can be incorporated when the suture is tied; this will allow for the reconstructed vein to expand without waisting. This may result in extravasation of blood initially, but usually resolves after few minutes.
- Place interrupted repair sutures as necessary to obtain a hemostatic anastomosis.
- Hemostatic agents such as cellulose may facilitate control of oozing from needle tracts.
- Release the remaining clamps.

Primary Longitudinal Closure

- Primary transverse closure is preferred over longitudinal closure due to lower thrombosis rate.
- The authors use primary longitudinal closure in very selected cases where the involvement of vein is only limited to a very short and lateral segment preventing significant narrowing.
- The advantage of this method is avoiding clamping the PV and the SMV minimizing bowel edema and decreasing operative time.
- A side bite clamp is placed longitudinal to the vein and the venotomy is repaired. The repair is done similar to what was described for a transverse repair except that one suture is placed on the superior aspect of the venotomy and the other on the inferior aspect. This can be done in an open fashion or in a robotic fashion (FIGURE 11).
- Alternatively, a 45 mm vascular stapler with an advanced placement tip can be used to resect the tumor off the vein. This is especially useful when the operation is done in a minimally invasive fashion (▶ Video 1, FIGURE 11).
- If there is a more than 25% narrowing of the vein, the authors recommend against a primary longitudinal closure.

Patch Closure

- When a lateral defect in the vein cannot be transversely closed without undue tension, employ a patch venoplasty using bovine pericardium (FIGURE 12).
- Cut the patch to size. Leaving the patch about 80% of the length of the defect and twice as wide as the defect will minimize the risk of narrowing the vessel.
- Initiate the double-armed suture line at the apex of the venotomy. The assistant retracts the patch caudally and laterally to expose the posterior suture line from the lumen side (FIGURE 12B).
- Use care to align the patch with the vein—bites of the vein should be spaced further apart to prevent a size mismatch.
- Place a second double-armed suture at the heel of the repair and then tie the posterior suture to this second suture.
- Alternatively, this suture can be placed at the same time as the apex suture and each suture can be run toward the middle. This approach reduces the risk of a significant size mismatch but limits the exposure.
- Run the anterior suture line to the midpoint of the repair and then use the heal suture to complete the anastomosis. Do not tie down the suture until retrograde restoration of blood flow has been accomplished.
- Release the remaining clamps; place repair sutures as needed.

Primary End-to-End Anastomosis

- When the vein has been circumferentially excised to obtain a margin, a primary repair can often be accomplished. Typically,

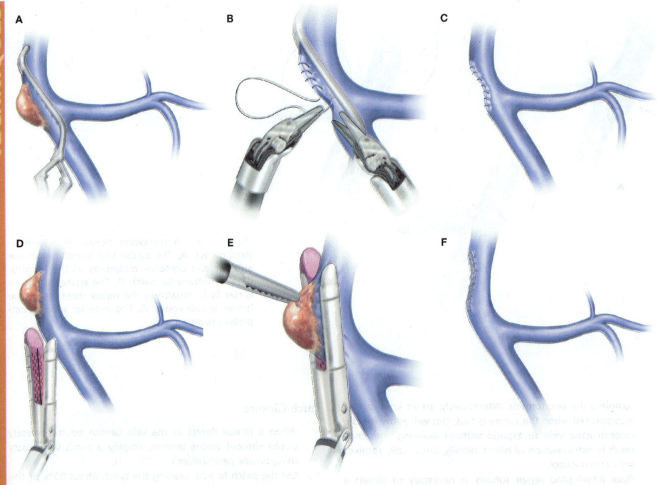

FIGURE 11 • A longitudinal closure. **A,** A side bite clamp is placed robotically. **B,** The venotomy created is closed with 6-0 Prolene robotically. **C,** The longitudinally closed venotomy shown with minimal narrowing. **D,** Tumor involving a short segment of the portal vein. **E,** A 45-mm vascular stapler with an advanced placement tip is used to resect the tumor off the vein. **F,** A longitudinal staple line causing minimal narrowing to the vein.

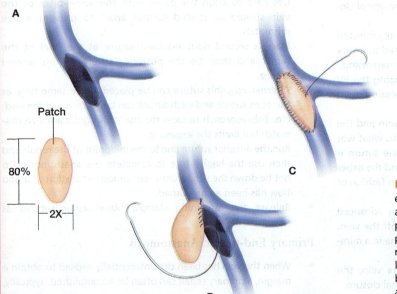

FIGURE 12 • A pericardial patch repair of a large lateral wall defect. **A,** Estimate the width of the patch and then double it to prevent narrowing. The authors prefer to also shorten the length of the defect by purposely shortening the patch. **B,** The lateral posterior suture line is placed first with exposure from the lumen side of the vein. The "heal" of the patch can be anchored to the proximal wall of the venotomy to assist in alignment (not shown). **C,** The anterior suture line is then placed to complete the patch repair.

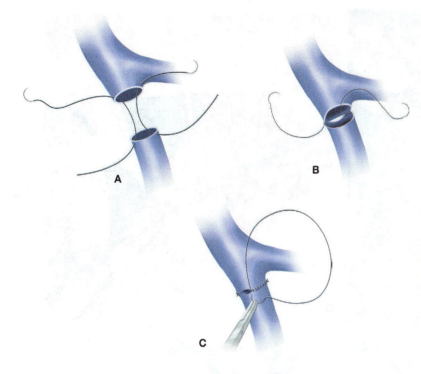

FIGURE 13 • End-to-end native vein reconstruction. Size mismatch is often an issue; the authors recommend interrupted sutures in this clinical setting. When compared to interrupted sutures, a running suture takes less time and is more hemostatic but puts the anastomosis at risk for narrowing by producing a purse-string effect. **A,** Double-armed, 6-0 Prolene sutures are placed at the 3-o'clock and 9-o'clock positions. **B,** The posterior suture line is placed under visualization from inside the lumen. The suture line is completed at the 9-o'clock position by tying the sutures together. **C,** The anterior suture line is then placed.

gaps of up to 4 to 5 cm can be closed by cephalad mobilization of the root of the mesentery and mobilizing the liver.
- Begin by placing double-armed sutures at the 3- and 9-o'clock positions (FIGURE 13). If there is a significant size mismatch, consider using interrupted sutures. The vein can usually be "rolled" 180° to expose the posterior wall so that these sutures can be placed with good exposure.
- Begin a running suture line using one of the 3-o'clock position strands. Pass this outside in the distal (hepatopedal) vein orifice. Then, run the suture using exposure from the lumen side. At the 9-o'clock position, pass the suture outside the lumen on the proximal side (hepatofugal) and tie it to one of the 9-o'clock position suture arms. Use care not to "purse-string" this posterior suture line. Some surgeons advocate not tying this suture until portal blood flow has been restored, thus allowing the suture line to "parachute" open and minimize the risk of narrowing the lumen.
- Run the anterior suture line from both the 3- and 9-o'clock positions so that the anastomosis is completed at the 12-o'clock position.

- Release the proximal clamp to degas the vessel and allow the suture line to parachute. Then, tie the sutures to complete the anastomosis and place repair sutures as needed.

Interposition Graft

- When the gap cannot be closed without undue tension, an interposition graft is indicated (FIGURE 14).
- Do not cut the conduit to length until the proximal anastomosis is completed.
- Each anastomosis is fashioned as described for the primary repair. The assistant maintains cephalad tension on the graft to facilitate the exposure.
- Minimize trauma to the endothelium of the conduit. When possible, only grasp the adventitia of the conduit with fine, atraumatic forceps.
- If the defect involves the splenoportal confluence, oversewing the SV is a reasonable option with acceptable morbidity. Reimplantation can be considered to avoid sinister portal hypertension and augment flow through the conduit, thus theoretically reducing the risk of thrombosis.

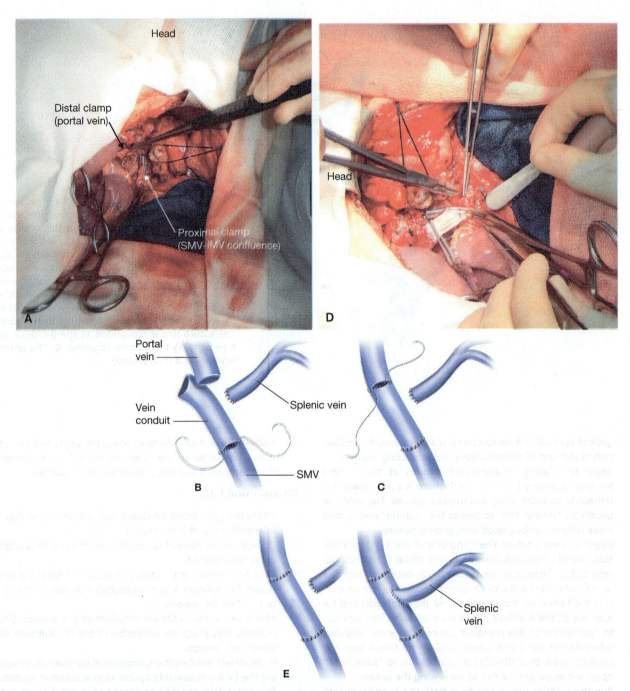

FIGURE 14 • An interposition graft repair of the superior mesenteric vein (SMV)/portal vein (PV) using a deep femoral vein conduit. In this example, the SMV/PV confluence has been resected. **A,** Intraoperative photograph of proximal and distal control with vascular clamps prior to placement of an interposition graft. The splenic vein (SV) has been oversewn and is not visualized. As nearly 5 cm of vein was resected, an interposition graft will be required but will only be 2 cm in length. This is facilitated by the mobilization of the retroperitoneal attachments of the mesentery. **B,** Reconstruction begins with the proximal anastomosis using identical technique to that depicted in **FIGURE 12**. **C,** The distal anastomosis is then constructed. **D,** Intraoperative photograph during performance of a proximal anastomosis. **E,** Reimplantation of the SV is at the surgeon's discretion. If it is performed, portal flow can be re-established prior to beginning the anastomosis by placing a side-biting clamp on the conduit. **F,** Reperfused interposition graft—the SV has been ligated by oversewing with Prolene.

Chapter 37 PORTAL VEIN RESECTION AND RECONSTRUCTION

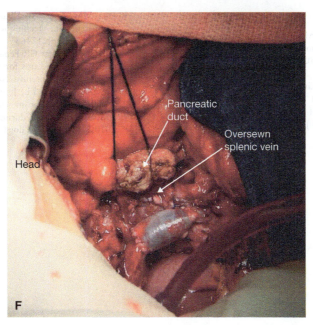

FIGURE 14 • Continued

PEARLS AND PITFALLS

Preoperative planning	■ Preoperative planning is paramount for a successful vein resection and reconstruction. ■ Determine the need of a vascular conduit based on imaging and prepare the left neck and the left thigh before starting the procedure.
Operative technique	■ Dissect the uncinate process from the SMA prior to controlling and dividing the vein. This provides superior exposure to the posterior aspect of the vein, minimizes clamp time, and avoids the tedious and occasionally bloody dissection of the uncinate while the PV is clamped. ■ Gain early control of the SMV and PV. ■ Procure the reconstruction conduit prior to clamping the mesoportal vessels and completing the resection.
Postoperative care	■ Prescribe antiplatelet therapy.

POSTOPERATIVE CARE

- Postpancreatectomy patients with venous resection are usually admitted to a monitored environment with the capacity of frequent assessment of vital signs and drain output.
- A standardized postpancreatectomy pathway should be implemented providing clear expectations for recovery on a daily basis.
- Instruct nursing team to immediately contact the service for a sudden increase in drain output; this can be the first sign of spontaneous thrombosis of the graft—early recognition of thrombosis is essential for any reasonable attempt at surgical revision.
- Bedside ultrasound with Doppler assessment is the first diagnostic modality to assess flow in the PV. Portal venous-phase CT can reliably assess patency of the PV.
- Thrombosis of the vascular reconstruction rarely occurs in the acute postoperative setting unless there is a technical error. However, it can occur over time in up to 10% to 20% of the cases. It occurs more often with patch closure and interposition graft.
- While there are no clear guidelines on the optimal pharmacological management of patients after vascular resection and reconstruction, the authors start 300 mg aspirin rectally and prophylactic heparin on postoperative day zero. Once the patient starts taking oral intake, enteric-coated oral aspirin (81 mg) is started and continued indefinitely.
- Return to the operating room or angiographic maneuvers to restore patency of a thrombosis have been reported but are rarely employed—reported patency rates of PV reconstruction exceed 90%.

OUTCOMES

- In well-selected patients, the morbidly, mortality, and oncologic outcomes of the operation are almost equivalent to standard pancreaticoduodenectomy.

COMPLICATIONS[1]

- Clinically relevant pancreatic fistula is ≤14%.
- In-hospital mortality rate is ≤4%.
- Major complication rate is ≤36%.
- PV thrombosis rate is ≤14%.
- Five-year survival rate for patients with pancreatic ductal adenocarcinoma is ≥9%.

REFERENCES

1. Raptis DA, Sánchez-Velázquez P, Machairas N, et al. Defining benchmark outcomes for pancreatoduodenectomy with portomesenteric venous resection. *Ann Surg.* 2020;272(5):731-737. doi:10.1097/sla.0000000000004267
2. Porembka MR, Hawkins WG, Linehan DC, et al. Radiologic and intraoperative detection of need for mesenteric vein resection in patients with adenocarcinoma of the head of the pancreas. *HPB.* 2011;13(9):633-642. doi:10.1111/j.1477-2574.2011.00343.x
3. Dua MM, Tran TB, Klausner J, et al. Pancreatectomy with vein reconstruction: technique matters. *HPB.* 2015;17(9):824-831. doi:10.1111/hpb.12463
4. Smith ST, Clagett GP. Femoral vein harvest for vascular reconstructions: Pitfalls and tips for success. *Semin Vasc Surg.* 2008;21(1):35-40. doi:10.1053/j.semvascsurg.2007.11.007
5. Lee DY, Mitchell EL, Jones MA, et al. Techniques and results of portal vein/superior mesenteric vein reconstruction using femoral and saphenous vein during pancreaticoduodenectomy. *J Vasc Surg.* 2010;51(3):662-666. doi:10.1016/j.jvs.2009.09.025

Chapter 38 Open Distal Pancreatectomy

Roberto J. Vidri and Rebecca M. Minter

DEFINITION

- Distal pancreatectomy is defined as the resection of the body and tail of the pancreas with a pancreatic transection point distal to (left of) the superior mesenteric vessels, with or without an *en bloc* splenectomy. As most elective distal pancreatectomies are precipitated by confirmed or suspected malignant or premalignant lesions, this chapter will discuss contemporary techniques and indications commonly applied to open distal pancreatectomy with a focus on oncological principles of resection.

PATIENT HISTORY AND PHYSICAL FINDINGS

- A detailed past medical history, in the setting of a known lesion of the pancreas, must explore known risk factors for pancreatic cancer, including a history of chronic pancreatitis, diabetes, obesity, exposure to heavy metals, heavy alcohol consumption, and smoking.[1] Character, duration, and mitigating factors of any acute or chronic abdominal or back discomfort or complaints should be explored, as should any sudden and unintended weight loss or recent onset or worsening dysglycemia. If a neuroendocrine tumor is suspected, signs or symptoms related to functional tumors such as rash, diarrhea, hypoglycemia, and peptic ulcer disease should be discussed. A detailed surgical history with special attention to previous abdominal operations is crucial.
- Medical comorbidities, as well as cardiovascular and pulmonary functional status, should be evaluated; any relevant testing required for preoperative clearance, such as stress echocardiograms or pulmonary function tests, should be performed in accordance with current anesthesia guidelines.[2]
- A thorough family history may help identify patterns of hereditary malignant disease, which in turn can guide preoperative decision making, postoperative surveillance, and genetic testing for the patient and their families.
- The physical examination must evaluate for any abdominal abnormalities such as organomegaly, hernias, and previous surgical incisions. Splenomegaly should raise concerns for sinister portal hypertension, which could be precipitated by tumor thrombosis or vascular invasion. Hepatomegaly can imply the presence of hepatic metastases. Special attention should be paid to a patient's nodal basins, specifically left supraclavicular and periumbilical nodes. Lymphadenopathy in these areas could imply the presence of an advanced, metastatic malignancy.

IMAGING AND OTHER DIAGNOSTIC STUDIES

- Laboratory testing should include a complete blood count, a comprehensive metabolic panel, liver enzymes, lipase, and amylase. A preoperative carbohydrate antigen 19-9 (CA 19-9) level is important for diagnosis and postoperative surveillance. When an endocrine tumor is suspected based upon symptoms or an underlying hereditary syndrome, functional urine and relevant hormone stimulation tests should be performed. If a patient has experienced substantial weight loss, prealbumin and albumin levels can help establish nutritional status and guide recommendations for preoperative nutritional rehabilitation and/or perioperative supplemental alimentation.
- Preoperative workup of a pancreatic mass or injury must include a contrasted, cross-sectional imaging study. Computed tomography (CT) using the "pancreas protocol," which produces triple-phase images and allows for evaluation of arterial, pancreatic, and portal venous phases, is currently the preferred imaging modality. This allows for determination of resectability and development of an appropriate operative plan. Three-dimensional reconstruction, where available, can be a valuable adjunct. **FIGURE 1** demonstrates a lesion with adrenal involvement that would be appropriate for radical antegrade modular pancreatico-splenectomy (or RAMPs, see below).
- In case of a cystic neoplasm of the pancreas, magnetic resonance cholangiopancreatography with contrast may be preferred to further characterize the cystic nature of the lesion and its communication with the main pancreatic or side branch ducts. MRI can also delineate focal fat within the pancreas and can determine if a lesion is cystic or solid.
- Endoscopic ultrasound (EUS) can elucidate possible lymph node metastases and confirm spatial relationships between a mass and the peripancreatic vasculature. Furthermore, it allows sampling of tissue and fluid from suspicious masses, lymph nodes, or cystic lesions. Multidisciplinary collaboration between surgeons and gastroenterologists is important to ensure that appropriate information is gathered and conveyed.
- The role of positron emission tomography (PET-CT) has not been completely defined, but it serves as an adjunct in selected patients.

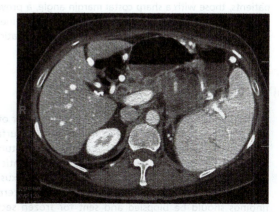

FIGURE 1 • CT scan showing distal pancreatic mass with adrenal involvement.

Table 1: Indications for Distal Pancreatectomy	
Indications for open distal pancreatectomy	**Contraindications for minimally invasive procedure**
• Malignancy with concern for vascular involvement or substantial retroperitoneal local invasion • Trauma/pancreatic duct disruption • Sequelae of acute/chronic pancreatitis (eg, stricture or disconnected pancreatic tail)	• Unable to tolerate pneumoperitoneum (ie, severe cardiopulmonary disorder) • Untreated coagulopathy or liver failure • Documentation of hostile abdomen

SURGICAL MANAGEMENT

- Whenever possible, minimally invasive techniques for distal pancreatectomy should be pursued. Indications for open distal pancreatectomy are dictated by the clinical circumstance mandating resection or the presence of a comorbidity or contraindication to laparoscopy. Patients suffering ductal rupture as a result of trauma, those with known or suspected adhesions or anatomic anomalies resulting from prior surgery, a history of peripancreatic inflammation in the setting of acute or chronic pancreatitis, a malignant diagnosis with known vascular involvement, or locally advanced disease involving the retroperitoneum should be considered for an open operative approach (**TABLE 1**).

Preoperative Planning

- Preoperative imaging typically guides the surgical approach. The planned resection margins must be carefully considered, as they relate to surrounding organs and vasculature. Particular attention must be given to the retroperitoneal margin, major mesenteric and celiac vessels, left adrenal gland, and left renal vasculature and kidney. If a portion of the colon appears involved, a bowel preparation must be considered in anticipation of an *en bloc* resection.
- Asplenic and hyposplenic patients are at risk of severe sepsis and death secondary to polysaccharide encapsulated bacteria, particularly *Streptococcus pneumoniae*, *Neisseria meningitidis*, and *Haemophilus influenzae* type b (Hib). The risk of infection and sepsis, termed "overwhelming postsplenectomy infection," is predominantly during the first 3 months post splenectomy. Thus, prophylactic vaccination against these bacteria is recommended at least 2 weeks before elective splenectomy, including influenza virus if not up to date.[3,4]
- The anesthesiology team should be informed in advance if a surgeon anticipates a difficult dissection or significant hemorrhage. A type and screen should be drawn on all patients to facilitate blood availability.
- In addition to adequate peripheral or central intravenous access, a Foley catheter, nasogastric tube, and arterial line are recommended.
- Perioperative antibiotics should be administered within 1 hour of incision. Coverage should be broad and include gram-positive skin flora, gram-negative, and anaerobic intestinal bacteria.
- The entire abdomen, from nipples to pubis, should be cleared of hair and prepped in the standard sterile manner. To facilitate subcostal and perixiphoid incisional extension, the flank area should be included in the operative field, even if a midline incision is anticipated.

Positioning

- The patient is positioned supine with arms extended out, unless precluded by patient shoulder mobility. The secure placement of the post(s) of a self-retaining retractor should be considered; a single post is ideally placed on the patient's left side.

INCISION

- Both a left subcostal and midline incision are appropriate; obesity and costal margin angularity can affect exposure. Incision location varies based on the patient's body habitus, tumor location, and surgeon preference. Generally, slender patients, those with a sharp costal margin angle, a previous midline incision, or tumors located closer to the midline are candidates for a midline incision. In case of obese patients, those with a particularly high splenic flexure, or a tumor that is relatively distal on the pancreas, a subcostal incision may provide enhanced visualization and exposure of the left upper quadrant.
- A midline incision typically extends from the xiphoid to just below the umbilicus. A left subcostal incision is made two fingerbreadths below the costal margin and carried from the midline, obliquely, to approximately the anterior axillary line.

INITIAL SURVEY AND EXPOSURE

- The abdomen is explored for signs of metastases or other unexpected pathology. The liver and peritoneal surfaces are visually examined and palpated, the omentum is examined for caking or nodularity, the gastrohepatic ligament and lymphatic tissues around the celiac plexus are inspected for any evidence of metastasis. Any concerning findings should be biopsied and sent for frozen section analysis prior to proceeding with resection. When a distal pancreatectomy is anticipated, the head of the pancreas must be examined and palpated to confirm the absence of abnormalities. In patients with high suspicion of metastatic disease, a diagnostic laparoscopy should precede open exploration.
- A self-retaining Omni-Trak or Bookwalter retractor should be placed. The Omni-Trak retractor allows for superior exposure in the upper abdomen using the sternal retractors to elevate the costal margin. If the Omni-Trak retractor is utilized, a third post is required for optimal exposure through a left subcostal incision. Some surgeons prefer the Thompson retractor.

- The splenic flexure is mobilized and reflected downward. In select patients, one may consider laparoscopic mobilization of the splenic flexure and division of the short gastric vessels prior to open distal pancreatectomy to allow for a smaller incision.

EXPOSURE OF THE PANCREAS

- The gastrocolic ligament is divided to access the lesser sac. The transverse colon is gently retracted inferiorly, with care not to avulse the middle colic vein as it inserts into the superior mesenteric vein (SMV) at the inferior neck of the pancreas.
- Unless splenic preservation using the Warshaw technique is planned, the short gastric vessels are divided with an energy device or between clamps and ties. Any posterior gastric attachments to the pancreas are divided, and the stomach is retracted superiorly to expose the anterior surface of the pancreas.
- In case of a small pancreatic lesion that is not readily identified, the inferior attachments of the pancreas can be freed to facilitate posterior palpation. The splenic vein is identified and isolated just to the left of its union with the portal vein (PV), usually beneath the pancreas. Use care to identify the inferior mesenteric vein as its insertion into the splenic vein is variable.
- Intraoperative ultrasound can be used as an adjunct to locate small lesions in the tail of the pancreas.
- Typically, the celiac trunk is located at the superior border of the pancreas. The hepatic and splenic arteries are then identified and followed to their origins. The splenic artery is then ligated and divided using either a vascular stapler or silk ties and secured with a stick tie (3-0 silk or Prolene) followed by free tie (**FIGURE 2**).

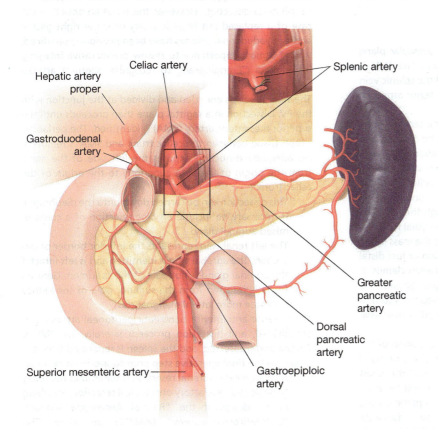

FIGURE 2 • Splenic artery division.

CHOICE OF PANCREATIC DISSECTION TECHNIQUE

- There are several, well-described, techniques to achieve a distal pancreatectomy. Preoperative planning must include a determination on surgical approach; this may include a lateral-to-medial (retrograde) or a medial-to-lateral (antegrade) dissection and whether a spleen-preserving procedure or *en bloc* splenectomy is appropriate. In the setting of malignancy, we prefer a radical antegrade resection with N1 dissection.

Splenectomy With Lateral to Medial (Retrograde) Dissection

- Beginning at the inferior pancreatic border, the posterior pancreatic attachments to the retroperitoneum are divided until the inferior mesenteric vein (IMV) and SMV are visualized (**FIGURE 3**). The pancreas is gently retracted anteriorly,

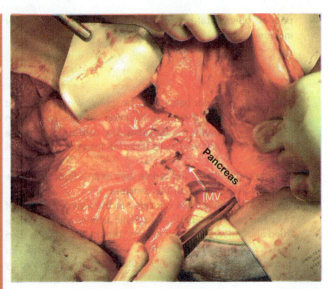

FIGURE 3 • Exposure of inferior pancreatic border—SMV and IMV.

which should facilitate development of the avascular plane between the pancreas and retroperitoneum. The IMV is divided if it inserts into the splenic vein, and the splenic vein is elevated with the specimen along the posterior aspect of the pancreas.

- With the body and tail of the pancreas mobilized, the splenorenal and splenophrenic attachments can be divided, and the spleen is mobilized from the posterior abdominal wall. At this point, posterior mobilization should be complete and the spleen and distal pancreas can be reflected medially. The splenic artery is identified, typically running along the superior border of the pancreas, although there can be anatomic variability, including an intraparenchymal location. The splenic artery is isolated 2 cm proximal to the mass lesion at the site of planned parenchymal transection or just distal to its origin from the celiac and divided between clamps. It is doubly secured with a stick tie and a simple ligature. The splenic vein can then be identified and followed to its confluence with the PV; it is then divided and ligated or oversewn or stapled at the insertion into the PV.
- With the distal pancreas entirely mobilized, palpation of the gland is performed to ensure that the anticipated point of transection is free from the lesion of interest. If the point of transection needs to occur proximal to the splenic vein–PV confluence, and the PV is free of tumor, a plane on the anterior surface of the vein can be developed to facilitate pancreatic parenchymal transection closer to the pancreatic neck. If needed, the gastroduodenal artery can be ligated to achieve a more proximal margin toward the pancreatic head.
- Pancreatic transection is now performed (see "Pancreatic Transection" for details).

Splenectomy With Medial to Lateral (Antegrade) Dissection

- This is our preferred approach for patients with locally advanced disease in the body or tail of the pancreas. This procedure facilitates early vascular isolation and enhanced lymph node procurement, as well as early and safe establishment of margin status. Early pancreatic transection is performed with this approach.
- Once the greater omentum is elevated and the colon retracted inferiorly, the lesser sac is accessed and the common hepatic artery is traced to the proper hepatic artery. The gastroduodenal artery is identified and typically preserved, unless a more proximal point of transection at the neck of the pancreas is required.
- Lymph nodes are dissected free of the left border of the proper hepatic artery, PV, and common hepatic artery. The avascular plane between the PV and posterior pancreatic neck is developed and the pancreatic neck is divided.
- The celiac trunk is identified and a celiac lymph node dissection is carried out from the superior border of the pancreas, ultimately exposing the origin of the splenic artery, which is then ligated as previously shown (**FIGURE 2**). The artery is typically ligated with a 2-0 silk and reinforced with a 3-0 silk stick tie but can be stapled if the angle is appropriate and no compromise to the celiac trunk exists. Rarely, the left gastric artery warrants ligation at this juncture to facilitate complete lymph node dissection. However, this is not an option in the case of a replaced left hepatic artery or if the right gastric and gastroduodenal arteries have been previously sacrificed. It is of utmost importance to review preoperative imaging, including a CT angiogram, to recognize aberrant arterial anatomy.
- The splenic vein is encircled and divided at the junction with the PV. Dissection in a sagittal plane then proceeds until the superior mesenteric artery (SMA) is identified. The periaortic lymph tissue between the celiac trunk and SMA is removed. An adequate dissection exposes the left side of the aorta from the origin of the SMA superiorly to the origin of the celiac trunk (**FIGURE 4**).
  - This dissection can be carried down onto the diaphragm, if necessary, to include *en bloc* resection of a compromised adrenal gland.
  - The left renal vein represents the inferior border of dissection. The adrenal vein is identified and is left intact if the adrenal gland is not part of the specimen. Gerota's fascia is resected from the superior pole of the kidney for those more lateral malignancies.
- The superior and inferior pancreatic peritoneal attachments are divided, and dissection proceeds laterally. The IMV is ligated and transected, and the spleen is separated from the kidney as the final operative step prior to specimen removal.
  - Although rare, adrenal resection is sometimes necessary to achieve a satisfactory oncological resection. Strasberg et al. described the "Radical Antegrade Modular Pancreaticosplenectomy" (RAMPS) procedure. This technique proceeds in antegrade fashion and provides improved visibility, early control of the vasculature, and the ability to follow one of two posterior surgical planes, which may include the left adrenal gland.[5]

Spleen-Preserving Distal Pancreatectomy

- Splenic preservation can be considered in cases involving cystic lesions or small, well-differentiated, neoplasms for which a radical resection is oncologically unnecessary.
- There are several techniques described for splenic preservation:

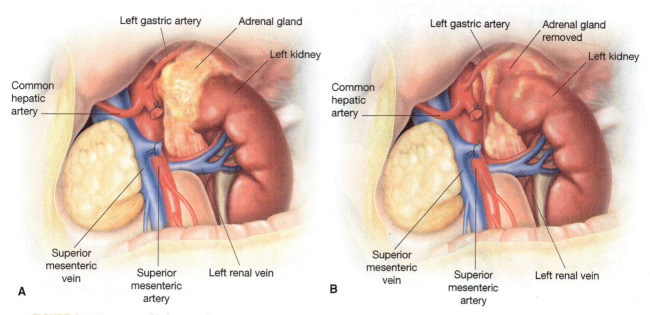

FIGURE 4 • Exposure of left aorta from SMA to celiac trunk (A) with left adrenal in place, (B) with left adrenal removed.

- The Warshaw technique involves dividing the splenic artery and vein proximal to the tumor and then, again, at the splenic hilum.[6] The short gastric arteries are left intact and become the primary blood supply to the spleen. Although thoroughly described, this approach is less commonly performed due to the severity of the complications that can occur. These include splenic hypoperfusion leading to infarcts and pain, splenic abscesses, and development of gastric varices.[7]
- The more common method of splenic preservation involves preserving the splenic vessels through careful dissection off the posterior pancreas up to the splenic hilum. The small arterial and venous branches are isolated between clamps and ligated or controlled with a surgical energy device. **FIGURE 5** shows the resection bed following a spleen preserving distal pancreatectomy.

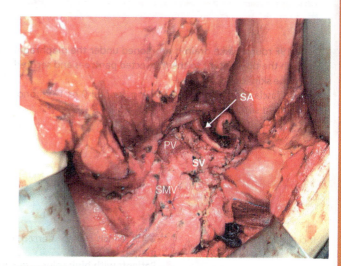

FIGURE 5 • Resection bed following spleen preservation. SA, splenic artery; SV, splenic vein.

PANCREATIC TRANSECTION

- For glands with relatively nonedematous or nonfibrotic parenchyma, and not greater than 1.5 cm in thickness, an Endo GIA stapler with a 3.0-mm load can be used to transect the pancreas. In cases of pancreatic edema or a thicker gland, an energy device can be used for parenchymal transection, with subsequent oversewing using a running and locking 3-0 polydioxanone stitch. **FIGURE 6** illustrates pancreatic transection using a thoracoabdominal (TA) stapler. The specimen is removed and marked for margins on a back table.
- The transected specimen should be sent to pathology for margin assessment—the pancreatic margin should be evaluated unless it will not change your management in the operating room (eg, no further resection can be performed). If in question, a frozen section on the retroperitoneal margin can be performed. Serial sections may be required to establish adequate margins.
- Surgeons are encouraged to orient and/or mark the specimen personally for the pathologist to ensure proper orientation and identification of surgical margins.
- The resection bed may be marked with clips for postoperative radiation, especially if there is concern of compromised margins following a radical resection.
- A closed suction drain is placed over the resection bed near the pancreatic stump. The size and type of drain are based on surgeon preference; a 10F flat Jackson-Pratt drain is commonly used. The colon and stomach are returned to their usual anatomic position.

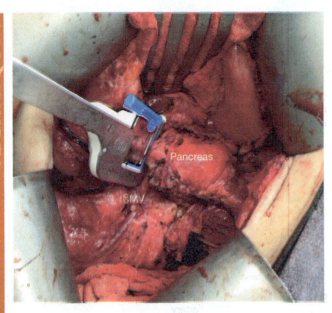

FIGURE 6 • Pancreas division using TA stapler.

CLOSURE

- A 19F round Blake drain is positioned under the diaphragm with the tip adjacent to the transected pancreas and secured to the skin (optional).
- The fascia is closed using a running, looped 0 or 1-0 monofilament suture.
- The skin is reapproximated using interrupted 3-0 braided polydioxanone deep dermal sutures and 4-0 poliglecaprone in a running subcuticular fashion or staples.
- For subcostal incisions, the fascia is closed in one or two layers using 0 or 1-0 polydioxanone suture depending on surgeon preference.

PEARLS AND PITFALLS

Incision	• Midline incision is preferred for more slender patients or those with a sharply angled costal margin. • Patients with high splenic flexure or those undergoing a splenic-preserving procedure may benefit from left subcostal incision.
Initial survey and exposure	• Retractor placement (Omni-Trak) • Any unanticipated lymphadenopathy outside the planned plane of dissection or unexpected suspected metastases should be biopsied and sent for frozen section prior to any dissection. This may be performed laparoscopically prior to opening. • Be certain to examine the head of the pancreas.
Exposure of the pancreas	• When mobilizing the posterior stomach away from the anterior pancreas, vessels encountered between the stomach and mesocolon should be ligated with care taken not to injure the middle colic vessels. • Do not apply undue tension in retracting the colon down as the middle colic vein can be avulsed off the SMV.
Lateral to medial (retrograde) dissection	• If the point of transection needs to occur proximal to the splenic vein–PV confluence and the PV is free of tumor, a plane on the anterior surface of the vein can be developed to facilitate pancreatic parenchymal transection closer to the pancreatic neck. This may require ligation of the gastroduodenal artery.

Medial to lateral (antegrade) dissection	▪ During splenic arterial ligation, control is obtained proximal to the anticipated site of ligation prior to tie or stapler placement. ▪ Before ligating the splenic artery, encircle and temporarily occlude it; identify the proper hepatic artery and verify that it is patent and pulsatile. ▪ If needed, secondary to extensive posterior involvement, dissection can be carried down onto the diaphragm to include *en bloc* resection of the adrenal gland. ▪ If transverse colon involvement is suspected, a full bowel preparation is recommended in anticipation of possible *en bloc* resection.
Splenic preservation	▪ Splenic preservation can be considered in the case of cystic lesions where occult malignancy is not suspected or small well-differentiated neoplasms.
Pancreatic transection	▪ In cases of severe edema or fibrosis or a thicker gland (>1.2 to 1.5 cm), hemostasis and pancreatic duct closure can be incomplete with the use of a stapler. In this instance, using an energy device to transect the pancreas is recommended. ▪ Regardless of transection method, consider oversewing the pancreatic stump using a running, locking 4-0 Prolene suture.
Specimen analysis	▪ It is important to work with the pathologist to ensure specimen orientation and appropriate nodal harvest. ▪ Orientation of the specimen and inking of margins by the surgeon is encouraged.

POSTOPERATIVE CARE

- Blood glucose should be closely monitored in the immediate postoperative period and at subsequent outpatient follow-up visits. Development of diabetes in the postoperative setting is variable, ranging from 14% to 39%. The risk is increased for those with a history of chronic pancreatitis and decreased in those undergoing distal pancreatectomy for benign or suspected malignant lesions.[8]
- A transient elevation of pancreatic enzymes may occur and generally normalizes within days. Closed suction drainage should remain in place until the patient's diet has been advanced. Drain output should be monitored for signs of a pancreatic fistula. Although there is a trend toward drainless pancreatic surgery, it remains our preference to use a closed suction drain. The reported incidence of fistula formation is 10% to 30%, regardless of pancreatic transection technique.[9] If there is persistent amylase-rich output after 4 weeks; patients may be treated with pancreatic duct stenting, which typically resolves the fistula and allows for drain removal. If a drain is not utilized, then it is important to have access to high-quality interventionalists as colleagues, both advanced endoscopists and interventional radiologists who can perform rescue drainage procedures as needed. This can be performed transgastrically or percutaneously for fluid collections that develop following distal pancreatectomy.
- A clear liquid diet is typically provided on postoperative day 2. The diet is advanced based on patient status and comfort level. Postoperative nasogastric tubes are not regularly used, although in case of prolonged operative times with retraction of the stomach upward and extensive dissection, it may be left in place for 24 to 48 hours.
- Once normal feeding is achieved, providers should be vigilant for symptoms of pancreatic insufficiency, even if blood glucose control remains adequate. Most patients benefit from perioperative pancreatic enzyme supplementation, particularly if previously diagnosed with chronic pancreatitis. Approximately 18% may benefit from supplementation in the long term (3 months) until normal exocrine function is regained.[10]
- Patients should be monitored for vitamin D deficiency and osteoporosis. These may result from long-standing pancreatic exocrine insufficiency. Primary care physicians should be involved, to ensure adequate supplementation is provided.
- In case of emergency, or unplanned splenectomy during an elective procedure, patients should receive vaccination against *S. pneumoniae*, *N. meningitidis*, *H. influenzae* type b, and the influenza virus at least 2 weeks after surgery; a booster dose of the tetanus-diphtheria-pertussis (dTaP) is also recommended. Patients with no measurable immunity should also receive vaccination against measles-mumps-rubella (MMR) and varicella.[3,4]

OUTCOMES

- Overall, the prognosis for patients diagnosed with left-sided pancreatic cancer is poor, with an estimated 5-year survival rate of 6.9%.[11] For patients diagnosed with tumors of the body or tail of the pancreas, who undergo resection, reported estimates from single and multi-institutional data remain heterogeneous, with 5-year survival ranging from 10% to 25% and median survival estimates ranging between 17 and 26 months.[11-14] It is our preference to treat all patients diagnosed with pancreatic adenocarcinoma with neoadjuvant chemotherapy. This allows for improved patient selection of those who are most likely to benefit from surgical resection and will also prevent the delay of important adjuvant chemotherapy for this disease if they develop a pancreatic fistula.
- Long-term results for distal pancreatectomy vary significantly, based on pathology, disease stage, baseline patient characteristics, and administered treatment. However, surgical resection with adequate margin clearance remains a prerequisite to achieve long-term survival. More contemporary dissection techniques, like the RAMPS, have reported

negative tangential margins in 89% of the specimens, with an overall R0 resection rates of 81%.[13]

COMPLICATIONS

- The overall rate of complications reported for open, distal pancreatectomies range from 14% to 70%.
- Postoperative pancreatic fistulas remain a significant cause of morbidity for patients undergoing distal pancreatectomies; the incidence of clinically significant fistulas ranges from 6.5% to 38%.[11-13,15-17]
- Perioperative mortality remains relatively low, ranging between <1% and 3% at 30 days and up to 6% at 90 days.[11,12,15]

REFERENCES

1. National Comprehensive Cancer Network. Pancreatic Adenocarcinoma (Version 2.2021). 2021. Accessed June 20, 2021. https://www.nccn.org/professionals/physician_gls/pdf/pancreatic_blocks.pdf
2. Fleisher LA, Fleischmann KE, Auerbach AD, et al. 2014 ACC/AHA guideline on perioperative cardiovascular evaluation and management of patients undergoing noncardiac surgery: a report of the American College of Cardiology/American Heart Association Task Force on practice guidelines. *J Am Coll Cardiol*. 2014;64(22):e77-e137.
3. Bonanni P, Grazzini M, Niccolai G, et al. Recommended vaccinations for asplenic and hyposplenic adult patients. *Hum Vaccin Immunother*. 2017;13(2):359-368.
4. Centers for Disease Control and Prevention. *Altered Immunocompetence*. 2021. Accessed July 12, 2021. https://www.cdc.gov/vaccines/hcp/acip-recs/general-recs/immunocompetence.html
5. Strasberg SM, Drebin JA, Linehan D. Radical antegrade modular pancreatosplenectomy. *Surgery*. 2003;133(5):521-527.
6. Warshaw AL. Conservation of the spleen with distal pancreatectomy. *Arch Surg*. 1988;123(5):550-553.
7. Warshaw AL. Distal pancreatectomy with preservation of the spleen. *J Hepato-Biliary-Pancreatic Sci*. 2010;17(6):808-812.
8. De Bruijn KM, van Eijck CH. New-onset diabetes after distal pancreatectomy: a systematic review. *Ann Surg*. 2015;261(5):854-861.
9. Zhang H, Zhu F, Shen M, et al. Systematic review and meta-analysis comparing three techniques for pancreatic remnant closure following distal pancreatectomy. *Br J Surg*. 2015;102(1):4-15.
10. Speicher JE, Traverso LW. Pancreatic exocrine function is preserved after distal pancreatectomy. *J Gastrointest Surg*. 2010;14(6):1006-1011.
11. Ruess DA, Makowiec F, Chikhladze S, et al. The prognostic influence of intrapancreatic tumor location on survival after resection of pancreatic ductal adenocarcinoma. *BMC Surg*. 2015;15:123.
12. de Rooij T, Tol JA, van Eijck CH, et al. Outcomes of distal pancreatectomy for pancreatic ductal adenocarcinoma in The Netherlands: a nationwide retrospective analysis. *Ann Surg Oncol*. 2016;23(2):585-591.
13. Mitchem JB, Hamilton N, Gao F, et al. Long-term results of resection of adenocarcinoma of the body and tail of the pancreas using radical antegrade modular pancreatosplenectomy procedure. *J Am Coll Surg*. 2012;214(1):46-52.
14. Strasberg SM, Linehan DC, Hawkins WG. Radical antegrade modular pancreatosplenectomy procedure for adenocarcinoma of the body and tail of the pancreas: ability to obtain negative tangential margins. *J Am Coll Surg*. 2007;204(2):244-249.
15. Bashir MU, Kandilis A, Jackson NM, et al. Distal pancreatectomy outcomes: perspectives from a community-based teaching institution. *Ann Hepatobiliary Pancreat Surg*. 2020;24(2):156-161.
16. Hutchins RR, Hart RS, Pacifico M, et al. Long-term results of distal pancreatectomy for chronic pancreatitis in 90 patients. *Ann Surg*. 2002;236(5):612.
17. Kooby DA, Gillespie T, Bentrem D, et al. Left-sided pancreatectomy: a multicenter comparison of laparoscopic and open approaches. *Ann Surg*. 2008;248(3):438-446.

Chapter 39 Minimally Invasive Distal Pancreatectomy

Jon M. Gerry, Jared A. Forrester, and Nathania M. Figueroa Guilliani

DEFINITION

- Minimally invasive distal pancreatectomy includes both laparoscopic and robotic methods.[1]
- The extent of resection includes the tail of the pancreas, and can include the more proximal body and neck of the pancreas. For oncological resection, the splenic artery and vein, with an adjacent regional lymphadenectomy, and the spleen are all removed *en bloc* with the removed portion of pancreas.
- The decision to attempt splenic preservation, either with the splenic vessel preservation (Kimura) or without (Warshaw) is dictated by the underlying pathology, the size and location of the lesion, and the tumor's relationship to the spleen and splenic vasculature.

DIFFERENTIAL DIAGNOSIS

- Pancreatic adenocarcinoma
- Pancreatic neuroendocrine tumors
- Cystic pancreatic lesions
- Pancreatic metastases
- Sequelae of chronic pancreatitis

PATIENT HISTORY AND PHYSICAL FINDINGS

- Resectable tumors of the pancreatic body and tail can be asymptomatic. Therefore, they may manifest as incidental findings on imaging. New-onset diabetes or worsening dysglycemia often precede diagnosis. Unintentional weight loss is an ominous feature associated with pancreatic cancer.
- In more advanced stages of disease, patients may present with symptoms such as back pain from invasion of the celiac plexus, nausea, and early satiety from invasion or compression of the stomach or duodenum, and splenomegaly caused by splenic vein thrombosis.

IMAGING AND OTHER DIAGNOSTIC STUDIES

- The primary imaging modality is a pancreatic protocol, multiphase computed tomography (CT) scan including pre contrast, arterial, and portal venous phases. One- to 3-mm cuts with coronal and sagittal reconstructions allow a detailed analysis of the pancreas, the lesion, and its relationship to the surrounding vasculature and viscera (**FIGURE 1A**). National Comprehensive Cancer Network (NCCN) guidelines also recommend a CT chest, CT pelvis, and serum CA 19-9 level, in patients with known or suspected pancreatic adenocarcinoma to evaluate for metastatic disease and to establish a baseline for future comparison.[2]
- Abdominal magnetic resonance imaging (MRI) is slightly more sensitive in identifying liver metastases but provides less anatomic soft tissue detail regarding the pancreas and vasculature (**FIGURE 1B**). Magnetic resonance cholangiopancreatography (MRCP) with intravenous contrast can be helpful in grossly examining pancreatic ductal anatomy particularly when evaluating a cystic lesion's mural nodularity or relationship to the main pancreatic duct. MRIs require a higher degree of patient cooperation. They may be used as an alternative imaging modality in patients with contrast allergies or other contraindications to contrast-enhanced CT.
- Endoscopic ultrasound (EUS) is an operator-dependent imaging modality that is routinely used preoperatively to obtain an accurate assessment of solid lesion size and relationship to the portal vein and superior mesenteric vein (SMV) (**FIGURE 1C**). It is also used to assess for worrisome features in cystic lesions. Tissue sampling via ultrasound-directed fine needle aspiration (FNA) of the primary tumor or regional lymph nodes may provide a tissue diagnosis. EUS-guided sampling of fluid from pancreatic cystic lesions may help distinguish between serous and mucinous lesions.
- Endoscopic retrograde cholangiopancreatography (ERCP) should only be employed with therapeutic intent.
- Intraoperative ultrasound (IOUS) is used routinely to define the relevant pathology, to identify important vascular structures, and to determine resectability during operative staging (**FIGURE 1D**).

SURGICAL MANAGEMENT

Preoperative Planning

- A plan for the resection should be determined preoperatively based on cross-sectional imaging and EUS. We use NCCN guidelines for resectability based on the relationship of the tumor to the SMA and celiac trunk.[2] Tumor invasion of major vascular structures such as portal vein, SMV, and celiac trunk, but not invasion of the splenic vein, is associated with an increased use of neoadjuvant treatment with about 10% of surgical cases undergoing minimally invasive distal pancreatectomy after neoadjuvant treatment.[3]
- The extent of gland resection is variable and should be directed by tumor location within the pancreas and its relationship with major blood vessels. Lesions in the tail of the pancreas can be resected with preservation of the neck and body, whereas more proximal lesions may require division of the gland closer to the portal vein. The gastroduodenal artery (GDA) is generally considered the landmark for the proximal limit of transection, as division of the pancreas more proximally risks injuring the intrapancreatic bile duct.
- The decision to remove the spleen is typically made preoperatively based on surgeon preference and the characteristics of the tumor. If malignancy is suspected, the spleen and lymphatic tissue along the splenic vessels should be resected *en bloc* with the pancreas. Cystic lesions that are

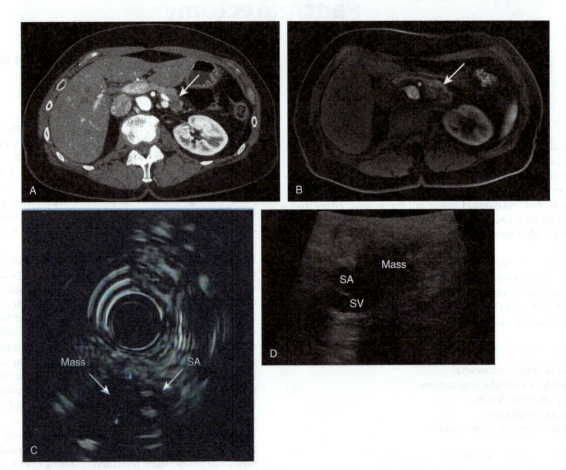

FIGURE 1 • **A,** Arterial-phase CT showing a hypodense mass (white arrow) in the pancreatic body adjacent to the splenic artery and vein. **B,** Corresponding contrast-enhanced T1 MR showing the mass (white arrow). **C,** EUS showing the pancreatic body mass with direct abutment with the splenic artery (SA). **D,** IOUS showing the mass adjacent to the splenic artery (SA) and splenic vein (SV).

- considered low risk for malignancy can be considered for a spleen-preserving approach. Postsplenectomy vaccinations include vaccination against pneumococcus, meningococcus ACWY, meningococcus B, and Haemophilus influenzae B.[4] Ensure asplenia vaccinations have been administered, ideally at least 2 weeks preoperatively or 2 weeks postoperatively.[5]
- Central venous access is typically not necessary as long as reliable, large-bore peripheral intravenous (IV) lines are established. An arterial line can be placed at the discretion of the anesthesiologist.

Positioning

- The patient is positioned supine or, in some cases, in a gentle right semilateral decubitus position on a padded mattress. The arms are supported on arm boards at just under 90° to prevent stretch of the brachial plexus. Alternatively, the arms may be tucked at the patient's side to facilitate placement of fixed retractors.
- During the dissection, the operating table is positioned in reverse Trendelenburg with the left side slightly elevated so that the hollow viscera fall caudad and to the right, away from the operative field.
- The position of the operating surgeon depends on the position of the tumor within the pancreas and may change during the procedure. During mobilization of the stomach and colon, the surgeon is typically on the patient's right with the assistant on the patient's left. Once the body and tail of the pancreas are exposed, the surgeon's position depends on tumor location. If the tumor is distal and the transection of the pancreas will be in the body, the surgeon stays on the patient's right. If the tumor is in the proximal body and the point of transection will be at the pancreatic neck, the dissection may be easier by having the surgeon stand on the patient's left. This facilitates the surgeon's ability to dissect along the superior mesenteric and portal veins and create the window behind the neck of the pancreas.

DIAGNOSTIC LAPAROSCOPY

Port Placement

- For exploratory laparoscopy, we start with two ports. The first is typically a 12-mm port and placed just below the umbilicus. This port facilitates the intraoperative ultrasound probe. The second port is 5 mm and placed lateral to the right or left rectus muscle and cephalad to the umbilicus.
- Two or three additional ports are placed, depending on the complexity of the procedure and on the position of the tumor within the pancreas (**FIGURE 2**).
- A high, right 5-mm subcostal port will ultimately serve to retract the stomach cephalad to expose the pancreas. Additional 5-mm ports may be placed just lateral to the right rectus muscle above the level of the umbilicus or laterally along the left subcostal margin.
- A hand port may be used at the surgeon's discretion. Hand assistance can be very useful for large tumors that invade the surrounding viscera, inflammatory masses, and proximal tumors that abut the celiac axis. The optimal position of the port is variable. Right-handed surgeons will prefer to have the left hand in the port, and a lower midline position is preferred. Left-handed surgeons typically prefer to have their right hand in the port, which should be positioned laterally beneath the left costal margin.
- We use a 30°, 10-mm high-definition (HD) laparoscope to ensure optimal visualization. Alternatively, a 5-mm HD laparoscope may be used.
- We use dual carbon dioxide (CO_2) insufflation devices to prevent decompression of pneumoperitoneum if suction is required for bleeding.

Examination of Peritoneum and Viscera

- The peritoneal surface is examined for carcinomatosis. Suspicious lesions are biopsied and sent for immediate pathologic analysis.
- The abdominal viscera are likewise examined and any suspicious lesions are sampled. Although we look at the omentum and easily accessible viscera, we typically do not "run the bowel" unless otherwise indicated.
- The root of the small bowel mesentery and the undersurface of the transverse mesentery are examined in case of large malignant tumors and those located in the central pancreas.

Intraoperative Ultrasound

- The liver is systematically examined for evidence of metastases. Surface lesions are wedged out and deeper lesions are biopsied by core needle. Specimens are sent for immediate pathologic analysis by frozen sectioning.

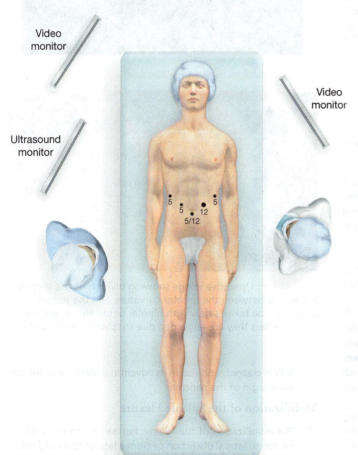

FIGURE 2 • Illustration showing port positions. The patient is positioned supine with the left side bumped slightly with a padded wedge. The arms can be tucked or extended. The surgeon can stand on either side; typically, patient's right for distal tumors and patient's left for proximal tumors.

- The pancreatic parenchyma is examined. The tumor size, location, and the relationship of the tumor to the SMA, SMV, IMV, splenic vein, and left renal vein are determined. The anticipated transection margin of the pancreas is determined.
- In case of anticipated enucleation, proximity of the tumor to the main pancreatic duct is also determined (FIGURE 3A and B).
- Para-aortic lymph nodes as well as those along the origins of the celiac trunk and the SMA are examined. Suspicious lymph nodes beyond the planned regional lymphadenectomy should be biopsied and sent for frozen section.
- The resection is aborted if diagnostic laparoscopy reveals metastatic or locally unresectable disease.

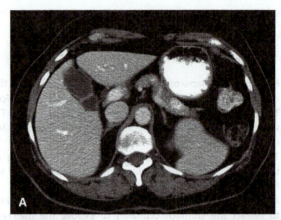

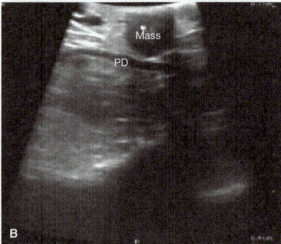

FIGURE 3 • A, Venous-phase CT showing a rounded hypervascular mass in the pancreatic tail. The patient presented with symptomatic hypoglycemia. The tumor was proven to be an insulinoma by EUS/FNA. The patient was treated with a spleen-preserving distal pancreatectomy. B, IOUS showing the insulinoma at the time of resection. The deep margin was within 2 mm of the pancreatic duct (PD).

LAPAROSCOPIC DISTAL PANCREATECTOMY AND SPLENECTOMY

Entry into the Lesser Sack and Division of the Short Gastric Vessels

- Preserving the right gastroepiploic arcade, the lesser sac is traditionally entered through the gastrocolic ligament just below the greater curve of the stomach. The gastrocolic and gastrosplenic omentum are then divided from right to left using ultrasonic shears or a bipolar electrocautery device.
- Enlarged venous collaterals may be present in this area if the splenic vein is invaded or thrombosed. A linear stapler or individual vessel ligation with clips or ties is often preferred for division of varices greater than 3 mm in diameter.
- Mobilization of the fundus continues all the way to the left crus, dividing the short gastric vessels (FIGURE 4). The posterior wall of the stomach is mobilized anteriorly to completely expose the body and tail of the pancreas. Avascular congenital adhesions are frequently present between the stomach and pancreas and can be divided bluntly or with electrocautery (FIGURE 5).
- For proximal tumors of the pancreatic body, the dissection continues toward the patient's right. The transverse mesocolon is swept caudally in an avascular plane that exposes the middle colic and gastroepiploic vein, which are followed to their confluence with the SMV. The anterior surface of the

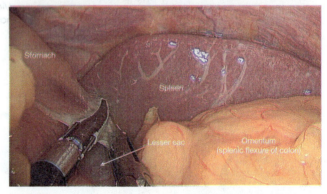

FIGURE 4 • Operative image showing division of the short gastric vessels between the greater curvature and the spleen. These vessels can be taken safely with bipolar or ultrasonic coagulating devices unless they are engorged due to splenic vein thrombosis.

SMV is cleared cephalad in its adventitial plane up to the caudal margin of the pancreas.

Mobilization of the Splenic Flexure

- The mobilization of the splenic flexure can be done from a medial to lateral dissection or from a lateral to medial dissection. The medial to lateral dissection begins within the lesser sac and follows the inferior border of the pancreas to the

Chapter 39 MINIMALLY INVASIVE DISTAL PANCREATECTOMY 323

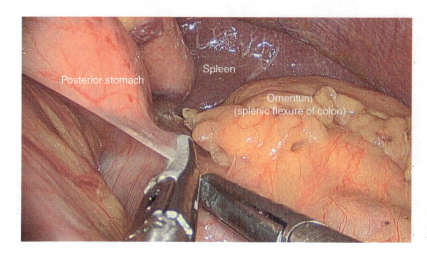

FIGURE 5 • Operative image demonstrating the division of the congenital adhesions from the posterior wall of the stomach to the pancreatic body.

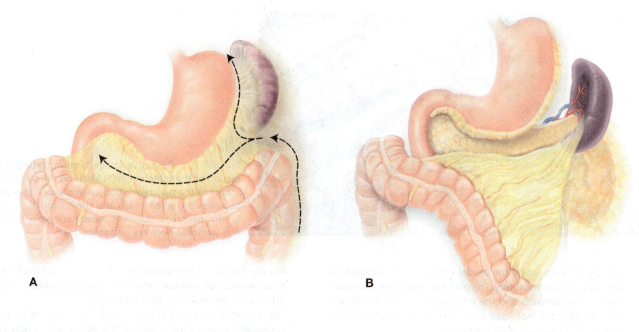

FIGURE 6 • Illustration showing "clockwise" technique for exposure of the distal pancreas. A, The left colon and splenic flexure are mobilized from left to right. The lesser sack is entered in the plane between the pancreatic tail and the transverse mesocolon. B, The gastrocolic and gastrosplenic ligaments are then divided to expose the pancreas and to drop the transverse colon out of the field of dissection.

- inferior pole of the spleen, clearing the mesocolon, colon, and omentum, caudally.
- The lateral to medial approach starts by medial and inferior mobilization of the lateral splenic flexure. The lesser sack can be entered anterior to the tail of the pancreas during this dissection. This "clockwise approach" is described by Asbun and Stauffer[6] and can be useful for exposure of the pancreatic body via a left to right division of the gastrocolic ligament.
- Whether the either approach, or a combination of both approaches are used, the goal is to completely expose the neck, body, and tail of the pancreas as needed (FIGURE 6A and B).

Mobilization of the Pancreatic Body and Tail

- The stomach is retracted anteriorly, away from the pancreas using a liver retractor or by suturing the greater curve to the abdominal wall (FIGURE 7).

- Using electrocautery or ultrasonic energy, the retroperitoneum is incised along the inferior border of the pancreas from medial to lateral. Gentle retraction is used on the pancreas, as it is prone to tearing and bleeding.
- Ultrasound is used to confirm the location of the tumor and to select an appropriate line of gland transection. A minimum 1-cm margin is desirable for malignant tumors. Tumors from the tail to the midbody can be resected with a generous margin by transecting the proximal pancreatic body. Tumors involving the proximal body require subtotal distal pancreatectomy with pancreas transection at the pancreatic neck anterior to the SMV. Tumors involving the pancreatic neck require transection to the right of the SMV. The most proximal resection plane is where the GDA passes anterior to the pancreatic head. Attempts to resect further to the right may result in injury to the intrapancreatic bile duct.

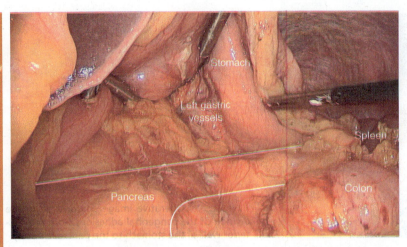

FIGURE 7 • Operative image showing excellent exposure of the pancreatic body after division of the gastrocolic omentum and elevation of the stomach with a retractor placed through a right upper quadrant port. The pancreas is outlined in white lines.

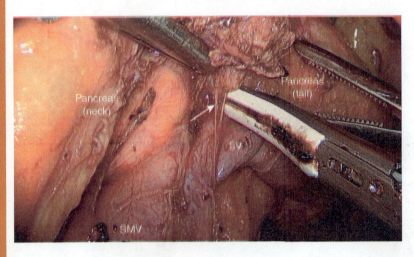

FIGURE 8 • Operative image demonstrating dissection of the splenic vein (SV) behind the posterior aspect of the pancreatic body. A window is created between the splenic vein and the posterior aspect of the pancreas. Superior mesenteric vein (SMV) and pancreas neck are also seen.

- The peritoneum along the caudal border of the pancreas is scored with electrocautery. The plane between the posterior wall of the pancreas and the retroperitoneal fat is entered and the gland is mobilized anteriorly off of Gerota's fascia with blunt dissection or electrocautery.
- The pancreatic tail is mobilized anteriorly along with the splenic vein when the posterior boundary of dissection is Gerota's fascia.

Isolation of the Splenic Vein

- For distal tumors, the vein is dissected behind the pancreatic body. For proximal tumors, the SMV/splenic vein confluence is dissected behind the pancreatic neck.
- With the pancreas reflected anteriorly and cephalad, the splenic vein is located behind the pancreas. The vein may be partially or completely enveloped in pancreatic tissue, particularly at the more distal aspects of the gland. Careful dissection is used to create a tunnel between the vein and pancreas (FIGURE 8).
- The splenic vein is dissected circumferentially and may be encircled with a vessel loop (FIGURE 9). The loop is used for retraction as the vein is mobilized away from the pancreas along a sufficient length to provide passage of a linear stapler.
- For proximal tumors, the anteromedial surface of the SMV is bluntly dissected away from the pancreatic neck to expose the confluence of the splenic vein (FIGURE 10), which can then be encircled and divided either proximal or distal to the inferior mesenteric vein (IMV) confluence.
- The tunnel is extended cephalad and anteriorly up to the cephalad margin of the pancreas. The splenic artery may be encountered and exposed during this dissection (FIGURE 11A and B).

Isolation of the Splenic Artery

- The splenic artery is typically encountered cephalad to the splenic vein along the superior edge of the pancreas, although it is a tortuous vessel and its course can be unpredictable. If its location is posterior to the pancreas, it can be approached from underneath the pancreas after creating space between the splenic vein and the posterior pancreas (FIGURE 11B). If the location is more anterior and cephalad to the pancreas, it can be approached over the top of the pancreas just cephalad to the superior edge of the pancreas (FIGURE 12).
- As with the splenic vein, the region of dissection and division of the splenic artery varies with tumor location. For tumors of the tail and midbody, the artery is divided distal to its origin from the celiac. For tumors of the proximal body and neck, the artery is divided at its origin.
- The artery is cleared circumferentially and encircled with a vessel loop. We recommend routine use of IOUS in proximal

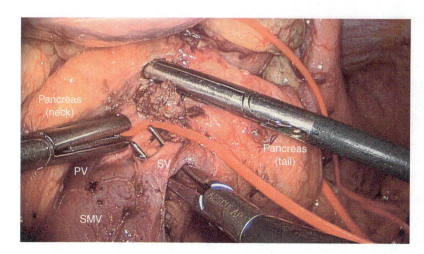

FIGURE 9 • Mobilization of the splenic vein (SV) away from the posterior wall of the pancreas, and encirclement of the vein with a vascular loop to facilitate retraction. The passage of the portal vein (PV) is seen under the neck of pancreas.

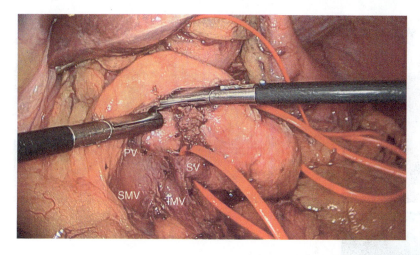

FIGURE 10 • Operative image showing the dissection of the superior mesenteric vein (SMV)/splenic vein (SV)/portal vein (PV)/inferior mesenteric vein (IMV) confluence behind the neck of the pancreas. This is the margin of pancreas transection for more proximal tumors of the pancreatic body. Pathology involving the pancreatic neck requires division of the pancreas even farther to the patient's right in the region of the GDA.

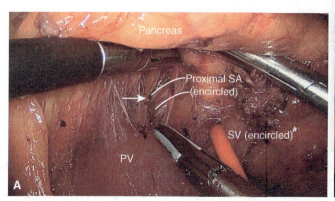 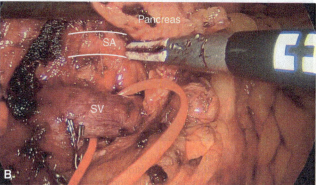

FIGURE 11 • **A,** Operative image demonstrating anterior retraction of the pancreas to expose the splenic vein (SV; looped and retracted posteriorly) and the splenic artery (SA; also looped and marked by white lines). The white arrow shows the window created for passage of a stapler to divide the pancreas. **B,** A second operative image showing the emergence of the splenic artery (SA, marked by white lines) when the portal/splenic confluence is freed from the posterior pancreas.

transections to confirm isolation of the splenic artery, as inadvertent division of the celiac trunk and common hepatic artery have been reported (**FIGURE 13A-C**).

Division of the Pancreas, Splenic Artery, and Splenic Vein

- Once sufficiently mobilized away from the adjacent vessels, the pancreas can be transected at any point in the operation. We prefer to divide the gland early on, as this will greatly enhance exposure of the underlying vascular structures.
- The perfect method of dividing the gland and controlling the pancreatic duct remains debatable. Numerous techniques have been applied with similar rates of leakage from the pancreatic stump.

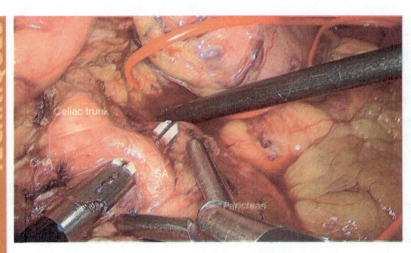

FIGURE 12 • Operative image showing the splenic artery (SA) just distal to its origin from the celiac axis.

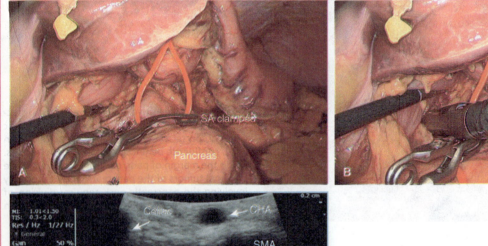

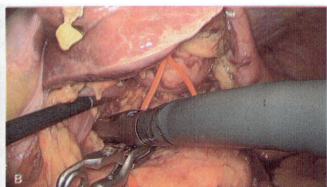

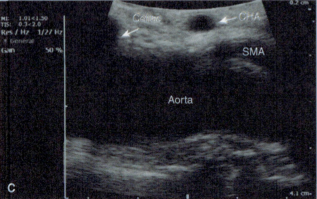

FIGURE 13 • **A,** Prior to ligation and division of the splenic artery, a bulldog clamp can be placed on the splenic artery (SA). **B,** IOUS is routinely performed prior to division of the splenic artery if the transection approaches the midline. The common hepatic artery can be mistaken for the splenic artery and divided accidently if care is not taken. **C,** IOUS image demonstrating the aorta, the superior mesenteric artery (SMA), the celiac axis, and the common hepatic artery (CHA). The bifurcation of these two vessels should be routinely visualized before dividing the splenic artery to ensure that the common hepatic is not inadvertently divided.

- Soft glands that are relatively thin (<1.5 cm in thickness) are best divided with a linear stapler (**FIGURE 14**). Reinforced staplers have been used with mixed results. We recommend slow compression of the gland for 3 minutes prior to division, as this minimizes parenchymal lacerations that can result in postoperative leaks. For neck and proximal body lesions, take care to ensure the stapler is not including the common hepatic artery with direct vision of the fixed anvil of the stapler along the posterior pancreas, yet anterior to the vessel.

- Fibrotic or thick glands can be divided with linear staplers, electrocautery, saline-enhanced monopolar cautery, or Harmonic scalpel. The pancreatic duct should be identified during the division.
- The pancreatic duct can be closed with a U-stitch if not divided with a reinforced stapler.
- The artery is divided with a linear vascular stapler, between locking vascular clips or between permanent suture ligatures (**FIGURE 15**).

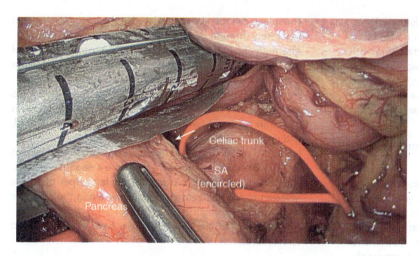

FIGURE 14 • The stapler placement to divide the neck or proximal body of the pancreas showing the anvil is anterior to the common hepatic artery (*white arrow*). Splenic artery (SA) is encircled with a vessel loop.

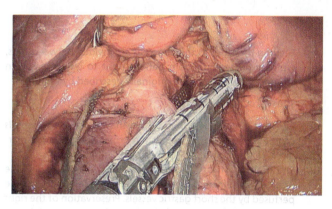

FIGURE 15 • Operative image showing placement of a vascular stapler across the splenic artery (SA) near its origin at the celiac axis. The common hepatic artery (CHA) and portal vein (PV) are seen.

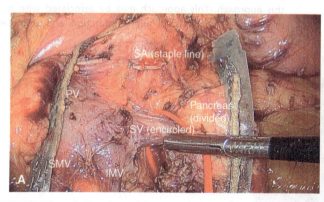 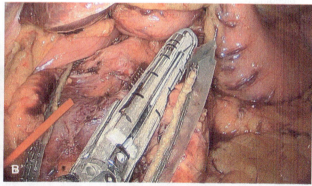

FIGURE 16 • **A,** The view of the typical operative field at the time of splenic vein division. The anticipated line of division of the splenic vein preserves the inferior mesenteric vein (IMV). **B,** Dividing the splenic vein with a vascular stapler.

- The vein is divided with a linear vascular stapler or between locking clips or nonabsorbable ties (**FIGURE 16A** and **B**). If the vein is closely opposed to the pancreas at the point of transection, it can be included in the staple load used to divide the pancreas.

Dissection of the Specimen off the Retroperitoneum

- After division of the pancreas and splenic vessels, the specimen is swept off the retroperitoneum in an avascular plane anterior to the left adrenal gland and Gerota's fascia, typically using hook electrocautery or an ultrasonic dissector.

- The remaining retroperitoneal and diaphragmatic attachments to the spleen are divided, completing the mobilization of the specimen.

Extent of Lymphadenectomy

- In the setting of suspected malignancy, en bloc distal pancreatectomy and splenectomy should be performed with the intention of harvesting the lymphatic tissue within the splenic hilum and along the splenic vessels.
- For pancreatic neuroendocrine tumors, cystic neoplasms, and small (<3 cm) pancreatic adenocarcinomas, the earlier description typically results in an adequate lymphadenectomy.

- For larger adenocarcinomas, a more extensive lymphadenectomy may be desired, which includes a lymph node dissection of the celiac trunk, SMA, and lateral aorta along with resection of the left adrenal gland (radical antegrade modular pancreaticosplenectomy [RAMPS] procedure) can be performed by experienced surgeons.[7] However, we recommend an open approach to these lesions as is warranted in most situations.

Specimen Extraction, Placement of Drains, and Port Site Closure

- The specimen is placed into a large extraction bag, spleen first with the pancreas on top. The wound is enlarged sufficiently for extraction of the entire specimen. Depending upon the clinical scenario and with the specimen oriented in this manner, the pancreas can be extracted through a smaller incision and then divided off the spleen extracorporeally. The spleen can then be morcellated in the bag and extracted separately through the same small incision.
- Alternatively, if the site of pathology is not in the distal pancreas, the spleen can be separated from the pancreas intracorporeally once the dissection is complete. The pancreas is placed in a separate bag from the spleen, and it is removed intact through the 12-mm port site. The spleen is placed in a second reinforced extraction bag, morcellated, and removed.
- In cases of malignancy, the transection margin should be sent for frozen section examination to ensure a negative margin.
- A closed suction drain is placed in the left upper quadrant adjacent to the pancreas staple line and along the posterior left hemidiaphragm.
- All port sites that are 10 mm or larger have the fascia closed with suture.

SPLEEN-PRESERVING LAPAROSCOPIC DISTAL PANCREATECTOMY

Splenic Vessel Preservation (Kimura) Technique

- The splenic vein is separated from the pancreas as described earlier and encircled with a vessel loop, which is used for both retraction and vascular control.
- Venous tributaries from the pancreas are skeletonized from patient right to left and divided between clips or with bipolar energy along the length of the splenic vein (FIGURE 17).
- Injury to small splenic vein tributaries can cause significant bleeding (FIGURE 18).
- The splenic artery is skeletonized along the superior border of the pancreas.
- Feeding branches to the pancreas are divided between clips, typically proceeding from patient right to left, which is in contrast to the technique originally described by Kimura.

Warshaw Technique

- In the technique described by Warshaw,[8] the splenic vessels can be ligated and divided at the proximal transection margin and again distally near the splenic hilum.
- The midportion of the splenic vessels is included with the resected specimen, whereas the spleen is left in situ to be perfused by the short gastric vessels. Preservation of the right gastroepiploic arcade and short gastrics are essential with this approach. This approach may be associated with left-sided portal hypertension, splenic infarction, and ultimately salvage splenectomy.[9]

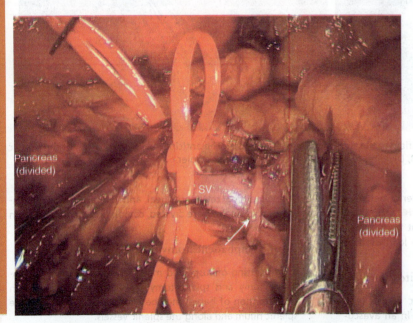

FIGURE 17 • Splenic vessel preservation during distal pancreatectomy. A venous tributary from the splenic vein (SV) is shown (white arrow).

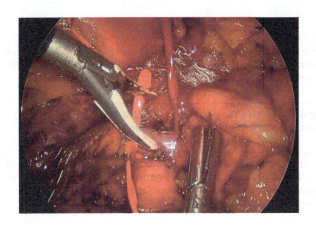

FIGURE 18 • Injury to the splenic vein during vessel-preserving technique can result in significant bleeding.

ROBOTIC DISTAL PANCREATECTOMY

General Concepts

- The robotic approach to a distal pancreatectomy is largely the same as the laparoscopic approach.
- The advantage of a robotic approach includes increased dexterity, which may prove beneficial in cases where splenic preservation is prioritized.[10] Cost may be similar to the laparoscopic technique in experienced centers.[11] The learning curve of robotic distal pancreatectomy may be similar to that of laparoscopic distal pancreatectomy.[12]
- The potential downside to a robotic approach includes limited access of surgeons to the robotic platform. However, once implemented at institutions, robotic surgery tends to steadily increase in frequency, even for complex oncological resections.[13] Another concern is access to the patient for urgent or emergent conversion to open surgery. However, recent evidence suggests that conversion for bleeding after robotic surgery is much less frequent than for laparoscopic surgery.[14] Patient selection may be a critical factor in reduced conversion rates for robotic distal pancreatectomy.

Patient Positioning

- The patient positioning is the same as a laparoscopic approach. Tucking the arms can help facilitate robot docking. Placing the patient supine with split legs or lithotomy are options for improving the assistant position.

Port Placement and Docking of the Robot

- Ports are placed slightly farther away from the target anatomy, about 20 cm, and slightly farther from each other, about 8 cm, in order to reduce the chance that ports will be inadvertently dislodged and reduce the chance that robotic arms will clash outside the patient.

- The optimal position for the camera during the dissection again depends on where the anticipated area of most difficult dissection lies. Most commonly, the camera will be in the infraumbilical port and the direction of surgical approach will be from the patient's right, looking toward the spleen.
- Retraction of the stomach may be performed with the third robotic arm or may be via a bed-mounted fixed retractor.
- The bedside assistant typically approaches from patient left.

Mobilization of the Colon and Pancreas

- The individual steps of colonic mobilization and exposure of the body and tail of the pancreas are the same as those described earlier for the laparoscopic approach.

Mobilization of the Pancreas and Control of the Vasculature

- The individual steps of pancreatic mobilization and control of the vasculature are the same as those described earlier for the laparoscopic approach.

Splenic Preservation Using a Robotic Approach to Distal Pancreatectomy

- The primary advantage of a robotic approach to a distal pancreatectomy is thought to be the increased dexterity by which the vasculature of distal pancreas and spleen can be dissected away from the tail of the pancreas.
- Using the three-dimensional (3-D) visualization, the small branches of the splenic vein and artery are identified, dissected, and individually divided using monopolar or bipolar technology.

Specimen Extraction

- The individual steps of specimen extraction are the same as those described above for the laparoscopic approach.

PEARLS AND PITFALLS

- Sequence and details of dissection can be altered based on individual anatomic characteristics. We typically divide pancreas, then splenic artery, and finally splenic vein.
- Dissection of the splenic vein deep to the superior pancreas margin may result in difficult-to-control bleeding. The vein is more safely approached inferiorly from below the pancreas.
- Bleeding from splenic vessels may be controlled with vascular loops, topical hemostatic agents, or nonabsorbable sutures.
- The distal pancreatic duct is suture ligated with a U-stitch if visualized when dividing the pancreas without duct-sealing technology.
- Individualized port placement based on abdominal length and body habitus. Ports should be moved cephalad in large and obese patients. A hand port is useful if mobilization is difficult.
- Method of gland transection should be individualized based on thickness and texture of the pancreas. Vascular staplers are generally appropriate for glands up to 2.0 cm in thickness. Saline-linked monopolar cautery and ultrasonic energy are alternative methods of transection.
- Consider dual insufflation systems to maintain pneumoperitoneum while suctioning.
- Placement of drains is optional and should be individualized based on texture of the pancreas and confidence in the closure of the pancreatic stump.
- Preserve as many short gastric vessels as possible when performing a spleen-preserving approach.
- The common hepatic artery should be visualized with IOUS prior to ligating the splenic artery to prevent inadvertent injury.

POSTOPERATIVE CARE

- Continuation of chemical and mechanical prophylaxis against deep vein thrombosis, which was initiated prior to incision.
- Clear liquid diet on postoperative day (POD) 1, advance as bowel function resumes.
- Early mobility commencing on the day of surgery.
- Drain amylase on POD 3 if a closed suction drain was used. Remove if within normal range of serum amylase. It can be rechecked on POD 5 if the initial drain amylase is elevated.
- CT scan if patient develops significant leukocytosis, fever, prolonged ileus, or other signs of pancreatic fistula or intra-abdominal infection.
- In almost all cases, percutaneous interventions are sufficient for management of intra-abdominal abscesses postoperative fistulas not controlled by surgical drains.
- Discharge from the hospital occurs between POD 3 and 7 in the absence of complications.

OUTCOMES

- Overall survival not related to minimally invasive surgery (MIS) vs open approach[15,16]
- Oncologic resection not compromised by MIS approach[16,17]
- Decreased blood loss compared to open resection[18,19]
- Increased length of surgery compared to open approach[19]
- Decreased average length of hospital stay compared to open approach[18]
- Morbidity and mortality equivalent or better than open surgery[18,19]

COMPLICATIONS

- Pancreatic fistula
- Intra-abdominal abscess
- Intraoperative/postoperative hemorrhage
- Pancreatic pseudocysts
- Splenic infarction
- Splenic vein thrombosis
- Overwhelming postsplenectomy infection (OPSI)
- Unplanned conversion to open surgery

REFERENCES

1. Asbun H, Moekotte AL, Vissers FL, et al. The Miami international evidence-based guidelines on minimally invasive pancreas resection. *Ann Surg.* 2020;271(1):1-14.
2. National Comprehensive Cancer Network. *Pancreatic Adenocarcinoma (Version 2.2021)*. Accessed December 6, 2021. http://www.nccn.org/professionals/physician_gls/pdf/pancreatic.pdf
3. Lof S, Korrel M, van Hilst J, et al. Impact of neoadjuvant therapy in resected pancreatic ductal adenocarcinoma of the pancreatic body or tail on surgical and oncological outcome: a propensity-score matched multicenter study. *Ann Surg Oncol.* 2020;27(6):1986-1996.
4. Centers for Disease Control and Prevention. *Asplenia and Adult Vaccination*. Centers for Disease Control and Prevention. Accessed December 17, 2021. http://www.cdc.gov/vaccines/adults/rec-vac/health-conditions/asplenia.html
5. Casciani F, Trudeau MT, Vollmer CM. Perioperative immunization for splenectomy and the surgeon's responsibility: a review. *JAMA Surg.* 2020;155(11):1068-1077.
6. Asbun HJ, Stauffer JA. Laparoscopic approach to distal and subtotal pancreatectomy: a clockwise technique. *Surg Endosc.* 2011;25(8):2643-2649.
7. Strasberg SM, Linehan DC, Hawkins WG. Radical antegrade modular pancreatosplenectomy procedure for adenocarcinoma of the body and tail of the pancreas: ability to obtain negative tangential margins. *J Am Coll Surg.* 2007;204(2):244-249. doi:10.1007/s00464-011-2141-z
8. Warshaw AL. Conservation of the spleen with distal pancreatectomy. *Arch Surg.* 1988;123(5):550-553.
9. Elabbasy F, Gadde R, Hanna MM, et al. Minimally invasive spleen-preserving distal pancreatectomy: does splenic vessel preservation have better postoperative outcomes? A systematic review and meta-analysis. *Hepatobiliary Pancreat Dis Int.* 2015;14(4):346-353.
10. Guerrini GP, Lauretta A, Belluco C, et al. Robotic versus laparoscopic distal pancreatectomy: an up-to-date meta-analysis. *BMC Surg.* 2017;17(1):105.
11. Magge DR, Zenati MS, Hamad A, et al. Comprehensive comparative analysis of cost-effectiveness and perioperative outcomes between open, laparoscopic, and robotic distal pancreatectomy. *HPB.* 2018;20(12):1172-1180.

12. Chan KS, Wang ZK, Syn N, et al. Learning curve of laparoscopic and robotic pancreas resections: a systematic review. *Surgery*. 2021;170(1):194-206.
13. Sheetz KH, Claflin J, Dimick J. Trends in the adoption of robotic surgery for common surgical procedures. *JAMA Netw Open*. 2020;3(1):e1918911.
14. Balduzzi A, van der Heijde N, Alseidi A, et al. Risk factors and outcomes of conversion in minimally invasive distal pancreatectomy: a systematic review. *Langenbeck's Arch Surg*. 2021;406(3):597-605.
15. Kooby DA, Hawkins WG, Schmidt CM, et al. A multicenter analysis of distal pancreatectomy for adenocarcinoma: is laparoscopic resection appropriate? *J Am Coll Surg*. 2010;210(5):779-785, 786-787.
16. Van Hilst J, Korrel M, de Rooij T, et al. Oncologic outcomes of minimally invasive versus open distal pancreatectomy for pancreatic ductal adenocarcinoma: a systematic review and meta-analysis. *Eur J Surg Oncol*. 2019;45(5):719-727.
17. Riviere D, Gurusamy KS, Kooby DA, et al. Laparoscopic versus open distal pancreatectomy for pancreatic cancer. *Cochrane Database Syst Rev*. 2016;4(4):CD011391.
18. Van Hilst J, de Rooij T, Klompmaker S, et al. Minimally invasive versus open distal pancreatectomy for ductal adenocarcinoma (DIPLOMA): a pan-European propensity score matched study. *Ann Surg*. 2019;269(1):10-17.
19. De Rooij T, van Hilst J, van Santvoort H, et al. Minimally invasive versus open distal pancreatectomy (LEOPARD): a multicenter patient-blinded randomized controlled trial. *Ann Surg*. 2019;269(1):2-9.

Chapter 40

Distal Pancreatectomy With Splenic Preservation

Patrick R. Carney, Adam S. Brinkman, and Sharon M. Weber

DEFINITION

- Distal pancreatectomy with splenic preservation (DPSP) is the complete removal of the distal pancreas (to the left of the superior mesenteric vein/portal vein [SMV/PV] confluence) while preserving the spleen via meticulous dissection and preservation of the splenic artery (SA) and splenic vein (SV), or with sacrifice of these vessels (Warshaw technique) with preserved blood flow to the spleen through the short gastric vessels.
- Indications for DPSP include benign tumors for which local excision is inadequate (neuroendocrine tumors), pancreatic cysts, chronic pancreatitis limited to the distal pancreas, and selected cases of distal pancreatic trauma. DPSP for distal pancreatic malignancies (adenocarcinoma) is controversial as body and tail lesions may have lymphatic drainage to the splenic hilum.
- The majority of cases performed in the United States are accomplished either open or laparoscopically (with or without a hand port). The robotic approach is becoming more common as more surgeons train in and adopt this technology. Variation in surgical technique with respect to preservation of the splenic vessels vs ligation of the vessels exists.

DIFFERENTIAL DIAGNOSIS

- Premalignant or malignant lesions a DPSP may be considered:
  - Solid pancreatic tumors
  - Functional and nonfunctional neuroendocrine tumors
  - Cystic pancreatic tumors
    - Intraductal papillary mucinous neoplasms (IPMNs)
    - Mucinous cystadenomas
    - Solid pseudopapillary tumors
  - Benign conditions
    - Congenital cysts
    - Serous cystadenomas
    - Chronic pancreatitis pancreatic pseudocysts can also be theoretically resected with a DPSP
- The location of the lesion and the anatomic relationships of the splenic vasculature are the major factors that should be evaluated before considering a DPSP as the surgical procedure of choice.

PATIENT HISTORY AND PHYSICAL FINDINGS

- Patients being considered for DPSP should be evaluated with a thorough history and physical examination. Specific considerations in the medical history include known risk factors for pancreatic malignancy such as a history of chronic pancreatitis, diabetes, obesity, exposure to heavy metals, heavy alcohol consumption, and smoking. Signs and symptoms of a functional neuroendocrine tumor such as rash, diarrhea, hypoglycemia, and peptic ulcer disease should also be evaluated. A detailed past surgical history and concomitant physical examination with particular attention to organomegaly, hernias, and prior surgical incisions is important. Splenomegaly, hepatomegaly, and the presence of lymphadenopathy should raise concern for malignancy that may preclude splenic preservation.
- Particular attention should be paid to symptoms of pancreatic insufficiency, nutritional status, and functional status with ability to tolerate a pneumoperitoneum of 15 mm Hg if a laparoscopic approach is chosen.
- Severely malnourished patients (more than 10%-15% of ideal body weight loss in the preceding 2 months) or serum albumin less than 3 g/dL should be considered for supplemental nutrition; enteral nutrition via Dobhoff tube or total parenteral nutrition through indwelling central venous catheter.

IMAGING AND OTHER DIAGNOSTIC STUDIES

- Pancreatic protocol computed tomography (CT) with triple-phase, contrast imaging to evaluate arterial, pancreatic, and portal venous phases is the preferred imaging modality for pancreatic diseases. The thin cuts through the pancreas allows for ideal delineation of vasculature, size of the lesion, involvement of surrounding structures, and evidence of local disease progression (**FIGURE 1**). Three-dimensional reconstruction may also aid in visualization and surgical planning. Careful attention should be paid to the arterial and venous phases as well as the arterial blood flow to the spleen, as this can determine feasibility of splenic preservation.

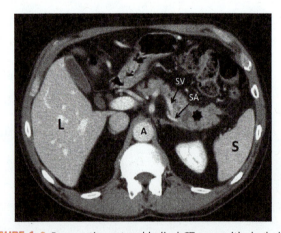

FIGURE 1 • Pancreatic protocol helical CT scan with dual phase intravenous contrast of the abdomen and pelvis demonstrating a solid 3.6 × 2.9-cm complex cystic lesion *(star)* in the tail of the pancreas concerning for malignant transformation of IPMN amenable for a DPSP. *A,* aorta; *L,* liver; *S,* spleen; *SA,* splenic artery; *SV,* splenic vein.

- The relationship of the mass, cyst, or stricture should be noted, and its anatomic relationship to the SV, inferior mesenteric vein (IMV), and SA should be noted in anticipation of potential intraoperative pitfalls.
- In addition to using CT, consideration can also be given to endoscopic ultrasound (EUS) to better evaluate the pancreatic lesion and its relationship to the surrounding structures. In addition, sampling of the mass with fine-needle aspiration for diagnostic purposes or aspiration of a cyst fluid for evaluation of carcinoembryonic antigen, amylase concentration, and mucin analysis may assist with diagnosis and operative planning. Next-generation sequencing analysis of pancreatic cyst fluid for common drivers of pancreatic cancer is becoming more commonly used to risk stratify lesions. EUS may be indicated if local disease is discovered on CT as it allows for further investigation and sampling of suspicious masses (often lymph nodes).
- Additional pathology can also be identified, including isolated gastric varices indicative of SV thrombosis and sinistral portal hypertension.
- Additional diagnostic testing that may be considered prior to a DPSP includes magnetic resonance imaging or magnetic resonance cholangiopancreatography, which may better define the pancreatic ductal anatomy.
- Consideration can also be extended to endoscopic retrograde cholangiopancreatography, the gold standard to define pancreatic ductal anatomy, which also offers an opportunity for evaluation of communication with the main pancreatic duct for cystic lesions, which is diagnostic for IPMN.
- Additional imaging including a chest radiograph or chest CT scan may be obtained for complete staging and preoperative evaluation in patients with suspected malignancy.

SURGICAL MANAGEMENT

Preoperative Planning

- Prior to proceeding to the operating room (OR), all patients should be evaluated with a full history and physical examination with cardiovascular and pulmonary testing as medically needed. Patients scheduled to undergo laparoscopic or robotic distal pancreatectomy should be made aware of the potential need to convert to an open approach during the operation.
- Consideration should also be given to vaccinating against encapsulated bacteria including *Neisseria meningitidis*, *Haemophilus influenzae* type B, and *Streptococcus pneumoniae*.[1]
- These vaccines should be given 1 to 2 weeks prior to operative intervention in the event splenic preservation is not possible.
- Should a splenectomy be required in a nonvaccinated patient then vaccines should be administered within 2 weeks following surgical intervention to mitigate postsplenectomy sepsis.
- Seasonal influenza vaccination is also recommended, further recommendations regarding SARS-CoV-2 immunization and boosters are still pending.
- Patients should also obtain baseline laboratory function including type and screen, serum electrolytes, hemoglobin, and hematocrit, as well as pregnancy testing in reproductive-aged females.
- Preoperative antibiotics covering gram-positive, gram-negative, and anaerobic organisms and deep venous thrombosis (DVT) prophylaxis should be ordered prior to patient arrival to the OR. Arterial lines and central venous catheters are placed selectively for high-risk patients.

Positioning

- Patients should be positioned supine on the OR table with arms extended wide with easy access to the OR table should a Bookwalter retractor need to be placed. Some surgeons may also prefer an Omni-Trak or Thompson retractor. Preoperative DVT prophylaxis with heparin should be administered subcutaneously prior to the induction of general anesthesia, bilateral lower extremity sequential compression devices should be placed, and a single dose of a second-generation cephalosporin should be administered within 60 minutes of skin incision.
- After the patient is intubated, a Foley catheter should be placed under sterile technique and a nasogastric tube should be placed for gastric decompression.
- The abdomen is shaved, prepped, and draped, with the xiphoid process, umbilicus, and right and left anterior superior iliac spines exposed.
- An adequate prep will allow for easy incision planning should there be a need to convert to the open technique.
- Some surgeons prefer a semilateral positioning in a relaxed right lateral decubitus position to assist with visualization of the left upper quadrant, whereas others prefer a split leg (Nissen) table to allow the surgeon to stand between the patient's legs.
- Standard laparoscopic instruments (including 0° and 30° laparoscopes), ultrasonic dissector or bipolar electrocautery, laparoscopic staplers (vascular and bowel staple loads), and clip appliers should be available.

LAPAROSCOPIC APPROACH

Port Placement

- Access to the abdominal cavity can be accomplished with either a supraumbilical Veress needle or Hassan trocar depending on surgeon preference, and a pneumoperitoneum is established at 15 mm Hg.
- Three to four additional ports are placed under direct visualization, usually with one in the upper midline or just right of midline, depending on the patient's anatomy. Two additional ports (a 5 mm and a 10 mm to accommodate the laparoscopic stapler) can be placed in the left middle or lower quadrant (FIGURE 2).
- Once all ports are placed, a thorough diagnostic laparoscopy is performed to rule out metastatic disease. If abnormal lesions are identified, they should be biopsied and sent for frozen sectioning. Adhesions are freed to allow full visualization of the left upper quadrant.

Opening the Lesser Sac

- The lesser sac is then opened along the greater curvature of the stomach inferior to the gastroepiploic vessels through the gastrocolic ligament. This allows visualization of the posterior stomach and the anterior surface of the pancreas (FIGURE 3).
- The short gastric vessels along the superior aspect of the fundus should be preserved, as they may be required for splenic preservation if the SA and SV are divided (Warshaw technique).
- If splenectomy is planned, all short gastric vessels will need to be transected.

Identification of the Pancreatic Lesion

- Every effort should be made to identify or palpate the pancreatic lesion and its relationship to the pancreatic neck. Lesions amenable to a DPSP are those to the left of the SMV/PV confluence (FIGURE 4). If the lesion cannot be identified then employment of the laparoscopic ultrasound or EUS can be performed to assist with localization.

Dissection of the Pancreas

- Dissection along the inferior border of the pancreas begins above the ligament of Treitz and should be extended toward the splenic hilum.
- Careful attention is paid to opening just the thin peritoneum inferior to the pancreas and to elevate the pancreas from the retroperitoneal tissue by assuring the plane of dissection stays within the fibroareolar plane. If this is done correctly, the SV will usually be elevated with the pancreas and will result in mobilization of the pancreas anteriorly (FIGURE 5).
- Careful attention is required to avoid lacerating or transecting the posterior SV.
- The IMV should be identified and ligated if it enters the SV to the left of the mass or preserved if it enters the SV to the right of the planned pancreatic transection plane. Neoplastic involvement of the IMV requires ligation and resection.
- Some surgeons advocate for placement of a hand port in the left upper quadrant to assist with tissue manipulation and aid with dissection during this step.

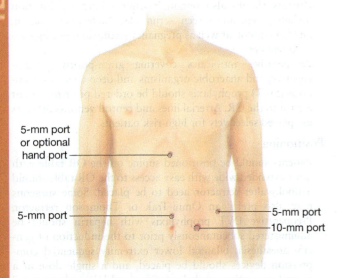

FIGURE 2 • Port placement for a laparoscopic DPSP includes three 5-mm ports, one 10-mm port, and an occasional hand port placed in the upper midline to assist with specimen retraction and dissection.

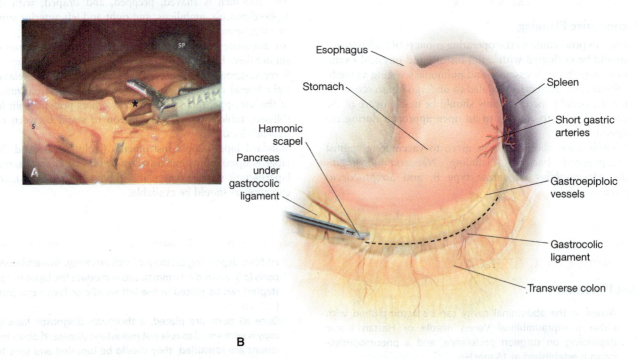

FIGURE 3 • A, The lesser sac is entered by opening the gastrocolic ligament (star) along the greater curve of the stomach (S). Care should be taken to avoid ligating all the short gastric arteries approaching the spleen (SP). B, Opening the lesser sac through the gastrocolic ligament. The gastroepiploic vessels are preserved during the dissection.

Dissection and Control of the Splenic Artery

- With splenic vessel preservation
  - Attention should then be focused on identification of the serpiginous SA located on the superior aspect of the pancreas. The SA can then be carefully dissected from the pancreas using suture ligation or clipping plus energy-assisted ligation and division of small arterial branches running to the pancreatic tail until the pancreas is completely separated from the SA.

- Without splenic vessel preservation (Warshaw technique)
  - The SA is dissected and controlled, followed by ligation using a vascular load of the laparoscopic stapler. The authors suggest additional, subsequent control of either ligation or clipping to minimize risk of pseudoaneurysm in the setting of pancreatic fistula. The SA (inflow) should be controlled before SV (outflow) to decrease bleeding.

Transection of the Pancreas

- With splenic vessel preservation
  - A tunnel should be created to the right of the lesion to free the pancreas from the vasculature for transection (**FIGURE 6**).
  - The pancreas can then be transected with a laparoscopic Endo GIA stapler, Harmonic scalpel, or LigaSure device.
    - In patients with thick pancreas, the pancreatic parenchyma can be thinned out with the ultrasonic

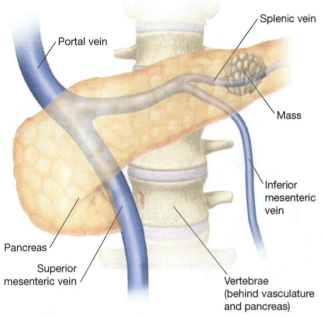

FIGURE 4 • Lesions amenable to a DPSP are those left of the SMV/PV confluence.

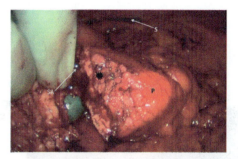

FIGURE 6 • Transection of the pancreas (P) at the confluence of the SV and portal vein left of midline using a hand port. The SA is dissected circumferentially and stapled. The cut edge of the pancreas (star) is reflected anteriorly and toward the spleen (S) to assist with further posterior dissection.

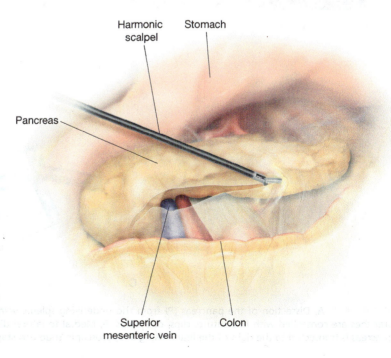

FIGURE 5 • Dissecting and opening the peritoneum along the inferior aspect of the pancreas in a medial to lateral direction. The SV is posterior to the pancreatic body and at risk for injury during dissection if the posterior fibroareolar plane is violated.

dissector while avoiding the pancreatic duct, which usually is positioned posteriorly in the pancreas approximately one-third inferior to the superior border. This enhances the ability of a stapler to appropriately control the pancreatic duct.
- Without splenic vessel preservation (Warshaw technique)
    - Alternatively, the pancreas can be transected with the laparoscopic stapler incorporating the SA and SV in the staple line. The pancreas, SA, and SV can also be dissected and transected individually. In most cases, it is simplest to ligate the SV with the pancreas using a stapler.

Dissection of the Distal Pancreas

- With splenic vessel preservation
    - The SV is identified and dissected off the pancreas posteriorly. This is often expedited by transection of the pancreatic parenchyma, with a right-to-left mobilization.
    - Small venous branches into the pancreas should be carefully dissected and divided between clips, ties, or with the ultrasonic dissector (FIGURE 7). Often, small bleeding veins can be controlled through direct pressure for a short time; however, persistent bleeding may require ligation with a Prolene suture.

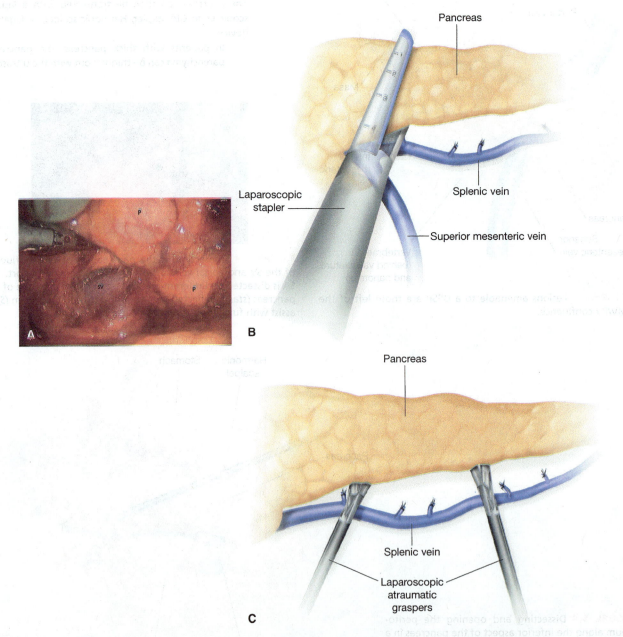

FIGURE 7 • **A,** Dissection of the pancreas (P) from the underlying splenic vein (SV) in a medial to lateral direction. Small venous branches are controlled with fine suture, clips, or staples. **B,** Medial to lateral dissection of the pancreas from underlying SV. **C,** The pancreas is transected to the right of the lesion using a laparoscopic Endo GIA stapler.

- Without splenic vessel preservation (Warshaw technique)
  - An additional fire of the laparoscopic stapler using a vascular load is needed to control the splenic vasculature at the splenic hilum.
  - Great care should be taken to avoid lacerating or puncturing the splenic parenchyma during control of the hilar vessels.
  - Once accomplished, the specimen can be removed from the abdomen using a specimen bag through the largest port site, leaving the spleen to obtain its vascular supply from the short gastric vessels.

Management of the Residual Gland

- Once the specimen is removed, careful attention should be paid to assuring meticulous hemostasis. The surgical bed should be irrigated with warm sterile saline, and the SA and SV should be investigated to ensure hemostasis. Attention should also be directed to the spleen to ensure adequate perfusion and no evidence of ischemia or bleeding.
- Placement of a soft closed suction drain to monitor for pancreatic leaks in the postoperative period is indicated.

Closure

- Following specimen removal, the spleen should be inspected to assess perfusion and bleeding. When using the Warshaw technique, if a completely ischemic or partially ischemic spleen is identified, a splenectomy should be performed, as ongoing ischemia will often result in significant left upper quadrant abdominal pain and bleeding.
- The fascia is closed for 10-mm or larger port sites, and the skin is closed with 4-0 dissolvable sutures. If a hand port is placed, the fascia is closed.

ROBOTIC TECHNIQUE

- The robotic approach to distal pancreatectomy with splenic preservation is increasingly favored over a laparoscopic approach by many surgeons for increased dexterity in vascular dissection, therefore potentially higher rates of splenic preservation. The major limitation of course is the increased cost of a robotic approach vs laparoscopic.[2,3]
- The main operative steps in the robotic approach are identical to those outlined above for the laparoscopic technique. Robotic port placement is slightly different from laparoscopic port placement to maximize exposure; however, this will vary based on surgeon preference.
- Access is typically obtained with a 5-mm Optiview port in the left upper quadrant, which will be upsized to an 8-mm working port. A periumbilical 12-mm camera port is placed. The remaining two 8-mm robotic ports are typically placed in the right upper quadrant, with additional 5-mm or 12-mm assist ports placed as necessary. The additional 12-mm assist port may aid with eventual specimen removal.
- As with the laparoscopic technique, placement of a soft closed suction drain to monitor for pancreatic leak is recommended.

OPEN TECHNIQUE

- The incision of choice for a DPSP depends on the patient's body habitus and previous abdominal surgery.
- Either an upper midline or left subcostal incision can be used. In patients with previous upper midline incisions these can be re-used, although it may be difficult to reach the pancreatic tail with a midline incision especially in obese patients and those with a narrow subcostal angle. In addition, locally advanced malignancies, large tumors, or those where oncologic endpoints may be compromised should be approached with the open technique.
- Once inside the peritoneal cavity, careful palpation of the abdominal cavity should be performed to ensure no evidence of metastatic disease. A self-retaining retractor (Bookwalter) can be placed with cephalad retraction of the left costal margin to allow for visualization.
- The remainder of the operative steps in the open technique are identical to those used for the laparoscopic technique, although sometimes it is easier to perform a left-to-right mobilization first, allowing the spleen to be elevated into the operative field. If performing the Warshaw technique, the SA and SV on the posterior aspect of the pancreas are transected, followed by pancreas transection. The transected edge of the pancreas should be investigated after the specimen is removed and the pancreatic duct ligated with a 2-0 or 3-0 polypropylene suture, or other techniques of pancreatic stump closure can be used, such as the stapler, ultrasonic dissector, or LigaSure.
- A soft closed suction drain should be placed along the cut edge of the pancreas and brought out through a separate stab incision on the abdominal wall. The fascia is then closed in several layers.

PEARLS AND PITFALLS

Preoperative considerations	• A complete history and physical examination should be performed to ensure the patient is a candidate for surgery. • Evaluate for pancreatic insufficiency and malnutrition; consider preoperative nutritional support. • Vaccination against encapsulated organisms. • If there is concern for malignancy the case may be appropriate for multidisciplinary tumor board presentation for planning.
Open vs laparoscopic technique	• Ability to tolerate pneumoperitoneum and previous foregut surgery. • Laparoscopic is the preferred approach for lesions amenable to this technique. • Consider placement of hand port to assist with dissection or specimen removal. • Midline or left subcostal incision can be used for the open approach.
Laparoscopic vs robotic technique	• Robotic approach is becoming more widely used by virtue of better vascular exposure. • Cost remains the major factor limiting implementation of robotic over laparoscopic approach.
Management of short gastric arteries (Warshaw technique only)	• Maintain short gastrics and avoid excessive traction.
Control of splenic artery and vein	• Small branches of the SV should be controlled with direct pressure, clips, or suture ligation. • IMV should be ligated and divided if it enters the SV to the left of the target lesion and preserved if it enters the SV to the right of the lesion or enters the SMV. • If the lesion involves the SA, SV, or IMV—ligate and resect the vessels with the specimen (Warshaw technique). • Careful dissection of the thin-walled SV can avoid bleeding and postoperative SV thrombosis.
Splenectomy	• Splenic preservation is an option except in cases of adenocarcinoma, unclear diagnosis, or direct involvement of the splenic hilum. • Unexpected bleeding or splenic ischemia may require unplanned splenectomy.
Management of the residual pancreas	• Soft closed suction drain placed and output monitored for several days.

POSTOPERATIVE CARE

- Following an uncomplicated DPSP, the patient should be admitted to the general care floor. Routine nasogastric decompression is per surgeon's discretion but may not be needed.
- Assuming stable hemodynamics and hematocrits, patients may begin a clear liquid diet the following day and diet may be advanced as tolerated.
- On postoperative day 1, drain amylase should be checked to assess the risk for pancreatic fistula formation. Attention should be paid to the volume, consistency, and color of the soft closed suction drain and changes in any of the three should prompt further investigation for a developing pancreatic fistula.
- Patients are encouraged to ambulate often and discharged home 4 to 5 days following surgery.

OUTCOMES

- With adequate laparoscopic training and a solid anatomic understanding, this approach can be safely performed with similar rates of morbidity, mortality, and pancreatic fistula development as compared with an open operation.[4,5] As with the majority of laparoscopic techniques, patients often experience less postoperative pain, narcotic use, shorter hospital stay, and nearly identical rates of operative blood loss.[6,7] Several studies have indicated that, when comparing splenic vessel ligation (Warshaw technique) with splenic vessel preservation, there was a greater incidence in splenectomy with splenic vessel ligation, although this technique is easier to perform with shorter operative times.[8] Despite similar outcomes compared with the open technique, a DPSP should be performed by those surgeons with advanced laparoscopic skills after careful patient selection.[9] The robotic approach so far has proven noninferior to laparoscopic with some studies suggesting higher rates of splenic preservation thought to be due to better vascular exposure.[2,3] Cost remains a limitation of the robotic approach, and additional analyses are needed to compare the approaches.

COMPLICATIONS

- Hemorrhage
- Infection—often subdiaphragmatic
- Pancreatic leak/fistula
- Splenic vein thrombosis
- Thrombocytosis
- Hyperglycemia—potential to develop diabetes mellitus
- Pancreatic exocrine insufficiency
- Splenic ischemia (Warshaw technique)

REFERENCES

1. Casciani F, Trudeau MT, Vollmer CM Jr. Perioperative immunization for splenectomy and the surgeon's responsibility: a review. *JAMA Surg.* 2020;155(11):1068-1077. doi:10.1001/jamasurg.2020.1463
2. Eckhardt S, Schicker C, Maurer E, Fendrich V, Bartsch DK. Robotic-assisted approach improves vessel preservation in spleen-preserving distal pancreatectomy. *Dig Surg.* 2016;33(5):406-413. doi:10.1159/000444269
3. Chen S, Zhan Q, Chen J, et al. Robotic approach improves spleen-preserving rate and shortens postoperative hospital stay of laparoscopic distal pancreatectomy: a matched cohort study. *Surg Endosc.* 2015;29(12):3507-3518. doi:10.1007/s00464-015-4101-5
4. Sherwinter DA, Lewis J, Hidalgo JE, Arad J. Laparoscopic distal pancreatectomy. *J Soc Laparoendosc Surg.* 2012;16(4):549-551. doi:10.4293/108680812X13462882736943
5. Cho CS, Kooby DA, Schmidt CM, et al. Laparoscopic versus open left pancreatectomy: can preoperative factors indicate the safer technique? *Ann Surg.* 2011;253(5):975-980. doi:10.1097/SLA.0b013e3182128869
6. Kneuertz PJ, Patel SH, Chu CK, et al. Laparoscopic distal pancreatectomy: trends and lessons learned through an 11-year experience. *J Am Coll Surg.* 2012;215(2):167-176. doi:10.1016/j.jamcollsurg.2012.03.023
7. Stauffer JA, Rosales-Velderrain A, Goldberg RF, Bowers SP, Asbun HJ. Comparison of open with laparoscopic distal pancreatectomy: a single institution's transition over a 7-year period. *HPB.* 2013;15(2):149-155. doi:10.1111/j.1477-2574.2012.00603.x
8. Partelli S, Cirocchi R, Randolph J, Parisi A, Coratti A, Falconi M. A systematic review and meta-analysis of spleen-preserving distal pancreatectomy with preservation or ligation of the splenic artery and vein. *Surgeon.* 2016;14(2):109-118. doi:10.1016/j.surge.2015.11.002
9. Weber SM, Cho CS, Merchant N, et al. Laparoscopic left pancreatectomy: complication risk score correlates with morbidity and risk for pancreatic fistula. *Ann Surg Oncol.* 2009;16(10):2825-2833. doi:10.1245/s10434-009-0597-z

Chapter 41 | Enucleation of Pancreatic Neuroendocrine Tumor

Morgan M. Bonds and Barish H. Edil

DEFINITION

- Pancreatic neuroendocrine tumors (PNETs) are neoplasms that arise from the islet cells of the pancreas or multipotent cells that have the ability to differentiate into endocrine and exocrine cells.[1,2]
- Functional PNETs produce hormones based on which islet cell type became neoplastic. Possible hormones produced by functional PNETs are as follows[2]:
  - Insulinomas produce insulin
  - Gastrinomas produce gastrin
  - Somatostatinomas produce somatostatin
  - VIPomas produce vasoactive intestinal polypeptide hormone
  - Glucagonomas produce glucagon
- Nonfunctional PNETs do not produce hormones. The majority of PNETs are nonfunctional.
- Enucleation refers to the surgical technique of removing a tumor from the surrounding normal tissue without formal, anatomic resection.
  - PNETs are eligible for enucleation if they are smaller than 2 cm due to the low risk of lymph node metastases at this size, although this remains an area of controversy.

DIFFERENTIAL DIAGNOSIS

- Functional PNET symptoms can overlap with other hormonal abnormalities such as serotonin-producing neuroendocrine tumors of the bowel or lung. Imaging will aid in making the correct diagnosis.
- Nonfunctional PNETs are typically found incidentally on imaging. Their appearance on cross-sectional imaging is similar to renal cell carcinoma metastases to the pancreas. Splenules in the tail of the pancreas can also be confused for PNETs.

PATIENT HISTORY AND PHYSICAL FINDINGS

- A thorough history and physical must be obtained to assess to determine whether the tumor is symptomatic. Symptoms can stem from tumor compression of adjacent structures (jaundice, early satiety) or tumor hormone production.
- A minority of PNETs are due to hereditary genetic syndromes. A detailed family history should be taken to evaluate for the presence of multiple endocrine neoplasia type 1, von Hippel-Lindau disease, neurofibromatosis type 1, and tuberous sclerosis complex to ensure the patient and their family are appropriately treated.[1,2]
- Physical examination is generally unremarkable. The patient should be examined for evidence of biliary obstruction, including pruritus and jaundice, as well as signs of distant lymphatic metastases.
- History and diagnostic findings of common functional PNETs:
  - Insulinoma: Whipple triad—documented low blood glucose levels when the patient experiences symptoms of hypoglycemia, and symptom relief with glucose administration.
    - Supervised 72-hour fast produces a plasma glucose of less than 45 mg/dL
    - Elevated C peptide more than 100 pmol/L to rule out exogenous insulin source
    - Negative sulfonylurea screen in urine
    - Negative insulin antibodies
  - Gastrinoma: Zollinger–Ellison syndrome—peptic ulcer disease refractory to prolonged medical/surgical therapy. Associated with secretory diarrhea.
    - Serum gastrin of more than 500 pg/mL while holding proton pump inhibitor therapy
    - Gastric pH less than 3
    - Positive secretin or calcium stimulation test
- **TABLE 1** shows symptoms associated with functional PNETs.

IMAGING AND OTHER DIAGNOSTIC STUDIES

- Computed tomography (CT) and magnetic resonance imaging (MRI) of the abdomen are the most commonly used imaging modalities to localize PNETs. The majority of nonfunctional PNETs are found using these modalities. PNETs tend to be hyperenhancing on arterial phase as seen in **FIGURE 1**.
- Endoscopic ultrasonography with fine needle aspiration (EUS/FNA) is utilized to confirm the diagnosis by obtaining tissue for pathologic evaluation. This is a critical step when considering enucleation as tumor characteristics like grade and proliferation rate may identify more aggressive pathology not amenable to enucleation.[3]
- Somatostatin receptor positron emission tomography (SSRT-PET), which uses ^{68}Ga-DOTATATE binding to somatostatin receptors to localize neuroendocrine tumors, has replaced somatostatin receptor scintigraphy (SRS) in the modern era. This modality has been shown to detect 95.1% of all neuroendocrine tumors compared with 45.3% and 30.9% of all tumors detected by cross-sectional imaging and SRS,

Table 1: Functional PNETs and Symptoms

PNET type	Symptoms
Insulinoma	Fatigue, anxiety, sweating, new cardiac arrhythmias, unsteadiness
Glucagonoma	Diabetes, weight loss, stomatitis, necrolytic migratory erythema
Gastrinoma	Recurrent gastric ulcers despite appropriate therapy, gastroesophageal reflux, secretory diarrhea
Somatostatinoma	Hypochlorhydria, steatorrhea, diabetes
VIPoma	Hypersecretory diarrhea

respectively.[4] Owing to this improved sensitivity and specificity, SSRT-PET is now used to localize and stage PNETs. A nonfunctional PNET in the neck of the pancreas on SSRT-PET is demonstrated in **FIGURE 2**.
- Rarely, percutaneous transhepatic portal venous sampling and arterial stimulation with venous sampling are needed localize small functional PNETs.
- As a part of EUS evaluation, small or deep lesions can be tattooed by the gastroenterologist to assist the surgeon with localization at the time of enucleation.[5] This is particularly helpful with enucleation as anatomic pancreatic resection does not require as precise tumor localization.
- Intraoperative ultrasound can also assist the surgeon with intraoperative PNET localization.

SURGICAL MANAGEMENT

Preoperative Planning

- Enucleation of PNET is typically reserved for insulinomas as they have a low malignant potential and tend to be small at the time of diagnosis. Other functional PNETs behave more aggressively and should undergo formal resection.[6]
- Nonfunctional PNETs can be safely enucleated. Formal resection is recommended for PNETs larger than 2 cm as 50% of these tumors have been found to have nodal metastases at the time of resection compared with 25% of 1- to 1.9-cm PNETs.[7]
- North American guidelines recommend enucleation be reserved for tumors more than 3 mm from the main pancreatic duct to avoid high-grade postoperative pancreatic fistula (POPF).[6] Preoperative placement of a pancreatic duct stent can be used to mitigate this risk, although there are limited data to support this.
- Contraindications to PNET enucleation include recent pancreatitis, uncontrolled coagulopathy, significant comorbidities, and concern for malignant potential (functional PNETs with the exception of insulinoma, high Ki67, poorly differentiated or regional lymphadenopathy).

Positioning

- For minimally invasive or open pancreatic tumor enucleation, the patient should be placed supine on the operating room table. The abdomen, pelvis, and lower chest should be sterilely prepped and draped.

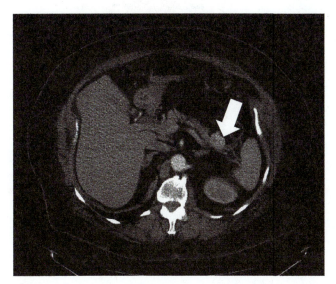

FIGURE 1 • CT scan of abdomen showing a PNET (*white arrow*) in the tail of the pancreas. This is the classic presentation with enhancement on arterial phase.

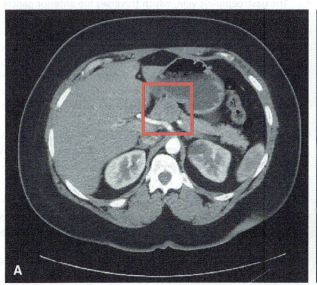 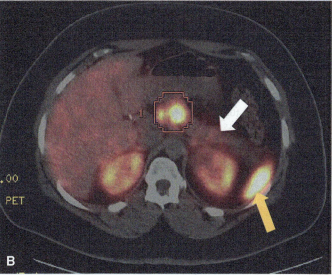

FIGURE 2 • **A,** CT image demonstrates a mass (*red box*) in the neck of the pancreas without enhancement on arterial phase. **B,** SSRT-PET imaging of the same mass is diagnostic of a PNET (*red box*). White arrow indicates the pancreatic tail. The yellow arrow demonstrates the normal physiologic uptake of the spleen.

PLACEMENT OF INCISION

- Open: An incision in the upper midline of the abdomen allows access to the entire pancreas gland.
- Laparoscopic: A 10-mm infraumbilical port is used to gain access to the abdomen. Two additional 10-mm ports are placed in the left upper quadrant and right lower quadrant, followed by two 5-mm ports in the right upper quadrant and left lower quadrant as shown in FIGURE 3.
- Robotic: An 8-mm robotic port is placed in the supraumbilical region. The additional three 8-mm robotic ports are placed with two in the right upper quadrant and one in left upper quadrant. A 12-mm assistant port is placed in the left lower quadrant.

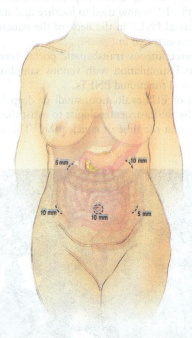

FIGURE 3 • Illustration of port site placement for laparoscopic enucleation of PNET. (Illustration by Frank Corl.)

ABDOMINAL EXPLORATION

- Complete examination of the abdomen and pelvis should be done prior to proceeding with enucleation to ensure there is no visible evidence of locoregional or distant metastases.

PANCREATIC DISSECTION

- An extensive Kocher maneuver should begin dissection if the target lesion is located in the head of the pancreas.
- Exposure of the pancreatic tail requires division of the gastrosplenic ligament and short gastric vessels.
- For lesions in the head, body, or tail of the pancreas, the surgeon next enters the lesser sac through the greater omentum.
- The right gastroepiploic and middle colic vein can be traced posteriorly to the superior mesenteric vein (SMV). Early identification of the SMV helps avoid inadvertent injury.
- Developing a tunnel between the neck of the pancreas and the portal vein–SMV confluence allows for the surgeon to perform a hanging maneuver, wherein an umbilical tape is passed through this space and tagged. The hanging maneuver decreases the trauma caused by direct handling of the pancreas and is particularly useful in minimally invasive pancreatic enucleations.
- The gastroepiploic vein, which traverses the anterior pancreatic head, may be divided to achieve adequate exposure.
- Once the pancreas has been exposed, the gland should be inspected. Intraoperative ultrasound is used to localize small or deep lesions and to confirm the location of superficial lesions. The distance of the tumor from the pancreatic duct is evaluated when enucleation is planned. This step also ensures there is not additional disease in the remainder of the gland.
- Mobilization of the superior and inferior borders of the pancreas using electrocautery allows for access to the posterior pancreas if necessary.

DISSECTING THE MASS

- PNETs, especially insulinomas, are well circumscribed and well encapsulated making them amenable to enucleation from the surrounding parenchyma. A dissection plane generally becomes clear as dissection begins. FIGURE 4 demonstrates a well-encapsulated insulinoma and dissection plane.
- The dissection plane can be developed with the surgeon's preference of energy devices. Traction is necessary in order to maintain a clear dissection plane.
- Should traction prove challenging, place a figure-of-8 suture through the tumor to act as a handle that allows for control of tumor position and areas of countertraction necessary to proceed with mass dissection.
- The authors advocate that bridging structures greater than 1 mm in diameter be surgically ligated.

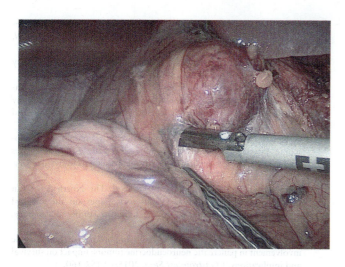

- Hemostasis must be ensured once the mass is completely excised. This can be done with monopolar or bipolar energy devices. Hemostatic agents can also be used.
- Routine duodenotomy should be considered for gastrinomas as they present with multiple tumors that can be located in the duodenum or pancreas.

FIGURE 4 • This image demonstrates how the lesion should be easily dissectable from the pancreatic parenchyma.

CLOSURE AND DRAIN PLACEMENT

- A drain is placed near the surgical resection bed in order to monitor for POPF. If the case was performed minimally invasive, the drain can be brought through an upper abdominal port site as shown in **FIGURE 5**.
- All fascial incisions larger than 10 mm should be closed to avoid future incisional hernias.

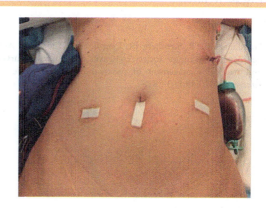

FIGURE 5 • A photograph of the closed abdomen after minimally invasive PNET enucleation; the upper abdominal port sites are ideal for drain extraction.

PEARLS AND PITFALLS

EUS with tattooing of the lesion	• Tattoo very small PNETs for intraoperative localization.
Intraoperative ultrasound	• Liberal use of intraoperative ultrasound should be done so the lesion of interest is not missed.
Deep PNETs/PNETs that approximate the main pancreatic duct	• PNETs that abut the main pancreatic duct or prove challenging for enucleation that are located in body/tail of the gland should undergo laparoscopic or open distal pancreatectomy.
Technique	• Avoid grasping the pancreas or PNET with instruments as this leads to avoidable blood loss. • Hanging maneuver can help manipulate the pancreas without trauma. • A suture through the PNET can aid in retraction of the mass in challenging cases.
Drain	• The rate of POPF after enucleation is high, so drainage of the surgical bed should be utilized routinely.

POSTOPERATIVE CARE

- Diet can be advanced as tolerated by the patient.
- Pain control should be carried out per institutional protocols.
- If an insulinoma or glucagonoma is removed, plasma glucose should be monitored every 15 minutes until stabilized.
- The drains should be monitored to ensure there is no postpancreatectomy hemorrhage. Routine drain amylase should be monitored to ensure there is no POPF prior to removing the drain.

OUTCOMES

- The advantage of PNET enucleation over formal resection is the preservation of pancreatic endocrine and exocrine function.[6]

- Disease-free and overall survival are similar for enucleation and pancreatic resection of nonfunctional PNETs with low malignant potential.[8] These patients and patients with non-insulinoma functional PNETs should undergo routine surveillance. Resection of insulinomas is usually curative.

COMPLICATIONS

- Common early complications include:
  - POPF
    - Managed with percutaneous drainage
  - Acute pancreatitis
  - Superficial or deep space infection
  - Postpancreatectomy hemorrhage
- Late complications
  - Chronic POPF resulting in a cutaneous fistula, pancreatic ascites, or pseudocyst
    - May require endoscopic placement of pancreatic duct stent
  - Disease recurrence

REFERENCES

1. Halfdanarson TR, Strosberg JR, Tang L, et al. The North American neuroendocrine tumor society consensus guidelines for surveillance and medical management of pancreatic neuroendocrine tumors. *Pancreas.* 2020;49:863-881.
2. Burns WR, Edil B. Neuroendocrine pancreatic tumors: guidelines for management and update. *Curr Treat Options Oncol.* 2012;13(1):24-34.
3. Bonds M, Rocha F. Neuroendocrine tumors of the pancreatobiliary and gastrointestinal tracts. *Surg Clin N Am.* 2020;100:635-648.
4. Sadowski SM, Neychev V, Millo C, et al. Prospective study of ^{68}Ga-DOTATATE positron emission tomography/computed tomography for detecting gastro-entero-pancreatic neuroendocrine tumor and unknown primary sites. *J Clin Oncol.* 2016;34(6):588-596.
5. Newman NA, Lennon AM, Edil BH, et al. Preoperative endoscopic tattooing of pancreatic body and tail lesions decreases operative time for laparoscopic distal pancreatectomy. *Surgery.* 2010;148(2):371-377.
6. Howe JR, Merchant NB, Conrad C, et al. The North American neuroendocrine tumor society consensus paper on the surgical management of pancreatic neuroendocrine tumors. *Pancreas.* 2020;49(1):1-33.
7. Curran T, Pockaj BA, Gray RJ, et al. Importance of lymph node involvement in pancreatic neuroendocrine tumors: impact on survival and implications. *J Gastrointest Surg.* 2015;19:152-160.
8. Yang Z, Gao H, Lu J, et al. Comparison of clinical outcomes between enucleation and regular pancreatectomy in patients with non-functional pancreatic neuroendocrine tumors: a retrospective multicenter and propensity score-matched study. *Jpn J Clin Oncol.* 2021;51(4):595-603.

Chapter 42

Operative Treatment of Gastrinoma

Kelly Lynn Koch, Julie Gail Grossman, and Nipun B. Merchant

DEFINITION

- Zollinger–Ellison syndrome is a rare etiology of ulcer disease that is defined by gastrin secretion of neuroendocrine tumors (gastrinomas) typically found in the duodenum and pancreas. These tumors may be sporadic or associated with multiple endocrine neoplasia type 1 (MEN1). Although the gastrin-mediated gastric acid hypersecretion can be controlled with modern antacid and proton pump inhibitor medications, the potentially malignant nature of the gastrinoma is the main determinant of patient survival. Therefore, surgical management remains critical in the care of patients with gastrinomas.

DIFFERENTIAL DIAGNOSIS

- **TABLE 1** summarizes the potential etiologies of hypergastrinemia.

PATIENT HISTORY AND PHYSICAL FINDINGS

- Patients with gastrinomas present with abdominal pain, diarrhea, weight loss, gastroesophageal reflux disease, peptic ulcer disease (often refractory), and complications from acid hypersecretion (bleeding, stricture, and perforation) (**TABLE 2**). Typically, patients have a small, solitary ulcer (<1 cm in diameter) in the first portion of the duodenum, although they may also have a history of recurrent ulcers in atypical locations such as the jejunum (11%) and distal duodenum (14%). Up to 20% of patients do not have an ulcer at presentation.[1,2]
- About 75% to 80% of gastrinomas occur sporadically, with the bulk of the remainder associated with MEN1. There is a slight male preponderance. In the sporadic form, tumors are usually singular, >2 cm, and located in the pancreas and have high malignant potential. MEN1-associated tumors, by contrast, are frequently multiple, <2 cm, and located in the duodenum and have low malignant potential.[3]
- It is important to differentiate the etiology as this dictates the clinical and surgical management of these patients. In addition to gastrinomas, patients with MEN1 may develop parathyroid adenomas, pituitary adenomas, and other neuroendocrine tumors.

IMAGING AND OTHER DIAGNOSTIC STUDIES

- If a gastrinoma is suspected, a serum fasting gastrin level should be obtained. Prior to this test, the patient should be instructed to hold antacid medication (proton pump inhibitors held for 7 days; histamine receptor blockers held for at least 30 hours). Of note, patients can develop esophageal strictures and perforations when proton pump inhibitor therapy has been interrupted.[4]
- An elevated gastrin level greater than 10 times the upper limit of normal (>1000 pg/mL) should be followed by a gastric pH probe in order to rule out achlorhydria. A gastric pH of <2 confirms the diagnosis of gastrinoma if other etiologies have been ruled out.
- A gastrin level that is elevated but < 10 times the upper limit of normal should be followed by a secretin stimulation test. Although normal G-cell gastrin secretion is inhibited by secretin, gastrin release by gastrinoma cells is paradoxically increased. Secretin is infused intravenously over 1 minute after baseline gastrin measurements are obtained; gastrin is then measured at 2, 5, 10, 15, and 20 minutes after infusion. A positive test, typically defined by a rise in serum gastrin of 200 pg/mL or greater, confirms diagnosis of gastrinoma.
- If these tests do not confirm the diagnosis but a high clinical suspicion remains, then basal acid output can be measured. A basal acid output of >15 mEq/h is consistent with the diagnosis of gastrinoma.[5] Serum chromogranin A levels have also been used as a tumor marker in patients with neuroendocrine tumors (**FIGURE 1**).

Table 1: Differential Diagnosis of Hypergastrinemia

Elevated gastric acid secretion	Normal/decreased gastric acid secretion
Helicobacter pylori infection	Pernicious anemia
Retained gastric antrum	Atrophic gastritis
Gastrinoma	Proton pump inhibitor or H₂ blocker use
Antral G-cell hyperplasia	
Renal failure	Postvagotomy
Short bowel syndrome	

Table 2: Signs and Symptoms of Gastrinoma

Abdominal pain (75%)
Diarrhea (73%)
Peptic ulcers (>90%)
Reflux esophagitis (44%)
Nausea (33%)
Emesis (25%)
Weight loss (17%)
Complications of hyperacidity
    Bleeding (25%)
    Perforation
    Obstruction
    Stricture (pylorus, duodenum, esophagus) (<10%)
Physical/Endoscopic findings
    Hypertrophic gastric rugal folds (94%)
    Multiple ulcers
    Unusual ulcer locations
        Distal duodenum (14%)
        Jejunum (11%)
    Pancreatic mass

Data from Roy PK, Venzon DJ, Shojamanesh H, et al. Zollinger-Ellison syndrome. Clinical presentation in 261 patients. Medicine. 2000;79:379-411; Meko JB, Norton JA. Management of patients with Zollinger-Ellison syndrome. Annu Rev Med. 1995;46:395-411.

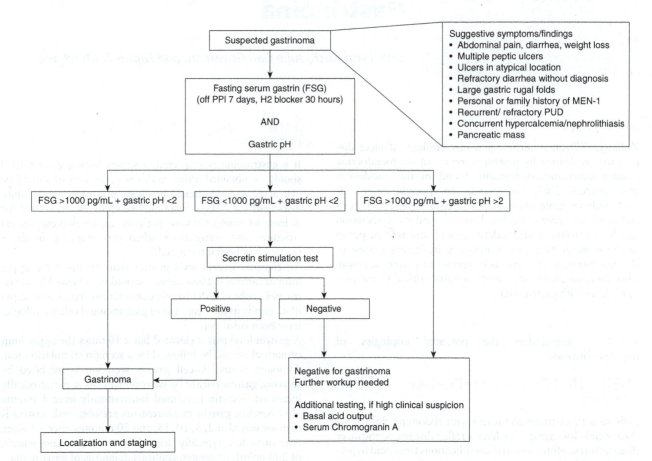

FIGURE 1 • Diagnosis of suspected gastrinoma. MEN1, multiple endocrine neoplasia; PPI, proton pump inhibitor; PUD, peptic ulcer disease; ULN, upper limit of normal.

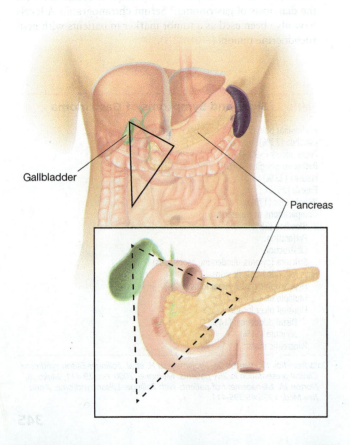

- After obtaining a biochemical diagnosis of gastrinoma, attention is turned to preoperative localization and staging. Up to 90% of gastrinomas can be located in the area bounded by the junctions of the cystic and common bile ducts, second and third portions of the duodenum, and neck and body of the pancreas—the so-called gastrinoma triangle. For patients with MEN1, 60% to 90% of tumors are located in the duodenum. Tumors in the pancreas are more likely to be associated with metastatic disease than those found in the duodenum[6] (**FIGURE 2**).
- Initial localization studies include contrast-enhanced triple-phase pancreas protocol computed tomography (CT) or magnetic resonance imaging (MRI), and endoscopic ultrasonography (EUS). Oral contrast can be used to help delineate intraluminal lesions. The decision to use CT vs MRI should be determined by the clinician based on institutional expertise and availability. Although the accuracy of these modalities continues to improve, the sensitivity for detection of tumors < 2 cm in diameter is decreased, although lesions as small as 4 mm have been detected.[7] EUS can detect smaller lesions (up to 2-3 mm, depending on operator experience) and also has the advantage of being able to obtain a cytologic specimen.
- Somatostatin analogue imaging, performed with a combination of positron emission tomography (PET)/CT and

FIGURE 2 • The gastrinoma triangle. Up to 90% of gastrinomas are located in this region.

68Ga/64Cu-Dotatate radiotracers, can help augment localization of the primary tumor, as well as identify metastatic disease. This modality offers 92% sensitivity and 95% specificity for neuroendocrine tumors disease. Improved detail and sensitivity with dotatate-PET imaging has allowed it to replace the more historical somatostatin receptor single-photon emission computerized tomography (SPECT)-CT (OctreoScan). FDG-PET has limited role in assessment of disease but can be useful to evaluate higher-grade tumors, which are less likely to express somatostatin receptors.[8]
- Patients determined to have MEN1-related gastrinoma should be evaluated for hyperparathyroidism. If a primary hyperparathyroidism is present, it should be addressed prior to further surgical treatment as hypercalcemia may increase anesthetic risk and elevates gastrin and acid production.
- If the etiology is sporadic and no metastases are detected, then surgical exploration is indicated even if a tumor is not localized by preoperative imaging, as these tumors can often be found with careful intraoperative exploration. Long delays related to attempts at localization can increase risk of metastases.
- The risk of liver metastases is increased when tumors are larger than 2 cm.[9]
- Patients who present with metastatic disease should be considered for resection, if possible, as chemotherapy has limited efficacy in the treatment of gastrinomas. Per National Comprehensive Cancer Network (NCCN) guidelines, cytoreductive surgery for distant metastatic disease is recommended in patients where >90% of disease can be safely resected by surgery with or without ablation as this also helps for symptom control.[10] Other options for systemic control include octreotide, radiolabeled somatostatin analogues (Lutathera), and conventional chemotherapy. Liver-directed therapies, such as radiofrequency ablation, stereotactic body radiation therapy, hepatic artery embolization, and liver transplantation can also be considered (FIGURE 3).

SURGICAL MANAGEMENT

Positioning

- Patients should be placed in the supine position for exploratory laparotomy to identify gastrinomas.

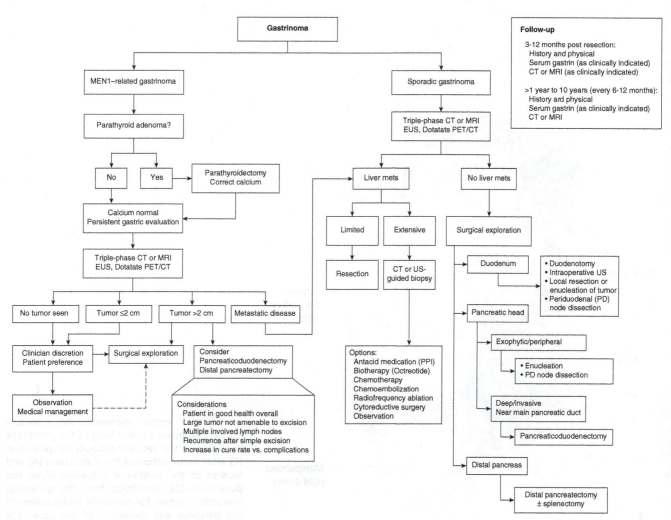

FIGURE 3 • Localization and treatment of gastrinoma.

PLACEMENT OF INCISION

- Either a bilateral subcostal incision or an upper midline incision may be used to approach the duodenum and pancreas for exploration.

Exploration and Kocher Maneuver

- After incision and entry into the peritoneal cavity and initial exploration, the hepatic flexure and ascending colon are mobilized (FIGURE 4A), the peritoneal reflection of the duodenum is incised along the second and third portion of the duodenum, and an extended Kocher maneuver is performed in order to expose and mobilize the duodenum and head of the pancreas (FIGURE 4B).
- After exposure is obtained, the surgeon may palpate the duodenum and pancreatic head (FIGURE 4C).
- It is important to also palpate the pancreatic body and tail. To accomplish this, the lesser sac is opened and the avascular inferior pancreatic border incised; this can be aided by mobilizing the splenic flexure if necessary. Once exposed, the pancreatic body and tail may be carefully palpated to detect any additional tumors (FIGURE 4D).

Intraoperative Ultrasound

- After mobilization of the duodenum and pancreas and detection of visible and palpable tumors, an ultrasound probe is used to visualize small tumors in the duodenum and pancreas. The relationship of any tumor to the pancreatic duct should be noted if an enucleation is to be performed (FIGURE 5).
- The type of probe used should be dictated by surgeon experience and preference. We prefer a fingertip transducer in our institution.
- During ultrasound examination, the surgeon's left hand is generally placed posterior to the duodenum and pancreas, while the right hand handles the probe.
- At this time, the liver is also examined for any possible metastatic lesions, and suspicious lesions should be biopsied.

Intraoperative Endoscopy

- Next, a gastroscope is used to perform intraoperative endoscopy. The gastroscope is advanced orally into the stomach and then duodenum where transillumination is used to identify any remaining gastrinomas. These lesions, located in the submucosa of the duodenum, will appear as shadows upon transillumination (FIGURE 6).

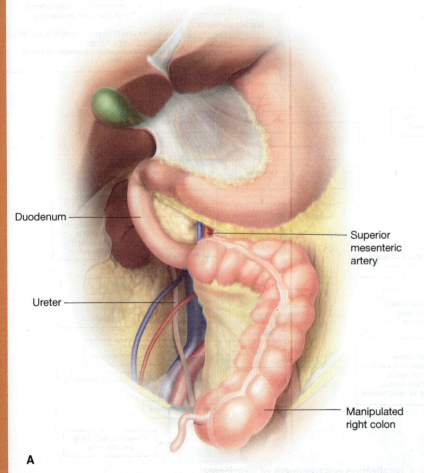

FIGURE 4 • Kocher maneuver. An extended Kocher maneuver allows lifting of the pancreatic head out of the retroperitoneum for palpation (C) after mobilization of the right colon (A) and incision of the peritoneal reflection along the duodenum (B). Separation from the transverse mesocolon allows for complete mobilization of the pancreas and palpation of the pancreatic body and tail (D).

Chapter 42 OPERATIVE TREATMENT OF GASTRINOMA   349

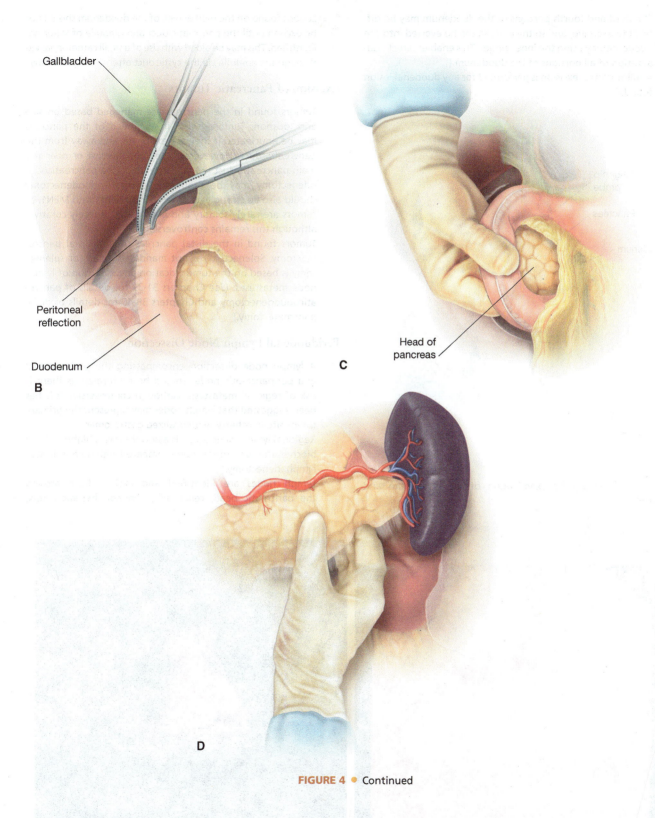

FIGURE 4 • Continued

Duodenotomy

- If duodenal lesions were identified during exploration prior, a longitudinal duodenotomy on the antimesenteric aspect is made to enable excision of the lesion.

- If the location of the lesion remains undetermined, a 2- to 3-cm longitudinal duodenotomy is created on the antimesenteric aspect of the second portion of the duodenum.
- Once the duodenotomy is made, the duodenal wall is palpated carefully with the index finger and thumb (FIGURE 7).

- The third and fourth portions of the duodenum may be difficult to examine, and so the mucosa can be everted into the duodenotomy using the index finger. This enables direct visualization of all portions of the duodenum (FIGURE 8).
- A full-thickness excision is performed for any duodenal lesion found.[11]

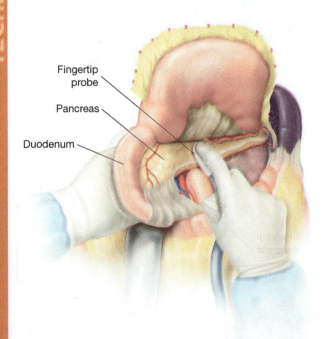

FIGURE 5 • Ultrasound examination of the duodenum and pancreas.

- Lesions found on the medial wall of the duodenum should not be excised until the pancreatic duct and ampulla of Vater are identified. This may be aided with use of a small catheter passed through the ampulla via the cystic duct after cholecystectomy.

Excision of Pancreatic Tumors

- Tumors found in the pancreas are managed based on size and location. Tumors found in the head of the pancreas may be enucleated if they are exophytic and away from the pancreatic duct. However, if they are invasive or near the main pancreatic duct (<3 mm from duct),[12] a pancreaticoduodenectomy may be required. Pancreaticoduodenectomy should also be strongly considered in patients with MEN1, as tumors are rarely solitary and enucleation is rarely curative, although this remains controversial.[6,13]
- Tumors found in the distal pancreas require distal pancreatectomy. Splenectomy is not mandated; need for splenectomy is based on the tumor location and suspicion of lymph node metastases. (See Chapters 31-39 for details of pancreaticoduodenectomy and Chapters 38-40 for details of distal pancreatectomy.)

Periduodenal Lymph Node Dissection

- A lymph node dissection encompassing the periduodenal and peripancreatic nodes should be performed as there is risk of regional metastasis. Although controversial, it is has been suggested that lymph nodes may represent the primary tumor site in otherwise unlocalized gastrinomas.
- Regional lymphadenectomy is associated with higher rate of biochemical cure after surgery compared with no or selective lymphadenectomy.[14]
- Lymph nodes are identified and excised from around the pancreatic head, celiac axis, common hepatic artery,

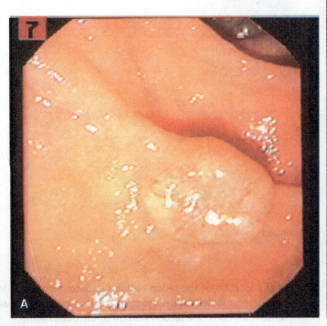
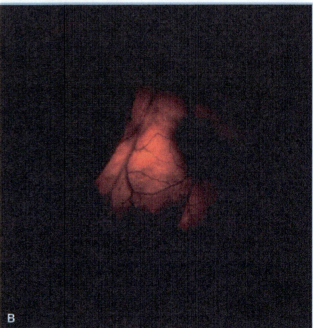

FIGURE 6 • Intraoperative endoscopy. The endoscope is advanced into the duodenum where submucosal tumors may be visualized directly (A) or through transillumination (B).

Chapter 42 OPERATIVE TREATMENT OF GASTRINOMA   351

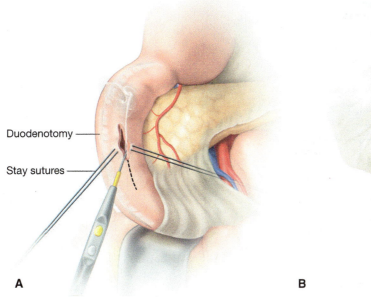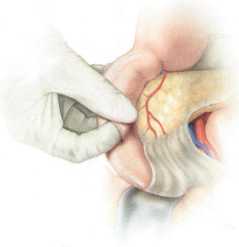

FIGURE 7 • The duodenotomy is made on the antimesenteric aspect of the second portion of the duodenum. **A,** This enables palpation of the duodenum with the thumb and index finger **(B)** so that small tumors may be detected.

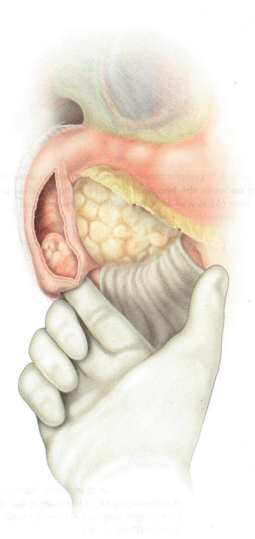

superior mesenteric artery, common bile duct, and portal vein. Lymphadenectomy should begin in the hepatoduodenal ligament and proceed from porta hepatis to celiac axis, followed by excision of all lymph nodes from the anterior and posterior aspects of the pancreatic head (**FIGURE 9**).

Closure of Duodenotomy

- After completion of exploration and excision of gastrinomas, the duodenotomy is closed transversely if possible in order to prevent narrowing of the lumen.
- This is not always possible when a long duodenotomy is required. If this is the case, then a careful longitudinal closure may be used (**FIGURE 10**).
- The duodenum is closed in two layers. Either interrupted or a running closure may be performed based on surgeon's preference.
- A Jackson–Pratt (JP) drain is placed adjacent to the closed duodenotomy in order to monitor output in the postoperative setting. If pancreatic tumors have been enucleated, then an additional drain may be placed overlying the resected lesion.

Management of Liver Lesions

- Solitary, localized lesions can be excised with a negative margin.
- For larger lesions, clusters of lesions, or those near vascular or biliary structures, formal resection can be considered.[15]

FIGURE 8 • Eversion of the mucosa of the third and fourth portions of the duodenum into the duodenotomy.

SECTION III SURGERY OF THE PANCREAS

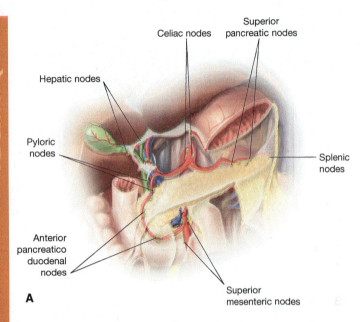

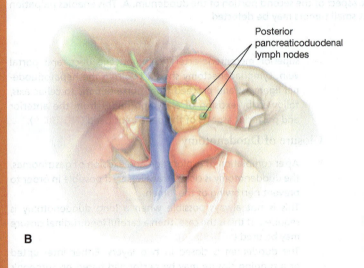

FIGURE 9 • Lymphadenectomy for gastrinoma should encompass nodes in the hepatoduodenal ligament, celiac axis, and anterior (A) as well as posterior (B) pancreatic head.

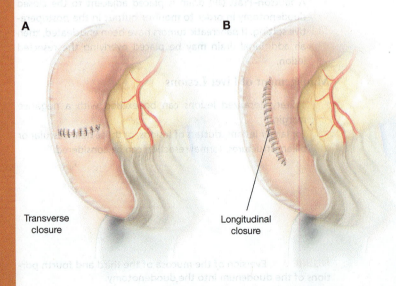

FIGURE 10 • A transverse closure of the duodenotomy (A) is preferable, but the incision length may make a careful longitudinal closure (B) necessary.

Chapter 42 OPERATIVE TREATMENT OF GASTRINOMA   353

PEARLS AND PITFALLS

Operative indications	▪ Biochemical diagnosis of sporadic gastrinoma. ▪ Gastrinoma >2 cm in patients with MEN1.[16] ▪ No evidence of unresectable or extensive metastatic disease. ▪ Reasonable surgical candidate.
Surgical exploration	▪ Intraoperative ultrasound and endoscopy with transillumination greatly aid detection of tumors. ▪ Duodenotomy should be performed in all patients as duodenal tumors are the most frequently missed.[3] ▪ Duodenal tumors require full-thickness excision. ▪ Avoid enucleation of pancreatic tumors if invasive or near main pancreatic duct; formal resection is indicated.
Lymphadenectomy	▪ Exploration and excision of regional lymph nodes is crucial.
Closure	▪ Close duodenotomy transversely, if possible.

POSTOPERATIVE CARE

- After exploration, the patient should be placed on a surgical floor and diet can be advanced as appropriate. Drain output should be monitored closely for character and volume until PO intake is resumed. If there is clinical concern of a leak, then a Gastrograffin swallow study should be obtained for confirmation. We remove the JP drain if the output is serosanguineous once patient is eating normally.
- Follow-up per the current NCCN guidelines includes history and physical exam, imaging (abdominal multiphasic CT or MRI), and biochemical tests (fasting gastrin level; consider stimulated gastrin level only if clinically indicated) starting 12 weeks after surgery and every 6 to 12 months up to 10 years post resection. A chest CT can be obtained if clinical suspicion is raised. Somatostatin receptor imaging and FDG-PET/CT do not have a role in routine surveillance at this time. Some centers include chromogranin A in their surveillance algorithm. Surveillance in MEN1-associated tumors also includes screening for other syndrome-associated neoplasms.[10]

OUTCOMES

- Mortality from this disease is due to metastasis, and it is thought that at least 60% of gastrinomas are metastatic at the time of diagnosis. Patients without liver metastases have a >95% survival at 10 years, whereas those with diffuse liver disease have a 10-year survival of only 15%. Those with solitary or few liver metastases have intermediate survival, about 60%.[17]
- Sporadic disease is potentially curable by surgical exploration. A large series comparing surgical vs medical treatment demonstrated a 41% cure rate at 12 years as well as significantly fewer liver metastases (5% vs 29%). Disease-related survival at 15 years was 98% with surgical intervention vs 74% with medical treatment.[18]
- Gastrinomas associated with MEN1 are associated with an increased risk of distant metastases, regardless of tumor size. However, metastatic gastrinomas in this setting were not significantly associated with a higher risk of death. Five-year survival in patients is reported as 88% to 100%, depending on aggressive vs nonaggressive subtype, regardless of metastatic status.[19] This is important given that >95% of patients with MEN1 show biochemical evidence of relapse within 3 years of surgery.[3]

COMPLICATIONS

- Failure to localize tumor during surgery
- Recurrence
- Residual tumor left after exploration
- Duodenal leak
- Pancreatic leak
- Infection (intra-abdominal abscess)
- Duodenal stricture

REFERENCES

1. Roy PK, Venzon DJ, Shojamanesh H, et al. Zollinger-Ellison syndrome. Clinical presentation in 261 patients. *Medicine*. 2000;79:379-411.
2. Meko JB, Norton JA. Management of patients with Zollinger-Ellison syndrome. *Annu Rev Med*. 1995;46:395-411.
3. Epelboym I, Mazeh H. Zollinger-Ellison syndrome: classical considerations and current controversies. *Oncologist*. 2013;19:44-50.
4. Poitras P, Gingras MH, Rehfeld JF. The Zollinger–Ellison syndrome: dangers and consequences of interrupting antisecretory treatment. *Clin Gastroenterol Hepatol*. 2012;10:199-202.
5. Campana D, Piscitelli L, Mazzotta E, et al. Zollinger-Ellison syndrome. Diagnosis and therapy. *Minerva Med*. 2005;96(3):187-206. PMID: 16175161.
6. Shao QQ, Zhao BB, Dong LB, Cao HT, Wang WB. Surgical management of Zollinger-Ellison syndrome: classical considerations and current controversies. *World J Gastroenterol*. 2019;25:4673-4681.
7. Khashab MA, Yong E, Lennon AM, et al. EUS is still superior to multidetector computerized tomography for detection of pancreatic neuroendocrine tumors. *Gastrointest Endosc*. 2011;73:691-696.
8. Pavel M, Öberg K, Falconi M, et al. Gastroenteropancreatic neuroendocrine neoplasms: ESMO clinical practice guidelines for diagnosis, treatment and follow up. *Ann Oncol*. 2020;31(7):844-860.
9. Norton JA, Jensen RT. Resolved and unresolved controversies in the surgical management of patients with Zollinger-Ellison syndrome. *Ann Surg*. 2004;240:757-773.
10. National Comprehensive Cancer Network. *Neuroendocrine and Adrenal Tumors (Version 3.2021)*. Accessed September 9 2021. https://www.nccn.org/professionals/physician_gls/pdf/neuroendocrine.pdf
11. Rossi RE, Elvevi A, Citterio D, et al. Gastrinoma and Zollinger Ellison syndrome: a roadmap for the management between new and old therapies. *World J Gastroenterol*. 2021;27(35):5890-5907.

12. Doi R. Determinants of surgical resection for pancreatic neuroendocrine tumors. *J Heparobiliary Pancreat Sci*. 2015;22:610-617.
13. Fendrich V, Langer P, Waldmann J, Bartsch D, Rothmund M. Management of sporadic and multiple endocrine neoplasia type 1 gastrinomas. *Br J Surg*. 2007;94:1331-1341.
14. Bartsch DK, Waldmann J, Fendrich V, et al. Impact of lymphadenectomy on survival after surgery for sporadic gastrinomas. *Br J Sur*. 2012;99:1234-1240.
15. Cisco R, Norton JA. Surgery for gastrinomas. *Adv Surg*. 2007;41:165-176.
16. Cingam SR, Botejue M, Hoilat G, Karanchi H. Gastrinoma. In: *StatPearls*. StatPearls Publishing; 2020. PMID:28722872.
17. Norton JA. Surgical treatment of neuroendocrine metastases. *Best Pract Res Clin Gastroenterol*. 2005;19:577-583.
18. Norton JA, Fraker DL, Alexander HR, et al. Surgery increases survival in patients with gastrinoma. *Ann Surg*. 2006;244:410-419.
19. Vinalult S, Mariet A, Le Bras M, et al. Metastatic potential and survival of duodenal and pancreatic tumors in multiple endocrine neoplasia type 1. *Ann For*. 2020;272:1094-1101.

Chapter 43

Lateral Pancreaticojejunostomy With (Frey) or Without (Puestow) Resection of the Pancreatic Head

Kevin E. Behrns

DEFINITION

- No consensus clinical definition exists for chronic pancreatitis.[1,2]
- Chronic pancreatitis is characterized by inflammation resulting in morphologic, histologic, and clinical features, which range from subclinical inflammatory infiltrates evident only in histologic specimens to marked gland destruction accompanied by atrophy, acinar cell dropout, prominent deposition of fibrous extracellular matrix, and pancreatic duct strictures.

DIFFERENTIAL DIAGNOSIS

- Acute pancreatitis
- Autoimmune pancreatitis
- Pancreatic adenocarcinoma
- Intraductal papillary mucinous neoplasm

PATIENT HISTORY AND PHYSICAL FINDINGS

- Advanced stages of chronic pancreatitis manifest clinically by disabling pain and pancreatic exocrine and endocrine insufficiency. The most prominent etiology of chronic pancreatitis is excess consumption of alcohol, but smoking, complex genotypes, and other factors contribute to the clinical features.[3]
- Important risk factors that exacerbate the development of chronic pancreatitis include alcohol use and smoking cigarettes.[4]
- Differentiating alcoholic chronic pancreatitis from autoimmune pancreatitis, especially focal autoimmune pancreatitis, and adenocarcinoma of the pancreas may require extensive evaluation and prove challenging.[5-7]
- A detailed history of alcohol consumption should be obtained; heavy alcohol use (>5 drinks per day) is present in the majority of patients with chronic pancreatitis.[8,9]
- The pain associated with chronic pancreatitis may be either episodic or persistent. Episodic abdominal pain has a duration of 1 to 2 weeks and is interposed by pain-free periods of a few months. Persistent pain occurs daily; however, on occasion pain may resolve spontaneously for a period of a month or more.[3,9]
- The weight loss seen in chronic pancreatitis typically occurs over many months to years, but it may be more rapid if morphologic changes such as pseudocyst formation induce gastroduodenal obstruction.
- Other complications of chronic pancreatitis include jaundice from biliary obstruction and upper gastrointestinal bleeding from gastric varices secondary to splenic vein thrombosis.

IMAGING AND OTHER DIAGNOSTIC STUDIES

- Computed tomography (CT) is the imaging procedure of choice. Intravenous contrast-enhanced, multiplanar, thin-slice CT provides excellent imaging of pancreatic parenchyma and ductal anatomy.[10] CT characteristics of chronic pancreatitis may include an enlarged pancreatic head with multiple calcifications, an atrophic tail, and a dilated pancreatic duct distally (**FIGURE 1**).
- Detection of early-stage disease may be improved by magnetic resonance (MR) with cholangiopancreatography (MRCP) with or without secretin administration. Morphologic

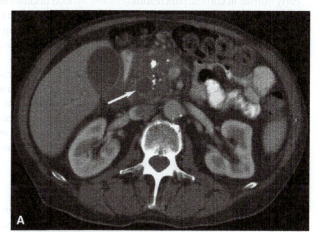

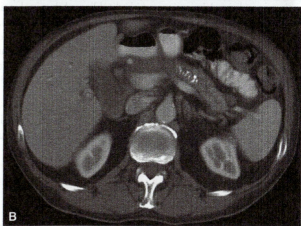

FIGURE 1 • **A,** CT of the abdomen demonstrating an enlarged head of the pancreas with multiple calcifications indicative of alcoholic chronic pancreatitis. A small pseudocyst is also noted in the head *(arrow)*. **B,** The distal pancreas contains calcifications and a dilated pancreatic duct.

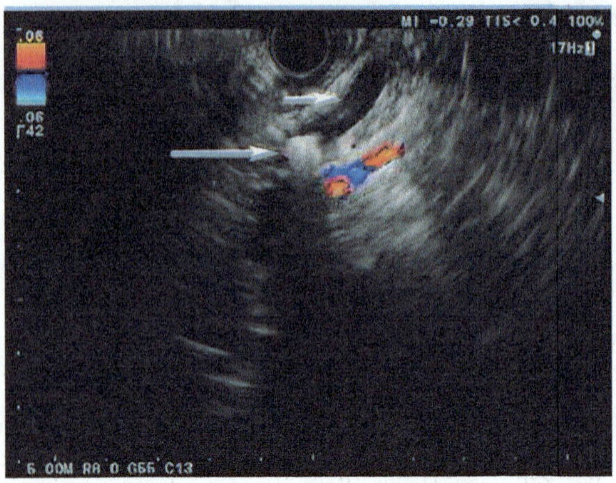

FIGURE 2 • Endoscopic ultrasound demonstrating a dilated pancreatic duct *(short arrow)* with a calculus *(long arrow)* in a patient with chronic pancreatitis.

Table 1: Preoperative Checklist for Patients Undergoing a Frey Procedure

Parameter	Assessment
Alcohol abstinence	Enrollment in substance abuse program with aftercare
Failed medical or endoscopic management	Detailed review of previous medical history
Laboratory evaluation	Blood chemistries, hematologic assessment, liver function tests including coagulation profile, pancreatic function test (fecal fat), nutrition assessment including albumin and prealbumin
Assessment of pancreatic parenchyma for fluid collections or mass lesions	CT or MRI
Assessment of pancreatic duct	MRCP, ERCP, and/or EUS
Assessment of biliary obstruction	Liver chemistries, cholangiogram

CT, computed tomography; ERCP, endoscopic retrograde cholangiopancreatography; EUS, endoscopic ultrasonography; MRCP, magnetic resonance with cholangiopancreatography; MRI, magnetic resonance imaging.

changes in the pancreatic duct and hydrodynamic-significant strictures may be evident on these images.[11]

- Endoscopic ultrasound (EUS) with or without functional testing by administration of secretin may aid in the diagnosis of early fibrosis in chronic pancreatitis (**FIGURE 2**). EUS findings in early chronic pancreatitis may predict the development of classic structural changes over time.[12] Furthermore, EUS is advantageous when mass lesions are present because EUS-guided biopsy is the most reliable method of confirming malignancy.
- Imaging of the pancreatic duct prior to surgical intervention is essential because all strictures and main duct calculi must be addressed by the operative approach. Ductal anatomy can be delineated by MRCP or endoscopic retrograde cholangiopancreatography (ERCP). ERCP is often performed in the context of pancreatic duct stenting as endotherapy often precedes operative management.

SURGICAL MANAGEMENT

- Operative management of chronic pancreatitis by lateral pancreaticojejunostomy with or without pancreatic head resection is indicated in patients with disabling abdominal pain, weight loss, and evidence of pancreatic duct obstruction.[13] Morphologic characteristics are associated with outcomes. An excellent response to pancreatic head resection with pancreaticojejunostomy is most likely in the setting of an enlarged head of the pancreas and a distally dilated pancreatic duct.[14]

Preoperative Planning

- Patients with alcohol-induced chronic pancreatitis typically are noncompliant and do not seek regular medical care; thus, a thorough evaluation of the patient prior to pancreatic head resection and duct drainage is essential.
- Patients should be alcohol-free for at least 6 months and enrolled in an alcohol cessation program with aftercare. Ideally, cigarette smoking would also be stopped prior to an operation, although this is difficult for most patients.
- Specific attention should be paid to the nutritional status of patients with chronic pancreatitis because they often meet criteria for severe protein-calorie malnutrition. Fat-soluble vitamin deficiency should also be considered. If malnutrition is evident, a nasojejunal feeding tube should be placed with the delivery of enteral feeds with pancreatic enzyme supplementation prior to operative intervention. Additional protein supplementation may also be necessary. Generally, 2 to 4 weeks of enteral nutrition prior to an operation will place the patient in an anabolic state, as measured by an increase in serum albumin and prealbumin.
- **TABLE 1** highlights the preoperative checklist of patients who are candidates for a Frey procedure with longitudinal drainage of the pancreatic duct.

Positioning

- The patient is placed on the operating room table in a supine position. General endotracheal anesthesia is required, and placement of an epidural catheter for postoperative pain control is desired. Because the risk for blood loss is moderately high, at least two large-bore intravenous cannulas should be established or a central line should be placed. Arterial monitoring is recommended for patients with comorbidities.

EXPOSURE OF THE PANCREAS

- A midline celiotomy is created to allow adequate exposure of the upper abdomen. After a thorough exploration of the abdomen, the pancreas is exposed by elevating the omentum off the transverse colon and pancreatic head back to the origin on the stomach. The hepatic flexure is mobilized as necessary, and the duodenum is widely Kocherized. Frequently, the posterior wall of the stomach is adherent to the pancreas and must be dissected free. At the inferior border of the pancreatic neck, the right gastroepiploic vein is circumferentially dissected and divided at the insertion into the superior mesenteric vein (SMV). The distal stomach and proximal duodenum are mobilized from the head of the pancreas to allow adequate exposure for resection of the pancreatic head. The SMV should not be dissected free from the posterior surface of the pancreas for fear of venous injury. These maneuvers should provide wide exposure of the pancreas from the duodenum to the tail of the pancreas (**FIGURE 3**).
- This approach and procedure may be accomplished with laparoscopic techniques and excellent outcomes.[15]

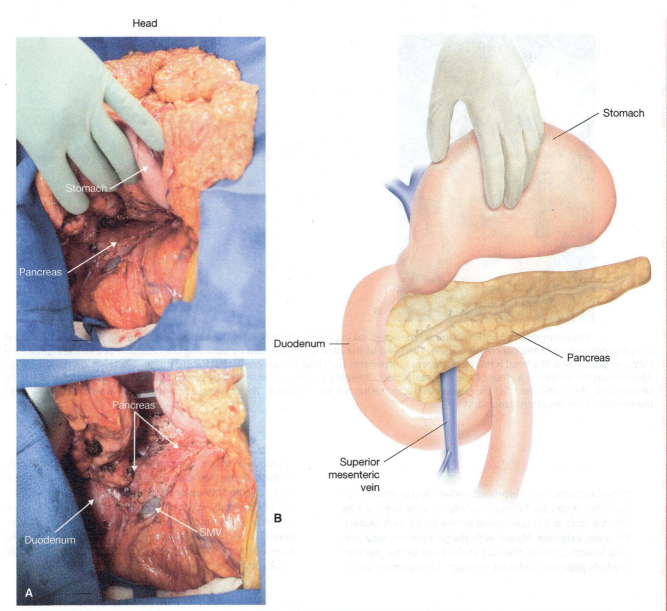

FIGURE 3 • The pancreas is exposed from the head of the gland to the tail. **A,** The omentum is dissected off the transverse colon and transverse mesocolon back to its origin on the stomach. The posterior gastric wall is freed from the anterior surface of the pancreas, and the duodenum is widely mobilized. **B,** The duodenum and anterior surfaces of the head, body, and tail of the pancreas are well exposed. The general location of the SMV inferiorly and portal vein superiorly are noted as anatomic landmarks.

PANCREATIC HEAD RESECTION

- The gastroduodenal artery is identified at the superior border of the pancreas and ligated with a figure-of-eight 4-0 Prolene suture. The resection of the pancreatic head should be mapped with care to avoid injury to the SMV. The pancreatic head is generously resected, leaving only a thin rim (3-5 mm) of tissue along the duodenal wall and posteriorly (**FIGURE 4**). Usually, the pancreatic duct is evident with excavation of the head, and the duct may be followed distally.

Resection of the pancreatic head should not be deeper than the posterior surface of the pancreatic duct. If this plane is not readily apparent, the duct should be identified in the body of the gland (described in the following text) and its course followed proximally to the head of the gland. Bleeding during the pancreatic head resection may be brisk and requires meticulous ligation with 5-0 Prolene sutures. The use of electrocautery to control arterial bleeding should be avoided because this often leads to temporary sealing of the vessel.

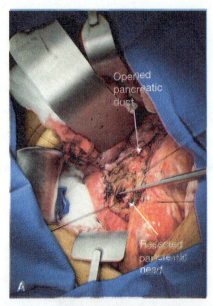
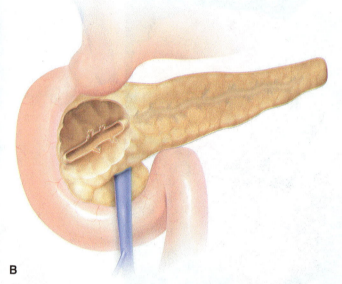

FIGURE 4 • The enlarged head of the pancreas is resected, taking care to identify safety landmarks including the SMV, portal vein, and the posterior surface of the pancreatic duct. **A,** The head of the pancreas is resected by outlining the resection bed to the right of the SMV and portal vein. The head is resected deeper in increments such that the pancreatic duct is identified. The resection should not go deeper than the posterior surface of the pancreatic duct. Bleeding should be controlled by suture ligation. All stone material should be removed. The probe identifies the pancreatic duct entering the duodenum. **B,** The drawing demonstrates excavation of the head of the pancreas with important landmarks.

LONGITUDINAL PANCREATIC DUCTOTOMY

- If the pancreatic duct is identified during the pancreatic head resection, it can be followed distally by inserting a probe into the duct and cutting down on the probe with cautery. However, extensive fibrosis with ductal strictures may prevent identification of the duct in the head of the gland or preclude proximal tracing of the duct. If the duct cannot be identified or traced, it can often be accessed well distal to its course over the SMV. Care should be taken not to identify the duct over the SMV–splenic vein confluence. Once the duct is identified distally, it should be opened from the tail of the pancreas to the junction of the pancreatic head and duodenum (**FIGURE 5**). All pancreatic stones should be removed from the main duct unless extraction of the stone would cause substantial parenchymal damage.

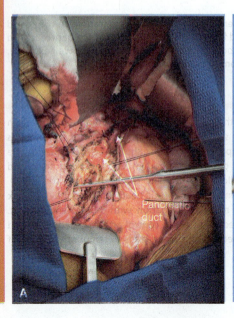
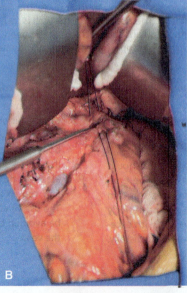

FIGURE 5 • The pancreatic duct is opened from the head of the pancreas to the tail. **A,** Once the pancreatic head is resected, the pancreatic duct can be followed distally and opened over a probe until the duct is opened out to the tail of the gland. **B,** If the pancreatic duct cannot be identified in the head of the gland, a dilated duct can be opened to the left of the SMV in the tail of the gland and followed distally to the pancreatic head resection. **C,** The drawing demonstrates the pancreatic duct opened from the duodenum to the head of the gland.

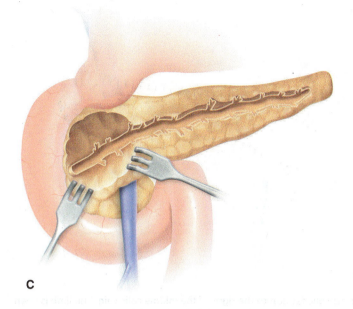

C

FIGURE 5 • Continued

INTRAPANCREATIC BILIARY SPHINCTEROPLASTY

- Patients with an accompanying biliary stricture are candidates for an intrapancreatic biliary sphincteroplasty, which is accomplished by identifying the bile duct along the duodenal wall in the depths of the excavated pancreatic head. This portion of the procedure is markedly aided by preoperative biliary stent placement. The intrapancreatic bile duct can be palpated by transduodenal compression on the biliary stent. The bile duct is opened over the stent with the longitudinal bile ductotomy extending up to the entrance of the bile duct into the pancreas. The stent is removed and not replaced. Once opened, the bile duct should accept at least a 6- to 8-mm probe. The bile duct is then circumferentially sewn with interrupted 6-0 polydioxanone (PDS) sutures to the surrounding pancreatic parenchyma such that the bile duct is widely opened (**FIGURE 6**).

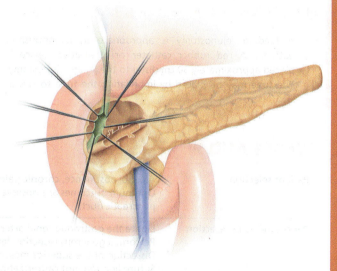

FIGURE 6 • An intrapancreatic biliary sphincteroplasty may be performed in patients with a bile duct stricture. A longitudinal bile ductotomy is performed. The bile duct should be opened superiorly to its entrance in the pancreas. The bile is secured circumferentially to the pancreas with interrupted 6-0 PDS sutures. The bile duct should accept a probe 6 to 8 mm in diameter.

ROUX-EN-Y PANCREATICOJEJUNOSTOMY

- A Roux-en-Y limb of jejunum is prepared by dividing the jejunum 25 to 30 cm distal to the ligament of Treitz. The mesentery is transected back toward its origin by dividing bridging vessels. The Roux-en-Y limb is delivered to the pancreas in a retrocolic position to the right of the middle colic vasculature. The divided end of the jejunum is oriented to the tail of the pancreas, and a two-layer side-to-side pancreaticojejunostomy is created with running 4-0 Prolene sutures (**FIGURE 7**). The epithelium of the pancreatic duct need not be incorporated with the inner layer of suturing. The jejunum should be opened in increments to avoid the creation of an overly long jejunotomy. A jejunojejunostomy is created 40 to 50 cm distal to the pancreaticojejunostomy to reestablish intestinal continuity.

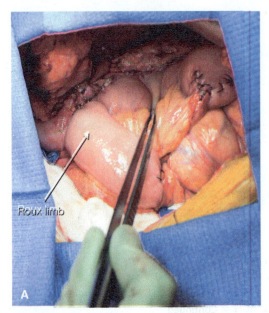 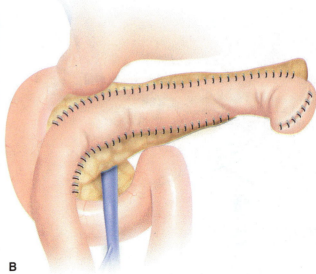

FIGURE 7 • **A,** A Roux-en-Y limb is delivered to the pancreas in retrocolic fashion to the right of the middle colic vein. The limb is sewn to the pancreas in two layers with running 4-0 Prolene. **B,** The drawing demonstrates the completed side-to-side pancreatojejunostomy.

PLACEMENT OF A FEEDING JEJUNOSTOMY

- A feeding jejunostomy is appropriate in malnourished patients. A red rubber catheter or alternative device is placed approximately 30 cm distal to the jejunojejunostomy. The tube may be placed by imbricating the tube to create a tunnel, and the tube should be tacked to the abdominal wall in four-quadrant fashion. Two closed suction drains are placed at the superior and inferior aspects of the pancreaticojejunostomy, and the abdomen is closed.

PEARLS AND PITFALLS

Patient selection	• Alcohol abstinence, chronic pain management • Optimum outcomes are observed in patients with an enlarged head of the pancreas and dilated pancreatic duct.
Pancreatic head resection	• Ligate the gastroduodenal artery first. • Perform a generous resection leaving only thin (3-5 mm) rim of pancreatic tissue. • Dissection of the superior mesenteric vein should be avoided. • Suture ligation, not cauterization, of bleeding vessels.
Pancreatic ductotomy	• Ductotomy should extend from duodenum to the far tail of pancreas.
Intrapancreatic biliary sphincteroplasty	• Assess biliary obstruction; place a biliary stent preoperatively if intrapancreatic biliary sphincteroplasty is anticipated.
Pancreaticojejunostomy	• Open the jejunum incrementally to avoid an overly large jejunotomy.

POSTOPERATIVE CARE

- Because of the risk of postoperative bleeding, the patient should be admitted to a monitored setting. The initial 24 to 48 hours require close observation for hemorrhage. If hemorrhage occurs, a CT arteriogram should be obtained to look for blood in the gastrointestinal lumen vs intra-abdominal hemorrhage. Bleeding into the gastrointestinal tract will require an operative approach, whereas intra-abdominal bleeding may be treated by angioembolization.
- Oftentimes, the exposure of the pancreas requires dissection of chronically inflamed adhesions and, therefore, the fluid requirements postoperatively may be high; close monitoring of the urine output is required.

- Early initiation of postoperative enteral nutrition is necessary because most of these patients are malnourished with low protein reserves.

OUTCOMES

- A randomized trial comparing endoscopic therapy with stents to surgical drainage confirmed superior results for surgical treatment.[16] Patients treated with pancreatic drainage procedures had better pain control, and 47% of patients initially managed by endoscopic therapy ultimately required surgery.
- Operative treatment of chronic pancreatitis may include resection with standard or pylorus-preserving pancreatoduodenectomy or a drainage procedure such as the Frey procedure. The merits of each of these operations have been debated, but a randomized, prospective trial demonstrated that the Frey operation was associated with better short-term outcomes, although the procedures were equivalent in terms of pain control and pancreatic function in long-term analysis.[17]
- Quality of life assessment demonstrated that global, physical, cognitive, and social functions had acceptable outcomes, but prevalent postoperative symptoms were persistent pain, insomnia, and digestive disturbances.[18]
- **TABLE 2** summarizes the results of patients undergoing the Frey procedure.
- The ESCAPE trial, a multicenter, randomized clinical superiority trial, demonstrated that early surgery compared favorably with the endoscopy first approach for the management of pain in patients with chronic pancreatitis.[19]

COMPLICATIONS

- Postoperative hemorrhage.
- Pancreatic fistula is distinctly uncommon.
- Delayed gastric emptying.
- Recurrent biliary stricture following intrapancreatic biliary sphincteroplasty if alcohol consumption is resumed.
- **TABLE 3** includes the anticipated frequency of other complications, which may occur following pancreatic head resection and lateral pancreaticojejunostomy.

Table 2: Outcomes Following Local Pancreatic Head Resection With Longitudinal Pancreaticojejunostomy

Parameter	Frequency (%)
Reintervention required	8
Exocrine insufficiency	86
Endocrine insufficiency	61
Return to work	42
Continued alcohol consumption	21

Adapted from Strate T, Bachmann K, Busch P, et al. Resection versus drainage in treatment of chronic pancreatitis: long-term results of a randomized trial. Gastroenterology. 2008;134:1406-1411.

Table 3: Complications Following Local Pancreatic Head Resection With Longitudinal Pancreaticojejunostomy[18]

Complication	Frequency (%)
Major complications	23
Biliary stricture	11
Pancreatic fistula	7

REFERENCES

1. Andersson R, Lohr JM; Working Group for Chronic Pancreatitis Guidelines (Sweden). Swedish national guidelines for chronic pancreatitis. *Scand J Gastroenterol.* 2021;56:469-483.
2. Whitcomb DC, Shimoseegawa T, Chari ST. International consensus statement on early chronic pancreatitis: recommendations from the working group for international consensus guidelines for chronic pancreatitis in collaboration with the International Association of Pancreatology, American Pancreatitive Association, Japan Pancreas Society, PancreasFest working group and European Pancreatic Club. *Pancreatology.* 2018;18:516-527.
3. Anderson MA, Akshintala V, Albers KM. Mechanism, assessment, and management of pain in chronic pancreatitis: recommendations of a multidisciplinary study group. *Pancreatology.* 2016;16:83-94.
4. Yadav D, Whitcomb DC. The role of alcohol and smoking in pancreatitis. *Nat Rev Gastroenterol Hepatol.* 2010;7:131-145.
5. Chari ST, Longnecker DS, Kloppel G. The diagnosis of autoimmune pancreatitis: a Western perspective. *Pancreas.* 2009;38:846-848.
6. Ha J, Choi SH, Byun JH. Meta-analysis of CT and MRI for differentiation of autoimmune pancreatitis from pancreatic carcinoma. *Eur Radiol.* 2021;31:3427-3438.
7. Whitcomb DC. Genetics of alcoholic and nonalcoholic pancreatitis. *Curr Opin Gastroenteol.* 2012;28:501-506.
8. Yadav D, Hawes RH, Brand RE, et al. Alcohol consumption, cigarette smoking, and the risk of recurrent acute and chronic pancreatitis. *Arch Intern Med.* 2009;169:1035-1045.
9. Ammann RW, Muelhaupt B. The natural history of pain in alcoholic chronic pancreatitis. *Gastroenterology.* 1999;116:1132-1140.
10. Siddiqi AJ, Miller F. Chronic pancreatitis: ultrasound, computed tomography, and magnetic resonance imaging features. *Semin Ultrasound CT MR.* 2007;28:384-394.
11. Madzak A, Olesen SS, Halderson IS. Secretin-stimulated MRI characterization of pancreatic morphology and function in patients with chronic pancreatitis. *Pancreatology.* 2017;17:228-236.
12. Monachese M, Lee PJ, Harris J. EUS and secretin endoscopic pancreatic function test predict evolution to overt strucgtural changes of chronic pancreatitis in patients with non-diagnostic baseline imaging. *Endosc Ultrasound.* 2021;10:116-123.
13. Behrns KE. Local resection of the pancreatic head for pancreatic pseudocysts. *J Gastrointest Surg.* 2008;12:2227-2230.
14. Amudhan A, Balachander TG, Kannan DG, et al. Factors affecting outcome after Frey procedure for chronic pancreatitis. *HPB (Oxford).* 2008;10:477-482.
15. Senthilnathan P, Babu NS, Vikram A. Laparoscopic longitudinal pancreatojejunostomy and modified Frey's operation for chronic calcific pancreatitis. *BJS Open.* 2019;24:666-671.
16. Cahen DL, Gouma DJ, Laramee P, et al. Long-term outcomes of endoscopic vs surgical drainage of the pancreatic duct in patients with chronic pancreatitis. *Gastroenterology.* 2011;141:1690-1695.
17. Strate T, Bachmann K, Busch P, et al. Resection vs drainage in treatment of chronic pancreatitis: long-term results of a randomized trial. *Gastroenterology.* 2008;134:1406-1411.
18. Fischer TD, Gutman DS, Warner EA. Local pancreatic head resection: the search for optimal indications through quality of life assessments. *Am J Surg.* 2015;210:417-423.
19. Issa Y, Kempeneers MA, Bruno MJ. Effect of early surgery vs endoscopy-first approach on pain in patients with chronic pancreatitis: the ESCAPE randomized clinical trial. *JAMA.* 2020;323:237-247.

Chapter 44

Enteric Drainage of Pancreatic Pseudocysts: Pancreatic Cyst Gastrostomy and Cyst Jejunostomy

Kenneth K. W. Lee

DEFINITIONS

- Collections of fluid or solid material may arise from episodes of acute pancreatitis. Although frequently referred to collectively as pancreatic pseudocysts, the 2012 revision of the Atlanta classification of acute pancreatitis distinguishes among several types of local collections that arise in acute pancreatitis based on their pathogenesis and imaging characteristics.[1] An understanding of these different collections is important as their management differs.
    - **Acute peripancreatic fluid collections** (APFCs) (**FIGURE 1A** and **B**) arise early in the course of interstitial edematous acute pancreatitis. APFCs lack a wall, are confined by fascial planes, and rarely require intervention as the risk of complications such as infection is very low and they usually resolve spontaneously (**FIGURE 2A** and **B**).
    - APFCs that fail to resolve may become **pancreatic pseudocysts** with well-defined walls. **Pancreatic pseudocysts** (**FIGURE 3A**) are encapsulated, well-defined peripancreatic or intrapancreatic fluid collections that arise from focal disruption of the pancreatic ductal system in the setting of acute or chronic pancreatitis or trauma. In contrast to cystic neoplasms of the pancreas, pseudocysts lack true epithelial walls and instead have walls composed of fibrous tissue containing histiocytes, giant cells, granulation tissue, and rarely eosinophils. The fluid within a pseudocyst is characteristically amylase-rich as it arises from disruption of the pancreatic ductal system. The 2012 revision of the Atlanta classification of acute pancreatitis also emphasizes that pseudocysts are not associated with detectable amounts of pancreatic or peripancreatic necrosis and do not contain a solid component. Magnetic resonance imaging (**FIGURE 3B**) or ultrasound may be useful for identification of solid material not distinguishable on computed tomography.
- In contrast to APFCs and pancreatic pseudocysts, acute necrotizing pancreatitis is defined by the presence of pancreatic and/or peripancreatic tissue necrosis. In the early stages of acute necrotizing pancreatitis, the necrotic

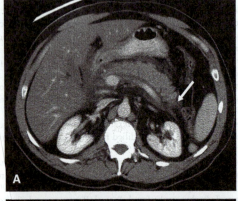

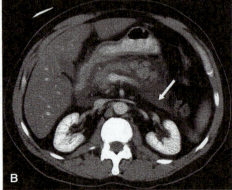

FIGURE 1 • Acute peripancreatic fluid collection. **A,** The pancreas appears edematous with small amounts of fluid surrounding it. **B,** Peripancreatic fluid tracks laterally anterior to the kidney but remains confined by fascial planes.

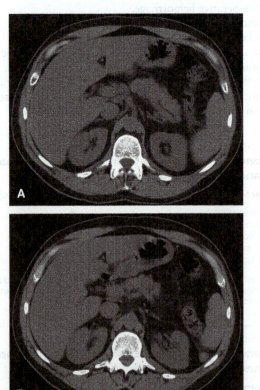

FIGURE 2 • **A and B,** Acute peripancreatic fluid collection. The acute fluid collections are resolved 3 weeks later.

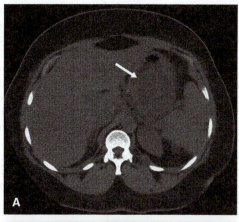
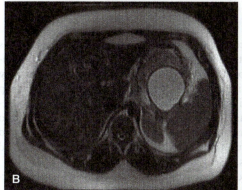
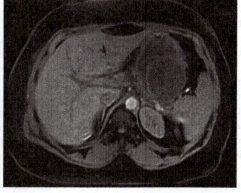

FIGURE 3 • Pancreatic pseudocyst. **A,** A homogeneous fluid collection is surrounded by a discrete wall that is apparent despite the absence of intravenous contrast. **B,** Magnetic resonance imaging confirms the absence of solid material (necrotic debris) within the pseudocyst.

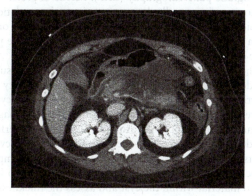

FIGURE 4 • Acute necrotic collection. Areas of pancreatic and peripancreatic necrosis surround portions of viable (enhancing) pancreas.

tissue is described as an **acute necrotic collection** (ANC) (**FIGURE 4**). Such collections may additionally contain fluid leaking from the pancreatic duct or resulting from liquefaction of necrotic tissue. The natural history of ANCs is variable. Such collections may persist or absorb, remain solid or liquefy, remain sterile or become infected.
- Fibrous walls form around necrotic collections that are not absorbed or do not require early surgical debridement. As with acute necrotic collections, areas of **walled-off necrosis** (**WON**) (**FIGURE 5**) may contain fluid in addition to solid material.

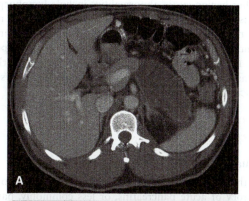
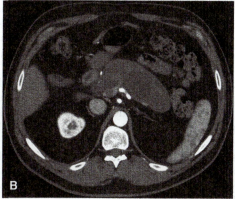

FIGURE 5 • **A** and **B,** Walled-off necrosis.

- Although the pathogenesis and contents of WON differ from pancreatic pseudocysts, their management is similar to pseudocysts, particularly if communication with the pancreatic ductal system is suspected.

DIFFERENTIAL DIAGNOSIS

- **Pancreatic pseudocyst**
- **Walled-off necrosis**
- **Pancreatic cystic neoplasms** possess a true epithelial lining and thereby differ from pseudocysts that are lined by fibrous tissue (see earlier discussion). Cystic neoplasms primarily fall into two categories. **Microcystic (serous) cystadenomas** contain serous fluid and carry minimal if any risk of malignant transformation. Treatment by means of surgical resection is reserved for those that are symptomatic. **Macrocystic (mucinous) cystadenomas (mucinous cystic neoplasms)** contain mucinous material, are characterized by the presence of ovarian stroma, and have the potential for malignant transformation. Surgical resection is therefore usually recommended for such lesions.
- **Neoplasms with cystic morphology.** Adenocarcinomas of the pancreas may have cystic components. Areas of tumor necrosis, for example, may liquefy and appear cystic on imaging studies. Pancreatic ductal adenocarcinomas may also cause proximal ductal obstruction that may resemble cysts in the pancreas. **Pancreatic endocrine tumors** may also occasionally be predominantly cystic.
- **Intraductal papillary mucinous neoplasms (IPMNs)** may arise in the main pancreatic duct or in side branch ducts and on imaging appear as solitary or multiple pancreatic cysts.
- Other benign cystic abnormalities include **lymphoepithelial cysts** and **inclusion cysts**. If diagnosed, treatment is reserved for those that are symptomatic. **Mucinous cysts** that do not contain ovarian stroma and do not appear to have potential for malignant transformation may also occur in the pancreas. Differentiation of such benign mucinous cysts from mucinous cystadenomas may be difficult.

PATIENT HISTORY AND PHYSICAL FINDINGS

Evaluation

- A thorough medical history must be taken to confirm **a history of acute pancreatitis**, or less commonly, pancreatic trauma. In the absence of such a history, the diagnosis of a pancreatic pseudocyst should be questioned, and the diagnosis of a neoplasm should be considered. As several weeks are required for a pseudocyst to form, the diagnosis of a pseudocyst should also be questioned if the clinical history of acute pancreatitis or pancreatic trauma is very recent and a cystic abnormality with an already well-formed wall is seen.
- The history should also attempt to identify the etiology of the patient's pancreatitis, as treatment of the etiology (eg, cholecystectomy, lipid- and triglyceride-lowering medications, and abstinence from alcohol consumption) should be considered.
- Symptoms potentially attributable to a pseudocyst should be elicited. Most frequently, these will include abdominal or back pain, abdominal pressure or fullness, early satiety, nausea, vomiting, or obstructive symptoms. If a complication of the pseudocyst such as infection, bleeding, or rupture has occurred, symptoms relating to the complication such as fever, light-headedness, or diffuse abdominal pain may also be present.
- The general medical history and overall health of the patient are important in determining the manner of treatment appropriate for the patient. Past surgical history should be reviewed with particular emphasis on prior operations on the stomach or small intestine and incisions that may impact on laparoscopic or open access to the abdomen.
- An abdominal mass or fullness should be sought on physical exam, and if found, its location should be noted in planning subsequent surgical procedures. Abdominal surgical scars should also be noted.

IMAGING AND OTHER DIAGNOSTIC STUDIES

- The presence and location of cystic changes of the pancreas are best determined by means of contrast-enhanced **computed tomography (CT)** or **magnetic resonance imaging (MRI)**. The imaging characteristics on these studies may help to differentiate among the various types of cystic pancreatic abnormalities listed earlier. Cross-sectional imaging also demonstrates the relationship of the cyst to the stomach and other structures as well as the thickness of the cyst wall and thereby aids in treatment planning.
- Pancreatic ductal abnormalities that may influence treatment decisions can be identified by means of **magnetic resonance cholangiopancreatography (MRCP)** or **endoscopic retrograde pancreatography (ERP)**. MRCP is preferred as it is noninvasive, usually does not require patient sedation, and avoids the risks of procedure-induced pancreatitis or infection of fluid collections in communication with the pancreatic duct.
- If the clinical history and imaging findings are not sufficient to determine the specific type of cystic abnormality and in particular to exclude the diagnosis of a neoplastic cyst with potential for malignant transformation, further imaging by means of **endoscopic ultrasound (EUS)** can be performed. Under EUS guidance, fine-needle aspiration of the cyst contents and cyst wall can be performed to obtain samples for biochemical and pathologic analysis. EUS can also identify solid material within the cyst and assess the thickness of the cyst wall.
- Biochemical and genetic analysis of cyst fluid obtained by means of EUS may also help to determine the specific type of cystic abnormality. As pseudocysts arise from disruption of the pancreatic ductal system, cyst fluid typically has an elevated amylase level. Fluid associated with WON is also frequently amylase-rich. Intraductal papillary mucinous neoplasms also are frequently amylase-rich.
- A limited set of genetic alterations is useful in the diagnosis of pancreatic cysts. Genetic alternations are absent in pseudocysts, WON, and other benign non-neoplastic cysts such as lymphoepithelial or retention cysts. In contrast, IPMNs are characterized by mutations in KRAS, GNAS, RNF43, BRAF, and CTNNB1. KRAS, RNF43, BRAF, and CTNNB1 mutations are also found with mucinous cystic neoplasms, but GNAS alterations are absent. VHL mutations and/or deletions are found in 90% of microcystic

(serous) cystadenomas, but neither KRAS nor GNAS mutations are present.
- ERP is not routinely performed for evaluation of pseudocysts, but in selected cases may be performed to evaluate ductal anatomy when MRCP cannot be performed or is inconclusive. Because of the potential for introducing infection into a sterile pseudocyst, ERP should be limited to patients selected for treatment (see the following text) and should be performed shortly before treatment.
- Although the pathogenesis and pathology of pancreatic pseudocysts and WON differ, their management is similar and therefore differentiating between pseudocysts and WON is not always required. In the discussion that follows, the term pseudocyst is used to describe both pseudocysts and WON as defined in the 2012 revision of the Atlanta classification of acute pancreatitis.

SURGICAL MANAGEMENT

Indications for Treatment
- Treatment should be considered for symptomatic pseudocysts or enlarging pseudocysts.
- Emergency treatment of complications such as infection, rupture, or bleeding into the pseudocyst may be required.
- Small, asymptomatic, nonenlarging pseudocysts do not require treatment as the risk of developing acute complications is low. However, as the risk of complications arising in large asymptomatic, nonenlarging pseudocysts is uncertain and may be greater, treatment of such large pseudocysts can be considered.
- Treatment should be considered if the diagnosis of a neoplasm with malignant potential cannot be excluded.

Treatment Options
- Surgical resection can be performed for removal of a pseudocyst.
- External drainage may be achieved by percutaneous or surgical means.
- Internal drainage of a pseudocyst creates a communication between the pseudocyst and the gastrointestinal tract.
  - Drainage into the stomach is achieved by creating a communication between the posterior wall of the stomach and a pseudocyst known as a **cyst gastrostomy**. This may be achieved by endoscopic means, surgical means, or a hybrid combination of these methods. The anastomosis can be fashioned within the stomach via an anterior gastrotomy, outside the stomach via the lesser sac, or within the stomach via endolaparoscopic means.
  - Drainage into the small intestine is achieved by surgical creation of an anastomosis between a defunctionalized segment of the small intestine (Roux limb) and a pseudocyst known as **a cyst jejunostomy**.
  - Pseudocysts arising in the head of the pancreas are infrequently drained by creation of an anastomosis between the descending duodenum and the pseudocyst known as a **cyst duodenostomy**.

Choice of Procedure
- Surgical resection should be considered when the diagnosis of a cystic-appearing neoplasm such as a mucinous cystadenoma cannot be excluded or selectively by means of a distal (left) pancreatectomy for a pseudocyst or WON involving the tail of the pancreas. Distal (left) pancreatectomy is discussed elsewhere in this text. Because of the greater morbidity and mortality of a pancreaticoduodenectomy (Whipple procedure), resection should not be considered for pseudocysts in the head of the pancreas.
- As pseudocysts arise as a result of disruption of the pancreatic ductal system and WON is also commonly associated with pancreatic duct disruption, external (percutaneous) drainage of pseudocysts or WON may give rise to a pancreatic fistula. Therefore, when treatment is necessary, internal drainage into the gastrointestinal tract is generally preferred. However, external drainage may be preferred if treatment of the pseudocyst is required before a wall suitable for construction of an anastomosis has formed. Temporary relief of symptoms may be achieved by large volume fine-needle aspiration. Infection of an evolving pseudocyst is treated by placement of a drainage catheter. External drainage may also be considered if internal drainage does not appear safe for treatment of acute complications such as pseudocyst rupture or infection that arise in mature pseudocysts.
- Surgical drainage is most commonly performed into either the stomach or the small intestine. Cyst jejunostomies have a lower incidence of pseudocyst recurrence and perioperative bleeding compared to cyst gastrostomies but require creation of a Roux limb and an intestinal anastomosis (see below). Additionally, pseudocyst recurrence after creation of a cyst gastrostomy may be amenable to endoscopic treatment. Therefore, if the stomach suitably abuts the pseudocyst, a cyst gastrostomy is usually created. Otherwise, a Roux-en-Y cyst jejunostomy is created.
- Endoscopic cyst gastrostomy (discussed in detail elsewhere in this text) is especially well suited for treatment of true pseudocysts containing only fluid and no necrotic tissue.
- Open and minimally invasive (laparoscopic or robot-assisted) techniques of creating cyst gastrostomies and Roux-en-Y cyst jejunostomies are fundamentally identical.

Preoperative Preparation
- Patients should be prepared in routine fashion for major abdominal surgery.
- Comorbidities such as hypertension and cardiopulmonary disease should be optimized.
- Patients should be evaluated and treated for pancreatic endocrine and exocrine insufficiency.
- Coagulation disorders if present should be corrected.
- Routine antibiotic and thromboembolic prophylaxis should be administered.
- In malnourished patients, surgery should be delayed and preoperative nutritional support should be given when possible. Enteral nutrition is preferred but may not be possible due to the mass effects of the pseudocyst.

Positioning
- For either open or minimally invasive procedures, the patient is placed in a supine position. Arms may either be tucked or extended outward.
- Table-mounted retractors are used as needed for open procedures.

DESCRIPTION OF PROCEDURES

- Gastric drainage procedures
  - Transgastric cyst gastrostomy
  - Extragastric cyst gastrostomy
  - Intragastric cyst gastrostomy
- Jejunal drainage procedure
  - Roux-en-Y cyst jejunostomy

TRANSGASTRIC CYST GASTROSTOMY

- See ▶ Video 1.
- A midline incision provides excellent exposure for **open transgastric cyst gastrostomies**. Palpation of the abdomen after induction of anesthesia and review of the patient's preoperative imaging studies will guide placement of the incision.
- A wound protector is placed, thorough exploration of the abdomen is performed, and the fullness posterior to the stomach caused by the pseudocyst is palpated and localized. If necessary, the pseudocyst can be further localized using ultrasound (FIGURE 6).
- Port placement for **minimally invasive transgastric cyst gastrostomy** will vary according to the size and position of the pseudocyst. In general, however, one midabdominal 5-mm port, two right upper abdominal 5-mm ports, and two left upper abdominal 5-mm ports will suffice. These ports are upsized as necessary for insertion of staplers and ultrasound probes.
- Stay sutures are placed over the epicenter of this fullness (FIGURE 7), and a longitudinal anterior gastrotomy is made using electrocautery (FIGURE 8). This incision should be centered between the lesser and greater curvatures of the stomach to facilitate subsequent closure of the anterior gastrotomy. The anterior gastric wall is usually mobile and, consequently, the anterior gastrotomy can usually be made short. The longitudinal orientation of the gastrotomy allows it to be lengthened proximally or distally if needed.
- Through the posterior wall of the stomach, the pseudocyst is palpated. The location of the pseudocyst can be confirmed by means of intraoperative ultrasound (FIGURE 9) or passage of a needle through the posterior wall of the stomach into the pseudocyst and aspiration of fluid from the pseudocyst (FIGURE 10). Both measures also provide an estimate of the distance between the stomach and the pseudocyst

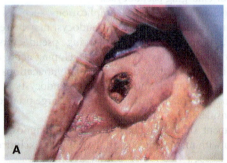

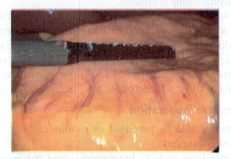

FIGURE 6 • Ultrasound can be used to localize the pseudocyst and assist in positioning of the anterior gastrotomy (laparoscopic cyst gastrostomy).

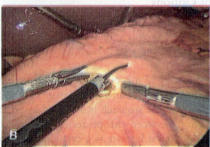

FIGURE 8 • A longitudinal anterior gastrotomy is made. **A,** Open cyst gastrostomy. **B,** Laparoscopic cyst gastrostomy.

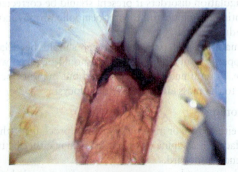

FIGURE 7 • Stay sutures placed into the anterior wall of the stomach may facilitate creation of the anterior gastrotomy (open cyst gastrostomy).

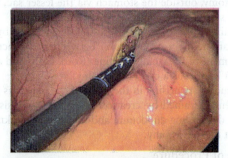

FIGURE 9 • Ultrasound examination through the posterior wall of the stomach assists in localization of pseudocyst and positioning of the cyst gastrostomy incision (laparoscopic cyst gastrostomy).

Chapter 43 ENTERIC DRAINAGE OF PANCREATIC PSEUDOCYSTS 367

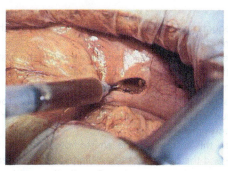

FIGURE 10 • Transgastric aspiration of the pseudocyst confirms the location of the pseudocyst and distance from the gastric wall and assists in positioning of the cyst gastrostomy incision (open cyst gastrostomy).

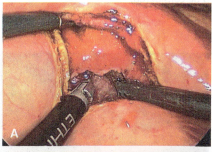

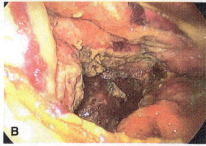

FIGURE 11 • The pseudocyst is entered (A) and its contents including any necrotic material are removed (B).

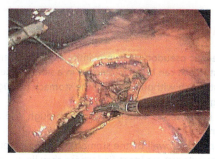

FIGURE 12 • A portion of the cyst wall is excised and sent for frozen section examination to confirm the presence of a fibrous wall consistent with a pseudocyst and absence of an epithelial lining suggestive of a cystic neoplasm (laparoscopic cyst gastrostomy).

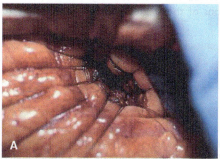

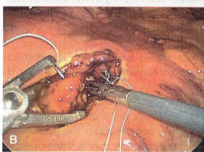

FIGURE 13 • A and B, Sutures are placed circumferentially along cyst gastrostomy to reinforce the adherence of the stomach to the pseudocyst wall and to ensure satisfactory hemostasis along the cyst gastrostomy. A, Open cyst gastrostomy. B, Laparoscopic cyst gastrostomy.

cavity. Fluid obtained by aspiration can be sent for biochemical, microbiologic, cytologic, and pathologic studies as indicated.
- The pseudocyst is entered through the posterior wall of the stomach using electrocautery at the site determined by ultrasound or aspiration and the contents of the pseudocyst are evacuated (FIGURE 11). Any necrotic debris within the cavity is removed. A portion of the pseudocyst wall is excised and sent for frozen section evaluation to confirm the presence of a fibrous wall and to exclude the presence of an epithelial lining (FIGURE 12).
- The opening into the pseudocyst is enlarged using electrocautery or another type of energized device. A finger or ultrasound probe placed into the pseudocyst helps to define the extent to which the posterior wall of the stomach is adherent to the anterior wall of the pseudocyst. A cyst gastrostomy of 5 cm or more is desirable when possible. The pseudocyst cavity is explored and any loculations within it are opened.

- Absorbable 2-0 sutures are placed circumferentially that approximate the posterior gastric wall to the pseudocyst wall (FIGURE 13). These sutures reinforce the adherence of the pseudocyst to the stomach and promote hemostasis along the cyst gastrostomy.
- After the initial entry into the pseudocyst, the cyst gastrostomy can also be enlarged using a linear surgical stapler. However, it remains mandatory to excise a portion of the pseudocyst wall for histologic evaluation.
- After ensuring that hemostasis is satisfactory, a nasogastric tube is positioned in the stomach and the anterior gastrotomy is closed using sutures or staplers. Depending on the length and position of the gastrotomy and the size of the stomach, the closure is oriented longitudinally or transversely.
- A final exploration of the abdomen is performed, and the midline incision is closed. Drains are not routinely placed.

EXTRAGASTRIC CYST GASTROSTOMY

- Lesser sac pseudocysts in proximity to the posterior wall of the stomach can be anastomosed in a side-to-side fashion to the stomach without entering the stomach through an anterior gastrostomy.
- The lesser sac is widely entered through the gastrocolic omentum.
- The posterior wall of the stomach and the anterior wall of the pseudocyst are identified where they lie in close proximity but are not adherent to one another.
- Small openings are made in the posterior wall of the stomach and the anterior wall of the pseudocyst where they lie in close proximity to one another, and a linear stapler is inserted into these openings and fired. Additional applications of the stapler are used as necessary to create an adequate anastomosis. The common opening is then closed using staplers or sutures.
- Alternatively, parallel incisions are made in the posterior wall of the stomach and the anterior wall of the pseudocyst and a hand-sewn anastomosis is fashioned.
- This technique of anastomosis between the stomach and pseudocyst can be performed as either an open or minimally invasive procedure.
- With this technique, the anastomosis between the stomach and the pseudocyst is not limited by the extent of their adherence to one another. Complications arising from the anterior gastrotomy are also eliminated.
- However, a leak at the cyst gastrostomy will result in extraluminal extravasation of gastrointestinal contents and a gastric fistula. Placement of a drain adjacent to the cyst gastrostomy should be considered.

LAPAROENDOSCOPIC INTRAGASTRIC CYST GASTROSTOMY

- See Video 2.
- Laparoscopic access into the peritoneal cavity is achieved in the usual manner. Three right-sided 5-mm ports are initially placed. The mobility of the anterior wall of the body of the stomach is assessed to determine if it will reach to the abdominal wall. To do so, the pneumoperitoneum may need to be decreased. Once confirmed, traction sutures are placed into the stomach at this location, and passed out through the abdominal wall at the previously determined site.
- The jejunum is followed from the duodenojejunal junction to a site where the jejunum is mobile. A noncrushing bowel clamp is applied across the jejunum to prevent distention of the intestine during subsequent insufflation of the stomach.
- A 12-mm port is inserted at the previously determined site. A small gastrotomy is made at the center of the traction sutures, and the 12-mm port is advanced through this opening into the stomach. The traction sutures are used to hold the stomach upward against the abdominal wall. This is facilitated by also using a cuffed 12-mm port (FIGURE 14).
- The stomach is insufflated through the intragastric port, and laparoscopic examination of the inside of the stomach is performed. The bulge in the posterior wall of the stomach caused by the retrogastric pseudocyst is visible (FIGURE 15).
- An endoscope is the passed via the mouth into the stomach, providing intragastric visualization and allowing for laparoscopic instrumentation to be passed into the stomach through the single intragastric port (FIGURE 16).
- After localization of the pseudocyst by means of aspiration or ultrasound evaluation, an incision is made through the posterior wall of the stomach into the pseudocyst using electrocautery or other types of energy devices (FIGURE 17).

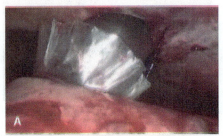
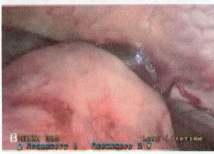

FIGURE 14 • **A and B,** Assisted by traction sutures, a cuffed 12-mm port is inserted into the stomach **(A)**, and the stomach is pulled upward against the abdominal wall.

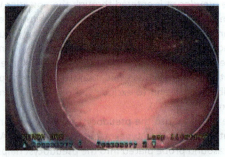

FIGURE 15 • After passage of a laparoscope into the stomach through the intragastric port, a bulge in the posterior wall of the stomach caused by the retrogastric pseudocyst is visible.

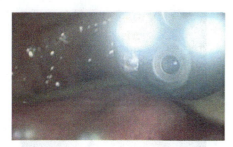

FIGURE 16 • An endoscope passed through the mouth into the stomach provides intragastric visualization and permits passage of laparoscopic instruments through the single intragastric port.

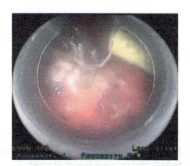

FIGURE 17 • Under endoscopic visualization and after localization of the retrogastric pseudocyst, a small incision is made in the posterior wall of the stomach and the pseudocyst is entered.

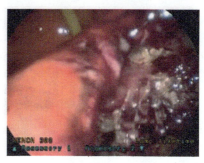

FIGURE 18 • The cyst gastrostomy is enlarged using staplers or energy devices, and drainage and debridement of the pseudocyst are completed.

- A small portion of the pseudocyst wall is excised for frozen section evaluation, and the cyst gastrostomy is enlarged using either stapling or energy devices. Particular attention is given to ensuring satisfactory hemostasis. Through the cyst gastrostomy drainage and debridement of the cyst cavity are completed (**FIGURE 18**). Small amounts of residual debris will subsequently pass through the cyst gastrostomy. A nasogastric tube is positioned in the stomach, the port is removed from the stomach, and the gastrotomy is closed using either sutures or staplers. The bowel clamp is removed from the intestine and the remaining laparoscopic ports are removed. A drain is not routinely placed.

ROUX-EN-Y CYST JEJUNOSTOMY

- See ▶ Video 3.
- A midline incision provides excellent exposure for **open Roux-en-Y cyst jejunostomies**. Palpation of the abdomen after induction of anesthesia and review of the patient's preoperative imaging studies will guide placement of the incision. As the operation is performed predominantly below the transverse mesocolon, the incision is usually slightly more inferior than the incision used for creation of a cyst gastrostomy.
- A wound protector is placed and thorough exploration of the abdomen is performed. The pseudocyst typically presents as fullness bulging into the transverse mesocolon, and the fullness caused by the pseudocyst is palpated and localized.
- Port placement for **minimally invasive Roux-en-Y cyst jejunostomy** will vary according to the size and position of the pseudocyst. In general, however, ports are positioned lower in the abdomen than for creation of a minimally invasive cyst gastrostomy. Port placement is selected not only for creation of the cyst jejunostomy but also for creation of the Roux limb and subsequent enteroenterostomy.
- The transverse colon is elevated upward, allowing visualization of the transverse mesocolon and the bulging resulting from the pseudocyst. The location of the pseudocyst can be confirmed by aspiration. If the location of the pseudocyst is not readily apparent, intraoperative ultrasound can be used with reference to the patient's preoperative imaging studies (**FIGURE 19**). Ultrasound evaluation may also assist in identifying mesenteric vessels overlying the pseudocyst that should be avoided in fashioning the cyst jejunostomy. Adhesions

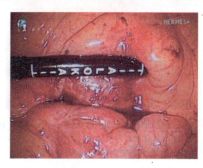

FIGURE 19 • Intraoperative ultrasound localization of pancreatic pseudocyst bulging through the transverse mesentery.

overlying the pseudocyst are then taken down using sharp and blunt dissection (**FIGURE 20**).

- With the pseudocyst identified and exposed, a defunctionalized Roux limb is then prepared. The consequences of a leak subsequently occurring at the cyst jejunostomy are mitigated by use of a Roux limb rather than a functional loop of jejunum. The jejunum is followed from the duodenojejunal junction to a site where the mobility of the jejunum and the configuration of its vascular arcades are suitable. As the cyst jejunostomy is positioned below the mesocolon, mobility of the Roux limb is rarely an issue. However, occasionally, the jejunal mesentery may be very foreshortened or thickened as a result of the prior episode(s) of pancreatitis. The intestine is divided using a linear stapler, and the mesentery is divided, taking care to ensure that hemostasis is meticulous and that the blood supply to both ends of the jejunum is satisfactory (**FIGURE 21**).

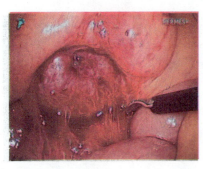

FIGURE 20 • Dissection and exposure of pseudocyst bulging through the transverse mesentery.

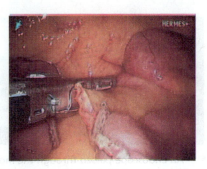

FIGURE 21 • Creation of Roux limb using a linear stapler to divide the jejunum and its mesentery.

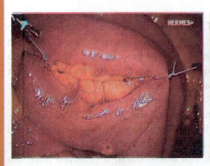
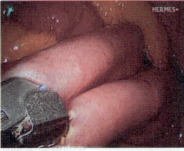

FIGURE 22 • Creation of side-to-side enteroenterostomy using a linear stapler.

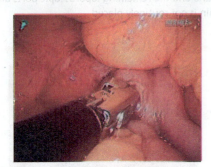

FIGURE 23 • Creation of side-to-side Roux-en-Y cyst jejunostomy using a linear stapler. The jaws of the stapler are positioned in the Roux limb (*right*) and pseudocyst (*left*).

- Gastrointestinal continuity can be reestablished before or after creating the cyst jejunostomy and can be performed using staplers, sutures, or a combination of both (FIGURE 22). The anastomosis can be performed in either a side-to-side or end-to-side fashion. A Roux limb measuring 40 to 50 cm should be created. In some instances, a longer Roux limb may be created if the patient's history or imaging results suggest the possible need for an additional cyst jejunostomy or biliary reconstruction in the future. In this case, the manner in which the enteroenterostomy is made and the positioning of the Roux limb should be carefully considered. After completing the enteroenterostomy, the resulting mesenteric defect is closed with sutures to prevent hernias.
- The Roux limb is positioned next to the pseudocyst and a side-to-side anastomosis measuring 3 to 5 cm in length is then created between the pseudocyst and the Roux limb. As with the extragastric cyst gastrostomy, this anastomosis

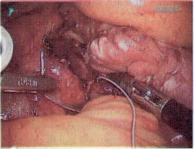
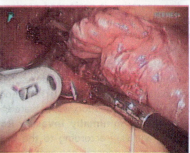

FIGURE 24 • Creation of side-to-side Roux-en-Y cyst jejunostomy using sutures. Suture has been passed through the Roux limb (**top**) and is now being passed through the pseudocyst (**bottom**).

  can be performed using staplers (FIGURE 23) and/or sutures (FIGURE 24). Stapler and suture choice is determined by the thickness of the pseudocyst wall.
- A drain is placed adjacent to the anastomosis, and after confirming that hemostasis is satisfactory, the incision or ports are closed.

Chapter 44 ENTERIC DRAINAGE OF PANCREATIC PSEUDOCYSTS

PEARLS AND PITFALLS

Differential Diagnosis	▪ Cystic neoplasm must always be considered.
Imaging and other diagnostic studies	▪ Management is driven by high-quality imaging. The anatomic relationships, presence of necrotic debris, and involvement of pancreatic duct must be well determined to implement appropriate therapy. ▪ Be mindful of a potential disconnected pancreatic duct.
Preoperative planning	▪ Timing of intervention is key. The goal is to allow the process to adequately mature while minimizing the duration of disability. ▪ Anatomic relationships drive management. ▪ Cyst gastrostomy is technically least demanding but associated with higher recurrence rates. ▪ Approach the pseudocyst from the transverse mesocolon for cyst jejunostomy. ▪ Consider laparoscopic approach or endoscopic assistance. ▪ Look for venous thrombosis and varices.
Surgical management	▪ Debride all necrotic material. ▪ Respect varices. Be liberal with ligation. ▪ Running or locking sutures to fashion the anastomosis are advised to minimize the risk of postoperative bleeding.

POSTOPERATIVE CARE

- A nasogastric tube is routinely placed in patients who undergo creation of a cyst gastrostomy and left in place until gastric emptying appears satisfactory.
- Drain output is evaluated for the presence of amylase and lipase. If present, the drain is left in place until output has ceased.
- Routine antibiotic and thromboembolic prophylaxis are administered. Other aspects of routine postoperative care are followed.
- Patients are evaluated for resolution of symptoms previously attributed to the pseudocyst. If symptoms persist, follow-up imaging (CT or MRI) is performed. Otherwise, routine follow-up imaging is obtained after 3 months to confirm resolution of the pseudocyst. Thereafter, further evaluations are dictated by the development of new symptoms.
- If symptoms persist after a cyst gastrostomy and imaging confirms the presence of a residual pseudocyst, endoscopy should be performed to evaluate the patency of the cyst gastrostomy. If narrowed, the cyst gastrostomy can be endoscopically dilated. The residual pseudocyst can be accessed, debrided, and drained endoscopically. Additionally, a nasocystic catheter can be placed for irrigation of the cavity.
- If symptoms persist after a Roux-en-Y cyst jejunostomy and imaging confirms the presence of a residual pseudocyst, the cyst jejunostomy can occasionally be evaluated and if necessary be dilated endoscopically. However, the Roux construction often prevents this from being accomplished. Although revision of the cyst jejunostomy may need to be considered, if imaging studies demonstrate evidence of patency of the cyst jejunostomy (eg, air in the pseudocyst), consideration should be given to allowing additional time for resolution of the pseudocyst before proceeding with surgery. Additionally, careful evaluation of the patient's symptoms should be performed to ensure that they are caused by the residual pseudocyst before embarking on further surgery.

COMPLICATIONS

- In addition to intraperitoneal bleeding, bleeding may occur from gastrotomies used to access the stomach and from any of the anastomotic sites. The cyst gastrostomy is particularly prone to bleeding because of the inherently rich blood supply of the stomach and the inflammation associated with the episode of pancreatitis and pseudocyst formation. Endoscopy is useful not only for evaluating the cyst gastrostomy but also for evaluating for bleeding within the pseudocyst cavity. However, accumulation of blood, fluid, and debris within the cavity may hinder thorough evaluation and consideration should be given to early angiography. Angiography should also be strongly considered for evaluation of bleeding from a Roux-en-Y cyst jejunostomy, as this anastomosis cannot be readily evaluated endoscopically.
- Leakage can occur at anastomotic and gastric closure sites. Leakage from an anterior gastrotomy closure or enteroenterostomy is managed as with any gastrointestinal leak. Leakage from a Roux-en-Y cyst jejunostomy can be managed nonoperatively if controlled satisfactorily by the drains placed at the time of surgery. Additional drains can be inserted percutaneously if needed. As the Roux limb is defunctionalized, surgical exploration is not required if adequate drainage is established. If leakage occurs from an extragastric cyst gastrostomy, the patient should initially be made nil per os (NPO). With adequate drainage from the surgically placed drains, leaks from either type of anastomosis will usually heal spontaneously.

REFERENCE

1. Banks PA, Bollen TL, Dervenis CL, et al. Acute Pancreatitis Working Group. Classification of acute pancreatitis—2012: revision of the Atlanta classification and definitions by international consensus. *Gut.* 2012;62(1):102-111.

Chapter 45 Pancreatic Necrosectomy

Nicholas J. Zyromski

DEFINITION

- Nearly 300,000 patients are admitted to US hospitals yearly with the primary diagnosis of acute pancreatitis. Among these patients, 10% to 15% will develop severe acute pancreatitis with variable necrosis of the peripancreatic soft tissue and pancreatic parenchyma.
- Necrotizing pancreatitis (NP) is a serious problem; despite improved disease understanding and critical care advances, NP mortality remains approximately 20%.
- Once pancreatic and peripancreatic necrosis have been established, one of the three outcomes will present itself. **FIGURE 1** illustrates these potential outcomes. A small percentage of patients will resolve their necrosis with no intervention. Another portion of patients will develop infection in the necrosis; this typically demands treatment. A third group of patients will have persistent necrosis. If the necrosis causes no symptoms, no intervention is necessary. However, symptomatic necrosis remains an indication for intervention. Symptoms may include fullness/early satiety, general malaise, and back pain. These symptoms are related to mass effect of the necrosis as well as to the inflammatory response.

PATIENT HISTORY AND PHYSICAL FINDINGS

- The etiology of pancreatitis should be investigated. Patients with biliary pancreatitis should be considered for cholecystectomy with cholangiography at the time of pancreatic debridement. A significant number of patients with NP will have idiopathic cause; current data implicate microlithiasis and/or sludge in many of these cases. Therefore, strong consideration should be given to cholecystectomy if technically possible and safe at the time of debridement.
- Patients with NP have widely variable physiologic condition prior to necrosectomy. On two ends of the spectrum, a patient may be acutely ill with systemic sepsis and require debridement urgently for infectious control. On the other hand, many patients may be "walking wounded"—that is to say, they are home from the hospital managing some oral alimentation and are in reasonable physical health; however, they remain moderately to profoundly symptomatic.
- All efforts should be made to optimize nutritional and physical condition prior to pancreatic debridement. The clinician should understand that objective nutritional values will never normalize with a volume of necrotic tissue in the retroperitoneum generating a persistent inflammatory response. Enteral alimentation is ideal; parenteral nutrition is often necessary to supplement caloric and protein intake. Many patients with NP receive alimentation as combination of TPN and enteral calories.
- It must be emphasized that multiple approaches are available to treat patients with NP. The disease is extremely heterogeneous, and no one intervention fits all patients. Ideally, an experienced multidisciplinary team consisting of surgeons, interventional endoscopists, and interventional radiologists are invested in evaluating these patients. One doctor must be responsible for the long-term care of these patients as the recuperation typically encompasses 6 to 12 months or longer.

IMAGING AND OTHER DIAGNOSTIC STUDIES

- A current cross-sectional image—that is, computed tomography (CT) or magnetic resonance imaging (MRI) scan—of the abdomen and pelvis is critically important to use as a road map guiding debridement.
- An important diagnostic consideration involves estimating the volume of solid material (as opposed to fluid) in the peripancreatic collection. MRI is more accurate than CT in making this estimation. Ultrasound may be most accurate; however, transabdominal ultrasound is plagued by artifact from hollow viscus. Endoscopic ultrasound (EUS) is an excellent modality; however, it requires sedation and is moderately invasive. **FIGURE 2** illustrates MRI and ultrasound images.
- Endoscopic retrograde pancreatography (ERP) is the most accurate in defining pancreatic ductal anatomy and, specifically, the presence of disrupted main pancreatic duct. If ERP is undertaken in the setting of NP, it should be done a short time before planned debridement, as ERP has a high chance of contaminating what otherwise may be sterile necrosis. Fine needle aspiration of the pancreatic and peripancreatic necrosis is relatively sensitive in diagnosing infection. This modality is not commonly necessary or used in contemporary practice.
- Transabdominal ultrasound of the gallbladder should be performed to diagnose stones or sludge and inform the need for cholecystectomy.
- Broad-spectrum empiric antibiotic treatment is not recommended currently. Antibiotic therapy should be reserved for documented infections with a discrete endpoint in treatment.
- Patients with NP have an extremely high (56%) incidence of venous thromboembolic events. Screening duplex ultrasonography should be considered in all patients with NP.

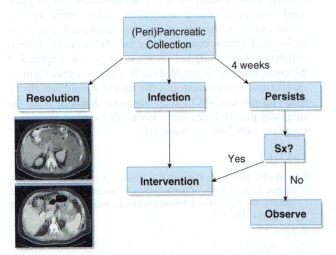

FIGURE 1 • Necrosis outcomes. *Sx*, symptoms.

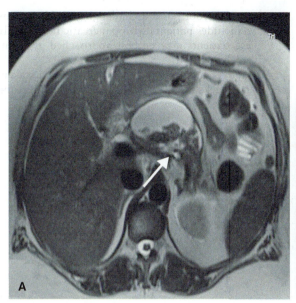
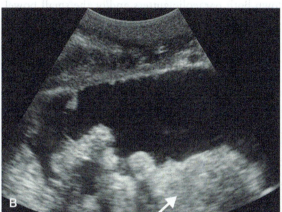

FIGURE 2 • **A,** MRI showing solid and fluid components *(arrow)* of peripancreatic collections. **B,** IOUS image of the same collection. Solid necrosis is highlighted with *arrow*.

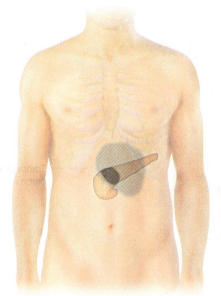
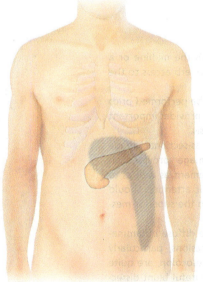
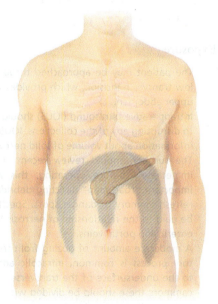

FIGURE 3 • Necrosis patterns.

SURGICAL MANAGEMENT

- In contemporary practice, most patients with NP are managed by minimally invasive approaches such as percutaneous drains, endoscopic debridement, or a combination of these techniques. Operative surgical debridement is currently reserved for patients refractory to minimally invasive approach (ie, the last step in the "step-up" approach) or those with concern for ischemic viscera (gallbladder, colon). Necrosis localized to the lesser sac should be approached surgically in biliary pancreatitis patients, in whom cholecystectomy may be performed concomitantly. Certain patients with multifield necrosis may be best treated by primary operative debridement.

- Perhaps the most important concept regarding NP is that this disease is extremely heterogeneous. The intervention/operative approach is dictated primarily by anatomic distribution of necrosis, involvement of the pancreatic parenchyma by necrosis, and specific individual clinical situation.
- Treatment approaches include percutaneous drainage, endoscopic drainage, a combination of percutaneous and endoscopic approaches, retroperitoneal debridement (videoscopic-assisted retroperitoneal debridement [VARD] or sinus tract necrosectomy), surgical transgastric approach, or traditional open operative debridement with external drainage.
- **FIGURE 3** illustrates typical patterns of necrosis. The image on the left with necrosis confined to the lesser

sac may be approached through the posterior stomach either endoscopically or surgically. The middle image with necrosis extending down the left paracolic gutter may be best approached from the retroperitoneum (VARD). The image on the right with necrosis extending down both paracolic gutters and/or the small bowel mesentery root poses a challenging problem. This group also includes patients with pancreatic head involvement. These patients may be best approached by open operative debridement.

- Definitive intervention should not be undertaken earlier than 4 weeks from the incident episode of pancreatitis.

Goals of pancreatic debridement are shown in **TABLE 1**. See also ▶ Video 1.

Table 1: Goals of Debridement

1. Debride as much solid necrotic tissue as possible safely.
2. Provide wide drainage of the pancreas (externally or into the alimentary tract if possible).
3. Establish enteral access.
4. Perform cholecystectomy and cholangiography if indicated.
5. Perform all the above with as little physiologic derangement as possible.

OPEN NECROSECTOMY

Exposure

- The patient may be approached through the midline or a low transverse incision, which provides superb access to the upper abdomen.
- Intraoperative ultrasound (IOUS) should be performed prior to disrupting any of the collections. IOUS provides important information about volume of solid necrosis.
- The surgeon should review recent cross-sectional image immediately before operating; this image provides an important "road map" directing debridement as well as to refresh memory of danger spots. Specific attention should be paid to the relationship of necrosis to the superior mesenteric and portal veins.
- A moderate amount of oozing from the diffuse inflammatory process is common. Infracolic adhesions, particularly to the undersurface of the transverse mesocolon, are quite common; these should be divided with careful blunt dissection as well as sharp dissection.
- The gastrocolic ligament should be divided. The inflammatory response commonly foreshortens the gastrocolic ligament, and care should be taken not to injure either the gastroepiploic vessels or the transverse colon wall.
- Lesser sac necrosis is always more cranial than it may seem.
- If necrosis extends down the paracolic gutters, these provide a reasonable and safe point of entry into the retroperitoneum. Debridement should progress from lateral to medial, paying special care to the known position of the superior mesenteric vein and portal vein around the pancreatic head (**FIGURE 4**).
- Catastrophic hemorrhage may occur from inadvertent vigorous debridement in the area of the superior mesenteric vein/portal vein (SMV/PV). The wall of the vein is weak from the inflammatory process. Proximal and distal vascular control is challenging because of the inflammatory process, and in a desperate circumstance, applying a long straight vascular clamp across the porta hepatis and root of the small bowel mesentery may be a life-saving maneuver, allowing time to ligate the SMV/PV.
- It is important to release the colic flexures to provide full exposure of the upper retroperitoneum.

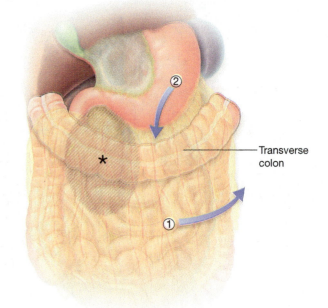

FIGURE 4 • If necrosis extends down the right paracolic gutter, (1) this route provides safe access to the retroperitoneum. When dividing the gastrocolic ligament (2), attention should be focused to preserving the gastroepiploic vessels and avoiding transverse colon injury. The *asterisk* highlights the danger zone with underlying SMV/PV.

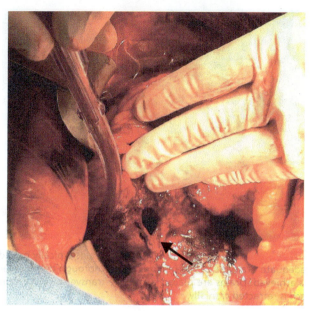

FIGURE 5 • Intraoperative photograph of right transverse mesocolon vessels skeletonized by adjacent necrosis (arrow). The transverse colon is reflected cranially in the surgeon's hand.

- Samples of the peripancreatic collection are commonly sent for Gram stain and aerobic, anaerobic, and fungal cultures.

Debridement

- The best tool for debriding pancreatic necrosis is the experienced surgeon's "educated finger." A ring forcep also is an excellent instrument.
- It is critical to only debride the necrosis that is freely mobile. Vigorous debridement of immature necrosis, particularly along the area of major veins, is fraught with hazard.
- A reasonable approach is to debride one field at a time and to pack that area before moving onto the next area of debridement. For example, debride the left paracolic gutter, then pack this area with laparotomy sponges, and then move into the lesser sac or other areas in a stepwise fashion. Oozing from the retroperitoneum is very common; however, the vast majority of this bleeding will stop with a short period of tamponade.
- Vigorous irrigation of the retroperitoneum helps dislodge small-volume necrosis.
- It is common to see skeletonized vessels both in the mesocolon as well as the retroperitoneum. These are quite friable; it is preferable to ligate these vessels if any question about their integrity exists. Many of these veins are already thrombosed (**FIGURE 5**).

Cholecystectomy

- Cholecystectomy may be performed at this point in the procedure if indicated and if the patient is physiologically stable. Obviously, the decision to perform cholecystectomy is a judgment call. A patient who is septic, requiring vasopressor support during debridement, is not the ideal candidate for a cholecystectomy, which is typically not a straightforward procedure and may involve substantial hemorrhage.
- Cholecystectomy is typically performed in the retrograde fashion. If the inflammatory process is too dense,

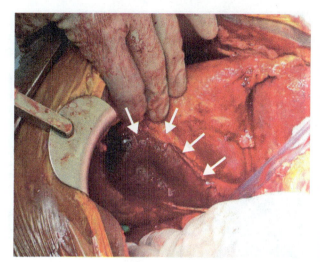

FIGURE 6 • Intraoperative photograph showing densely inflamed gallbladder/right upper quadrant (arrows) in the setting of biliary acute NP.

cholecystectomy may be deferred, although it should not be abandoned and completely forgotten as a significant number of patients (35%) will have recurrent biliary symptoms (either cholecystitis or pancreatitis) if cholecystectomy is not performed within the next several months.
- In the setting of a densely inflamed right upper quadrant, subtotal cholecystectomy (Thorek procedure) is acceptable (**FIGURE 6**).
- Cholangiography should be performed for all patients with biliary pancreatitis. Common bile duct exploration is potentially quite hazardous in this situation, and experienced judgment should be sought before undertaking common duct exploration in the setting of NP. However, documenting the presence of common bile duct stones is important to direct further management.

Enteral Access

- Many patients with retroperitoneal necrosis have gastric ileus and/or small bowel ileus. Our preference is to place gastrojejunostomy feeding tubes liberally (**FIGURE 7**). This tube is easy to place and permits decompression of the stomach and feeding distal to the ligament of Treitz to provide enteral nutrition in the immediate postoperative period. The tube is then easily removed in the office once the patient has recuperated completely.
- The gastrostomy tube is placed in the anterior body in the fashion of Stamm.
- The stomach should be tacked securely to the anterior abdominal wall with heavy suture to permit replacement of the gastrojejunostomy tube should dislodgement occur.

Drains

- Debridement beds are drained widely.
- Our preference is to use closed suction large-caliber (19-mm) drains (**FIGURE 8**). Three-way drains, although attractive in theory, are extremely challenging to manage in the intensive care unit and on the hospital ward.
- If disconnected pancreatic duct is suspected and external drainage employed, it is critical to maintain this drain, which controls the pancreatic fistula externally.

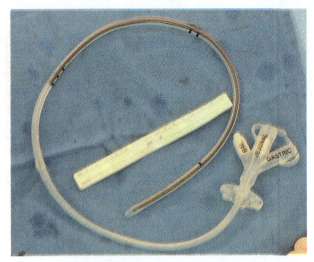

FIGURE 7 • Gastrojejunostomy feeding tube permits feeding downstream of ligament of Treitz while simultaneously decompressing the stomach.

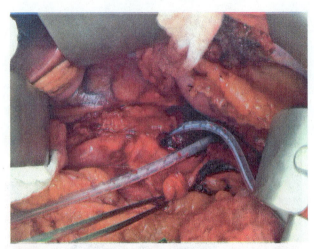

FIGURE 8 • Large-caliber closed suction drains typically provide adequate drainage of the necrosis bed if thorough debridement is achieved. Drains are placed above the transverse colon; stomach is retracted cranially.

Abdominal Closure

- The fascia is most often able to be closed primarily, although the operator should pay close attention to the peak airway pressures at the time of closure.

- The need for true retention sutures is unusual; however, a combination of running and interrupted slowly reabsorbable monofilament sutures seems prudent.
- The incidence of ventral hernia after open pancreatic debridement is substantial (42%).
- The skin is typically left open to close by secondary intention.

TRANSGASTRIC NECROSECTOMY

- Transgastric necrosectomy is appropriate for patients with necrosis confined to the lesser sac (**FIGURE 3**, left image), who comprise about 20% to 25% of all patients with NP. This approach may be endoscopic or surgical; patients with biliary etiology should be offered surgical approach as cholecystectomy may be accomplished at the same time as complete debridement.
- Transgastric necrosectomy may be approached laparoscopically or through a short upper midline incision (**FIGURE 9**). This technique is selectively applied to patients with necrosis

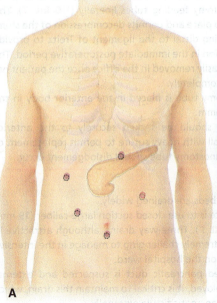
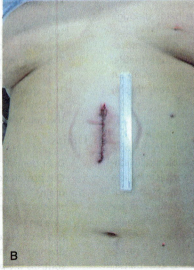

FIGURE 9 • **A**, Diagram showing port placement for laparoscopic transgastric debridement. **B**, Postoperative photograph: even with heavy body habitus, open transgastric debridement may be achieved through a short (6 cm) upper midline incision.

Chapter 45 PANCREATIC NECROSECTOMY **377**

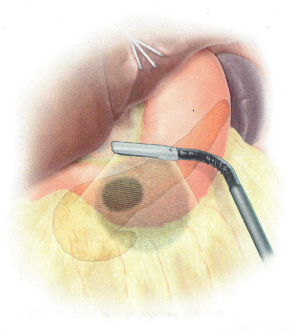

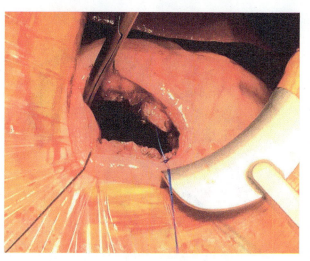

FIGURE 11 • Intraoperative photograph showing anterior gastrotomy and large posterior cystogastrostomy. Note stay sutures on posterior gastric wall.

FIGURE 10 • IOUS is critical, particularly in the laparoscopic approach.

- isolated in the lesser sac; it may be particularly effective for patients with a disconnected pancreatic tail. Clinicians should be aware that necrosis extending down the small bowel mesenteric root or paracolic gutter may not be appropriate for this technique.
- IOUS is a critical adjunct, especially if the majority of the necrosis is solid as opposed to liquid. Ultrasound should be applied through the front wall of the stomach and particularly through the back wall of the stomach to help localize posterior gastrotomy (**FIGURE 10**).
- The surgeon should be aware of the potential for hemorrhage from varices in the gastric wall in the setting of left-sided (sinistral) portal hypertension.
- Stay sutures in the posterior gastric wall are extremely helpful in the laparoscopic approach, delivering this opening into the operative field (**FIGURE 11**). Wide posterior gastrotomy is created either with cautery or a linear stapling device. The posterior gastrotomy is sutured to the cyst with permanent suture. This suture aids in hemostasis as well as in durably maintaining this ostomy. Gentle debridement and copious irrigation are applied. The conduct of debridement is similar to that in the open situation (**FIGURE 12**).
- Anterior gastrotomy is closed with suture or stapler (**FIGURE 13**). Often, the stomach is thick and suturing provides a more secure closure.
- If gastrostomy or gastrojejunostomy feeding tube is indicated, placing this tube prior to closing the anterior gastrotomy affords visualization of the tube passing through the duodenum. Care should be taken to place the gastrostomy entrance site at a distance away from the gastrotomy closure site.
- Drains are typically not necessary with transgastric necrosectomy, except in patients with necrosis extending to the small

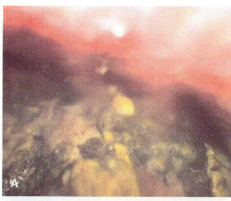

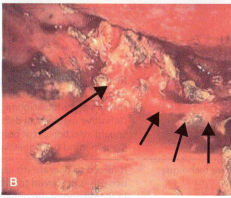

FIGURE 12 • Intraoperative photographs of laparoscopic transgastric debridement. **A**, Camera is in necrosis cavity. **B**, After debridement. *Long arrow* shows disconnected pancreatitis tail; *short arrows* show splenic artery.

bowel mesentery or down a paracolic gutter—drainage of these potential dead spaces may help avoid recurrent retroperitoneal collection.
- Cholecystectomy and cholangiography may be performed if indicated.

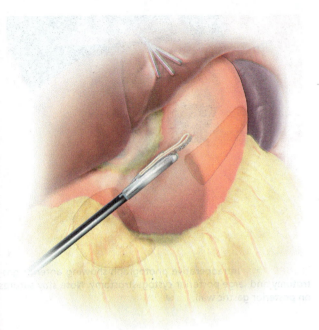

FIGURE 13 • Anterior gastrotomy may be closed with suture or stapler (shown).

DISTAL PANCREATECTOMY ± SPLENECTOMY

- In the setting of major body necrosis with a very small amount of viable pancreatic tail, the surgeon may consider distal pancreatectomy at the time of operative debridement.

This operation should be reserved for highly select cases. It is almost always necessary to perform splenectomy in this setting due to the significant inflammatory response and frequent incidence of gastric varices.

PEARLS AND PITFALLS

Surgical decision making	• NP is an extremely heterogeneous disease. Appropriate treatment must be based on the underlying necrosis anatomy as well as the patient's general condition. Ideally, treatment decisions are made in the context of multidisciplinary review. • Definitive mechanical debridement should not be applied before 4-6 weeks' time. • Should infection occur before 4 weeks' time, percutaneous drainage is the most appropriate intervention. • Keep in mind the potential for colon ischemia at any point in the course of this disease.
Operative technique	• If forced to operate (to prove or exclude colon ischemia) prior to 4 weeks, wide drainage of immature necrosis is preferred to attempts at debriding immature necrosis. • In the setting of disconnected pancreatic tail, the transgastric approach may be most appropriate. Alternatively, distal pancreatectomy plus splenectomy may be considered in highly select patients. • Be aware of the potential for visceral arterial pseudoaneurysm. • When manually debriding pancreatic necrosis, only remove the necrosis that comes easily. • In biliary pancreatitis, cholecystectomy and cholangiography should be performed if technically possible at time of debridement. Cholecystectomy may be hazardous, and clinical judgment regarding extent of operation is important.
Postoperative care	• Do not be afraid to reoperate if the patient is not following the expected course. It is important to regain control of a poorly controlled or uncontrolled pancreatic fistula. It is also important to exclude ischemic colitis in the early postoperative period following the first debridement.

POSTOPERATIVE CARE

- Optimal nutritional support is critical for expedient recuperation. Oftentimes, this requires some combination of parenteral and enteral nutrition. While recognizing the crucial importance of enteral alimentation, the surgeon should be cognizant of small bowel and gastric ileus that are very common in the setting of NP and post debridement. Increasing tube feeding volume too rapidly may be detrimental.
- Aggressive physical rehabilitation is also critical. Early planning for discharge to an extended-care treatment facility is prudent; direct communication with health care providers at these facilities is important to maintain the continuity of care.
- Venous thromboembolism is a very common occurrence (>50%) in the setting of NP. Patients should be observed carefully. Serial ultrasound screening permits early detection and prompt treatment of deep vein thrombosis and prevents pulmonary emboli.
- Bright red blood in the surgical drain should be considered visceral arterial pseudoaneurysm until proven otherwise. Often, a small amount of blood is from retroperitoneal venous hemorrhage; however, visceral arterial pseudoaneurysm is a potentially lethal problem that should not be missed. Cross-sectional imaging with computed tomography angiography (CTA) is rapid and widely available; CTA is an excellent first-line test with which to diagnose or exclude pseudoaneurysm.
- Appropriate duration of antibiotic treatment after satisfactory source control is important. However, no clear data exist to inform this treatment decision. Antibiotic treatment of no shorter than 7 days should be employed. We have tried to cut down antibiotic treatment and had recurrent retroperitoneal infected collections. It is noteworthy that retroperitoneal collections infected with resistant bacteria and yeast are extremely hard to clear. Consideration should be given to extended-duration antibiotic treatment in these cases.
- The patient should be observed for the presence of external pancreatic fistula. Measurement of amylase and surgically placed drains will diagnose this condition.
- Enterocutaneous fistulas may occur. These should be managed in a similar fashion to enterocutaneous fistulas developing from other conditions. Duodenal fistula is extremely challenging. Percutaneous transhepatic drainage with diversion of the biliopancreatic secretion will usually allow these fistulas to close with nonoperative management.
- Patients dismissed from the hospital with controlled external pancreatic fistula and/or supplemental enteral and parenteral nutrition should have early and frequent postoperative follow-up.
- Patients who fail to progress as expected should have early cross-sectional imaging. Additional percutaneous drainage or reoperation may be necessary to regain control of an uncontrolled pancreatic fistula.
- Long-term follow-up is crucial for patients undergoing transgastric debridement, as long-term outcomes from this relatively new approach are unknown. A small number of patients will manifest recurrent pancreatitis (FIGURE 14) or recurrent retroperitoneal fluid collections (pseudocyst) after transgastric debridement.

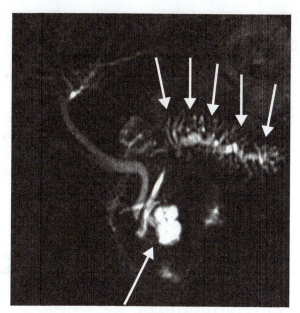

FIGURE 14 • MRI 2 years after transgastric debridement showing dilated main and side branch pancreatitis ducts *(short arrows)* in the disconnected tail. The etiology of this patient's pancreatitis was the side-branch IPMN *(long arrow)*.

OUTCOMES

- Mortality after pancreatic debridement in contemporary series ranges from 5% to 10% at specialized centers. Although this mortality is relatively high, these outcomes represent substantial improvement from historical mortality figures and is likely most related to improved operative selection. Patients and family members should be educated from the start of this disease process that NP is a long-term problem and that even in the best of circumstances, patients should expect a recuperation period measured in months.
- In general, reports of long-term outcomes for patients with NP and operative debridement are scarce. Recent data suggest that over 80% of closely followed patients with NP will experience one or more long-term sequelae, highlighting the importance of durable follow-up in this population.
- Ideally, patients will have long-term follow-up with primary physician and/or gastroenterologist attentive to exocrine and endocrine functions as well as digestive function.
- A small number of patients with NP will have intraductal papillary mucinous neoplasm (IPMN) or pancreatic adenocarcinoma as the cause. Unfortunately, prognosis in this subgroup of patients is uniformly poor.
- A small subgroup of patients with NP is too well to die but too sick to recuperate with reasonable quality of life. This is an extremely challenging group of patients to care for. However, in a highly select number of these patients, hospice care may be appropriate. These patients, for example, have protracted immobilization, protracted organ failure, and unreconstructable enteric fistulas.
- A highly select number of patients may be candidates for intestinal or multivisceral transplant. Obviously, this is decision making that must be undertaken in conjunction with the organ transplant group.

Table 2: Complications of Necrotizing Pancreatitis	
Short-term	**Long-term**
Pancreatic fistula (particularly with disruption of the main pancreatitis duct)	Recurrent retroperitoneal collections/infection
Colonic ischemia	Bile duct or duodenal obstruction from stricture
Venous thromboembolism	Exocrine and endocrine insufficiency
Enteric fistula	Chronic pain
Visceral arterial pseudoaneurysm	Recurrent acute pancreatitis progressing to chronic pancreatitis in the remnant pancreas
	Ventral hernia

COMPLICATIONS

- Complications after pancreatic necrosectomy may be related to disease progression or operation. **TABLE 2** highlights these complications.

SUGGESTED READINGS

1. Banks PA, Bollen TL, Dervenis C, et al. Classification of acute pancreatitis--2012: revision of the Atlanta classification and definitions by international consensus. *Gut.* 2013;62(1):102-111.
2. Baron TH, DiMaio CJ, Wang AY, Morgan KA. American gastroenterological association clinical practice update: management of pancreatic necrosis. *Gastroenterology.* 2020;158(1):67-75 e61.
3. Driedger M, Zyromski NJ, Visser BC, et al. Surgical transgastric necrosectomy for necrotizing pancreatitis: a single-stage procedure for walled-off pancreatic necrosis. *Ann Surg.* 2018;271(1):163-168.
4. Forsmark CE, Vege SS, Wilcox CM. Acute pancreatitis. *N Engl J Med.* 2016;375(20):1972-1981.
5. Gluck M, Ross A, Irani S, et al. Dual modality drainage for symptomatic walled-off pancreatic necrosis reduces length of hospitalization, radiological procedures, and number of endoscopies compared to standard percutaneous drainage. *J Gastrointest Surg.* 2012;16(2):248-256; discussion 256-247.
6. Guo Q, Li A, Xia Q, et al. The role of organ failure and infection in necrotizing pancreatitis: a prospective study. *Ann Surg.* 2014;259(6):1201-1207.
7. Gupta R, Kulkarni A, Babu R, et al. Complications of percutaneous drainage in step-up approach for management of pancreatic necrosis: experience of 10 years from a tertiary care center. *J Gastrointest Surg.* 2020;24(3):598-609.
8. Horvath K, Freeny P, Escallon J, et al. Safety and efficacy of video-assisted retroperitoneal debridement for infected pancreatic collections: a multicenter, prospective, single-arm phase 2 study. *Arch Surg.* 2010;145(9):814-825.
9. Maatman TK, Flick KF, Roch AM, Zyromski NJ. Operative pancreatic debridement: contemporary outcomes in changing times. *Pancreatology.* Published online 2020.
10. Maatman TK, Heimberger MA, Lewellen KA, et al. Visceral artery pseudoaneurysm in necrotizing pancreatitis: incidence and outcomes. *Can J Surg.* 2019;63(3):E272-E277.
11. Maatman TK, Mahajan S, Roch AM, et al. Disconnected pancreatic duct syndrome predicts failure of percutaneous therapy in necrotizing pancreatitis. *Pancreatology.* 2020;20(3):362-368.
12. Maatman TK, McGreevy KA, Sood AJ, et al. Improved outpatient communication decreases unplanned readmission in necrotizing pancreatitis. *J Surg Res.* 2020;253:139-146.
13. Maatman TK, McGuire SP, Flick KF, et al. Outcomes in endoscopic and operative transgastric pancreatic debridement. *Ann Surg.* 2021;274(3):516-523.
14. Maatman TK, McGuire SP, Lewellen KA, et al. Prospective analysis of the mechanisms underlying ineffective deep vein thrombosis prophylaxis in necrotizing pancreatitis. *J Am Coll Surg.* 2021;232(1):91-100.
15. Maatman TK, Roch AM, Ceppa EP, et al. The continuum of complications in survivors of necrotizig pancreatits. *Surgery.* 2020;168(6):1032-1040.
16. Maatman TK, Roch AM, Heimberger MA, et al. Disconnected pancreatic duct syndrome: spectrum of operative management. *J Surg Res.* 2020;247:297-303.
17. Maurer L, Maatman TK, Luckhurst CM, et al. Risk of gallstone-related complications in necrotizing pancreatitis patients treated with a step-up approach: the experience of two tertiary care centers. *Surgery.* 2021;169:1086-1092.
18. Nealon WH, Bhutani M, Riall TS, Raju G, Ozkan O, Neilan R. A unifying concept: pancreatic ductal anatomy both predicts and determines the major complications resulting from pancreatitis. *J Am Coll Surg.* 2009;208(5):790-799; discussion 799-801.
19. Petrov MS, Shanbhag S, Chakraborty M, Phillips AR, Windsor JA. Organ failure and infection of pancreatic necrosis as determinants of mortality in patients with acute pancreatitis. *Gastroenterology.* 2010;139(3):813-820.
20. Roch AM, Maatman T, Carr RA, et al. Evolving treatment of necrotizing pancreatitis. *Am J Surg.* 2018;215(3):526-529.
21. Roch AM, Maatman TK, Carr RA, et al. Venous thromboembolism in necrotizing pancreatitis: an underappreciated risk. *J Gastrointest Surg.* 2019;23(12):2430-2438.
22. Trikudanathan G, Tawfik P, Amateau SK, et al. Early (<4 Weeks) versus standard (>/= 4 Weeks) endoscopically centered step-up interventions for necrotizing pancreatitis. *Am J Gastroenterol.* 2018;113(10):1550-1558.
23. van Baal MC, Bollen TL, Bakker OJ, et al. The role of routine fine-needle aspiration in the diagnosis of infected necrotizing pancreatitis. *Surgery.* 2014;155(3):442-448.
24. Van Santvoort H, Besselink M, Bakker O, et al. A step-up approach or open necrosectomy for necrotizing pancreatitis. *N Engl J Med.* 2010;362:1491-1502.
25. Working Group IAP/APA Acute Pancreatitis Guidelines. IAP/APA evidence-based guidelines for the management of acute pancreatitis. *Pancreatology.* 2013;13(4 suppl 2):e1-15.
26. Zyromski NJ, Nakeeb A, House MG, Jester AL. Transgastric pancreatic necrosectomy: how I do it. *J Gastrointest Surg.* 2016;20(2):445-449.

Chapter 46 Laparoscopic Pancreatic Necrosectomy

O. Joe Hines and Stephanie S. Kim

DEFINITION
- Laparoscopic pancreatic debridement is a minimally invasive technique for pancreatic resection and is indicated for infected pancreatic necrosis and symptomatic sterile necrosis. Additional options for pancreatic debridement include other minimally invasive methods, such as percutaneous catheter drainage and endoscopic drainage, and open necrosectomy. Methods of laparoscopic debridement will be the focus of this chapter.

DIFFERENTIAL DIAGNOSIS
- The differential diagnosis of acute pancreatitis includes biliary colic, peptic ulcer disease, cholecystitis, acute mesenteric ischemia, small bowel obstruction, visceral perforation, vascular catastrophes such as ruptured aortic aneurysm, and intra-abdominal infection.
- In the setting of recent severe acute pancreatitis, the differential for a fluid collection in the setting of acute pancreatitis includes acute peripancreatic fluid collection, acute necrotic collection, pseudocyst, and walled-off necrosis. Characteristic computed tomography (CT) findings and patient history and physical examination can help characterize whether fluid collections are infected or necrotic.

PATIENT HISTORY AND PHYSICAL FINDINGS
- Acute pancreatitis has a broad range of clinical symptoms. The majority of cases can be mild and self-limiting; however, about 20% of these patients will develop severe acute pancreatitis.[1] Severe acute pancreatitis is associated with high mortality and morbidity; these patients are at risk for pancreatic necrosis, infection, multisystem organ failure, and death.[2]
- Signs and symptoms of pancreatic necrosis include a recent history of acute pancreatitis and continued abdominal pain, chronic low-grade fever, nausea, lethargy, and anorexia. Signs of infection in the setting of pancreatic necrosis include tachycardia, hypotension, fever, and deteriorating organ function.
- Pancreatic necrosis can be classified as sterile or infected. Secondary infection of pancreatic necrosis occurs by bacterial or fungal translocation through the gastrointestinal tract or by hematogenous spread from transient bacteremia resulting from intravenous (IV) catheters, endotracheal intubation, or urinary catheters. Infection usually occurs 2 to 6 weeks after the initial onset of acute pancreatitis, but can occur as early as 10 days.

IMAGING AND OTHER DIAGNOSTIC STUDIES
- Plain radiographs are nonspecific. Ultrasound (US) may show a diffusely enlarged, hypoechoic pancreas and can be important in identification of the etiology of pancreatitis (eg, gallstones).
- Appropriate imaging for acute pancreatitis includes contrast-enhanced CT scan. CT imaging in the case of mild acute pancreatitis will show pancreatic enlargement, edema, peripancreatic fat stranding, and effacement of the normal contours of the organ. When complications are clinically suspected, serial CT scans should be obtained. Complications of pancreatitis evolve with time, and impending necrosis may not be appreciated on CT imaging obtained within the first 24 to 48 hours of symptoms.
- In the setting of pancreatic necrosis, IV contrast can help delineate areas of poor perfusion, assess the extent of necrosis, and predict the severity of disease. Visualization of air bubbles within necrotic tissue is diagnostic of infection (FIGURE 1).
- CT scan can also identify pancreatic collections, which can be classified into four categories based on the Revised Atlanta Classification. Fluid collections that occur early (less than 4 weeks after onset of pain) without evidence of necrosis are classified as acute peripancreatic fluid collections and can be managed conservatively. Early fluid collections with evidence of necrosis are classified as acute necrotic collection. Late fluid collections (occurring greater than 4 weeks after onset of pain) are classified as a pseudocyst if there is no evidence of necrosis, but are classified as walled-off necrosis if there is evidence of necrosis (TABLE 1).[3]
- If infected pancreatic necrosis is suspected, the diagnosis is confirmed with radiologic confirmation of air bubbles in a collection that has not been instrumented or culture results from CT-guided fine needle aspiration or from specimens collected during necrosectomy.

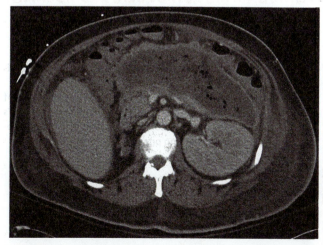

FIGURE 1 • Infected pancreatic necrosis. Computed tomography scan showing a hypoenhancing pancreas, indicating necrosis, with gas bubbles indicating bacterial infection of the necrotic material. This is likely necrosis mixed with peripancreatic phlegmon.

Table 1: Pancreatic Collections After Pancreatitis

Pancreatic collection	Time after the onset of pain	Evidence of necrosis	Management
Acute peripancreatic fluid collection	Less than 4 wk	No	Conservative
Acute necrotic collection	Less than 4 wk	Yes	Conservative unless infected—percutaneous drainage with or without surgical debridement
Pseudocyst	Greater than 4 wk	No	Conservative vs minimally invasive drainage if symptomatic
Walled-off necrosis	Greater than 4 wk	Yes	Conservative unless infected or symptomatic—percutaneous drainage with or without surgical debridement

SURGICAL MANAGEMENT

Preoperative Planning

- Conservative management is recommended in the case of sterile necrosis. Surgical management can be considered in symptomatic sterile necrosis; not infrequently, occult infection proves to be present. In the setting of infected pancreatic necrosis, drainage and/or debridement is the preferred method of treatment.
- A step-up approach involving percutaneous drainage and proceeding to minimally invasive necrosectomy only if needed has been shown to reduce morbidity in patients with infected necrotizing pancreatitis, when compared to early open necrosectomy.[4]
- Cross-sectional imaging as described earlier is necessary to determine the presence and location of necrosis, evaluate for infection, and help plan the surgical approach.
- The surgical approach is driven largely by the anatomy of the walled-off necrosis, combined with the clinical status of the patient. Not all patients are eligible for minimally invasive approaches to necrosectomy, particularly video-assisted retroperitoneal debridement (VARD).
- If possible, outcomes are better if surgical debridement is delayed for at least 4 weeks. This delay allows for organization of the necrosis and clearer delineation between live and dead tissue, as well as clinical stabilization of the patient, resolution of any signs of organ failure, and decreased inflammatory reaction.[5,6]
- For patients undergoing surgery, standard preoperative antibiotics are recommended prior to incision even for patients without evidence of infection. However, the ongoing use of prophylactic antibiotics in sterile pancreatitis remains controversial, given concerns for antibiotic resistance and fungal infection. A 2010 Cochrane review found no mortality benefit with prophylactic antibiotics, except for IV imipenem, which was associated with a decreased rate of infection of pancreatic necrosis.[7]
- Access: large-bore IV and/or central access for rapid volume resuscitation and vasopressor infusion; Foley catheter and nasogastric tube placement. Consider arterial line monitoring in the case of hemodynamic instability.

Positioning

- For a transperitoneal approach, the patient should be supine and the abdomen should be prepped from nipple to midthigh. For the retroperitoneal approach, the patient should be placed in lateral position.

RETROGASTRIC RETROCOLIC DEBRIDEMENT (TRANSPERITONEAL)

First Step

- The initial trocar should be placed in the periumbilical position (FIGURE 2).
- A 30° angled laparoscope is used to guide the insertion of two right paramedian trocars and an additional assistant's trocar in the left lateral abdomen. Start with exploratory laparoscopy after establishing pneumoperitoneum.

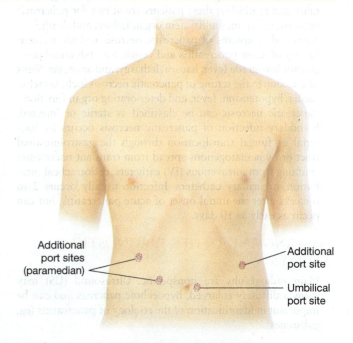

FIGURE 2 • Port placement for transperitoneal debridement. Transumbilical port placement and two or more paramedian ports are placed with respect to the location of greatest pancreatic necrosis.

Chapter 46 **LAPAROSCOPIC PANCREATIC NECROSECTOMY** 383

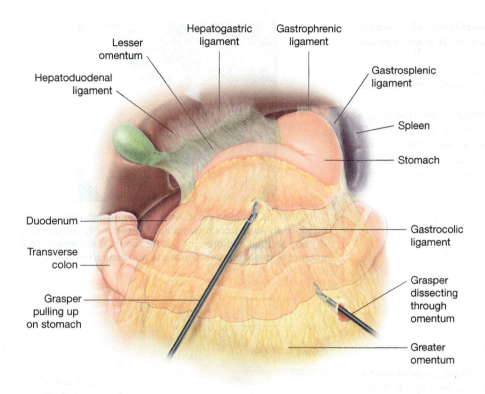

FIGURE 3 • Access to the body and distal pancreas can be obtained transperitoneally through the gastrocolic ligament and the left mesocolon.

Second Step

- The area of necrosis can be approached through the gastrocolic ligament or the transverse mesocolon (**FIGURE 3**). Dissection can be performed with a harmonic scalpel or bipolar electrocautery device. If a percutaneous drainage catheter is in place, this can be used as a guide to identify the necrosis. The left side of the pancreas may be drained by mobilization of the splenic flexure. If necrosis extends above the pancreas, the lesser sac may be entered through the gastrohepatic ligament, taking care to safeguard the right and left gastric arteries.

Third Step

- Debridement is accomplished under direct vision with the use of a grasping instrument (**FIGURES 4** and **5**). A 10-mm stone extractor instrument is often most efficient. Necrotic material should be sent for histology and microbiology.

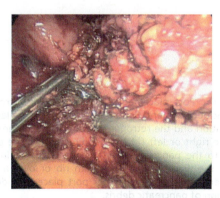

FIGURE 4 • Debridement of necrotic pancreas. The pancreas has been accessed laparoscopically through the gastrocolic omentum using a harmonic scalpel. In this case, two drains had been placed preoperatively into fluid collections in the head and tail of the pancreas, respectively. Access was gained to the poorly draining tail collection by following the drain into the lesser sac. After draining purulent fluid, debridement was achieved with the use of blunt forceps.

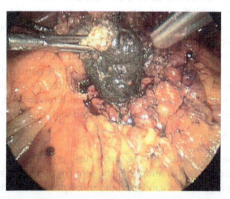

FIGURE 5 • Removal of necrotic pancreas. A 6-cm piece of necrotic pancreas was removed through the anterior abdominal wall with the use of an Endo Catch bag.

- Consider intraoperative US for localization of retroperitoneal necrosis and the identification of major vascular anatomy.
- The suction irrigator can be used to break down and aspirate pancreatic debris. An endobag is a useful tool for further removing debris.
- The cavity can be inspected by introducing the laparoscope into the debridement bed. Referring to the preoperative CT scan helps to ensure all areas of necrosis have been removed. Sump drains are placed through the trocar sites for continuous lavage of the debridement bed in the postoperative period (FIGURE 6).

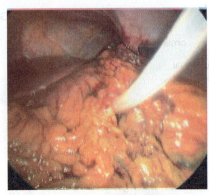

FIGURE 6 • Drain placement. After adequate debridement and irrigation, an Axiom drain was placed in the cavity surrounding the body and tail and brought out through the abdominal wall through the midabdominal trocar site and secured in place.

VIDEO-ASSISTED RETROPERITONEAL DEBRIDEMENT (VIDEO 1)

First Step

- Retroperitoneal debridement may be used in early necrotizing pancreatitis, especially if there is minimal fibrotic tissue, inflammation, or edema. This approach allows for the examination of the posterior pancreas (FIGURE 7).
- This approach can be aided by preoperative access to the retroperitoneal space with catheter placement by interventional radiology into the dominant fluid collection.
- The patient is placed in the lateral decubitus position, and the retroperitoneum is entered from the right or left side, depending on the site of most inflammation and damage to the pancreas.

Second Step

- A 0° laparoscope is inserted in the flank between the iliac crest and the 12th rib posteriorly. Alternatively, a videoscope may be inserted directly over the drain site.
- An angled, rigid, therapeutic thoracoscope facilitates debridement under visualization through a single access point.
- After insufflation, the right and left kidneys can be used as landmarks toward the head or tail of the pancreas.
- Mechanical debridement may be limited by access and visualization and may require multiple interventions; however, peritoneal contamination is limited with this approach.

Third Step

- The remainder of the procedure proceeds as previously described, with samples being sent for pathology and microbiology. Drains can be placed through the port sites for continuous lavage.

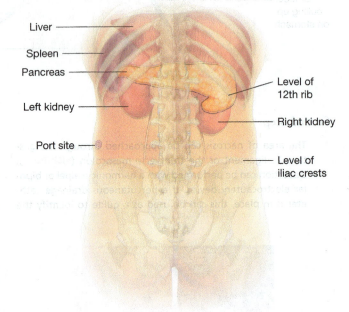

FIGURE 7 • Port placement and anatomy of retroperitoneal pancreatic debridement. Patient placement is in the lateral decubitus position and the retroperitoneum can be entered through either the right or left side, depending on the site of greatest damage to the pancreas. A videoscope is placed in the flank between the iliac crest and the 12th rib or over a previously placed percutaneous drain. Other port placement depends on the location of pancreatic debris.

PEARLS AND PITFALLS

Indications	• Indications for laparoscopic pancreatic debridement include infected pancreatic necrosis and symptomatic sterile necrosis.
Imaging	• Contrast-enhanced CT imaging is required for determining preoperative planning. • Anatomic relationships to the necroma should drive the surgical approach.
Choice of approach	• Retroperitoneal approach may limit the ability to adequately debride tissues, but is suitable for multiple interventions and limits peritoneal contamination. • Transperitoneal approach may be limited by potential peritoneal contamination and limited reintervention.
Timing	• The optimal timing of operative intervention is 4-6 weeks following the onset of acute pancreatitis.
Drain placement	• Preoperative drain placement can aid in initial management and intraoperative dissection and identification of necrotic material. • Place large drains at the time of surgery; consider continuous lavage with isotonic saline.
Indications for reimaging or relook laparoscopy	• Reimaging and/or reoperation is indicated in cases of clinical deterioration or incomplete debridement.

POSTOPERATIVE CARE

- Immediate postoperative care will depend on the status of the patient perioperatively. However, all patients with necrotizing pancreatitis are at risk of multi-organ dysfunction and may benefit from close surveillance in an intensive care unit.
- Close attention must be paid to volume status, blood glucose control, maintenance of normothermia, and adequate pain control.[8]
- Because of massive third space fluid losses and fluid shifts postoperatively, some patients will require continued intubation postoperatively in the initial 24 to 36 hours while receiving aggressive fluid resuscitation.
- Early aggressive enteral feeding can be started after the first 48 hours of resuscitation postoperatively.

OUTCOMES

- In a meta-analysis comparing interventional strategies for necrotizing pancreatitis, both retroperitoneal and transperitoneal pancreatic debridement were found to be effective. Laparoscopic debridement had a 79% success rate, 33% morbidity, and 0% mortality, and retroperitoneal debridement carried a 64% success rate, 47% morbidity, and 14% mortality, though heterogeneous data and small sample size limited direct comparison of the two methods.[9]
- Recent prospective feasibility studies of VARD show a reasonable safety and efficacy profile for VARD, although the authors were unable to establish that VARD techniques are superior to open necrosectomy.[10]
- There are no controlled trials comparing open necrosectomy to laparoscopic methods.

COMPLICATIONS

- The most common postoperative complication is a residual fluid collection, which can usually be managed with percutaneous drainage.[11]
- Other acute complications include bleeding, sepsis, acute pancreatitis, pancreatic duct leak, need for repeat debridement, exocrine insufficiency, endocrine deficiency, and enteric leak.
- Long-term complications include pancreatic pseudocyst formation, chronic pancreatitis, enterocutaneous fistula, pancreatic fistula, and chronic abdominal/back pain.

REFERENCES

1. Whitcomb DC. Clinical practice. Acute pancreatitis. *N Engl J Med*. 2006;354(20):2142-2150. doi:10.1056/NEJMcp054958
2. Popa CC, Badiu DC, Rusu OC, Grigorean VT, Neagu SI, Strugaru CR. Mortality prognostic factors in acute pancreatitis. *J Med Life*. 2016;9(4):413-418. Accessed June 12, 2021. http://www.ncbi.nlm.nih.gov/pmc/articles/pmc5141403/
3. Foster BR, Jensen KK, Bakis G, Shaaban AM, Coakley FV. Revised Atlanta classification for acute pancreatitis: a pictorial essay. *Radiographics*. 2016;36(3):675-687. doi:10.1148/rg.2016150097
4. van Santvoort HC, Besselink MG, Bakker OJ, et al. A step-up approach or open necrosectomy for necrotizing pancreatitis. *N Engl J Med*. 2010;362(16):1491-1502. doi:10.1056/nejmoa0908821
5. Hines OJ, Pandol SJ. Management of severe acute pancreatitis. *BMJ*. 2019;367:l6227. doi:10.1136/bmj.l6227
6. Wysocki AP, McKay CJ, Carter CR. Infected pancreatic necrosis: minimizing the cut. *ANZ J Surg*. 2010;80(1-2):58-70. doi:10.1111/j.1445-2197.2009.05177.x
7. Villatoro E, Mulla M, Larvin M. Antibiotic therapy for prophylaxis against infection of pancreatic necrosis in acute pancreatitis. *Cochrane Database Syst Rev*. 2010;2010(5):CD002941. doi:10.1002/14651858.cd002941.pub3
8. Hasibeder WR, Torgersen C, Rieger M, Dünser M. Critical care of the patient with acute pancreatitis. *Anaesth Intensive Care*. 2009;37(2):190-206. doi:10.1177/0310057x0903700206
9. Bradley EL, Howard TJ, Van Sonnenberg E, Fotoohi M. Intervention in necrotizing pancreatitis: an evidence-based review of surgical and percutaneous alternatives. *J Gastrointest Surg*. 2008;12(4):634-639. doi:10.1007/s11605-007-0445-z
10. Horvath K, Freeny P, Escallon J, et al. Safety and efficacy of video-assisted retroperitoneal debridement for infected pancreatic collections: a multicenter, prospective, single-arm phase 2 study. *Arch Surg*. 2010;145(9):817-825. doi:10.1001/ARCHSURG.2010.178
11. Werner J, Feuerbach S, Uhl W, Büchler MW. Management of acute pancreatitis: from surgery to interventional intensive care. *Gut*. 2005;54(3):426-436. doi:10.1136/gut.2003.035907

Chapter 47 Endoscopic Pancreatic Debridement and Drainage

Samuel Han and Georgios Papachristou

DEFINITION

- Endoscopic pancreatic debridement or necrosectomy is performed in patients with pancreatic necrosis, specifically walled-off pancreatic necrosis (WON).
- Pancreatic necrosis is defined by the lack of enhancement of the pancreatic parenchyma on cross-sectional imaging after intravenous contrast administration.
- Pancreatic necrotic collections are classified by the revised Atlanta classification as acute necrotic collections and WON depending on the time (4 weeks) from the diagnosis of pancreatitis, and presence or lack of encapsulated wall.[1]
- Acute necrotic collection is defined as a collection containing various amounts of fluid and necrotic tissue involving the pancreatic parenchyma and/or the peripancreatic tissues occurring within the first 4 weeks of acute pancreatitis (**FIGURE 1**).[1]
- WON is a mature, encapsulated collection of pancreatic and/or peripancreatic necrosis that has developed a well-defined wall. WON usually occurs more than 4 weeks after the onset of necrotizing pancreatitis (**FIGURE 2**).

DIFFERENTIAL DIAGNOSIS

- Differentiating WON from a pseudocyst remains an important component in management. A pseudocyst is a fluid collection in the pancreatic and/or peripancreatic tissue surrounded by a well-defined wall that contains no or minimal solid material. Diagnosis can be typically made using these morphologic criteria. Should the fluid content of a pseudocyst be sampled, the amylase level will be elevated. Disruption of the main pancreatic duct or side branches without necrosis usually leads to pseudocyst formation.[1]
- Cystic lesions of the pancreas such as intraductal papillary mucinous neoplasms, mucinous cystic neoplasms, and serous cystic adenomas can mimic WON. A previous history of acute pancreatitis helps differentiate between the two conditions; fine needle aspiration (FNA) can be performed for pancreatic fluid analysis so as to better characterize the collection before endoscopic drainage.

PATIENT HISTORY AND PHYSICAL FINDINGS

- A large proportion of patients with pancreatic necrosis in the setting of necrotizing pancreatitis have sterile necrosis, which can be managed conservatively without any intervention if patients remain relatively symptom-free.[2] In a prospective registry from the United States, interventions for drainage/debridement of necrotic collections were performed in 68 out of 155 patients with necrotizing AP (44%) with a median intervention time of 45 days from presentation.[3]

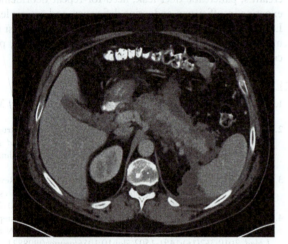

FIGURE 1 • Acute necrotizing pancreatitis seen in patient admitted with severe abdominal pain with fevers and leukocytosis. CT demonstrates areas of nonenhancement in the body and tail.

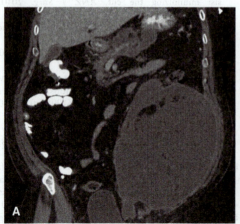 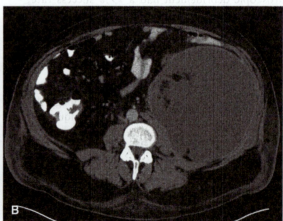

FIGURE 2 • **A** and **B**, CT revealing WON in a patient who presented with abdominal pain and nausea/vomiting 6 weeks after initial episode of necrotizing pancreatitis.

- Indications for drainage of sterile pancreatic necrosis include signs of gastric outlet obstruction (nausea, vomiting, early satiety, and inability to resume oral intake) and signs of biliary obstruction (elevated liver function tests and a dilated bile duct). Recurrent acute pancreatitis, pancreatic fistulae, and/or persistent systemic inflammatory response syndrome represent other indications for drainage in sterile necrosis.[2]
- The primary indication for endoscopic drainage and debridement is suspected or confirmed infected pancreatic necrosis with concomitant clinical deterioration.
- Typically, debridement should be avoided in the early, acute period (first 2 weeks) and optimally delayed until the necrosis is walled-off and a well-defined capsule is present, which typically takes around 4 weeks.
- The goals of therapy must be well defined and a multidisciplinary approach (medical pancreatologist, therapeutic endoscopist, surgeon, and interventional radiology) offers the highest chance of success.

IMAGING AND OTHER DIAGNOSTIC STUDIES

- The morphologic features of acute pancreatitis and resultant complications are diagnosed by high-resolution cross-sectional imaging such as multidetector contrast-enhanced computed tomography (CT) and MRI, which can detect most local complications as reported in the revised Atlanta classification.[1]
- The diagnosis of necrosis is based on imaging features of a heterogeneous collection with liquid and nonliquid density with varying degrees of loculations.[1]
- WON is defined based on the presence of a heterogeneous collection with a well-formed wall and complete encapsulation.
- CT may not readily distinguish with high sensitivity solid from liquid content to distinguish pseudocysts from necrosis.
- WON may be better diagnosed when performing magnetic resonance imaging (MRI) or endoscopic ultrasound (EUS) that can identify necrotic debris within the collection.
- The diagnosis of infected necrosis is based on the presence of gas within the collection on CT (**FIGURE 2**). The extraluminal gas is present in areas of necrosis. This diagnosis is suspected in patients with persistent organ failure, fevers, and leukocytosis. Should the diagnosis be unclear, EUS or CT-guided FNA for grain stain and culture may be performed.

SURGICAL (ENDOSCOPIC) MANAGEMENT

Preoperative Planning

In addition to careful patient selection, preoperative considerations including any underlying coagulopathy has been treated. In general, a platelet count >50,000 platelets/mL and an international normalized ratio <1.6 is recommended prior to the procedure. Given the need for electrocautery, the presence of a pacemaker or a defibrillator should be accounted for and a ring magnet may be required for the brief period of electrocautery. A type and cross should also be obtained preprocedure should a patient develop bleeding that requires blood transfusions. Intraoperative antibiotics should be given during the procedure. Antibiotic therapy is typically continued for 10 to 14 days postendoscopic intervention.

Positioning

- While the positioning of the patient needs to be selected based on the patient and nature of the WON, in patients who are clinically unstable, the supine position is generally better tolerated compared to prone. The prone position (ERCP position) allows for better gravitational drainage of WON and is the preferred starting position when feasible.
- General anesthesia is recommended for these procedures given the risk of aspiration with large volume of fluid being released from the collection into the gastrointestinal lumen.
- Carbon dioxide is now the standard of care during endoscopy and should be used during these procedures because it reduces the risk of air embolism and is more quickly absorbed by the body.

TECHNIQUES

ENDOSCOPIC ULTRASOUND-GUIDED DRAINAGE

- EUS-guided drainage is the current standard of care for endoscopic transmural drainage of WON. It allows for selection of an appropriate site for drainage from the stomach or duodenum that is free from intervening blood vessels.
- EUS-guided drainage is favored for well-encapsulated collections that are adjacent to the stomach or duodenum.
- There are two primary modalities for maintaining the cystenterostomy tract (either cystgastrostomy or cystduodenostomy) during EUS-guided drainage: (1) Multiple double pigtail plastic stent placement and (2) Single lumen-apposing metal stent (LAMS) placement.
- Double pigtail stent placement entails initial puncture of the collection with a 19-gauge FNA needle. A long angled guidewire is then advanced into the collection and is coiled within the collection several times to maintain a stable position. Dilation is then performed of the enterocyststomy tract using a variety of devices including a needle-knife catheter, cystotome, passage dilator, and/or a balloon dilator. A minimum of two double pigtail stents (7 or 10 Fr) are placed into the cavity with the distal pigtail in the collection and the proximal pigtail in the gastric/duodenal lumen (**FIGURE 3**).
- LAMS placement (**FIGURE 4**, ▶ **Video 1**) has become a widely used approach, primarily due to its easy deployment and ability to place a large-diameter metal stent (6-20 mm in inner diameter). Placed either over a guidewire (after puncture with a 19-gauge needle) or using a freehand technique, the LAMS has an electrocautery-enhanced tip that allows for direct placement of the 10.8-Fr catheter into the collection. The distal end of the dumbbell-shaped stent is first deployed and used to bring the wall of the collection toward the stomach/duodenum. The proximal end of the stent is then deployed in the stomach/duodenal lumen. The stent is then

typically balloon dilated to enhance drainage/permit necrosectomy. While not necessary, many endoscopists will then place a single or two double pigtail stents through the LAMS to prevent migration of the LAMS into the collection and also theoretically reduce the risk of bleeding by keeping a buffer between the opposite wall of the collection and the distal flange of the LAMS.[4]

- The multiple-gateway technique refers to performing the above technique in two or more sites of a large necrotic cavity (typically transgastric and transduodenal) to facilitate drainage (FIGURE 5, ▶ Video 2). While data are limited, retrospective series appear to demonstrate high success rates in treating large walled-off collections with low recurrence rates.[5,6]

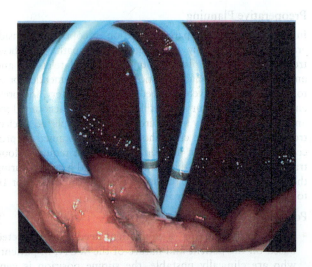

FIGURE 3 • Placement of two double pigtail stents into a WON via transgastric route.

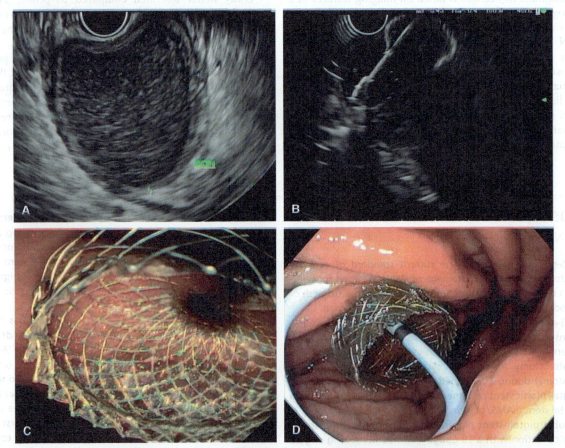

FIGURE 4 • A and B, Visualization of WON on EUS (A) with deployment of distal flange of lumen-apposing metal stent into WON (B). This is followed by deployment of the proximal flange (C) and after aspiration of liquid contents, a double pigtail stent is placed coaxially into the WON through the lumen-apposing metal stent (D).

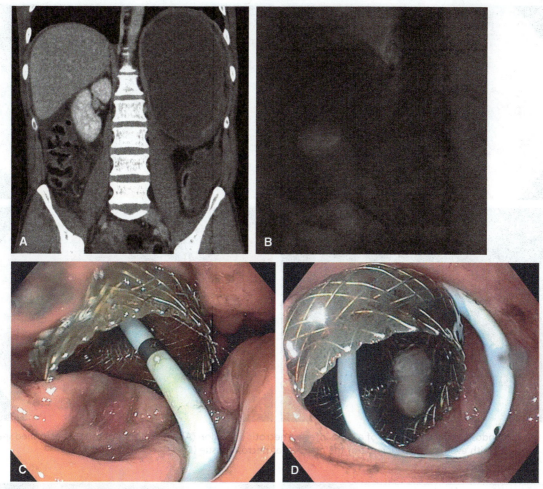

FIGURE 5 • Placement of two lumen-apposing metal stents into different sites of a large WON **(A)** for multigateway drainage as seen on fluoroscopy **(B)** and endoscopically with stents placed in the stomach **(C)** and duodenum **(D)**.

DIRECT ENDOSCOPIC NECROSECTOMY

- Direct endoscopic necrosectomy (DEN) entails entering the necrotic collection with the endoscope to directly access and remove necrotic tissue and debris within a WON (**FIGURE 6**, ▶ Video 3). The technique will vary depending on the type of stent placed, and evidence to guide the optimal timing of DEN is lacking at this time. Furthermore, this process is typically labor-intensive due to a lack of specialized endoscopic accessories that could facilitate necrosectomy.
- Nearly 30% to 50% of patients who receive transmural drainage alone will not require DEN and have good resolution of the WON.[7-9]
- In a randomized trial comparing LAMS and DPS for the treatment of WON, LAMS-related adverse events typically occurred ≥3 weeks after initial stent placement.[10] For this reason, cross-sectional imaging is typically performed 2 to 3 weeks after LAMS placement to assess the size of the cavity and whether the LAMS can be removed.
- If DEN is performed through a LAMS, the endoscope (typically a standard gastroscope or a therapeutic gastroscope) can enter directly into the necrotic cavity through the LAMS.
- If DEN is performed after index placement of double pigtail stents, the cystenterostomy tract will typically need to be dilated first (minimum of 10 mm) to allow passage of the gastroscope into the cavity.
- Fluid contents are typically drained first via suction through the gastroscope while simultaneously irrigating the cavity with water.
- Debridement is then performed, which can be performed with a myriad of devices including hot (typically for adherent debris) and cold snares, wide-jaw forceps, baskets, and retrieval nets.
- Extraction of necrotic debris entails the removal of necrotic tissue, which is typically performed by simply exiting the necrotic cavity with the gastroscope and releasing the necrotic contents into the stomach/duodenum. This can also be performed with snares, wide-jaw forceps, and retrieval nets.
- Irrigation with gentamicin or hydrogen peroxide at the end of the procedure may facilitate resolution of the cavity with a large multicenter retrospective series demonstrating higher clinical success rates with the use of diluted hydrogen peroxide.[11]
- An automated morcellator device (EndoRotor, Interscope Medical, Inc, Worcester, MA) is the first device approved by the FDA for performing DEN and involves simultaneously sucking, cutting, and removing necrotic tissue through a

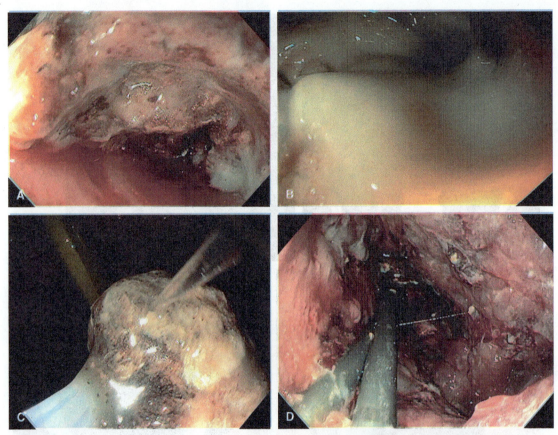

FIGURE 6 • Direct endoscopic necrosectomy of a large infected necrotic collection **(A)** with pockets of pus **(B)** performed snare removal of necrotic debris **(C)** with eventual debridement of the majority of necrotic tissue **(D)**.

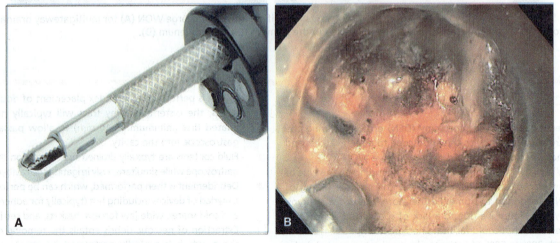

FIGURE 7 • Use of an automated morcellator device **(A)** that simultaneously cuts, sucks, and removes necrotic tissue to facilitate endoscopic necrosectomy **(B)**.

catheter that rotates between 1000 and 17,000 revolutions per minute (FIGURE 7, Video 4). Several case series have demonstrated its safety and effectiveness in removing necrotic tissue in particularly challenging cases.[12-14]

- Given the risk for bleeding due to adherent blood vessels and pseudoaneurysms during DEN, hemostasis devices should be available, including a coagulation grasper hemostatic forceps, bipolar hemostasis catheters, and hemostatic powder.

- In cases where a large amount of necrotic tissue occupies the cavity, multiple sessions of DEN may be required to clean the cavity adequately. While there is no formal endpoint to what constitutes a successful necrosectomy, in general, is to result in no visible necrotic tissue remaining, and pink, viable tissue being visible throughout the cavity.

- Factors that support performing DEN include WON measuring ≥10 cm, paracolic extension, and ≥30% solid necrosis.[15]

PERCUTANEOUS ENDOSCOPIC NECROSECTOMY

- Percutaneous endoscopic necrosectomy (PEN) combines percutaneous drainage with endoscopic necrosectomy by using the percutaneous tract after initial drain placement to advance the flexible endoscope into the cavity and perform debridement.
- PEN may offer an effective step-up therapy after percutaneous drain placement in patients with collections not amenable to endoscopic drainage, clinically unstable patients with sepsis, or poorly encapsulated collections.
- When performing PEN, a retroperitoneal approach is favored as an anterior transperitoneal approach carries the risk of peritonitis via spread of infected material into the abdominal cavity.
- The percutaneous tract must be mature (typically a mean of 17 days) before PEN can be attempted, but this modality can be performed at the bedside using moderate sedation.[16]
- Upon initial PEN, a pediatric gastroscope (4.9-5.5 mm diameter) can be used, gradual upsizing of the percutaneous tract is performed with insertion of larger drains (up to 28-30 Fr) until a standard gastroscope can be inserted into the tract to perform debridement similar to a DEN. An alternative approach is to replace the percutaneous drain with a self-expanding metal stent (18-20 mm diameter), which can then be sutured to the skin to be left in place until resolution of the cavity.[17,18] This facilitates insertion of larger therapeutic gastroscopes and removes the need for gradual upsizing of the percutaneous drain.

ENDOSCOPIC VS SURGICAL APPROACH

- The management of infected pancreatic necrosis requires a dedicated multidisciplinary team with expertise in medical pancreatology, therapeutic endoscopy, interventional radiology, critical care, nutrition, and pancreaticobiliary surgery. The landmark PANTER trial demonstrated that a step-up approach, in which percutaneous or endoscopic drainage is performed first, results in lower rates of major adverse events such as multiple-organ failure compared to open necrosectomy.[7] Long-term results of this study also demonstrated that patients receiving a step-up approach had a lower rate of incisional hernias, pancreatic exocrine and endocrine insufficiency without an increased need for reinterventions.[19] A pooled analysis of 1980 patients with necrotizing pancreatitis found that in high-risk patients, minimally invasive surgical and endoscopic necrosectomy are associated with reduced mortality rates compared to open necrosectomy, further arguing against open necrosectomy as the primary approach for necrotizing pancreatitis.[20]
- A subsequent randomized study comparing endoscopic drainage with a surgical step-up approach, in which percutaneous drainage was followed by video-assisted retroperitoneal debridement (VARD) when needed, found that the endoscopic approach had a lower rate of pancreatic fistulas and a shorter length of hospitalization (by 16 days) without any difference in mortality.[8]
- A single-center randomized trial compared endoscopic treatment with minimally invasive surgery (video-assisted or laparoscopic-assisted) for infected necrotizing pancreatitis and found that endoscopic treatment had a lower adverse event rate with improved quality of life and a lower overall cost.[9] Another randomized trial compared endoscopic cystgastrostomy with laparoscopic cystgastrostomy, finding that endoscopic drainage required fewer reinterventions and a shorter time to resuming oral feeding with similar clinical success rates.[21]
- The above trials support a step-up approach using minimally invasive techniques, either endoscopic or surgical based on local expertise.

PEARLS AND PITFALLS

Indications	- The management of patients with WON requires a multidisciplinary team approach. - Two-thirds of patients with pancreatic necrosis have sterile necrosis and often can be managed conservatively without any intervention.
Endoscopic preparation	- A type and cross should be obtained prior to the procedure in case blood transfusions are required. - Antibiotic therapy is typically continued for 10-14 days post–endoscopic intervention.
Site of access	- The appropriate site of access needs to be established via EUS guidance. - Endoscopic drainage should only be performed when the WON is well-encapsulated and within 1 cm from the stomach or duodenum.

Stent placement	• Double pigtail stents are often placed coaxially through the lumen-apposing metal stent to reduce the risk of bleeding and help prevent migration of the stent. • Cross-sectional imaging should be obtained 2-3 weeks after index stent placement to assess resolution of the necrotic cavity and plan removal of the stent as soon as possible.
Necrosectomy	• Hemostasis devices and expertise are needed to manage bleeding encountered during necrosectomy
Failure of endoscopic procedures	• Large or complex collections may benefit from a multiple-gateway technique and/or a multimodality approach including endoscopic and percutaneous drainage. Endoscopic necrosectomy can also be performed via percutaneous route at the bedside once a percutaneous tract has become mature.

POSTOPERATIVE CARE

- Symptoms leading to the procedures rapidly resolve after successful therapy.
- Most patients are able to start a clear liquid diet and rapidly advance to a low-fat diet soon after successful drainage.
- Proton pump inhibitors should be discontinued to allow for gastric acidity to aid in the dissolution of necrotic debris.[22]
- Cross-sectional imaging is typically performed 2 to 3 weeks after index stent placement.
- If the collection fails to resolve or reaccumulates, disconnected pancreatic duct syndrome should be considered and leaving several double pigtail stents in the collection indefinitely should be considered in addition to other treatment options.[23]
- Treatment of disconnected pancreatic duct syndrome includes ERCP with transpapillary pancreatic duct stenting across or into the cavity. Surgical resection of the distal remnant should also be considered.

OUTCOMES

- A single-center randomized trial compared the use of LAMS with double pigtail stents for the treatment of WON, finding no difference in treatment success (94% LAMS vs 97% double pigtail stents) and no difference in recurrence rates (3% LAMS vs 0% double pigtail stents).[10] The same study group compared endoscopic drainage with minimally invasive surgery, finding that endoscopic treatment had a significantly lower rate of major adverse events (12%) than surgery (41%).[9] Endoscopic treatment also had lower costs ($76,000) compared to surgery ($117,000).
- In a multicenter randomized study comparing endoscopic drainage with minimally invasive surgery for the treatment of infected necrotizing pancreatitis, there was no difference in major adverse events (43% endoscopy vs 45% surgery). Endoscopic treatment had a lower rate of pancreatic fistula formation (5% vs 32%) and a lower length of stay (median of 35 days vs 65 days).[8]
- A meta-analysis including 3 randomized trials (190 patients) comparing endoscopic with surgical treatment for infected necrosis found no difference in mortality, but found that endoscopic treatment had lower odds of developing new-onset multiple-organ failure (OR: 0.31) or pancreatic fistulae (OR: 0.09) and resulted in a shorter mean length of hospitalization (mean difference of 8 days).[24]
- These results suggest that endoscopic treatment of WON is safe and effective with the potential to reduce costs and decrease hospital stay compared to surgery.

Adverse Events

- Endoscopic treatment of WON is associated with potential adverse events. A multidisciplinary approach is required to determine candidacy for endoscopic drainage and surgical back-up is always recommended.
- Major bleeding remains a significant adverse event of endoscopic drainage, particularly with the use of lumen-apposing metal stents, occurring in up to 10% of cases.[10,25]
- The overall adverse event rate of endoscopic transmural drainage is reported between 15% and 25%.[8-10,26]

REFERENCES

1. Banks PA, Bollen TL, Dervenis C, et al. Classification of acute pancreatitis–2012: revision of the Atlanta classification and definitions by international consensus. *Gut*. 2013;62:102-111.
2. Baron TH, DiMaio CJ, Wang AY, et al. American Gastroenterological association clinical practice update: management of pancreatic necrosis. *Gastroenterology*. 2020;158:67-75.e1.
3. Koutroumpakis E, Slivka A, Furlan A, et al. Management and outcomes of acute pancreatitis patients over the last decade: a US tertiary-center experience. *Pancreatology*. 2017;17:32-40.
4. Puga M, Consiglieri CF, Busquets J, et al. Safety of lumen-apposing stent with or without coaxial plastic stent for endoscopic ultrasound-guided drainage of pancreatic fluid collections: a retrospective study. *Endoscopy*. 2018;50:1022-1026.
5. Varadarajulu S, Phadnis MA, Christein JD, et al. Multiple transluminal gateway technique for EUS-guided drainage of symptomatic walled-off pancreatic necrosis. *Gastrointest Endosc*. 2011;74:74-80.
6. Binda C, Dabizzi E, Anderloni A, et al. Single-step endoscopic ultrasound-guided multiple gateway drainage of complex walled-off necrosis with lumen apposing metal stents. *Eur J Gastroenterol Hepatol*. 2020;32:1401-1404.
7. van Santvoort HC, Besselink MG, Bakker OJ, et al. A step-up approach or open necrosectomy for necrotizing pancreatitis. *N Engl J Med*. 2010;362:1491-1502.
8. van Brunschot S, van Grinsven J, van Santvoort HC, et al. Endoscopic or surgical step-up approach for infected necrotising pancreatitis: a multicentre randomised trial. *Lancet*. 2018;391:51-58.
9. Bang JY, Arnoletti JP, Holt BA, et al. An endoscopic transluminal approach, compared with minimally invasive surgery, reduces complications and costs for patients with necrotizing pancreatitis. *Gastroenterology*. 2019;156:1027-1040.e3.
10. Bang JY, Navaneethan U, Hasan MK, et al. Non-superiority of lumen-apposing metal stents over plastic stents for drainage of walled-off necrosis in a randomised trial. *Gut*. 2019;68:1200-1209.

11. Messallam AA, Adler DG, Shah RJ, et al. Direct endoscopic necrosectomy with and without hydrogen peroxide for walled-off pancreatic necrosis: a multicenter comparative study. *Am J Gastroenterol.* 2021;116:700-709.
12. van der Wiel SE, May A, Poley JW, et al. Preliminary report on the safety and utility of a novel automated mechanical endoscopic tissue resection tool for endoscopic necrosectomy: a case series. *Endosc Int Open.* 2020;8:E274-e280.
13. Rizzatti G, Rimbas M, Impagnatiello M, et al. Endorotor-based endoscopic necrosectomy as a rescue or primary treatment of complicated walled-off pancreatic necrosis. A case series. *J Gastrointestin Liver Dis.* 2020;29:681-684.
14. Stassen PMC, de Jonge PJF, Bruno MJ, et al. Safety and efficacy of a novel resection system for direct endoscopic necrosectomy of walled-off pancreas necrosis: a prospective, international, multicenter trial. *Gastrointest Endosc.* 2021;95(3):471-479.
15. Chandrasekhara V, Elhanafi S, Storm AC, et al. Predicting the need for step-up therapy after EUS-guided drainage of pancreatic fluid collections with lumen-apposing metal stents. *Clin Gastroenterol Hepatol.* 2021;19(10):2192-2198.
16. Jain S, Padhan R, Bopanna S, et al. Percutaneous endoscopic step-up therapy is an effective minimally invasive approach for infected necrotizing pancreatitis. *Dig Dis Sci.* 2020;65:615-622.
17. Thorsen A, Borch AM, Novovic S, et al. Endoscopic necrosectomy through percutaneous self-expanding metal stents may be a promising additive in treatment of necrotizing pancreatitis. *Dig Dis Sci.* 2018;63:2456-2465.
18. Saumoy M, Kumta NA, Tyberg A, et al. Transcutaneous endoscopic necrosectomy for walled-off pancreatic necrosis in the paracolic gutter. *J Clin Gastroenterol.* 2018;52:458-463.
19. Hollemans RA, Bakker OJ, Boermeester MA, et al. Superiority of step-up approach vs open necrosectomy in long-term follow-up of patients with necrotizing pancreatitis. *Gastroenterology.* 2019;156:1016-1026.
20. van Brunschot S, Hollemans RA, Bakker OJ, et al. Minimally invasive and endoscopic versus open necrosectomy for necrotising pancreatitis: a pooled analysis of individual data for 1980 patients. *Gut.* 2018;67:697-706.
21. Garg PK, Meena D, Babu D, et al. Endoscopic versus laparoscopic drainage of pseudocyst and walled-off necrosis following acute pancreatitis: a randomized trial. *Surg Endosc.* 2020;34:1157-1166.
22. Powers PC, Siddiqui A, Sharaiha RZ, et al. Discontinuation of proton pump inhibitor use reduces the number of endoscopic procedures required for resolution of walled-off pancreatic necrosis. *Endosc Ultrasound.* 2019;8:194-198.
23. Bang JY, Mel Wilcox C, Arnoletti JP, et al. Importance of disconnected pancreatic duct syndrome in recurrence of pancreatic fluid collections initially drained using lumen-apposing metal stents. *Clin Gastroenterol Hepatol.* 2021;19:1275-1281.e2.
24. Haney CM, Kowalewski KF, Schmidt MW, et al. Endoscopic versus surgical treatment for infected necrotizing pancreatitis: a systematic review and meta-analysis of randomized controlled trials. *Surg Endosc.* 2020;34:2429-2444.
25. Brimhall B, Han S, Tatman PD, et al. Increased incidence of pseudoaneurysm bleeding with lumen-apposing metal stents compared to double-pigtail plastic stents in patients with peripancreatic fluid collections. *Clin Gastroenterol Hepatol.* 2018;16:1521-1528.
26. Gardner TB, Coelho-Prabhu N, Gordon SR, et al. Direct endoscopic necrosectomy for the treatment of walled-off pancreatic necrosis: results from a multicenter U.S. series. *Gastrointest Endosc.* 2011;73:718-726.

Chapter 48: Pancreas: Drainage, Distal Pancreatectomy/Splenectomy

Kojo Wallace, Randi N. Smith, and Christopher J. Dente

DEFINITIONS

- Blunt and penetrating abdominal trauma can be associated with injuries to the pancreas.
- While nonoperative management of minor pancreatic injuries is generally straightforward, the management of major pancreatic injuries which involve the pancreatic duct often requires more complex surgical intervention.
- For major injuries outside the head of the pancreas, both simple pancreatic drainage and resection in the form of distal pancreatectomy are surgical options for management.
- For the latter technique, both splenectomy and splenic preservation have been described.

INDICATIONS

- While there are multiple considerations in the management of distal pancreatic injuries, the two most important are the presence of pancreatic duct disruption and the hemodynamic status of the patient. For patients in extremis or with multiple injuries, pancreatic drainage is an option for all grades of injury, although this will likely commit the patient to a pancreatic fistula. Therefore, distal pancreatectomy for AAST Grade III and higher injuries is generally preferred (**TABLE 1**).
- Preservation of the spleen may be considered in the setting of trauma, assuming the patient's injury is relatively isolated and the patient's hemodynamic status is reasonable. Preservation of the spleen adds a layer of technical difficulty and a significant amount of time to the procedure. In a patient with multiple injuries that require active management and those who are requiring ongoing resuscitation, a splenectomy is indicated. In adults, the risk of overwhelming postsplenectomy infection (OPSI) is sufficiently low to warrant this life saving maneuver.

PATIENT HISTORY, PHYSICAL FINDINGS, AND DIAGNOSIS

- A high index of suspicion is required for diagnosis given the significant morbidity of a missed injury.
- With penetrating trauma, pancreatic injury is generally diagnosed on laparotomy. A thorough examination of the lesser sac is imperative during exploration. After blunt injury, diagnosis may be made during emergent operative intervention or on cross-sectional imaging as discussed below. Generally, direct, high-energy transfer to the upper abdomen is the typical cause of injury to the pancreas, given its relatively protected retroperitoneal location.
- Once pancreatic injury is identified, either on imaging or during laparotomy, the surgeon must next determine the integrity of the pancreatic duct. Pancreatic duct disruption is best treated with resection if the injury is to the left of the superior mesenteric vein. This is discussed further below.
- Physical examination findings may include abdominal bruising such as "seatbelt sign," peritonitis, and hemodynamic instability.

IMAGING AND OTHER DIAGNOSTIC STUDIES

- Computed tomography (CT) with intravenous (IV) contrast is generally a reliable study for intraperitoneal or retroperitoneal injuries and is indicated in stable patients who do not require immediate surgical exploration. However, this modality may miss minor pancreatic injuries[1]; clues such as air and fluid collections in the lesser sac may aid in diagnosis (**FIGURE 1**). Major pancreatic injuries are generally visualized as pancreatic parenchymal lacerations with surrounding free fluid.
- Ultrasound/E-FAST examinations are commonly performed in initial trauma evaluations but are not useful to identify injuries to the pancreas, due to its retroperitoneal location.
- As mentioned earlier, the intraoperative evaluation of ductal integrity is one of the key aspects that determine management. Examination of the injury may allow a surgeon to determine an obvious injury to the duct (eg, complete transection of the parenchyma). Further examination under loupe magnification in a stable patient may allow for identification of clear pancreatic fluid drainage from the injured organ. Unfortunately, intraoperative pancreatography is often impractical during laparotomy for trauma. Either endoscopic or direct transduodenal ampullary cannulation may be considered in a hemodynamically stable patient but these are often difficult to organize and, in the latter case, require an otherwise unnecessary enterotomy. Finally, a needle cholecystocholangiogram

Table 1: Pancreatic Grading System and Recommended Management

Grade	Findings	Treatment
1	Superficial laceration or small hematoma without injury to pancreatic duct	Drainage
2	Major laceration or contusion without injury to pancreatic duct	Drainage
3	Distal parenchymal injury with injury to pancreatic duct	Distal pancreatectomy
4	Proximal parenchymal injury involving pancreatic duct	Distal pancreatectomy if left of superior mesenteric vein (SMV) Closed suction drainage if right of SMV
5	Extensive injury of pancreatic head	Drainage with or without pyloric exclusion Pancreaticoduodenectomy

Reprinted with permission from Moore EE, Cogbill TH, Malangoni MA, et al. Organ injury scaling, II: Pancreas, duodenum, small bowel, colon, and rectum. J Trauma. 1990;30(11):1427-1429. Table 1.

Chapter 48 PANCREAS: DRAINAGE, DISTAL PANCREATECTOMY/SPLENECTOMY

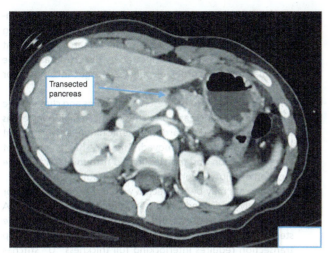

FIGURE 1 • Computed tomography scan image of a transected pancreas. This modality may miss minor pancreatic injuries; clues such as air and fluid collections in the lesser sac may aid diagnoses in such cases.

is another described and simpler technique, but often does not visualize the pancreatic duct.
- Postoperative MRCP and/or ERCP may be used if there is concern about a missed pancreatic ductal injury, such as in a patient with persistent abdominal pain, elevated pancreatic enzymes, and nonspecific CT findings. It may also be used to determine the extent of known injury or provide a therapeutic option for patients with persistent pancreatic fistulas.

SURGICAL MANAGEMENT

Preoperative Management
- The suspected injury, anticipated procedure, need for special equipment such as stapling devices, potential need for transfusion, and/or imaging should be communicated with the operating room team and anesthesiologists.

Positioning
- The patient should be supine with both arms extended to allow access for IVs; they should also be exposed and prepped from the chin to knees as per trauma protocols.

STEPS
- Exploratory laparotomy is indicated for patients with suspected pancreatic injury; this is performed through a generous midline incision in the acute setting; however, an upper midline incision may be considered with caudal extension of the incision as indicated. In the acute setting, all quadrants of the abdominal cavity are inspected on entry—per trauma protocols—to identify and control other potential causes of instability/peritonitis such as hemorrhage or leakage from a hollow viscus.
- The pancreas is located in the lesser sac; it must be completely exposed to perform adequate evaluation for potential injury. The gastrocolic ligament inferior to the gastroepiploic vessels is divided to enter the lesser sac; this is facilitated by elevating and retracting the stomach and transverse colon to place tension on the gastrocolic ligament (FIGURE 2). A relatively thinned portion of the ligament is usually a safe entry point and can be extended to widely open the lesser sac. The anterior surface of the pancreas and the borders of the body and tail can then be visualized. Any posterior adhesions between the posterior wall of stomach and the anterior surface of pancreas may be lysed, and a malleable retractor may be used to facilitate anterior retraction of the stomach.
- The splenic vessels may be quickly accessed at this point in the procedure, as needed, along the superior border of the pancreas.
- A generous Kocher maneuver will allow complete visualization of the pancreatic head and uncinate process. This should be performed to confirm there is no associated pancreatic head injury. In some instances, mobilization of the hepatic flexure may be indicated to achieve this goal.
- Exposure of the splenic hilum and subsequent medial mobilization allows visualization of both spleen and posterior aspect of the pancreatic tail. Alternatively, if pancreatic injury is obvious, transection of the pancreas may be performed prior to splenic mobilization.
- If a splenectomy is to be performed, mobilization of this organ proceeds with division of the gastrosplenic ligament and short gastric vessels, as well as the splenocolic, splenorenal, and splenodiaphragmatic ligaments. These vessels may be clamped and tied and or controlled with a vessel sealing

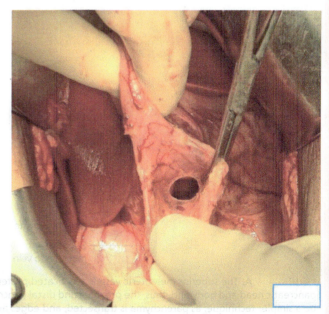

FIGURE 2 • The gastrocolic ligament inferior to the gastroepiploic vessels is divided to enter the lesser sac; this is facilitated by elevating and retracting the stomach and transverse colon to place tension on the gastrocolic ligament.

device. After traumatic injury, a dissecting hematoma along this plane may facilitate relatively rapid blunt dissection; this can be achieved by "cupping" along superolateral border of the spleen and gently pulling it inferiorly.
- At this stage, if there is no concern for a ductal injury (Grade 1 or 2), management consists of hemostasis and closed suction drainage (**FIGURE 3**).
- The superior mesenteric vessels are located posteriorly and are a landmark defining the junction of the pancreatic head and body and, thus, the proximal and distal pancreas (**FIGURE 4A**). The surgeon is usually able to slide their fingers posterior to the pancreas at this location, elevating pancreas from the major vessels and demarcating a point of resection. This can be facilitated by dissecting along the avascular inferior border of pancreas to get into posterior plane behind the gland.
- When the spleen is to be preserved, fine ties and clips may be used to ligate pancreatic branches of these major vessels as dissection is carried toward the splenic hilum, at which point the pancreatic tail is removed. The IMV has a somewhat variable location and may be ligated if found lateral to the location of injury/lesion; otherwise, it should be preserved.
- The pancreas may be transected with a GIA or TA stapler or may simply be divided sharply and the raw end oversewn. A stapling device transects and closes the parenchyma in one step and is probably a simpler technique (**FIGURE 4B**). Sharp transection requires interlocking full thickness "U" stitches with nonabsorbable sutures to close the parenchyma (**FIGURE 4C**). With either technique the pancreatic duct should be identified and suture ligated as well if possible (**FIGURE 4D**). Unfortunately, the distal pancreatic duct in a normal pancreas is oftentimes not well visualized. Leak rates are equivalent with either technique. The splenic artery and vein are typically stapled prior to pancreatic resection.
- Additional buttressing with omentum or surgical glue has failed to show any benefit in leak rates, which approach 20% regardless of technique.[2] Therefore, routine drainage is recommended. Once resection is complete, a final check for hemostasis should be performed. Postoperative bleeding complications are most common from the short gastric vessels if splenectomy has been performed.

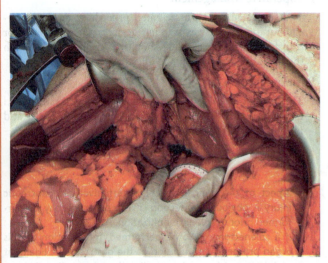

FIGURE 3 • Closed suction drain is placed in lesser sac, anterior to the pancreas, to drain any accumulated pancreatic fluid or blood.

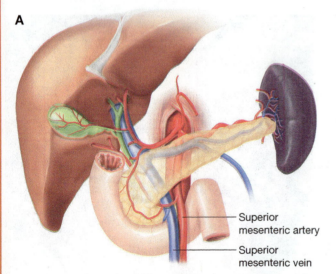
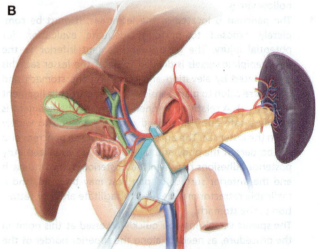

FIGURE 4 • **A,** The superior mesenteric vessels are located posterior to the pancreas and are a landmark defining the junction of the pancreatic head and body and, thus, the proximal and distal pancreas. **B,** A "TA stapler" may be used to transect the pancreas. This may be a simpler technique, as parenchyma is transected, and edges approximated in one step.

PEARLS AND PITFALLS

- The most important determinations of treatment of distal pancreatic injuries are the presence or absence of pancreatic duct injury and the patient's hemodynamic status.
- Resection for injuries left of the SMV is indicated whenever pancreatic ductal injury is discovered or strongly suspected.
- Splenic preservation is desirable if possible, but commonly splenectomy is performed to expedite patient management.
- Complete exposure of the pancreas should be performed to decrease incidence of missed injury.
- Closed suction drains are important in the management of pancreatic injuries, whether or not resection is performed, as fistula rates are high. Fistulas, should they occur, are most often self-limited.
- Carefully examine the short gastric vessel ligations to prevent postoperative hemorrhage. Consideration of using Lembert sutures to invaginate the vessel stumps into the stomach wall is recommended.
- Postsplenectomy vaccinations should be administered in effort to mitigate OPSI (if splenectomy is performed).

POSTOPERATIVE CARE

- Standard post laparotomy care is indicated. Gastric dilatation early after injury may contribute to postoperative short gastric hemorrhage and should be avoided.
- Drain care: Drain is usually kept for 7 to 10 days to monitor for leaks; it may also be kept until the patient is tolerating a diet. Drain amylase is measured on day 3 for evidence of a leak; defined by drain amylase >3× serum level.[3]
- Vaccinations: If splenectomy is performed, vaccinations for encapsulated bacteria are performed 2 weeks after surgery or at discharge.

COMPLICATIONS

- A fistula is the most common complication following pancreatic injury, with studies citing an incidence range of 5% to 37%.[4] These are usually minor and self-limited. A closed suction drain aids in diagnosis and may be the only treatment required.
- Abscess formation may cause significant morbidity and may be more likely in the setting of associated hollow viscus injuries.
- Acute pancreatitis occurs uncommonly and is usually self-limited.
- Secondary hemorrhage may occur in the setting of infections, abscess, or inadequate drainage; these bleeding complications may be amenable to IR embolization, but may require reexploration.
- Pseudocysts may form and require internal drainage and/or ERCP.

REFERENCES

1. Phelan HA, Velmahos GC, Jurkovich GJ, et al. An evaluation of multidetector computed tomography in detecting pancreatic injury: results of a multicenter AAST study. *J Trauma*. 2009;66:641Y64.
2. Peck GL, Blitzer DN, Bulauitan CS, et al. Outcomes after distal pancreatectomy for trauma in the modern era. *Am Surg*. 2016;82(6):526-532. PMID: 27305885.
3. International Study Group on Pancreatic Surgery (ISGPS); Bassi C, Marchegiani G, Dervenis C, et al. The 2016 update of the International Study Group (ISGPS) definition and grading of postoperative pancreatic fistula: 11 Years after. *Surgery*. 2017;161(3):584-591. doi:10.1016/j.surg.2016.11.014. Epub 2016 Dec 28. PMID: 28040257.
4. Agarwal H, Gupta A, Kumar S. An overview of pancreatic trauma. *J Pancreatol*. 2020;3(3):139-146. doi:10.1097/JP9.0000000000000044

SECTION IV: Surgery of the Spleen

Chapter 49: Elective Splenectomy (Open and Minimally Invasive Techniques)

Zachary J. Brown and Mary E. Dillhoff

DEFINITION
- Splenectomy is the surgical removal of the spleen either by traditional open surgery or minimally invasive (either laparoscopic or robotic) techniques.

DIFFERENTIAL DIAGNOSIS
- Hematologic disorders
  - Red blood cell disorders
    - Hereditary spherocytosis
    - Hereditary elliptocytosis
    - Hereditary pyropoikilocytosis
  - Lymphoma/leukemia/myeloproliferative disorders
  - Platelet disorders
    - Immune thrombocytopenia (ITP)
    - Thrombotic thrombocytopenic purpura (TTP)
- Hemaglobinopathies
  - Sickle cell
  - Thalassemia
- Autoimmune disorders
  - Autoimmune hemolytic anemia
- Genetic disorders
- Vascular disorders
- Idiopathic/iatrogenic
- Infection
- Cyst
- Tumors
  - Malignant
    - Angiosarcoma
  - Benign
    - Hemangioma
    - Hamartoma
    - Lymphangioma
  - Metastatic

PATIENT HISTORY AND PHYSICAL FINDINGS
- A comprehensive history should be performed prior to surgery. This includes a detailed past medical history including prior operations, signs and symptoms of abnormal bleeding, a history of liver failure, as well as a history of abdominal pain or constitutional symptoms. A list of all medications, allergies, in addition to a personal and family history of bleeding, clotting disorders, and cancers should be noted.
- A complete physical examination of the patient should be done, and all patients should be examined for signs of hepatomegaly, portal hypertension, or liver failure (jaundice, palmar erythema, spider angiomata, gynecomastia, caput medusa, or ascites), as well as the presence or absence of splenomegaly.
- Hematologic conditions may present with a history of purpura, epistaxis, petechiae, gingival bleeding, hematuria, gastrointestinal bleeding, myalgia, or fatigue.
- Although now a rare indication for splenectomy, patients with lymphomas and myeloproliferative disorders present with diffuse lymphadenopathy, constitutional symptoms (such as night sweats, weight loss, or fatigue), pancytopenia, abdominal pain, splenomegaly, or early satiety.
- Patients with hemoglobinopathies and hereditary disorders of red blood cells (RBCs) may present with jaundice, abdominal pain, or splenomegaly. Alternatively, they may be asymptomatic and incidentally identified due to an abnormal laboratory value obtained for a different indication.
- Patients with hereditary spherocytosis (HS), hereditary elliptocytosis (HE), or hereditary pyropoikilocytosis (HP) have molecular defects causing alterations in RBC membrane proteins causing misshaped RBCs. As such, the RBCs are often sequestered and degraded by the spleen, and thus patients often benefit from splenectomy. HS is the most common congenital anemia often requiring splenectomy. Splenectomy eliminates or improves anemia in patients with moderate HS and eliminates the need for regular transfusions in patients with the severe form of the disease.[1,2] These patients often receive splenectomies in childhood to alleviate symptoms and long-term sequela of the disease including skeletal abnormalities and repeated need for blood transfusion. In mild HS, the purpose of splenectomy is to prevent the production of bilirubin gallstones. As such, in these cases where splenectomy is performed for HS, splenectomy is often combined with a cholecystectomy. Patients with HE or HP usually have milder severity of anemia as these cells are generally more deformable than spherocytes. As such, splenectomy is usually reserved for patients with severe disease.
- Splenectomy for platelet disorders such as ITP or TTP is often a result of failed medical management to control thrombocytopenia or abdominal pain associated with splenomegaly. ITP results from autoimmune destruction of platelets as a result of antiplatelet antibodies and is a diagnosis of exclusion. Symptoms include bleeding, bruising, purpura and petechiae. Patients may be observed as long as platelet counts are above 20,000 to 30,000/mm^3. Medical management is the first-line treatment for ITP for persistently low platelet counts below 30,000/mm^3, and most patients initially respond to glucocorticoids. However, in one series, only 39% of prednisone-treated

patients achieve complete remission, and only half of these patients have sustained remission beyond 6 months of cessation of maintenance therapy.[3] Rituximab, and anti-CD20 monoclonal antibody, has also been shown to have benefit in patients with ITP. Intravenous immunoglobulin (IVIG) can also be used as first-line treatment and can increase the platelet count in over 75% of patients within 5 days of treatment.[4] IVIG is often reserved for those patients with life-threatening bleeding and intracranial hemorrhage and those preparing for splenectomy or other surgical procedures. Splenectomy is reserved for patients with symptomatic thrombocytopenia following glucocorticoid administration for at least 8 weeks and having a platelet count persistently less than 30,000/μL. Splenectomy is also indicated in patients in whom the condition recurs after cessation of therapy. TTP on the other hand is a result of a deficiency of the ADAMS13 protein and leads to platelet aggregation and microvascular thrombosis. Patients often have hemolytic anemia, thrombocytopenia, fever, renal failure, and neurologic symptoms such as headache, seizures, or coma. Initial therapy is often plasmapheresis. Second-line therapies include rituximab and glucocorticoids. Splenectomy is reserved for refractory thrombocytopenia or relapse.

- Splenectomies may be performed via open or minimally invasive technique. Minimally invasive splenectomy may be performed either laparoscopically or robotically. The approach is often determined by the disease process and clinical stability of the patient. Currently, many consider minimally invasive splenectomy to be the gold standard approach for patients undergoing elective splenectomy. Massive splenomegaly is considered a relative contraindication for a minimally invasive approach. As patients may be undergoing splenectomy for coagulopathic disorders, it is important to note that coagulopathy is not a contraindication for a minimally invasive approach and many patients often do better with minimally invasive surgery.
- Grading systems have been developed to predict the morbidity and difficulty of elective laparoscopic splenectomies with male gender, age, pathology and spleen weight significantly related with operative time, operative bleeding, and conversion to open surgery[5,6] (TABLE 1).

SURGICAL MANAGEMENT

Planning

- All patients with a known or suspected hematologic, autoimmune, or myeloproliferative disorder should have a hematologist fully involved in the patient's evaluation and treatment plan prior to and following surgery.
- Computed tomography (CT) scan is crucial part of operative planning. CT allows for determining the size of the spleen, the anatomy and size of the splenic vascular supply, the relationship of the spleen to surrounding organs, and potential locations of accessory spleens in the abdomen (FIGURE 1).
- Ultrasound is a noninvasive modality for the examination of splenomegaly and portal hypertension.
- Magnetic resonance imaging (MRI) of the spleen is an excellent method for evaluating focal lesions as well as aid in the detection and differential diagnosis of peri- and intrasplenic tumors.[7]

Preoperative Planning

- Patients who have been treated with prolonged courses of glucocorticoids should be considered to receive appropriate stress-dose steroids intraoperatively, with rapid tapering postoperatively in a multidisciplinary approach with anesthesiology and hematology.
- Blood products should be ordered and available intraoperatively. For patients with platelet disorders, platelet transfusion should be given after ligation of the splenic artery.
- For all elective cases, vaccinations against the encapsulated organisms (*Hemophilus influenza B*, *Streptococcus pneumoniae*, and *Neisseria meningitidis*) should be administered several weeks prior to surgery. For emergent cases, vaccinations should also be administered. Timing of vaccination is debated, but 2 to 4 weeks postoperatively is recommended. Vaccination against encapsulated organisms is to prevent overwhelming postsplenectomy infection (OPSI). OPSI is the development of a fulminant, rapidly fatal bacterial infection following the removal of the spleen. The incidence of OPSI in the first 2 years after splenectomy is estimated to be 0.9% for adults and 5% for children.[8] Current guidelines for

Table 1: Difficulty Score for Laparoscopic Splenectomy

Age	
≤40 y old	0
40-60 y old	1
≥60 y old	2
Gender	
Female	0.5
Male	1
Pathology group	
ITP	0.5
Other benign	1
Malignant	2
Spleen weight	
<400 g	1
400-1000 g	3
>1000 g	5
Difficulty grade	
Low	≤4
Medium	4.5-5.5
High	≥6

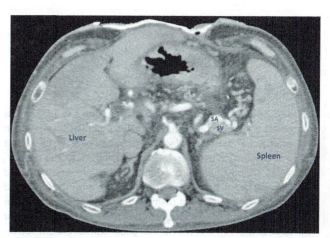

FIGURE 1 • CT image demonstrating splenomegaly. The volume of the spleen approaches that of the liver. *SA*, splenic artery; *SV*, splenic vein.

Table 2: Overwhelming Postsplenectomy Infection Prophylaxis

Vaccine	Recommendation
Pneumococcal	1 dose of Pneumococcal 13-valent conjugate (PCV13)
	≥8 wk after PCV13 administer pneumococcal polysaccharide (PPSV23)
	Revaccination of PPSV23 5 y after first dose
Meningococcal	4-valent conjugate (MenACWY) or polysaccharide (MPSV4)
	MenACWY: Two doses given ≥8 wk apart, revaccinate every 5 y
	MPSV4: Two doses administered ≥4 wk apart
Hemophilus influenza B	Single dose
	Titers can be followed to assess the need for booster dose
Influenza	Yearly
Elective cases: vaccinate 2 wk preoperatively	
Nonelective cases: discharge or 2 wk postoperatively	
Consider monitoring antibody titers of all three pathogens in immunocompromised patients	

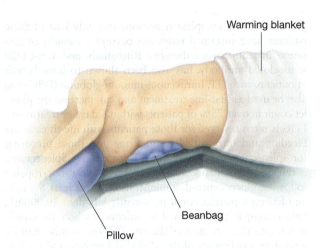

FIGURE 2 • Patient positioning in the right lateral decubitus position.

vaccination to prevent OPSI are listed in **TABLE 2**. In addition, patients at very high risk for OPSI (severely immunocompromised patients, patients who underwent splenectomy for hematologic malignancy, or those with graft-vs-host disease) may require antibiotic prophylaxis.[9]

- All patients should be given prophylactic antibiotics to cover skin flora within 60 minutes of making the skin incision in the OR. Nasal or oral gastric tubes should be inserted once the patient is under anesthesia to decompress the stomach and aid in visualization.
- Minimally invasive splenectomy (either robotic or laparoscopic) is the operation of choice for most elective splenectomies. However, other options include hand-assisted or open approaches. Indications for conversion from minimally invasive to an open procedure include intolerability or inability to insufflate the abdominal cavity, uncontrollable bleeding, or massive splenomegaly that is unable to be extracted.
- In cases of massive splenomegaly or portal hypertension, preoperative embolization of the splenic artery by interventional radiology will decrease the amount of blood loss and may aid in the technical aspects of the procedure. Embolization of the splenic artery causes decreased perfusion and thereby results in involution of the spleen, making mobilization of the spleen technically easier.

Positioning

- For open splenectomies, most patients are placed in a supine position, with both arms extended, and a midline laparotomy incision is made. An additional option in isolated nontraumatic open cases is to make a left subcostal incision.
- Patients undergoing a minimally invasive splenectomy can be positioned supine or in the right lateral decubitus position. In the right lateral decubitus position, the beanbag or kidney rest is placed to maximize the distance between the costal margin and iliac crest. The table may also be flexed to assist in widening this space. Ensure that all pressure points are properly padded and the shoulders, extremities, and spine are in comfortable, neutral positions (**FIGURE 2**).

Your Technique and Steps

OPEN SPLENECTOMY

Incision

- Prior to incision, ensure adequate monitoring and intravenous access is obtained in preparation for potential bleeding. An arterial line should be placed based upon patient risk factors and a discussion between the surgeon and anesthesia team.
- After endotracheal intubation and standard prepping and draping of the patient, a midline laparotomy incision is used to enter the peritoneal cavity. A supraumbilical incision can be made initially with extension inferiorly as needed for exposure (**FIGURE 3**). Without good exposure from retraction and adequate visualization, the propensity for bleeding will increase, making the operation much more technically difficult.

Mobilization

- The spleen resides high and posterior in the upper left abdomen. In order to remove the spleen, all peritoneal and visceral attachments must be divided. These include the splenorenal attachments to the kidney; the splenophrenic attachments to the diaphragm; the splenocolic attachments to the colon; and the gastrosplenic ligament attachments to the stomach, which contains the short gastric vessels (**FIGURE 4**).
- Splenic mobilization is accomplished using traction and countertraction. The operating surgeon places a splayed, nondominant hand (usually with the aid of a lap sponge for better grip) and applies dorsal and medial traction on the spleen. This will help clearly define the splenorenal and splenophrenic ligaments. Be mindful that the tendency for a lifting of the spleen out of the left upper quadrant often

Chapter 49 ELECTIVE SPLENECTOMY (OPEN AND MINIMALLY INVASIVE TECHNIQUES) 401

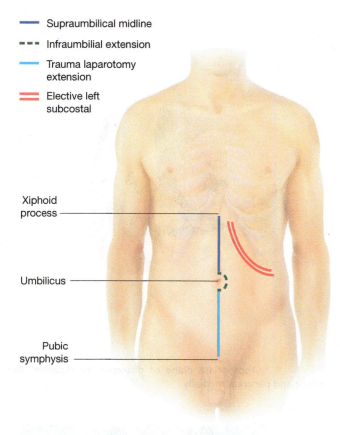

FIGURE 3 • Various incisions for an open splenectomy.

occurs, which can result in capsular tearing causing unnecessary bleeding. Be sure to first mobilize all attachments of the spleen to the anterior abdominal wall or you will find this maneuver cannot be done.

- Division of the splenocolic ligament allows for mobilization of the splenic flexure, which displaces the colon away from the spleen (FIGURE 5). This is best done sharply or by using electrocautery. Once this is done, continue laterally toward the splenorenal ligaments, which, when divided, separate the spleen from Gerota fascia of the kidney. Finally, continue superiorly to the splenophrenic ligaments. Again, the importance of traction and countertraction cannot be overemphasized. The first assistant provides countertraction with tissue forceps to divide the ligaments, whereas the surgeon continues to maintain midline traction on the spleen.

- Division of the ligaments should be made 1 to 2 cm from the spleen to avoid injury to both the spleen and other organs. As the spleen is mobilized anteriorly, deeper layers of connective tissue are brought into view and can be easily divided either bluntly or sharply.

- Once free from the retroperitoneal attachments, digital control of the hilar vessels can be accomplished and will stop any bleeding and improve visualization.

- As dissection continues lateral to medial, the left adrenal gland can be visualized and should be kept in its proper anatomic location. The tail of the pancreas and the splenic vein will also come into view. This visualization is crucial and paramount to avoid injury to the tail of the pancreas (FIGURE 6).

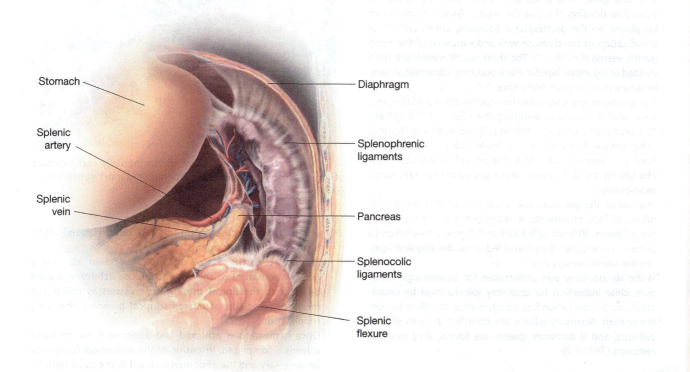

FIGURE 4 • Attachments of the spleen in the left upper quadrant.

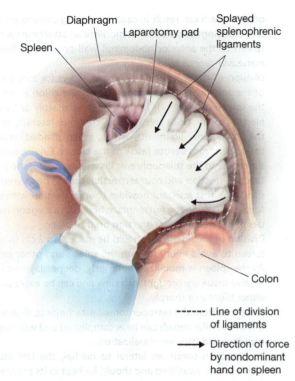

FIGURE 5 • Direction of force applied to the spleen and line of division of the splenic attachments.

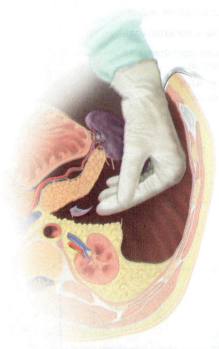

FIGURE 6 • Appropriate plane of dissection to mobilize the spleen and pancreas medially.

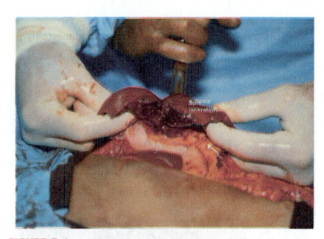

FIGURE 7 • Mobilization of the spleen medially and exposure of the gastrosplenic ligament, containing the short gastric vessels (arrow).

Ligation of Vessels and Excision

- With the spleen fully mobilized to the midline, attention is turned to dividing the vascular supply. Gentle traction can be placed on the gastrosplenic ligament, which will allow visualization of the stomach wall and exposure of the short gastric vessels (FIGURE 7). The short gastric vessels are then divided using either bipolar electrocautery, ultrasonic shears, or sutures per surgeon preference (FIGURE 8).
- The splenic artery is seen on the superior border of the pancreas and is visualized entering the hilum of the spleen. The artery and vein are individually isolated and ligated, using suture ligature (such as 0-silk), LigaSure (Valleylab, Boulder, Colorado, CA), or a stapler with a vascular load. The spleen is now free and can be passed off for pathologic examination.
- The tail of the pancreas will often extend into the splenic hilum. In 75% of patients, it lies within 1 cm of the hilum, and of these, 30% actually touch it.[10] Care must be taken to ensure a pancreatic injury is avoided when dividing and ligating the splenic vessels (FIGURE 9).
- If the splenectomy was undertaken for hematologic disorders, close inspection for accessory spleens must be undertaken, or the operation has a high chance of failure to cure the patient. Accessory spleens are identified in up to 30% of patients, and if accessory spleens are found, they must be removed (TABLE 3).

Closure

- Once the spleen is removed, attention must be paid to ensuring hemostasis is achieved. Oozing from the splenic bed can usually be controlled with selected cauterization, argon beam, or hemostatic agents.
- The short gastric vessels may be oversewn along the greater curvature of the stomach. Close attention should be paid to the apical short gastric vessels as this is the most frequent site of missed surgical bleeding requiring reoperation.
- Once hemostasis is achieved and assessment for accessory spleens is completed, irrigation of the abdominal cavity may be necessary and the abdomen is closed in the usual fashion.
- Selective drainage with a closed suction drain in the splenic bed may be performed if an injury of the tail of the pancreas is known or suspected.

Chapter 49 ELECTIVE SPLENECTOMY (OPEN AND MINIMALLY INVASIVE TECHNIQUES) 403

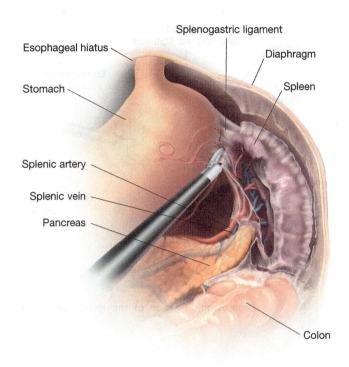

FIGURE 8 • Division of the short gastric vessels.

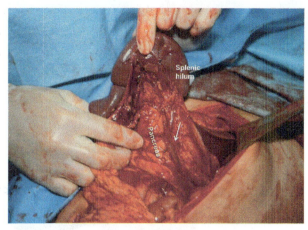

FIGURE 9 • The tail of the pancreas abuts the splenic hilum. *White arrow* indicates the splenic vein.

Table 3: Common Locations for Accessory Spleens

Splenic hilum
Splenorenal ligament
Greater omentum
Retroperitoneal area surrounding the tail of the pancreas
Splenocolic ligament
Small bowel mesentery

MINIMALLY INVASIVE SPLENECTOMY

Laparoscopic Splenectomy

- There are two main approaches for mobilization of the spleen, the supine (anterior) approach and the lateral decubitus approach. The lateral approach is the one most commonly used when performing laparoscopic splenectomies and is described below.
- The position of the operating surgeon and placement of the port sites for laparoscopic splenectomy can be seen in **FIGURE 10**.
- Once pneumoperitoneum is established, the operation is begun with a thorough exploration of the abdominal cavity, looking for accessory spleens. If found, all accessory spleens need to be excised.
- Dissection begins similar to an open procedure, with mobilization of the splenic flexure of the colon from the spleen. This is done using sharp dissection under direct visualization and can be done using hook electrocautery or an ultrasonic dissector. As with an open procedure, the technique of traction and countertraction is also employed with the laparoscopic technique. It is important to note that this division of the splenocolic ligament should be done without disturbing the spleen itself, decreasing the risk of a capsular tear (**FIGURE 11**).
- Dissection is approached in an inferior to superior counterclockwise direction. The superior splenophrenic attachments are left intact to help facilitate exposure for dissection of the splenic hilum.
- With the complete release of the splenocolic ligament and posterior dissection up to the splenophrenic ligament, dissection of the hilum can begin.

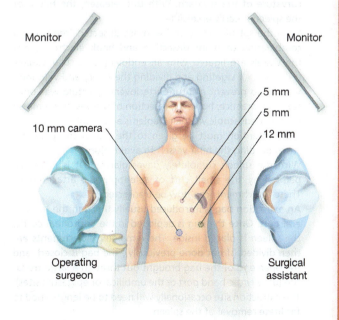

FIGURE 10 • Arrangement and port site placement for a laparoscopic splenectomy. Note that patient is drawn supine to clearly show port site placement.

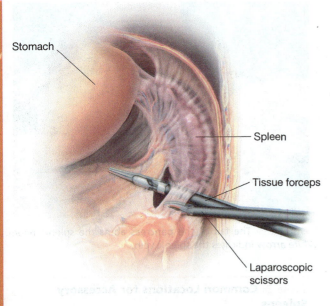

FIGURE 11 • Laparoscopic division of the splenocolic ligament.

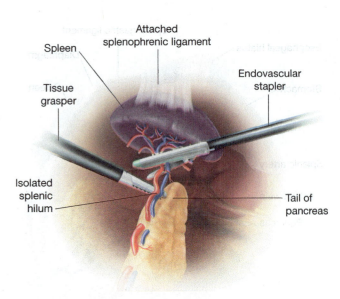

FIGURE 12 • Laparoscopic ligation of the splenic artery and vein.

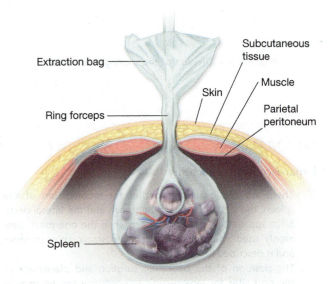

FIGURE 13 • Extraction and morcellation of the spleen.

- Similar to the open procedure, the lesser sac is entered and progression moves in a cephalad direction, exposing the anterior surface of the hilum. The posterior aspect of the hilum should already be cleared. This allows the surgeon to have quick access for any unexpected bleeding should it arise before isolating the vessels themselves.
- The short gastric vessels and main vascular pedicle are visualized. The short gastric vessels are divided using an ultrasonic or bipolar electrocautery dissector along the greater curvature of the stomach. With this released, the hilum of the spleen is easily accessible.
- Once the splenic artery and vein are dissected free using a combination of blunt dissection and hook electrocautery, the vessels are ligated with an endoscopic vascular stapler (**FIGURE 12**). Ligating and dividing the artery and vein individually to prevent a future arteriovenous fistula was once standard practice; however, resection of the vessels en masse with an endoscopic vascular stapler is acceptable.
- Close attention must be given to the tail of the pancreas when dividing the hilar vessels to avoid injury.
- With the spleen completely devascularized, it is now suspended by the small cuff of splenophrenic attachments. These attachments can now be transected.
- An extraction bag is introduced usually through the left lateral port. Once the bag is deployed in the peritoneal cavity, the spleen is placed inside. The remaining attachments are then divided (if not done previously), the bag is closed, and the open end of the bag brought out through a large trocar site (usually the hand port or the umbilical or epigastric sites). The extraction site occasionally will need to be lengthened to facilitate removal of the spleen.
- The spleen can often be removed piecemeal via finger fraction or morcellation with ring forceps (**FIGURE 13**). As the spleen is rarely excised in the setting of malignancy, this is an accepted practice. Although a rare occurrence, there have been case reports of splenic implants in the surgical wound and contamination should be avoided.
- The abdomen is then examined for hemostasis, pneumoperitoneum is stopped, and the port sites are closed. Fascial closure should be performed for all incisions measuring greater than 1 cm to avoid future hernias.
- Placement of a drain in the splenic bed is performed selectively, as stated earlier.

Robotic Splenectomy

- A robotic platform provides the advantage of improved optics and instrument articulation compared with laparoscopic surgery.
- The patient is placed in partial right lateral decubitus position; the left arm is tucked, and the patient is positioned in

Chapter 49 ELECTIVE SPLENECTOMY (OPEN AND MINIMALLY INVASIVE TECHNIQUES) 405

- either split leg with a foot board or modified lithotomy position to allow room for an assistant to stand.
- Once the abdominal cavity is accessed and pneumoperitoneum is established, port sites are placed in a linear diagonal fashion facing the left upper quadrant just superior to the umbilicus. An assistant port is placed in the right upper quadrant (FIGURE 14).
- The patient should be placed in reverse Trendelenburg position prior to docking the robot.
- The robot is docked on the patient's left side.
- A medial to lateral approach is used on the robotic platform. Dissection begins similar to the laparoscopic procedure, with mobilization of the splenic flexure of the colon from the spleen.
- Dissection continues toward the stomach exposing the gastrosplenic ligament opening the lesser sac with division of the short gastric vessels using the vessel sealer.
- The splenorenal ligament is then divided exposing the splenic vessels.
- Once the splenic artery and vein are dissected the vessels are ligated using an endoscopic vascular stapler, dividing the artery prior to the vein. Again, close attention must be given to the tail of the pancreas when dividing the hilar vessels to avoid injury.
- The remaining attachments can now be divided completely freeing the spleen.
- Similar to the laparoscopic approach, an extraction bag is introduced and the spleen is placed inside and then removed from the abdominal cavity.
- The abdomen is then examined for hemostasis, pneumoperitoneum is stopped, and the port sites are closed with fascial closure for all incisions measuring greater than 1 cm to avoid future hernias.
- Again, placement of a drain in the splenic bed is performed selectively.

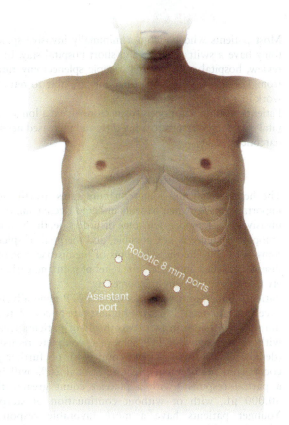

FIGURE 14 • Arrangement and port site placement for a robotic splenectomy. Note that patient is drawn supine to clearly show port site placement.

PEARLS AND PITFALLS

Imaging and other diagnostic modalities	■ Involvement of a hematologist is essential for proper diagnosis and preoperative medical management. ■ For elective splenectomies, CT of the abdomen is pivotal in the preoperative planning.
Preoperative planning	■ All elective splenectomy patients need vaccinations 2 weeks preoperatively. ■ Consider prophylactic embolization for splenomegaly or portal hypertension. ■ Have blood products with a current type and screen, type, and crossmatch readily available intraoperatively.
Technique—open resection	■ Quick mobilization to the midline is a key maneuver in a hemorrhaging spleen. ■ Keep dorsal and medial traction when mobilizing to avoid capsular tears. ■ Work lateral to medial. ■ Leave 1-2 cm cuff of peritoneum to prevent damage to surrounding organs or further injury to the spleen. ■ Ligate the splenic artery and vein, with close attention not to injure the pancreatic tail.
Technique—minimally invasive resection	■ Positioning the patient with the maximal exposure between the iliac crest and the costal margin is key. ■ Examine the entire abdomen for any accessory spleens. ■ Let gravity help with the dissection.
Technique—closure	■ No need to drain unless there is a known or suspected pancreatic injury or infection.

POSTOPERATIVE CARE

- Most patients who undergo a minimally invasive splenectomy have a swift recovery and short hospital stay. In one review, hospital stay for laparoscopic splenectomy ranged from 1.5 to 6.4 days.[11] Most patients are able to return to work in a week.
- Patients who undergo open splenectomy have a longer hospital stay, longer return to a full diet, and increased need for narcotics.[12,13]

OUTCOMES

- The hematologic and long-term cure rates are the most important factors when patients undergo elective minimally invasive splenectomies. For some disorders (ie, the hemoglobinopathies), cure is not possible, and the goal of splenectomy is to alleviate the symptoms of the disease. For other diseases, splenectomy offers the relief of pain and early satiety that can accompany splenomegaly.
- Patients undergoing splenectomy for ITP generally have excellent outcomes. It has the highest rate of complete and durable remission; in fact, two-thirds of patients treated with splenectomy for ITP achieve a complete remission (defined as a normal platelet count with no further glucocorticoid requirements). An additional 20% will have a partial response, with a platelet count greater than 50,000 µL, with or without continuation of steroids. Younger patients have a more favorable response.[14] Also, favorable response to splenectomy is also found in patients with a postoperative platelet count greater than 150,000 by postoperative day 3.
- Patients undergoing splenectomy for HS have reasonable outcomes. Coupling the splenectomy with a cholecystectomy obviates the need for a cholecystectomy later in life if pigmented stones are present. For severe HS, splenectomy eliminates the need for regular blood transfusions; however, anemia will still persist. Growth failure or skeletal changes from the high degree of erythropoiesis needed to compensate for the hemolytic anemia is reversed for children after the spleen is removed.[15]

COMPLICATIONS

- Bleeding 4% to 16% (most common)
- Thromboembolic events/thrombosis 2% to 4%
- Pancreatic injury
- Seroma
- Hematoma
- Incisional hernia
- Wound dehiscence
- OPSI

REFERENCES

1. Schilling RF. Risks and benefits of splenectomy versus no splenectomy for hereditary spherocytosis—a personal view. *Br J Haematol*. 2009;145(6):728-732.
2. Agre P, Asimos A, Casella JF, McMillan C. Inheritance pattern and clinical response to splenectomy as a reflection of erythrocyte spectrin deficiency in hereditary spherocytosis. *N Engl J Med*. 1986;315(25):1579-1583.
3. Stasi R, Stipa E, Masi M, et al. Long-term observation of 208 adults with chronic idiopathic thrombocytopenic purpura. *Am J Med*. 1995;98(5):436-442.
4. Godeau B, Chevret S, Varet B, et al. Intravenous immunoglobulin or high-dose methylprednisolone, with or without oral prednisone, for adults with untreated severe autoimmune thrombocytopenic purpura: a randomised, multicentre trial. *Lancet (London, England)*. 2002;359(9300):23-29.
5. Gonçalves D, Morais M, Costa-Pinho A, Bessa-Melo R, Graça L, Costa-Maia J. Validation of a difficulty grading Score in laparoscopic splenectomy. *J Laparoendosc Adv Surg Tech Part A*. 2018;28(3):242-247.
6. Rodriguez-Otero Luppi C, Targarona Soler EM, Balague Ponz C, et al. Clinical, anatomical, and pathological grading Score to predict technical difficulty in laparoscopic splenectomy for non-traumatic diseases. *World J Surg*. 2017;41(2):439-448.
7. Dujardin M, Vandenbroucke F, Boulet C, Op de Beeck B, de Mey J. Indications for body MRI Part I. Upper abdomen and renal imaging. *Eur J Radiol*. 2008;65(2):214-221.
8. Mourtzoukou EG, Pappas G, Peppas G, Falagas ME. Vaccination of asplenic or hyposplenic adults. *Br J Surg*. 2008;95(3):273-280.
9. Rubin LG, Schaffner W. Clinical practice. Care of the asplenic patient. *N Engl J Med*. 2014;371(4):349-356.
10. Beauchamp RD HM, Fabian TC, et al. In: Townsend CM. eds. *Sabiston Textbook of Surgery: The Biological Basis of Modern Surgical Practice*. 18th ed. Saunders; 2007:1624-1652.
11. Katkhouda N, Mavor E. Laparoscopic splenectomy. *Surg Clin*. 2000;80(4):1285-1297.
12. Curran TJ, Foley MI, Swanstrom LL, Campbell TJ. Laparoscopy improves outcomes for pediatric splenectomy. *J Pediatr Surg*. 1998;33(10):1498-1500.
13. Tanoue K, Okita K, Akahoshi T, et al. Laparoscopic splenectomy for hematologic diseases. *Surgery*. 2002;131(1 suppl):S318-S323.
14. Kojouri K, Vesely SK, Terrell DR, George JN. Splenectomy for adult patients with idiopathic thrombocytopenic purpura: a systematic review to assess long-term platelet count responses, prediction of response, and surgical complications. *Blood*. 2004;104(9):2623-2634.
15. Perrotta S, Gallagher PG, Mohandas N. Hereditary spherocytosis. *Lancet (London, England)*. 2008;372(9647):1411-1426.

Chapter 50 Splenorrhaphy

Shawn D. Larson and Saleem Islam

DEFINITION

- Splenorrhaphy literally translates to "suturing of the spleen." Broadly applied, splenorrhaphy encompasses numerous operative strategies aimed at preserving splenic tissue and maintaining normal physiologic function in the setting of injury. Other terms for splenorrhaphy include splenic salvage, splenic preservation, and partial splenectomy. Partial splenectomy may be preferred to control disease or repair injury in selected cases. Understanding various operative techniques for splenorrhaphy is a required component of the armamentarium of all general surgeons.

DIFFERENTIAL DIAGNOSIS

- Splenic trauma: grades I to IV (**TABLE 1**).[1]
    - Grade V splenic injuries are *not* amenable to splenorrhaphy (see Chapter 49).
- Iatrogenic injuries—commonly occur during retraction of the transverse colon/stomach or during left upper quadrant laparoscopic operations
- Hemoglobinopathies
    - Hereditary spherocytosis (HS)
    - Thalassemia/sickle cell disease
- Splenic cysts (eg, epithelial or epidermoid cysts)
- Splenic hamartomas

PATIENT HISTORY AND PHYSICAL FINDINGS

- Prior to elective surgery, a thorough history should be obtained, including an account of abdominal pain or constitutional symptoms, detailed past medical/surgical history, and all current medications and allergies. Particular attention should be directed to eliciting any symptoms of liver disease, clotting or bleeding disorders, and a blood product transfusion history.
- Patients presenting with splenic trauma require rapid assessment making use of the principles outlined in the American College of Surgeons Advanced Trauma Life Support (ATLS) protocol. Hemodynamic instability is a general contraindication to splenorrhaphy. A thorough history should be obtained as outlined earlier. Particular attention must be paid to associated injuries, as these will influence decisions regarding nonoperative management (NOM), splenorrhaphy, or splenectomy (**FIGURE 1**). In *pediatric patients*, NOM is the preferred treatment choice and early consultation with a pediatric surgeon is highly recommended. Adult trauma patients with low-grade splenic injuries may be managed with NOM (**TABLE 2**).
- Patients presenting with hemoglobinopathies have abnormal laboratory profiles and often present with abdominal pain/discomfort, a history of jaundice, or splenomegaly. Rarely, patients will be completely asymptomatic. Patients with HS often present with sequestration of abnormal red blood cells (RBCs) and may have splenomegaly.[2,3] Historically, these patients benefited from splenectomy. Recently, clinical evidence demonstrates that patients with HS are amenable to partial splenectomy (PS), eliminating the need for repeat transfusions and significantly reducing the risk of overwhelming postsplenectomy infection (OPSI). Additionally, patients with sickle cell anemia have shown improvement following PS.[2-4]
- A complete and thorough physical examination should be performed on *all* patients. The presence or absence of splenomegaly should be noted. All signs of portal hypertension or liver failure should be elicited. Presence or location of surgical scars must be considered prior to determining operative approach.
- Splenorrhaphy is best performed via an open technique, which allows full visualization of the injury. An open approach allows easy conversion to a splenectomy should the clinical situation warrant this. Elective PS may be performed via an open or laparoscopic technique. Laparoscopic PS requires substantial experience in minimally invasive surgery and therefore, we prefer an open or a laparoscopic-assisted technique.

IMAGING AND OTHER DIAGNOSTIC STUDIES

- All patients with a suspected or known hemoglobinopathy require input from a hematologist. Patients should have a blood smear and/or bone marrow analysis, a complete blood count (CBC), and specialized blood studies as indicated by the disease process.
- Computed tomography (CT) scanning should be performed for all hemodynamically stable patients with suspected splenic trauma. CT is an excellent modality for preoperative planning to evaluate injury extent and to delineate vascular

Table 1: American Association for the Surgery of Trauma Organ Injury Scaling: Spleen

Grade	Injury	Description
I	Hematoma	Subcapsular, <10% surface area
	Laceration	Capsular tear, <1 cm parenchymal depth
II	Hematoma	Subcapsular, 10%-50% surface area; intraparenchymal, <5 cm in diameter
	Laceration	Capsular tear, 1-3 cm parenchymal depth not involving trabecular vessel
III	Hematoma	Subcapsular, >50% surface area or expanding; ruptured subcapsular or parenchymal hematoma; intraparenchymal hematoma >5 cm or expanding
	Laceration	>3 cm parenchymal depth or involving trabecular vessels
IV	Laceration	Laceration involving segmental or hilar vessels producing major devascularization (>25% of spleen)
V	Laceration	Completely shattered spleen
	Vascular	Hilar injury with devascularized spleen

Adapted with permission from Moore EE, Cogbill TH, Jurkovich GJ, et al. Organ injury scaling: spleen and liver (1994 revision). J Trauma. 1995;38(3):323-324.

SECTION IV SURGERY OF THE SPLEEN

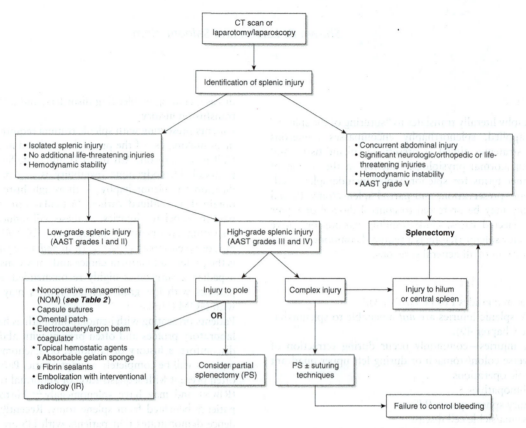

FIGURE 1 • Treatment algorithm for splenic injury outlining various options based on grade of injury. AAST, American Association for the Surgery of Trauma.

Table 2: Criteria and Contraindications to Nonoperative Management for Splenic Injury

Criteria for nonoperative management (NOM)
- Hemodynamic stability
- No additional comorbid injuries (eg, head injury, significant orthopedic trauma)
- Limitation of splenic-related blood transfusion (≤2 units)
- CT scan documenting splenic injury and grade
- Absence of active intrasplenic bleeding on CT
- Absence of other intra-abdominal injuries on CT requiring operative intervention

Contraindications for NOM
- Hemodynamic instability ± peritonitis
- Associated intra-abdominal/retroperitoneal organ injury
- Inability to perform reliable serial abdominal exams
- Need for anticoagulation
- Inability to correct coagulopathy
- Ongoing blood transfusion requirement
- AAST grade V splenic injury

AAST, American Association for the Surgery of Trauma; CT, computed tomography.

anatomy. CT is recommended for elective PS to determine the relationship of the spleen to adjacent organs, splenic size, and potential locations of accessory spleens (**FIGURE 2**).
- Ultrasound (US) is a noninvasive imaging modality to assess for splenomegaly, presence of splenic cysts/masses, and determination of portal hypertension in selected patients. US is particularly useful in assessing the spleen in children with the added advantage of minimizing ionizing radiation exposure. In the evaluation of trauma patients, focused abdominal sonography for trauma (FAST) is an accepted screening tool to diagnose intraperitoneal fluid or blood. Preoperative US should be performed for all patients with symptomatic biliary colic and patients with hemoglobinopathies to evaluate for cholelithiasis. Patients with cholelithiasis should be considered for concurrent cholecystectomy.
- Magnetic resonance imaging (MRI) is a recognized method for evaluating splenic lesions without the use of ionizing radiation. MRI is not recommended in the setting of splenic injury.

SURGICAL MANAGEMENT

Preoperative Planning

- Patients undergoing PS for elective indications should receive vaccinations for encapsulated organisms (*Haemophilus influenzae B*, *Streptococcus pneumoniae*, and *Neisseria meningitidis*) 2 to 4 weeks prior to surgery. Although PS should theoretically eliminate the risk of OPSI, vaccinations should be administered in the event that a total splenectomy is performed. Patients undergoing PS in the setting of splenic injury should receive vaccinations 2 to 4 weeks postoperatively. Current guidelines for OPSI prevention are outlined in Chapter 49, Table 2.
- Blood products should be ordered and available intraoperatively including packed red blood cells (PRBCs), platelets, and fresh frozen plasma (FFP).

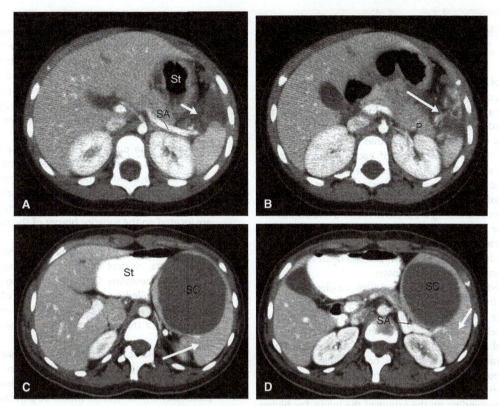

FIGURE 2 • CT scan of splenic laceration **(A, B)** and splenic cyst **(C, D)**. **A,** CT demonstrating isolated injury to the spleen *(white arrow)* from blunt abdominal trauma with hemoperitoneum. Note the proximity to the splenic artery (SA). **B,** CT from same patient demonstrating extent of splenic injury *(white arrow)* extending to inferior pole. Note the proximity of the spleen to the tail of the pancreas (P). **C,** CT demonstrating a large splenic cyst (SC) compressing normal splenic parenchyma *(white arrow)*. The cyst is compressing the stomach (St). **D,** CT image from same patient demonstrating the relationship of the SC to the SA. This patient underwent successful laparoscopic PS with preservation of normal splenic parenchyma. *Large white arrow,* splenic laceration; *narrow white arrow,* normal spleen.

- All patients should receive prophylactic antibiotics to cover skin flora within 60 minutes prior to the skin incision.
- Appropriate antithrombotic precautions should be instituted, including sequential compression devices (SCDs) for all patients aged 12 years and older. Appropriate anticoagulation medications (eg, low-molecular-weight heparin) should be administered preoperatively per hospital protocol.
- A nasogastric tube (NGT) should be inserted following induction of anesthesia to decompress the stomach and aid in visualization. Consideration should be given to leaving the NGT in situ for 24 to 48 hours postoperatively to prevent gastric distension.
- An open approach is recommended for patients undergoing splenorrhaphy for splenic injury. The human hand as a retractor to provide compressive hemostasis is invaluable in the successful performance of PS. This approach also provides good exposure and allows for possible splenectomy should attempts at splenorrhaphy prove unsuccessful.
- PS may be performed by a laparoscopic approach in the elective setting. Laparoscopic PS requires advanced laparoscopic skills and should only be undertaken by a surgeon familiar with the procedure.
- In adult splenic trauma patients, consideration should be given to preoperative splenic artery embolization (SAE) by interventional radiology. SAE has been demonstrated to improve the use of NOM, with improvement in splenic salvage, length of hospital stay, and mortality.[5] Pediatric patients with splenic trauma rarely require embolization and consultation with a pediatric surgeon is highly recommended before treatment with SAE is commenced.[6]

Positioning

- For open splenorrhaphy, patients are placed in a supine position with both arms extended. For patients with isolated splenic trauma, an upper midline incision from the xiphoid process to the umbilicus allows adequate exposure. This incision can be extended inferiorly if additional exposure is required or other intra-abdominal injuries are identified. For pediatric patients, a left subcostal incision or a transverse incision starting at the left 12th rib tip can be used (see Chapter 49, Figure 5).
- Patients undergoing laparoscopic PS can be positioned supine with both arms tucked at the side. A beanbag or kidney rest is placed under the left flank to increase exposure between the 12th rib and iliac crest. The table may be rotated to allow near-supine positioning for port placement and then rotated during the operation to achieve a right lateral decubitus position. As with all operations, all pressure points should be appropriately padded (see Chapter 49, Figure 4).

SPLENORRHAPHY

Incision

- A variety of incisions can be used to perform splenorrhaphy depending on the clinical situation.
  - Trauma patients. A midline incision extending from the xiphoid process to the pubis is used to enter the peritoneal cavity. This incision allows maximal exposure. A quick thorough inspection of each quadrant and the pelvis should be performed. Active bleeding should be immediately addressed. Retractors should be placed to maximize visualization and determine if additional sources of bleeding are present. All fluid and particulate matter should be quickly evaluated. Additional abdominal/retroperitoneal injuries discovered at the time of laparotomy should be prioritized and dealt with as outlined in corresponding chapters.
  - Isolated splenic injury. A midline incision extending from the xiphoid process to the level of the umbilicus can be used. Should additional exposure be required, the incision can be extended inferiorly. Retractors are placed to allow maximal exposure of the left upper quadrant. If a splenic injury occurs while performing an upper abdominal laparoscopic procedure, consideration should be made to convert to an open procedure depending on the extent of the injury. For higher grade injuries (American Association for the Surgery of Trauma [AAST] grades III and IV), a left subcostal incision can be made approximately 3 cm inferior to the costal margin (see Chapter 49, Figure 5).
  - Pediatric patients. A midline incision can be used similar to adult patients in the setting of trauma. For isolated splenic injuries, either a left subcostal incision or a transverse incision can be used. For a transverse incision, the tip of the 12th rib is identified and the incision is extended medially to allow for exposure of the spleen.

Mobilization

- Anatomically, the spleen resides superiorly and posteriorly in the left upper abdomen. For adequate assessment of a splenic injury and successful splenorrhaphy, the spleen must be completely mobilized by removing all peritoneal and visceral attachments. This includes the splenophrenic attachments to the diaphragm, the splenocolic ligament to the splenic flexure of the colon, the splenorenal ligaments, and the gastrosplenic ligament (see Chapter 49, Figure 6). The splenophrenic and splenorenal ligaments are avascular and can be divided sharply. Conversely, the gastrosplenic ligament (containing short gastric vessels) and the splenocolic ligament require careful attention to ensure excellent hemostasis. Vessels in these ligaments should be ligated with ties or an energy-based sealant device.
- Division of the ligaments begins first with the splenocolic ligament, allowing the splenic flexure of the colon to be mobilized away from the spleen. Splenic mobilization is further achieved by the operating surgeon placing their left hand posteriorly on the spleen (a laparotomy pad may improve the grip) and rotating it anteromedially. This maneuver will better expose the splenophrenic and splenorenal ligaments. Once the spleen is free of these attachments, it can be carefully mobilized into the wound. The gastrosplenic ligament is then carefully divided. Laparotomy pads can be carefully placed posteriorly to further aid in mobilization.
- Division of the ligaments should be made 2 to 3 cm from the spleen to avoid injury to both the spleen and adjacent organs (ie, pancreas).
- The tail of the pancreas extends to the splenic hilum in most patients. Care must be taken during mobilization of the spleen to avoid iatrogenic injury. The tail of the pancreas should be fully visualized, particularly as the spleen is rotated into the operative field. The splenic artery and vein are located on the superior border of the pancreas and must be carefully isolated to avoid injury.
- Once the spleen is mobilized from the retroperitoneal attachments, control of the hilar vessels can be quickly achieved if necessary to control bleeding. Active bleeding can be controlled by direct compression of the hilar vessels between the surgeon's thumb and forefinger. This maneuver allows for thorough assessment of the extent of splenic injury.
- Note: Full splenic mobilization may be unnecessary for small isolated injuries (eg, capsular tear) that occur intraoperatively and can be completely visualized. In all other situations, complete splenic mobilization should be performed.

Repair of Low-Grade Splenic Injuries (AAST Grades I and II)

- After mobilizing the spleen, a thorough inspection can be carried out to allow complete assessment of the injury (see **TABLE 1** and **FIGURE 1**). If necessary, vascular control can be obtained by compression of the hilar vessels as discussed earlier.
- Grade I and II injuries can generally be controlled by simple techniques including the following:
  - Direct compression (for minor capsular tears <1 cm)
  - Application of topical hemostatic agents
    - Absorbable gelatin sponge
    - Absorbable oxidized regenerated cellulose
    - Fibrin sealants
  - Electrocautery or argon beam coagulator (ABC) (**FIGURES 3** and **7**)
  - Absorbable sutures placed in the capsule (interrupted or running) (**FIGURES 3** and **8**). For most low-grade injuries, suture pledgets are not required.
- Following repair, the injury should be observed for 5 to 10 minutes to ensure that bleeding is controlled. Ongoing bleeding may require a combination of techniques listed earlier to repair the injury. Once the injury is controlled, the spleen is carefully returned to the left upper abdomen.

Repair of Moderate to High-Grade Splenic Injuries (AAST Grades III and IV)

- After complete mobilization of the spleen, a thorough inspection is performed. The vascular supply of the spleen is carefully inspected and if an injury is present, PS may be possible if 20% or more of the spleen can be salvaged (**FIGURE 1**). If significant injury to the splenic artery or vein

Chapter 50 SPLENORRHAPHY

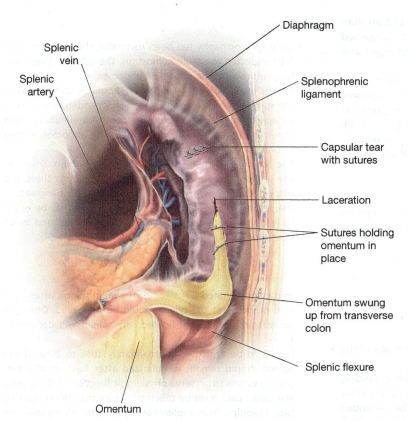

FIGURE 3 • Splenorrhaphy technique demonstrating (1) use of interrupted sutures for linear capsular tear and (2) patch with omentum mobilized and rotated upward. Sutures are placed into splenic capsule and around omentum to buttress injury.

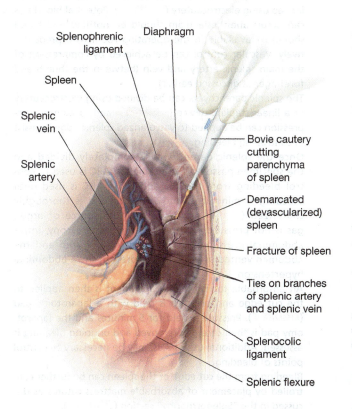

is present, then consideration for a splenectomy should be strongly considered (see Chapter 49). Vascular control is achieved by compression of hilar vessels as discussed earlier.
- Devitalized tissue should be debrided either sharply or with electrocautery to healthy splenic tissue (FIGURE 4).
  - Penetrating vessels to a devitalized segment should be ligated. If a line of demarcation is present, the splenic capsule can be incised with electrocautery. A linear stapling device can be used to transect a devitalized pole.
  - Clips can be applied to trabecular vessels. Gentle compression of the cut of the edge of the spleen will help control bleeding.
  - An ABC can be used to achieve hemostasis. Alternatively, mattress sutures can be placed along the cut edge. Pledgets are recommended to prevent further capsular damage (see FIGURES 7 and 8).

FIGURE 4 • Division of spleen using electrocautery. A splenic fracture of the lower pole is present. Branches of the splenic artery and vein have been ligated and divided with subsequent demarcation of the avascular lower pole. The splenic capsule is now divided along the line of demarcation. The splenic artery and vein can be compressed between the thumb and finger of the operative surgeon to control blood loss while the parenchyma is divided.

- Topical hemostatic agents can be applied and pressure held with a laparotomy pad for 10 minutes. Continued bleeding will require additional hemostatic agent and compression.
- Alternatively, omentum from the transverse colon can be swung up and placed in the splenic laceration. Mattress sutures can then be placed to compress the edges and secure the omentum in place (FIGURE 3). Hemostatic mesh can be used in place of omentum.
- PS can be considered for segmental injury and will be discussed in the following text.

AAST Grade V Splenic Injuries

- Splenorrhaphy is *not* indicated for AAST grade V injuries. Patients with these injuries require expeditious splenectomy (see Chapter 49)

Closure

- Once splenorrhaphy has been successful, the spleen is carefully inspected to ensure hemostasis. The spleen is then carefully returned to the upper left abdomen.
- Careful inspection of the abdomen should be undertaken by the surgeon and assistant surgeon independently to ensure all laparotomy pads have been removed. A preliminary count should be simultaneously performed. The abdomen is then irrigated to remove all blood clots.
- The abdomen is then closed in the usual fashion. Drains in the left upper abdomen are unnecessary unless there is a suspected or known injury to the tail of the pancreas. In the setting of abdominal trauma, a decision may be made to leave the abdomen open, allowing for a "second look" operation in 24 to 48 hours.

PARTIAL SPLENECTOMY

Incision

- For open PS, the incision will be dependent on the age of the patient and indications for surgery.
  - Adult patients. An upper midline incision extending from the xiphoid process to the umbilicus should allow adequate exposure. This incision can be extended inferiorly should additional exposure be required. Alternatively, a left subcostal incision can be used for isolated splenic lesions. Caution should be exercised in using this incision if splenomegaly is present.
  - Pediatric patients. A left upper abdominal transverse incision can safely be used, starting from the 12th rib tip and extending medially. Alternatively, a left subcostal incision can be used.
- For laparoscopic-assisted PS, ports are placed in a similar fashion to a laparoscopic splenectomy (see Chapter 49). After mobilization of the spleen, a left transverse or left subcostal incision can be used to perform the PS.

Mobilization

- The spleen should be completely mobilized by dividing the splenophrenic, splenorenal, splenocolic, and gastrosplenic ligaments (see earlier discussion).
  - For open PS, mobilization begins in a similar fashion to open splenectomy (see Chapter 49) and as discussed under the "Splenorrhaphy" section. The spleen needs to be completely mobilized.
  - For laparoscopic-assisted PS, mobilization begins in a similar fashion as discussed in preceding chapters (see Chapter 49). Once the spleen is completely mobilized laparoscopically, an open incision can be made as described in the preceding section. The spleen needs to be mobilized to allow it to be brought completely into the incision.

Division of Spleen

- Once the spleen is completely mobilized into the incision, the splenic vessels can be identified. Depending on the location of the lesion, branches of the splenic artery and splenic vein can be ligated (FIGURE 3). The main splenic artery and vein branches at the hilum should be preserved. Once the penetrating vessels are ligated, the spleen will demarcate (FIGURES 3-5).
- For PS to be effective, approximately 10% to 20% of the spleen should remain vascularized after ligation of penetrating vessels to preserve physiologic function of the splenic remnant.[4] Care must be taken to ensure that the remaining blood supply is from a splenic artery branch. Relying solely on short gastric arteries will not be adequate to maintain adequate blood flow to the splenic remnant.
- Once the spleen demarcates, the splenic capsule can be incised using electrocautery (FIGURE 4). Potential blood loss can occur; anesthesia team should be notified and blood should be available in the operating room (OR) preoperatively. Vascular control can be achieved by compression of the main splenic artery and vein (between the thumb and forefinger as discussed earlier).
- The splenic parenchyma can be divided using electrocautery or a linear stapling device (FIGURES 4 and 5). Gentle compression can be applied to vascularized splenic edge to assist in controlling bleeding.
- Once the splenic parenchyma is completely divided and the specimen passed off the table, an ABC is used to control bleeding from the cut edge. The ABC is used until bleeding is minimized and the cut edge is thoroughly cauterized (FIGURE 7). Note that the source of argon gas is not pressure regulated. During laparoscopy, intra-abdominal pressure must be closely monitored and the abdomen vented as indicated to prevent intra-abdominal hypertension.
- An absorbable topical hemostatic agent is then applied to the cut edge and pressure is held with a laparotomy pad (FIGURE 6). Pressure is held for 5 minutes and the laparotomy pad is then carefully removed and ongoing bleeding is assessed. Additional use of ABC may be necessary to control points of bleeding.
- Bleeding from the cut edge of the spleen can be further controlled by placement of absorbable mattress sutures as discussed in the "Splenorrhaphy" section (FIGURE 8).
- Once hemostasis is meticulously achieved, the remainder of the spleen is observed for adequate blood flow. Again,

10% to 20% of the total splenic tissue should remain viable to preserve splenic physiologic function. The splenic remnant is then carefully returned to the left upper abdomen.

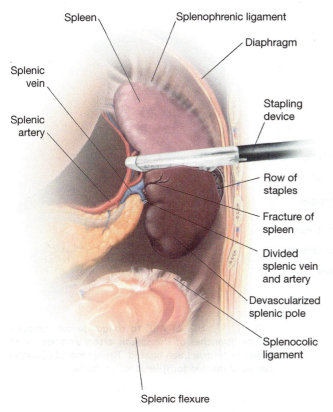

FIGURE 5 • Division of the spleen with a linear stapling device. Following ligation and division of branches of the splenic artery and vein to the lower pole, the demarcated spleen is then divided using multiple fires of a linear stapling device. Staple size is dictated by the size of the spleen. Vascular control can be achieved by compression of the main branch of the splenic artery and vein between the surgeon's thumb and index finger until the spleen is divided.

- To prevent torsion of the splenic remnant, consideration can be given to performing splenopexy. Sutures are carefully placed in the splenic capsule and then attached to the lateral abdominal wall or retroperitoneum for fixation. At least two points of fixation should be used. Once placed, these sutures should have minimal tension to avoid tearing the capsule.
- Depending on the site of PS, omentum can be placed against the cut surface of the spleen. Sutures can be placed to hold the omentum in place as discussed in the preceding section.
- In the case of PS for hemoglobinopathies (eg, HS), a thorough search for accessory splenic tissue should be performed. The incidence of accessory spleens is 10% to 30%. The most common location for an accessory spleen is at the splenic hilum (approximately 75%), followed by the tail of the pancreas (approximately 20%). The remainder is located along the splenic artery, in the mesentery, or in the omentum.[7] If accessory splenic tissue is located, it should be completely removed with careful attention to hemostasis.
- Consideration should be given to a concurrent cholecystectomy for patients with symptomatic biliary colic or preoperative US evidence of cholelithiasis.

Closure

- After returning the spleen to the left upper abdomen, a thorough inspection of the peritoneal cavity is performed to ensure there are no retained laparotomy pads. A preliminary count should be performed prior to closing.
- The abdomen is thoroughly irrigated with warmed normal saline. All blood should be removed from the abdomen. The spleen should be inspected to ensure exquisite hemostasis.
- The abdominal incision is then closed in the standard fashion. Drains are not necessary. If the procedure was performed with laparoscopic assistance, ports are removed and port sites are closed in the standard fashion.

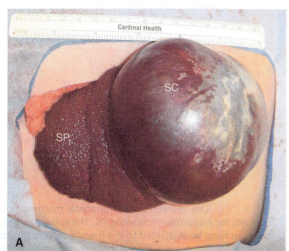
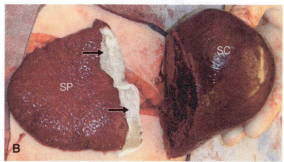

FIGURE 6 • **A.** Large epidermoid cyst *(SC)* of the lower pole of the spleen. **B.** Following division of the splenic parenchyma, the superior pole *(SP)* remains perfused. Absorbable hemostatic agent is applied to the cut edge following coagulation with an ABC *(arrows)*. SC, splenic cyst; SP, superior pole of spleen; arrows, absorbable hemostatic agent.

414 SECTION IV SURGERY OF THE SPLEEN

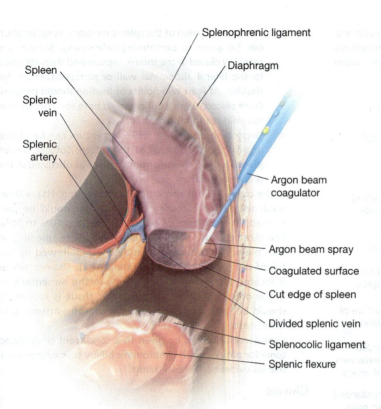

FIGURE 7 • Use of ABC to coagulate cut surface of spleen. Branches of the splenic artery and vein to the lower pole have been ligated. The splenocolic ligament has been divided for splenic mobilization.

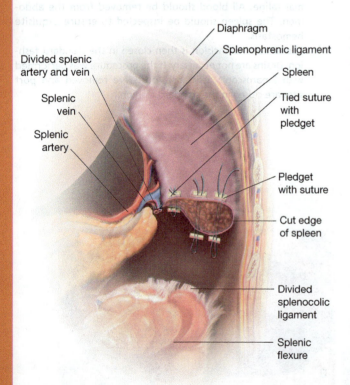

FIGURE 8 • Use of interrupted horizontal mattress sutures with pledgets for hemostasis following PS. The splenic artery and vein branches have been divided to the lower pole and the lower pole is removed. Sutures are placed in close proximity to reapproximate the capsule. The use of pledgets is recommended to prevent sutures from tearing the splenic capsule.

PEARLS AND PITFALLS

Indications	- Splenorrhaphy is used to repair an injured spleen (AAST grades I–IV). - Splenorrhaphy is *contraindicated* in AAST grade V injuries. - PS can be used as a splenorrhaphy technique or to treat various hemoglobinopathies (eg, HS), splenic cysts, or splenomegaly.
Imaging and other diagnostics	- CT scanning is recommended for hemodynamically stable patients with suspected intra-abdominal trauma. - Patients with hemoglobinopathies should have preoperative imaging to plan operative approach (ie, vessel location, splenic size) - Patients undergoing PS for hemoglobinopathies are recommended to have preoperative US evaluating for cholelithiasis. - Involvement of a hematologist is essential for patients with hemoglobinopathies for proper diagnosis and preoperative medical management.
Preoperative planning	- Vaccinations need to be administered 2 weeks prior to elective PS. - Crossmatched blood and blood products should be readily available intraoperatively. - Consideration of stress-dose steroids for patients with hemoglobinopathies (review past medication history) - CT imaging (see earlier discussion) available in the OR for intraoperative guidance - Placement of an NGT for gastric decompression
Technique—splenorrhaphy	- Hemodynamically *unstable* patients are not candidates for splenorrhaphy. - Complete mobilization of the spleen is key to assessing injury and performing splenorrhaphy. - Work lateral to medial for mobilization. - Leave a 1- to 2-cm cuff of peritoneum to prevent damage to surrounding organs. - Lower grade injuries can often be repaired with sutures. - Moderate to high-grade injuries may require a combination of techniques including PS. - Be prepared to proceed to total splenectomy should splenorrhaphy techniques fail.
Technique—PS	- May be performed via open or laparoscopic approach - Laparoscopic PS requires advanced minimally invasive skills and an elective setting. - Identify the splenic artery and vein. A viable splenic remnant requires blood supply from the artery. - Do not rely on short gastric blood supply for remnant. - After division of blood supply, allow spleen to demarcate prior to dividing spleen. - Approximately 30% of the spleen should remain viable for splenic function postoperatively. - A thorough search for accessory spleens should be undertaken (and removed if found). - Consider performing splenopexy to prevent torsion of remnant. - Consideration for concurrent cholecystectomy for patients with symptomatic biliary colic or preoperative US evidence of cholelithiasis.
Technique—closure	- Drains should not be used unless there is a known or suspected pancreatic injury.

POSTOPERATIVE CARE

- Patients undergoing splenorrhaphy will require ongoing hemodynamic monitoring in the immediate postoperative period. Hemodynamic instability should prompt further investigation for bleeding from the splenic repair.
- The NGT can be removed when evidence of bowel function is present. A diet can be initiated and advanced as tolerated.
- Careful attention to pulmonary toilet should be made, including the use of incentive spirometer, early mobilization, and pain control.
- Most patients undergoing splenorrhaphy will have concurrent injuries that will require continued attention.

OUTCOMES

Splenorrhaphy

- NOM should be considered the standard of care for low- to moderate-grade splenic injuries. NOM has demonstrated splenic preservation rates ranging from 81% to 91% for AAST grades I to III injuries.[8]
- Splenectomy has been demonstrated to be an independent risk factor for infectious complication following blunt splenic trauma. The authors recommend broader consideration for the use of splenic-preserving techniques.[9]
- Splenorrhaphy has been shown to be successful in 86% of patients with intraoperative splenic injury.[10] However, some caution is warranted in interpreting these findings as most reports of this nature are based on small sample sizes.
- The use of ABC dramatically improved rates of successful splenorrhaphy. ABC can be used for many splenic injury types/grades. The ABC can also be used successful with laparoscopic procedures.

Partial Splenectomy

- PS for HS leads to clinically significant improvements in hematologic profiles and symptoms in the pediatric

population. Hemoglobin levels significantly increased, whereas reticulocyte count and bilirubin levels decreased.[2]
- PS for other congenital hemolytic anemias (ie, sickle cell disease) has been demonstrated to control symptoms of hypersplenism and splenic sequestration. Splenic immune function also appears to be preserved in patients following PS who were followed for 4 years from surgery.[3,4]
- PS can be safely performed with few conversions to total splenectomy. Consideration should be given at the time of operation for cholecystectomy for children with symptoms of biliary colic and/or preoperative US demonstrating cholelithiasis.

COMPLICATIONS

Splenorrhaphy
- Bleeding (most common)
- Pancreatic injury/fistula
- Atelectasis/pneumonia/left pleural effusion
- Intra-abdominal abscess (3%-13%; higher rates with use of drains)
- Wound complications (higher rates with open procedures)
  - Seroma
  - Infection
  - Wound dehiscence

NOTE: Complication rates will be higher in multisystem trauma patients.

Partial Splenectomy
- Bleeding
- Splenic regrowth
- Disease recurrence (may occur when too large of a splenic remnant remains)
- Need for total splenectomy
- Splenic remnant torsion
- Pancreatic injury/fistula
- Wound complications (higher rates with open procedures)

REFERENCES

1. Moore EE, Cogbill TH, Jurkovich GJ, et al. Organ injury scaling: spleen and liver (1994 revision). *J Trauma*. 1995;38(3):323-324.
2. Buesing KL, Tracy ET, Kiernan C, et al. Partial splenectomy for hereditary spherocytosis: a multi-institutional review. *J Pediatr Surg*. 2011;46(1):178-183.
3. Vick LR, Gosche JR, Islam S. Partial splenectomy prevents splenic sequestration crises in sickle cell disease. *J Pediatr Surg*. 2009;44(11):2088-2091.
4. Rice HE, Oldham KT, Hillery CA, et al. Clinical and hematologic benefits of partial splenectomy for congenital hemolytic anemias in children. *Ann Surg*. 2003;237(2):281-288.
5. Sabe AA, Claridge JA, Rosenblum DI, et al. The effects of splenic artery embolization on nonoperative management of blunt splenic injury: a 16-year experience. *J Trauma*. 2009;67(3):565-572; discussion 71-72.
6. Zamora I, Tepas JJIII, Kerwin AJ, et al. They are not just little adults: angioembolization improves salvage of high grade IV-V blunt splenic injuries in adults but not in pediatric patients. *Am Surg*. 2012;78(8):904-906.
7. Impellizzeri P, Montalto AS, Borruto FA, et al. Accessory spleen torsion: rare cause of acute abdomen in children and review of literature. *J Pediatr Surg*. 2009;44(9):e15-e18.
8. Renzulli P, Gross T, Schnuriger B, et al. Management of blunt injuries to the spleen. *Br J Surg*. 2010;97(11):1696-1703.
9. Demetriades D, Scalea TM, Degiannis E, et al. Blunt splenic trauma: splenectomy increases early infectious complications – a prospective multicenter study. *J Trauma Acute Care Surg*. 2012;72(1):229-234.
10. Chung BI, Desai MM, Gill IS. Management of intraoperative splenic injury during laparoscopic urological surgery. *BJU Int*. 2011;108(4):572-576.

Chapter 51 Splenic Injury: Splenectomy and Splenorrhaphy

Lucy Ruangvoravat and Kimberly A. Davis

DEFINITION

- Splenic injury can be blunt or penetrating and involve injury to either the splenic parenchyma or hilar vessels.
- These injuries can cause hemorrhage and hematoma formation. Injuries are graded on a scale of severity and may require repair, splenectomy, or occasionally damage control techniques.
- Many splenic injuries may be managed nonoperatively or in conjunction with angioembolization depending on the hemodynamic status of the patient. However, on average, 30% of patients with splenic trauma will present with hemorrhagic shock and require urgent splenectomy.

DIFFERENTIAL DIAGNOSIS

- Splenic injury may be present any time there is impact to the torso with blunt trauma, often in association with left-sided rib fractures.
- Splenic injury also can be present in penetrating injuries with thoracoabdominal trajectory.

PATIENT HISTORY AND PHYSICAL FINDINGS

- Traumatic splenic injury can present in isolation or in combination with other solid organ injury such as the liver, kidney, or pancreas.
- The spleen is contained within the lower portion of the ribs and fractures of the lower left ribs should increase suspicion for splenic injury in blunt or penetrating mechanisms.
- Depending on the extent of hemorrhage, patient vital signs may be variable. However, tachycardia and hypotension should prompt a rapid evaluation for clinically significant hemorrhage.
- The abdominal examination is a crucial step in assessing for splenic injury. Tenderness in the left upper quadrant should increase suspicion. Peritonitis can be present due to bleeding from the splenic parenchyma or hilum but is absent in 30% of patients with hemoperitoneum. Physical examination cannot differentiate peritonitis from hemoperitoneum due to perforated viscus, however.

IMAGING AND OTHER DIAGNOSTIC STUDIES

- Ultrasound is often the first imaging modality utilized in splenic injury due to its ability to be performed at the bedside. This is typically within the focused assessment with sonography for trauma (FAST) examination, which assesses for free fluid within the peritoneum in four views. Any blunt injury patient with hemodynamic instability who has free fluid present within the abdomen should proceed to laparotomy without delay or further imaging.[2] If no signs of shock are present, patients with hemoperitoneum can undergo further workup prior to determining whether laparotomy is indicated. The presence of hemoperitoneum may be from a broad array of injuries, and further diagnostic testing is needed to determine the source of abdominal hemorrhage.
- Cross-sectional imaging with computed tomography (CT) imaging allows for the diagnosis and grading of splenic injuries (**TABLE 1**). CT is indicated in patients with abdominal pain or tenderness, patients who cannot participate in an abdominal examination, stable patients with blunt injury and free fluid seen on FAST examination, or patients who have penetrating wounds to the left thoracoabdominal area without other clear need for immediate laparotomy. Evaluation of splenic injury, as with all blunt injuries, is augmented with the use of arterial contrast to assess for active bleeding. If extravasation of contrast is present or a parenchymal pseudoaneurysm (**FIGURE 1**) is identified, angioembolization should be considered as a therapeutic modality (**TABLE 2**).

CT Image of Grade V Splenic Injury

- Angiography with embolization is utilized when the patient is hemodynamically normal and does not have other injuries that require immediate laparotomy.
- Angioembolization allows the patient to keep the immune function of the spleen. Nonoperative management has a reported success rate of >92% in the literature.[2] Failure of nonoperative management may occur in a small percentage of patients who will go on to require splenectomy (**FIGURE 2**).[3,4]

Table 1: American Association for the Surgery of Trauma Splenic Injury Scale

AAST grade	AIS severity	Imaging criteria
I	2	• Subcapsular hematoma <10% surface area • Parenchymal laceration <1 cm depth • Capsular tear
II	2	• Subcapsular hematoma 10%-50% surface area, intraparenchymal hematoma <5 cm • Parenchymal laceration 1-3 cm depth
III	3	• Subcapsular hematoma 10%-50% surface area, intraparenchymal hematoma ≥5 cm • Parenchymal laceration >3 cm depth
IV	4	• Any injury in the presence of a splenic vascular injury or active bleeding confined within splenic capsule • Parenchymal laceration involving segmental or hilar vessels producing >25% devascularization
V	5	• Any injury in the presence of splenic vascular injury with active bleeding extending beyond the spleen into the peritoneum • Shattered spleen

AAST, American Association for the Surgery of Trauma; AIS, Adjusted Injury Score.
Adapted from Kozar RA, Crandall M, Shanmuganathan K, et al. Organ injury scaling 2018 update: spleen, liver, and kidney. J Trauma Acute Care Surg. 2018;85(6):1119-1122.

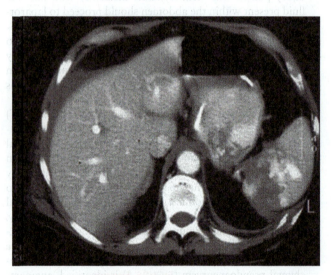

FIGURE 1 • Pseudoaneurysm.

Table 2: Predictors of Failure of Nonoperative Management on Cross-Sectional Imaging

Imaging finding	Failure rate (%)
Large hemoperitoneum	22.3
Moderate hemoperitoneum	19
Small hemoperitoneum	6
Pseudoaneurysm[5]	6
Arteriovenous fistula[6]	40

Adapted with permission from Peitzman AB, Heil B, Rivera L, et al. Blunt splenic injury in adults: multi-institutional study of the eastern association for the surgery of trauma. J Trauma. 2000;49(2):177-189.

SURGICAL MANAGEMENT

Preoperative Planning
- All patients should have an active type and crossmatch to facilitate rapid transfusion if needed.
- A nasogastric or orogastric tube should be placed for gastric decompression.
- The operating room should be prepped for a patient who may become unstable at any point.
- Nonoperative management of higher grade splenic injuries is feasible but mandates the immediate availability of a surgical team. Hospitals with limited access to operating rooms at night or on the weekend may consider a more liberal surgical approach to splenic injury, specifically for higher grade injuries.

Positioning
- Patient should be positioned supine with arms extended to allow for placement of self-retaining retractor posts and surgical team members. This also allows the anesthesia team to perform venous or arterial cannulation as needed.

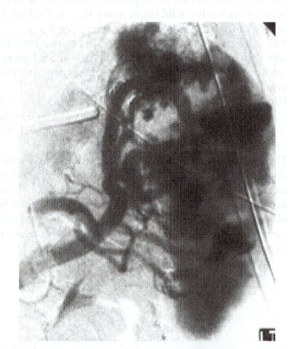

FIGURE 2 • Computed tomography image of Grade V splenic injury.

SKIN INCISION

- Laparotomy is performed through a midline incision.
- Elective splenectomy is sometimes performed through left subcostal incision, but this does not provide adequate flexibility for laparotomy in trauma as it may impede the management of associated intra-abdominal injuries.
- A midline incision can be extended to the xyphoid for better splenic exposure or inferiorly as needed for evaluation of the entire abdomen and pelvis.

EXPLORATION

- Exploration of the abdomen should be carried out in a systematic fashion to assess for sources of bleeding or contamination. Hemoperitoneum should be evacuated to facilitate visualization. Laparotomy pads should be packed in all four quadrants. These pads should be placed above and below the injured spleen to facilitate tamponade. Specifically for effective splenic packing, pads should be seated firmly between the spleen and both the diaphragm and abdominal sidewall. While these are in place, the bowel can be assessed for injury.
- If significant splenic injury is suspected, pads effectively providing tamponade in the left upper quadrant should be left in place until all others have been removed and injury in other quadrants evaluated. Conversely, if the left upper quadrant is not hemostatic while fully packed, splenectomy should be expedited.

SPLENIC MOBILIZATION

- The spleen sits against the diaphragm deep to the stomach in the abdomen. Avascular attachments suspend the spleen in its anatomic position: the splenophrenic and splenocolic ligaments. The splenocolic ligament attaches the spleen to the splenic flexure of the colon and merges with the splenophrenic as a thin attachment of the spleen to the lateral abdominal wall.
- The surgeon, standing at the patient's right, can use their right hand to slide up the left upper quadrant wall of the abdomen, encountering the spleen (**FIGURE 3**). From here it can easily be delivered toward the surgical field with the surgeon's right hand providing traction for cautery of those attachments if needed. After lateral attachments have been mobilized, there should be an avascular plane which can be manually dissected between the posterior spleen and the retroperitoneum, sometimes referred to as the splenorenal ligament.
- Once those attachments are divided, either with cautery or by finger fracture, the spleen should be mobile within the abdomen. Gentle retraction of the colon caudally and the stomach medially is helpful in these maneuvers.

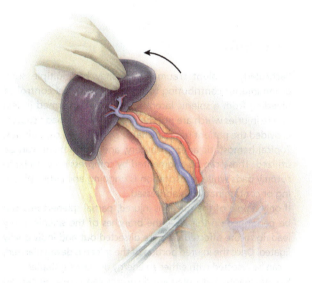

FIGURE 3 • Mobilization of the spleen from the left upper quadrant to the midline.

SPLENECTOMY

- Once the spleen has been mobilized up and into the midline wound, it can be better visualized and assessed. In cases of ongoing hemorrhagic shock with active splenic hemorrhage, manual compression should be applied to the splenic hilum at the organ's medial aspect to facilitate hemostasis. This will allow some time for resuscitation before the splenectomy is carried out.
- Ligation of the splenic artery can then easily be performed. Care should be taken to avoid the superior border of the pancreas.
- After ligation of the artery, the splenic vein can be ligated at the inferior border of the pancreas. Individual ligation of the vessels is preferred to decrease the theoretical risk of arteriovenous fistula formation.
- At this point the spleen will have the gastrocolic ligament as its remaining attachment. A clear area along the greater curve of the stomach can be identified and entered with cautery. Any visible short gastric vessels should then be divided, completing the splenectomy.
- There are several methods for vascular control. Clamps and ties have traditionally been used but often an energy device or vascular stapler is more efficient in dividing these vessels.

Care should be used to avoid the stomach wall and ensure adequate ligation, particularly along the more proximal portions of the stomach approaching the diaphragm. Here there is less anatomic space. Adequate ligation is necessary to prevent postoperative bleeding.

- The splenic bed should be inspected for hemostasis. The border of the stomach and pancreas should also be reinspected for injury. It is not our practice to leave any drains after splenectomy if there is no suspected pancreatic injury. However, if vessel ligation is proximate to the tail of the pancreas, or there is evidence of associated pancreatic contusion, drain placement is indicated. Inspection of the diaphragm should also be performed to avoid missed injury (FIGURE 4).

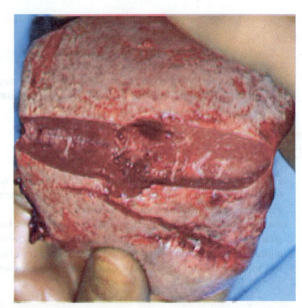

FIGURE 4 • Pathology specimen: Spleen with traumatic lacerations.

SPLENORRHAPHY

- Particularly in blunt trauma there may be multiple solid organ injuries contributing to hemorrhage. Local control of bleeding from a splenic laceration can be performed in less severe injuries which are not the primary hemorrhage source, provided the patient has reasonable coagulation capabilities. Topical hemostatic agents, cautery, and argon beam can be utilized. These can be augmented by compression with laparotomy pads while resuscitation is ongoing and other bleeding or contamination is addressed.
- If only a pole of the spleen is injured, partial splenectomy can be performed. In this case, the branches of the splenic artery leading to the affected pole are dissected out and individually ligated. Once the injured portion of the spleen is devascularized, it can be resected with either an energy device or a stapler.
- Splenorrhaphy with pledgeted sutures can rarely be carried out for injuries in an isolated pole of the spleen but we find little utility for this in the trauma patient (FIGURE 5).
- Mesh splenorrhaphy involves wrapping the injured spleen tightly in absorbable mesh and leaving a keyhole for the splenic artery and vein (FIGURE 6). This allows hemostasis via compression from the mesh and reapproximation of the lacerated parenchyma. This technique, however, is time-consuming and can be cumbersome. It is not commonly performed.
- In all cases, if hemorrhage is persistent despite splenic salvage maneuvers or if no other source of bleeding is identified in a patient with signs of hemorrhagic shock, splenectomy should be performed.

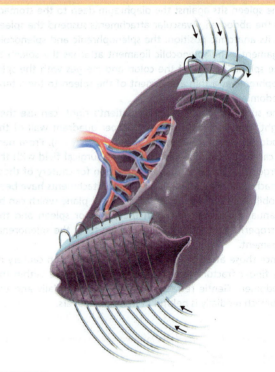

FIGURE 5 • Splenic repair using pledgets after splenic resection.

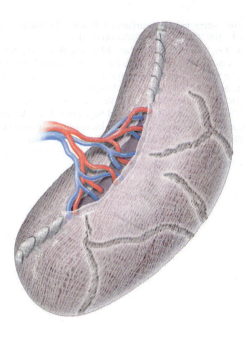

FIGURE 6 • Mesh splenorrhaphy.

PEARLS AND PITFALLS

- The patient in shock should immediately be taken for laparotomy. If the patient is hemorrhaging from the spleen, then splenectomy should be performed without hesitation or attempts at splenorrhaphy.
- Care should be taken to identify the pancreas. If there is a question of pancreatic injury, a drain should be left.
- Short gastric vessels should be re-examined for hemostasis prior to abdominal closure as they can be a source of postoperative bleeding and return to the operating room.

Postoperative Care

- Patients with splenic injury should be monitored for adequacy of resuscitation. Thrombocytosis due to splenectomy is normal.
- Splenectomy patients who do not have other contraindications can typically have chemical prophylaxis for venous thromboembolism begun within 24 to 48 hours after splenectomy.
- Ileus, particularly gastric, can be common in these patients and patients should be monitored for aspiration risk.
- Early mobilization should be carried out in splenectomy patients to mitigate against both ileus and thromboembolism as well as pulmonary compromise.[7]
- Postsplenectomy patients also need to receive immunizations against pneumococcus, meningococcus, and *Haemophilus influenzae* per CDC guidelines.[8] Common practice in the setting of trauma is to give the initial vaccines prior to the patient's discharge from the hospital.

Complications

- Overwhelming postsplenectomy sepsis is a much-feared complication in asplenic patients, although with low incidence after splenectomy for trauma. It most frequently does not occur for at least 2 years after splenectomy.[9] Risk is minimized by adherence to vaccination schedule and early recognition of asplenia in patients with upper respiratory tract infections.
- Postoperative bleeding after splenectomy should initially be treated with resuscitation and correction of coagulopathy in stable patients. Patients with hemodynamic compromise or lack of response to resuscitation should be returned to the operating room. Short gastric vessels can often be the culprit in postop bleeding secondary to vasodilation associated with postoperative gastric distension.
- Due to its close association with the splenic vessels, any fluid collection in the splenic cavity should raise concern for pancreatic tail injury. Percutaneous image-guided drainage of the collection can be performed. Pancreatic duct stenting has a role in the management of persistent or high-volume pancreatic fistulae.

REFERENCES

1. Kozar RA, Crandall M, Shanmuganathan K, et al. Organ injury scaling 2018 update: spleen, liver, and kidney. *J Trauma Acute Care Surg*. 2018;85(6):1119-1122. doi:10.1097/TA.0000000000002058
2. Requarth JA, D'Agostino Jr RB, Miller PR. Nonoperative management of adult blunt splenic injury with and without splenic artery

embolotherapy: a meta-analysis. *J Trauma*. 2011;71(4):898-903. doi:10.1097/TA.0b013e318227ea50
3. Rowell S, Biffl W, Brasel K, et al. Western trauma association critical decisions in trauma. *J Trauma Acute Care Surg*. 2017;82(4):787-793. doi:10.1097/TA.0000000000001323
4. Peitzman AB, Heil B, Rivera L, et al. Blunt splenic injury in adults: multi-institutional Study of the eastern association for the Surgery of trauma. *J Trauma*. 2000;49(2):177-189. doi:10.1097/00005373-200008000-00002
5. Haan J, Biffl W, Knudson M, et al. Splenic embolization revisited: a multicenter review. *J Trauma Inj Infect Crit Care*. 2004;56(3):542-547. doi:10.1097/01.TA.0000114069.73054.45
6. Davis KA, Fabian TC, Croce MA, et al. Improved success in nonoperative management of blunt splenic injuries: embolization of splenic artery pseudoaneurysms. *J Trauma*. 1998;44(6):1008-1015. doi:10.1097/00005373-199806000-00013
7. Fair KA, Connelly CR, Hart KD, Schreiber MA, Watters JM. Splenectomy is associated with higher infection and pneumonia rates among trauma laparotomy patients. *Am J Surg*. 2017;213(5):856-861. doi:10.1016/j.amjsurg.2017.04.001
8. "*CDC Recommendations for Vaccinations in Adults: Asplenia.*" Published May 2, 2016. Accessed September 2, 2021. https://www.cdc.gov/vaccines/adults/rec-vac/health-conditions/asplenia.html
9. Cullingford GL, Watkins DN, Watts AD, Mallon DF. Severe late postsplenectomy infection. *Br J Surg*. 1991;78(6):716-721. doi:10.1002/bjs.1800780626

Index

Note: Page numbers followed by "*f*" indicate figures and "*t*" indicate tables.

A

Ablation, of hepatic neoplasms, 132
  chemical, 133
  complications with, 136
  contraindications for, 133
  indications for, 132–133
  irreversible electroporation (IRE), 134
  microwave ablation (MWA), 133–134, 134*f*–135*f*, 136
  outcomes with, 135–136
  pearls and pitfalls of, 135, 135*f*
  radiofrequency ablation (RFA), 133, 133*f*–134*f*, 136
Ampullectomy, 36, 37*f*
Arteriography, for TACE and radioembolization, 139, 139*f*–140*f*, 141–142, 142*f*

B

Balloon dilation, of biliary ducts, 33, 33*f*, 47–48, 47*f*–48*f*
Balloon tamponade, for hepatic trauma, 241, 241*f*
Bile duct injuries, after laparoscopic cholecystectomy, 10
Biliary atresia, 103, 104*f*
  differential diagnosis of, 103
  operative management of
    cholangiogram for, 105, 105*f*
    complications with, 110
    hepatic mobilization for, 106, 106*f*
    imaging and diagnostic studies for, 103
    incision for, 104, 105*f*
    liver biopsy for, 105, 106*f*
    outcomes with, 110
    patient history and physical findings for, 103
    pearls and pitfalls of, 109
    portal dissection for, 107–108, 107*f*
    portoenterostomy for, 108*f*, 109
    positioning for, 103
    postoperative care for, 109–110, 110*t*
    preoperative planning for, 103
    Roux-en-Y hepaticojejunostomy for, 108, 108*f*
Biliary-enteric anastomosis, 63, 64*f*–65*f*
  after choledochal cyst excision, 98–99, 98*f*–99*f*
Biliary fistula/biloma, Roux-en-Y choledochojejunostomy, 60
Biliary leak, checking for, 128, 128*f*
Biliary stricture
  Roux-en-Y choledochojejunostomy, 60
  Strasberg classification, 82, 82*f*
Biliary system
  balloon dilation, 33, 33*f*, 47–48, 47*f*–48*f*
  brushings/biopsy, 49, 49*f*
  cannulation, 32–33, 32*f*
  in choledochoduodenostomy. *See* Choledochoduodenostomy
  in hilar cholangiocarcinoma (HC), 76–78
  liver anatomy, 117, 118*f*
  in radical cholecystectomy, 19, 19*f*
  sphincterotomy, 33, 33*f*
  stent insertion, 35–36, 35*f*
  strictures of
    ERCP dilation of, 34
    intrahepatic biliary-enteric anastomosis. *See* Intrahepatic biliary-enteric anastomosis
  tissue acquisition from, 36
Biopsy
  biliary system, 49, 49*f*
  of liver, in biliary atresia management, 105, 106*f*
Bismuth classification, 112
Bismuth-Corlette classification, 75, 75*f*
Blumgart anastomosis, 295–296, 295*f*–296*f*
  modified, 296
B-mode ultrasound, of liver, 122, 123*f*
Brisbane terminology, 112, 112*t*
Brushings, of biliary system, 49, 49*f*

C

Cannulation
  of biliary system, 32–33, 32*f*
  for percutaneous transhepatic cholangiography (PTC), 45–46, 46*f*
Caroli disease, 101
Catheter-based treatment, of hepatic neoplasms, 138
  complications with, 145
  imaging and diagnostic studies for, 138
  outcomes with, 145
  patient history and physical findings for, 138
  pearls and pitfalls of, 143–144
  positioning for, 138, 138*f*
  postoperative care for, 144–145, 145*f*
  preoperative planning for, 138
  radioembolization, 138, 141–143, 142*f*
  transarterial chemoembolization (TACE), 138–141, 140*f*–141*f*
Cattell-Braasch maneuver
  in pancreaticoduodenectomy, 247–248, 248*f*
Caudate, in HC resection, 78
Caudate lobe, 112–113, 113*f*, 117
  resection of, 150–151, 151*f*
Caudate tumors, 206
Celiac arteriogram, for TACE and radioembolization, 139, 139*f*–140*f*
Celiac axis, in pancreaticoduodenectomy, 245
Chemical ablation, of hepatic neoplasms, 133
Cholangiocarcinoma. *See* Hilar cholangiocarcinoma (HC)
Cholangiogram, 40, 40*f*
Cholangiography
  for biliary atresia, 105, 105*f*
  for biliary leak checks, 128, 128*f*
  ERCP. *See* Endoscopic retrograde cholangiopancreatography (ERCP)
  for hepatic trauma, 237
Cholangioscopy, 36
Cholangitis, Roux-en-Y choledochojejunostomy, 60
Cholecystectomy
  laparoscopic cholecystectomy, 1
    closure, 10, 10*f*
    complications, 10
    critical view, 7, 7*f*–8*f*
    cystic duct and artery division in, 8, 8*f*
    differential diagnosis, 1
    gallbladder dissection in, 8, 9*f*
    gallbladder extraction in, 9, 9*f*
    imaging and other diagnostic studies, 1–3
    patient history and physical findings for, 1
    pearls and pitfalls, 10
    peritoneal cavity entry in, 3–4, 4*f*
    port placement for, 4, 5*f*
    positioning, 3, 4*f*
    postoperative care for, 10
    preoperative planning, 3
    reverse triangle exposure in, 7, 7*f*
    triangle of Calot exposure in, 5–6, 5*f*–6*f*
  in left hepatic trisegmentectomy, 222, 222*f*
  open cholecystectomy
    abdominal wall opening for, 14
    closure for, 17
    complications with, 18
    cystic duct and artery ligation in, 15–16, 16*f*
    gallbladder dissection in, 15
    imaging and diagnostic studies for, 12–13
    incision for, 14, 14*f*
    indications for, 13
    outcomes with, 18
    patient history and physical findings for, 12
    pearls and pitfalls of, 17
    peritoneum incision for, 15, 15*f*
    positioning for, 13
    postoperative care for, 17
    preoperative planning for, 13
    retractor placement for, 14, 14*f*
  in pancreaticoduodenectomy, 251, 251*f*
  radical cholecystectomy, 19, 19*f*
    complications, 27
    extrahepatic biliary tree resection in, 25–26, 26*f*
    imaging and other diagnostic studies, 20–22
    incision and exposure, 24, 24*f*
    intraoperative ultrasound, 24, 24*f*

I-1

I-2 INDEX

Cholecystectomy (continued)
    outcomes, 27
    patient history and physical findings, 19–20
    pearls and pitfalls, 26
    portal lymphadenectomy in, 25–26, 26f
    positioning, 23, 23f
    postoperative care, 27
    preoperative planning, 22–23
    segment IVb/V resection in, 24–25, 25f
    subtotal, 16–17, 17f
Choledochal cyst, 92
    classification, 92–93, 92f
    differential diagnosis, 93
    imaging and diagnostic studies, 93–94, 94f
    operative management
        biliary–enteric reconstruction, 98–99, 98f–99f
        circumferential dissection, 97
        complications, 102
        cyst excision, 98, 98f–99f
        cyst types, 101
        gallbladder and arterial dissection, 96, 96f
        incision and exposure, 96
        laparoscopic approach, 99, 100f–101f
        pearls and pitfalls, 102
        positioning, 95, 95f
        preoperative planning, 95
        technique, 94–95
    outcomes, 102
    patient history and physical findings, 93
    postoperative care, 93
Choledochocele, 101
Choledochoduodenostomy
    complications, 72
    differential diagnosis, 67
    end to side, 71
    imaging and diagnostic studies, 67
    laparoscopic
        choledochoduodenal anastomosis for, 72
        initial dissection, 71–72
        patient positioning and port placement, 71
    outcomes, 72
    patient history and physical findings, 67
    pearls and pitfalls, 72
    preoperative planning, 68
    side-to-side
        choledochoduodenal anastomosis for, 69–70, 70f–71f
        incision and exposure, 68–69, 68f–69f
Choledochojejunostomy
    minimally invasive. See Minimally invasive choledochojejunostomy
    Roux-en-Y. See Roux-en-Y choledochojejunostomy
Choledocholithiasis
    biliary endoscopy, 41, 41f
    cholangiogram, 40, 40f
    ERCP for. See Endoscopic retrograde cholangiopancreatography (ERCP)
Cholestasis, 74
Cirrhosis, left hepatic lobectomy and, 188
Cisplatin, chemoembolization using, 140
Colon
    mobilization of
        in minimally invasive PD, 259–260, 259f–260f
        pancreaticoduodenectomy, 268, 268f
Colorectal liver metastases (CRLM)
    ablation of, 133, 136
    intraoperative ultrasound (IOUS) of, 121, 122f
Common bile duct (CBD)

CDD for obstruction of, 67
choledochal cyst of, 92–93
in choledochojejunostomy. See Choledochojejunostomy
in HC resection, 77
in laparoscopic cholecystectomy, 1
in pancreaticoduodenectomy, 251, 251f
surgical anatomy of, 117, 118f
Common hepatic arteriogram, for TACE and radioembolization, 139, 139f–140f
Common hepatic duct (CHD), 117, 118f
    in right hepatic trisegmentectomy, 218, 218f
Computed tomography (CT)
    biliary imaging with, 44, 44f–45f
    choledochal cyst, 94, 94f
    for choledochoduodenostomy (CDD), 67
    distal pancreatectomy with splenic preservation (DPSP), 332–333, 332f
    ex vivo hepatic resection, 229
    for hepatic trauma, 236, 236f
    for hepatic trisegmentectomy
        left, 221
        right, 214
    hilar cholangiocarcinoma (HC), 73
    for lobectomy, left hepatic, 187, 187f
    minimally invasive distal pancreatectomy, 319, 320f
    for minimally invasive right hepatectomy, 170
    open distal pancreatectomy, 311, 311f
    for pancreaticoduodenectomy, 245–246, 246f
    portal vein (PV) resection and reconstruction, 298, 298f
    radical cholecystectomy, 20, 21f–22f
    for robotic-assisted, pancreaticoduodenectomy, 266, 266f
    Roux-en-Y choledochojejunostomy, 55
Computed tomography abdomen/pelvis with IV contrast—triple phase (CT A/P)
    minimally invasive choledochojejunostomy, 61
Contact scanning, of liver, 124
Coronary ligament, 114, 114f
Couinaud's segments, 111, 111f
Critical view, in laparoscopic cholecystectomy, 7, 7f–8f
Cystic artery, 114
    in laparoscopic cholecystectomy, 8, 8f
    in open cholecystectomy, 15–16, 16f
Cystic duct
    dilation, 40–41
    in laparoscopic cholecystectomy, 8, 8f
    in open cholecystectomy, 15–16, 16f
    surgical anatomy of, 117, 118f

D

Direct endoscopic necrosectomy (DEN), 389–390, 390f
Distal pancreas dissection, 336–337, 336f
Distal pancreatectomy
    minimally invasive. See Minimally invasive distal pancreatectomy
    open. See Open distal pancreatectomy
Distal pancreatectomy with splenic preservation (DPSP)
    complications, 338
    computed tomography (CT), 332–333, 332f
    differential diagnosis, 332
    indications, 332
    laparoscopic approach
        closure, 337
        distal pancreas dissection, 336–337, 336f

lesser sac, 334, 334f
pancreas dissection, 334, 335f
pancreas transection, 335–336, 335f
pancreatic lesion, 334, 335f
port placement, 333, 333f
residual gland management, 337
splenic artery, dissection and control, 335
    open technique, 337
    outcomes, 338
    patient history and physical findings, 332
    pearls and pitfalls, 338
    positioning, 333
    postoperative care, 338
    preoperative planning, 333
    robotic technique, 337
    surgical management, 333
Doppler ultrasound, of liver, 123, 123f
Doxorubicin, chemoembolization using, 140
Drug-eluting microspheres, 140, 141f
Duct-to-mucosa, 287, 287f
    Blumgart anastomosis, 295–296, 295f–296f
    modified Blumgart anastomosis, 296
Duodenoscope, 29
Duodenotomy, 349–350, 351f
Duodenum
    in choledochoduodenostomy. See Choledochoduodenostomy
    division of, in minimally invasive PD, 258–259, 258f–259f
    mobilization of
        in minimally invasive PD, 259–260, 259f–260f
        pancreaticoduodenectomy, 268, 268f
    in pancreaticoduodenectomy, 252, 252f
    scope passage to, for ERCP, 31, 32f
Duplex ultrasound (DUS)
    of liver, 123, 123f
    in pancreaticoduodenectomy, 246

E

Endobiliary stent placement, 39
    imaging and diagnostic studies, 39
    indications, 42, 42t
    outcomes and complications, 43, 43t
    patient history and physical findings, 39
    postoperative care, 43
    preoperative planning, 39
    radiographic markers, 42, 42f
    stent retrieval, 43, 43f
Endoscopic pancreatic debridement and drainage
    acute necrotic collection, 386, 386f
    adverse events, 392
    differential diagnosis, 386
    direct endoscopic necrosectomy (DEN), 389–390, 390f
    endoscopic ultrasound-guided drainage, 387–389, 388f–389f
    endoscopic vs. surgical approach, 391
    imaging and diagnostic studies, 386f, 387
    outcomes, 392
    patient history, 386–387
    pearls and pitfalls, 391–392
    percutaneous endoscopic necrosectomy, 391
    physical findings, 386–387
    positioning, 387
    postoperative care, 392
    preoperative planning, 387
    surgical (endoscopic) management, 387
    walled-off pancreatic necrosis (WON), 386
Endoscopic retrograde, in pancreaticoduodenectomy, 246
Endoscopic retrograde cholangiography (ERC)

for hilar cholangiocarcinoma (HC), 73
intrahepatic biliary-enteric anastomosis, 81
Endoscopic retrograde cholangiopancreatography (ERCP), 29
  cholangioscopy and pancreatoscopy, 36
  choledochal cyst, 93, 93f
  for choledochoduodenostomy (CDD), 67
  complications, 38
  differential diagnosis, 29
  esophagus intubation for, 31, 32f
  imaging and diagnostic studies, 29
  indications, 30, 30t
  laparoscopic cholecystectomy, 2f
  major papilla cannulation, 32–33, 32f
  minimally invasive choledochojejunostomy, 61
  minimally invasive distal pancreatectomy, 319, 320f
  outcomes, 38
  patient history and physical findings, 29
  pearls and pitfalls of, 37
  positioning, 30, 31f
  postoperative care, 38
  preoperative planning for, 30, 30t
  risk factors, 30, 30t
  Roux-en-Y choledochojejunostomy, 55–56, 56f
  scope passage in, 31, 32f
  special uses of, 36–37
  sphincterotomy, 33, 33f
  stent insertion, 35–36, 35f
  stone extraction, 33–34, 34f
  stricture dilation, 34
  surgically assisted. See Surgically assisted endoscopic retrograde cholangiopancreatography (ERCP)
  tissue acquisition, 36
Endoscopic ultrasound (EUS)
  for choledochoduodenostomy (CDD), 67
  for hilar cholangiocarcinoma (HC), 74
  minimally invasive distal pancreatectomy, 319, 320f
  open distal pancreatectomy, 311
  of pancreas, for pancreaticoduodenectomy, 246, 266
End-to-side choledochoduodenostomy, 71
Enterotomies, in pancreaticojejunostomy, 277, 277f
ERCP. See Endoscopic retrograde cholangiopancreatography (ERCP)
Esophagus, intubation of, for ERCP, 31, 32f
Ethiodol, 140, 141f, 143, 144f
EUS. See Endoscopic ultrasound (EUS)
Ex situ liver resection, 232, 232f
Extended focused assessment with sonography for trauma (eFAST), for hepatic trauma, 236
Extragastric cyst gastrostomy, 368
Extrahepatic biliary tree
  choledochal. See Choledochal cyst
  in choledochoduodenostomy. See Choledochoduodenostomy
  in radical cholecystectomy, 25–26, 26f
Ex vivo hepatic resection, 229
  assessment, 231–232
  complications with, 235
  differential diagnosis, 229
  imaging and diagnostic studies for, 229
  incision and operability, 230–231
  indications for, 229
  intraoperative planning, 230
  liver resection and vascular reconstruction, 232–233, 232f, 233f
  patient history and physical findings for, 229

pearls and pitfalls for, 234
positioning, 230
postoperative care for, 235
preoperative planning, 230, 230f
reimplantation, 233–234, 234f

F
Falciform ligament, 114, 114f
Feeding jejunostomy, placement of, 360

G
Gallbladder
  in choledochal cyst management, 96, 96f
  surgical anatomy of, 117, 118f
Gallbladder cancer
  differential diagnosis of, 19
  open cholecystectomy, 13
  radical cholecystectomy. See Radical cholecystectomy
Gastric bypass, after surgically assisted endoscopic retrograde cholangiopancreatography (ERCP), 51
Gastric pexy, surgically assisted endoscopic retrograde cholangiopancreatography (ERCP), 52
Gastrinoma
  complications, 353
  differential diagnosis, 345, 345t
  duodenotomy, 349–350, 351f
    closure of, 351, 352f
  exploration, 348
  imaging and other diagnostic studies, 345–347, 346f–347f
  incision placement, 348
  intraoperative endoscopy, 348, 350f
  intraoperative ultrasound, 348, 350f
  Kocher maneuver, 348, 348f–349f
  liver lesions management, 351
  localization and treatment of, 347f
  outcomes, 353
  pancreatic tumors excision, 350
  patient history, 345
  pearls and pitfalls, 353
  periduodenal lymph node dissection, 350–351, 352f
  physical findings, 345
  positioning, 347
  postoperative care, 353
  signs and symptoms of, 345t
  surgical management, 347
Gastroduodenal arteriogram, for radioembolization, 142, 142f
Gastroduodenal artery (GDA), in pancreaticoduodenectomy, 246, 250, 250f, 266
Gastroepiploic vein, in pancreaticoduodenectomy, 248, 249f, 259, 259f
Gastrohepatic ligament, 114, 114f
Gastrostomy, after surgically assisted endoscopic retrograde cholangiopancreatography, 53, 53f
Goldsmith and Woodburne classification, 112

H
Hemangioma, liver, intraoperative ultrasound (IOUS) of, 121, 121f
Heparin, in hepatectomy, 147, 162
Hepatectomy
  hilar cholangiocarcinoma (HC), 78
  vena cava resection during

anatomic considerations for, 205–206, 206f
complications with, 212
imaging and diagnostic studies for, 205
incision for, 207
indications for, 205
for invasion of IVC wall without thrombus, 207–209, 207f–209f
for invasion of IVC wall with thrombus, 209–211, 210f, 211f
outcomes with, 212
patient history and physical findings for, 205
positioning for, 207
postoperative care for, 212
preoperative planning for, 205, 206f
Hepatic arteries
  in choledochal cyst management, 96, 96f
  hilar cholangiocarcinoma (HC) resection, 76, 77f
  in hilar hepaticojejunostomy, 84, 84f
  in left hepatic trisegmentectomy, 223–224, 223f
  in left lateral sectionectomy, 149–150, 150f
  replaced, 115, 115f
  in right hepatectomy, 172, 172f
  in right hepatic trisegmentectomy, 217, 217f
  in right posterior sectionectomy, 147–148, 148f
  surgical anatomy of, 114–115, 114f
  variations in, 139, 139f
Hepatic cystic disease, 121
Hepatic hilum, intraoperative ultrasound (IOUS) of, 128–129, 129f
Hepatic lesions and neoplasms
  ablation of, 132
    chemical, 133
    complications with, 136
    contraindications for, 133
    indications for, 132–133
    IRE, 134
    MWA, 133–134, 134f–135f, 136
    outcomes with, 135–136
    pearls and pitfalls of, 135, 135f
    RFA, 133, 133f–134f, 136
  catheter-based treatment of, 138
    complications with, 145
    imaging and diagnostic studies for, 138
    outcomes with, 145
    patient history and physical findings for, 138
    pearls and pitfalls of, 143–144
    positioning for, 138, 138f
    postoperative care for, 144–145, 145f
    preoperative planning for, 138
    radioembolization, 138, 141–143, 142f
    transarterial chemoembolization (TACE), 138–141, 140f–141f
  differential diagnosis of, 138
  intraoperative ultrasound (IOUS) of, 120–122, 121f–122f
Hepaticoduodenostomy, for choledochal cysts, 99
Hepaticojejunostomy, 61
  in biliary atresia management, 108, 108f
Hepatic trauma, 236t
  abdominal exploration, 237
  balloon tamponade, 241, 241f
  closure, 243, 243f
  complications with, 243–244
  damage control, 239
  deep parenchymal hemorrhage control, 239, 240f–241f
  differential diagnosis for, 236

INDEX

Hepatic trauma (continued)
  imaging and diagnostic studies for, 236–237, 236f
  manual compression, 237, 238f
  outcomes with, 243
  patient history and physical findings for, 236
  perihepatic packing, 238, 238f
  positioning for, 237
  postoperative care for, 243
  preoperative planning for, 237
  Pringle maneuver, 241, 241f
  resection, 242, 242f
  skin incision for, 237
  surgical management of, 237
  topical hemostasis, 239, 239f
  vascular isolation, 242, 242f
Hepatic veins
  ex vivo hepatic resection, 232, 233f
  in HC resection, 77, 77f
  intraoperative ultrasound (IOUS) of, 125
  in left hepatic trisegmentectomy, 222, 223, 225–226, 225f
  in left lateral sectionectomy, 150, 150f
  in right hepatectomy, 163–164, 164f, 172, 172f
  in right hepatic trisegmentectomy, 214, 215f
  surgical anatomy of, 116–117, 117f
  tumors near roots of, 206
Hepatobiliary iminodiacetic acid (HIDA) cholescintigraphy scan
  bile leak, 45, 45f
  for cholecystectomy, open, 13
  laparoscopic cholecystectomy, 2, 2f
Hepatocellular carcinoma (HCC)
  ablation of, 132–133, 136
  catheter-based treatment of, 138, 145
  IOUS of, 121, 122f
  IVC resection for, 205
Hepatoduodenal ligament, 114, 114f
Hepatorenal ligament, 114, 114f
Hepp-Couinaud approach. See Hilar hepaticojejunostomy
Hilar arterial anatomy, 75, 75f
Hilar cholangiocarcinoma (HC), 73
  differential diagnosis, 73
  resection of
    complications, 80
    imaging and diagnostic studies, 73–74
    laparotomy, 76–79
    outcomes, 80
    patient history and physical findings, 73
    pearls and pitfalls, 79
    positioning, 74, 78f
    postoperative care, 80
    preliminary laparoscopy, 76
    preoperative planning, 74, 75f
Hilar dissection
  in left hepatic trisegmentectomy, 223–225, 223f, 224f
  in left lateral sectionectomy, 150, 150f
  in right hepatectomy, 164–165, 165f
  in right hepatic trisegmentectomy, 217–218, 217f, 218f
  in right posterior sectionectomy, 148, 148f
Hilar hepaticojejunostomy
  exposure, 83–84, 85f
  hepatic duct incision, 85–86, 85f–86f
  hepaticojejunostomy, 86–88, 86f–88f
  hilar plate, 85, 85f
  incision, 83, 84f
  left hepatic duct, 85
  preparation, 83, 84f–85f
  Roux-en-Y jejunal limb construction, 86, 86f

Hilar hepatic structures, IOUS of, 128, 129f
Hilar palpation, for right hepatic trisegmentectomy, 216–217, 217f
Hilar plate, in hilar hepaticojejunostomy, 85, 85f
Hilum, inspection of, in left hepatic trisegmentectomy, 222, 222f

I
Infants
  biliary atresia of, 103, 104f
  choledochal cysts, 99
Inferior vena cava (IVC)
  anatomy of, 205–206
  ex vivo hepatic resection, 232–233
  hepatectomy with resection of, 205
    anatomic considerations for, 205–206, 206f
    complications with, 212
    imaging and diagnostic studies for, 205
    incision for, 207
    indications for, 205
    for invasion of IVC wall without thrombus, 207–209, 207f–209f
    for invasion of IVC wall with thrombus, 209–211, 210f, 211f
    outcomes with, 212
    patient history and physical findings for, 205
    positioning for, 207
    postoperative care for, 212
    preoperative planning for, 205, 206f
  intraoperative ultrasound (IOUS) of, 125, 125f
  in right hepatectomy, 163, 164f, 172, 172f
Inflow and outflow control
  left hepatectomy, 183, 183f
  in minimally invasive left hepatic lobectomy, 189, 190f, 191–192
In-plane and out-of-plane method, of liver IOUS, 125, 125f
Intrahepatic biliary-enteric anastomosis, 81
  complications, 91
  differential diagnosis, 81
  hilar hepaticojejunostomy, 83–88
  imaging and diagnostic studies, 81–82, 81f
  outcomes, 91
  patient history and physical findings, 81
  pearls and pitfalls, 90–91
  positioning, 83, 83f
  postoperative care, 91
  preoperative planning
    benign stricture, 82, 82f
    malignant stricture, 82–83
  segment 3 hepaticojejunostomy, 88–90, 89f–90f
Intraoperative cholangiography (IOC)
  choledochal cyst, 94, 95f
  Roux-en-Y choledochojejunostomy, 56, 56f
Intraoperative endoscopy, 348, 350f
Intraoperative ultrasound (IOUS), 348, 350f
  of liver, 120, 120f
    applications of, 120–121
    biliary leak checks with, 128, 128f
    equipment for, 122–123, 122f
    hepatic lesion diagnosis with, 121–122, 121f–122f
    hilum structures on, 128–129, 129f
    imaging examples of, 125–126, 125f–126f
    laparoscopic, 127, 127f
    lesion targeting in, 127, 127f
    liver parenchyma on, 121
    medical ultrasonography, 120

  methods of, 125, 125f
  modes used in, 123, 123f
  pearls and pitfalls of, 130
  prescan preparation for, 123–124, 124f
  for right hepatic trisegmentectomy, 215, 215f
  scanning during, 124–125
  radical cholecystectomy, 24, 24f
Intussuscepting anastomosis, 291–293, 292f–294f
Irinotecan, chemoembolization using, 141
Irreversible electroporation (IRE), of hepatic neoplasms, 134

J
Jejunum
  in choledochojejunostomy. See Choledochojejunostomy
  transection of, in minimally invasive PD, 261, 261f
Jugular vein, portal vein (PV) resection and reconstruction, 303

K
Kasai portoenterostomy, in biliary atresia management, 108f, 109
Kim's triangle, 259, 259f
Klatskin tumor. See also Hilar cholangiocarcinoma
  Bismuth-Corlette classification, 75, 75f
  liver-specific criteria, 74, 74t
Kocher maneuver, 348, 348f–349f
  in pancreaticoduodenectomy, 247–248, 248f

L
Laparoendoscopic intragastric cyst gastrostomy, 368–369, 368f–369f
Laparoscopic-assisted endoscopic retrograde cholangiopancreatography (LA-ERCP), 51
Laparoscopic cholecystectomy, 1
  closure, 10, 10f
  complications, 10
  critical view, 7, 7f–8f
  cystic duct and artery division in, 8, 8f
  differential diagnosis, 1
  gallbladder dissection in, 8, 9f
  gallbladder extraction in, 9, 9f
  imaging and other diagnostic studies, 1–3
  patient history and physical findings for, 1
  pearls and pitfalls, 10
  peritoneal cavity entry in, 3–4, 4f
  port placement for, 4, 5f
  positioning, 3, 4f
  postoperative care for, 10
  preoperative planning, 3
  reverse triangle exposure in, 7, 7f
  triangle of Calot exposure in, 5–6, 5f–6f
Laparoscopic choledochoduodenostomy
  choledochoduodenal anastomosis for, 72
  initial dissection, 71–72
  patient positioning and port placement, 71
Laparoscopic choledochojejunostomy, 63–64, 64f–65f
Laparoscopic common bile duct exploration and cholecystectomy, 39
  biliary endoscopy, 40–41
  cholangiography, 40
  cystic duct dilation, 40–41
  imaging and diagnostic studies, 39
  outcomes and complications, 43, 43t

INDEX I-5

patient history and physical findings, 39
positioning, 39, 39f
postoperative care, 43
preoperative planning, 39
transcholedochal exploration, 41, 41t
transcystic exploration, 40, 40f
trocar placement, 40
T-tube placement, 42
Laparoscopic distal pancreatectomy
  drains placement, 328
  lesser sack and short gastric vessels, 322, 322f–323f
  linear stapler, 326, 327f
  lymphadenectomy, 327–328
  pancreatic body and tail mobilization, 323–324, 324f
  port site closure, 328
  retroperitoneum, 327
  specimen extraction, 328
  spleen-preserving, 328, 329f
  splenic artery isolation, 324–325, 325f–326f
  splenic flexure, 322–323, 323f
  splenic vein division, 327, 327f
  splenic vein isolation, 324, 324f–325f
  vascular stapler, 326, 327f
Laparoscopic intraoperative ultrasound (IOUS), of liver, 127, 127f
Laparoscopic left hepatic lobectomy. See Minimally invasive left hepatic lobectomy
Laparoscopic pancreatic necrosectomy
  complications, 385
  differential diagnosis, 381
  imaging and diagnostic studies, 381, 381f, 382t
  outcomes, 385
  patient history, 381
  pearls and pitfalls, 385
  physical findings, 381
  positioning, 382
  postoperative care, 385
  preoperative planning, 382
  retrogastric retrocolic debridement, 382–384, 382f–384f
  surgical management, 382
  video-assisted retroperitoneal debridement, 384, 384f
Laparoscopic pancreatoduodenectomy (LPD), 257
  colon and duodenum mobilization in, 259–260, 259f–260f
  complications with, 265
  duodenum or stomach division in, 258–259, 258f–259f
  imaging and diagnostic studies for, 257
  indications for, 257
  jejunum transection in, 261, 261f
  outcomes with, 265, 265t
  pancreatic neck division in, 261, 261f
  patient history and physical findings for, 257, 257f
  pearls and pitfalls of, 264
  porta hepatis dissection in, 260–261, 260f
  positioning for, 258
  postoperative care for, 265
  preoperative planning for, 258
  PV identification in, 258–259, 258f–259f
  RPD, 264, 264f
  SMV identification in, 259–260, 259f–260f
  trocar placement for, 258, 258f
  uncinate process dissection from SMA in, 262–263, 262f, 263f

Laparoscopic right hepatectomy
  hand-assisted, 171–174, 171f–174f
  pure, 175, 175f
Laparoscopic splenectomy, 403–404, 404f
Laparoscopy
  for choledochal cysts, 99, 100f–101f
  hilar cholangiocarcinoma (HC), 76
  in left hepatic trisegmentectomy, 222
  minimally invasive distal pancreatectomy
    intraoperative ultrasound, 321–322, 322f
    peritoneum and viscera examination, 321
    port placement, 321, 321f
  in pancreaticoduodenectomy, 247, 266
  pancreaticojejunostomy (PJ), 289
    end-to-end intussuscepting anastomosis, 291–293, 292f–294f
    end-to-side, duct-to-mucosa (Blumgart) anastomosis, 295–296, 295f–296f
    surgical management, 289, 289f
    trocar placement, 290, 290f
Laparotomy (LAP)
  for hepatic trauma, 236
  for hilar cholangiocarcinoma (HC)
    biliary resection and reconstruction in, 78
    hepatectomy in, 78
    incision and abdominal inspection in, 76
    paraaortic node assessment and biliary dissection in, 76–78
    portal vein division in, 78–79, 79f
Lawn-mower method, of liver intraoperative ultrasound (IOUS), 124, 124f
LC beads, 141, 141f
Left hepatectomy, 179, 179f, 201, 201f
  bile duct division, 184
  cholangiogram in, 184
  closure for, 184
  complications with, 185
  drain placement in, 184
  imaging and diagnostic studies for, 179–180
  incision and exposure, 181, 181f–182f
  inflow control, 183, 183f
  mobilization, 182–183, 183f
  outcomes with, 185
  outflow control, 183, 183f
  parenchymal transection in, 184
  patient history and physical findings of, 179, 179t
  pearls and pitfalls of, 184–185
  positioning, 180
  postoperative care for, 185
  preoperative planning, 180, 180f–181f
Left hepatic artery (LHA)
  for choledochal cysts, 96
  in left hepatic trisegmentectomy, 223, 223f
  in left lateral sectionectomy, 150, 150f
  surgical anatomy of, 115, 115f
Left hepatic duct (LHD)
  in hilar hepaticojejunostomy, 85
  in left hepatic trisegmentectomy, 223–224
  in right hepatic trisegmentectomy, 218, 218f
  surgical anatomy of, 117
Left hepatic trisegmentectomy, 221, 221f
  cholecystectomy in, 222, 222f
  closure for, 227
  complications with, 228
  diagnostic laparoscopy in, 222
  hepatic vein dissection in, 222, 223, 225–226, 225f
  hilar dissection in, 223–225, 223f, 224f
  hilum inspection in, 222, 222f
  imaging and diagnostic studies for, 221, 221f
  incision for, 222, 222f

liver mobilization in, 222–223
  outcomes with, 228
  parenchyma transection in, 226, 227f
  patient history and physical findings for, 221
  pearls and pitfalls of, 227
  positioning for, 221
  postoperative care for, 228
  preoperative planning for, 221
Left hepatic vein (LHV), 117, 117f
  in left hepatic trisegmentectomy, 225–226, 225f
  in left lateral sectionectomy, 150, 150f
  in right hepatic trisegmentectomy, 215, 215f
Left lateral sectionectomy, 149–150, 150f
  robotic-assisted, 201, 201f
Left portal vein (LPV), 115–116, 116f
  intraoperative ultrasound (IOUS) of, 126, 126f
  in left hepatic lobectomy, 189, 190f
  in left hepatic trisegmentectomy, 223–224
  in left lateral sectionectomy, 150, 150f
Lesser sac, distal pancreatectomy with splenic preservation (DPSP), 334, 334f
Ligament of Treitz (LT), in pancreaticoduodenectomy, 252
Ligamentum teres, 114, 114f. See Segment 3 hepaticojejunostomy
Ligamentum venosus, 114
Liver
  biopsy of, in biliary atresia management, 105, 106f
  intraoperative ultrasound (IOUS) of, 120, 120f
    applications of, 120–121
    biliary leak checks with, 128, 128f
    equipment for, 122–123, 122f
    hepatic lesion diagnosis with, 121–122, 121f–122f
    hilum structures on, 128–129, 129f
    imaging examples of, 125–126, 125f–126f
    laparoscopic, 127, 127f
    lesion targeting in, 127, 127f
    liver parenchyma on, 121
    medical ultrasonography, 120
    methods of, 125, 125f
    modes used in, 123, 123f
    prescan preparation for, 123–124, 124f
    for right hepatic trisegmentectomy, 215, 215f
    scanning during, 124
  mobilization of, in biliary atresia management, 106, 106f
  surgical anatomy of
    biliary system, 117, 118f
    Bismuth classification, 112
    blood supply, 114–117, 115f–117f
    Brisbane terminology, 112, 112t
    caudate lobe, 112–113, 113f, 117
    conclusions about, 119
    Couinaud's segments, 111, 111f
    Goldsmith and Woodburne classification, 112
    innervation, 118
    lymphatics, 118–119, 119f
    size and position, 121, 121t
    surface anatomy, 113–114, 114f
Liver cirrhosis, in open cholecystectomy, 13
Liver lesions management, 351
Longitudinal pancreatic ductotomy, 359, 359f
Lymphadenectomy, portal, in radical cholecystectomy, 25–26, 26f

M

Magnetic resonance cholangiopancreatography (MRCP)
  choledochal cyst, 93–94, 94f
  for choledochoduodenostomy (CDD), 67
  for hilar cholangiocarcinoma (HC), 73
  intrahepatic biliary ductal dilation, 44, 45f
  intrahepatic biliary-enteric anastomosis, 81, 82f
  laparoscopic cholecystectomy, 2, 2f
  Roux-en-Y choledochojejunostomy, 55, 56f
Magnetic resonance imaging (MRI)
  hilar cholangiocarcinoma (HC), 73
  intrahepatic biliary-enteric anastomosis, 81, 81f
  minimally invasive distal pancreatectomy, 319, 320f
  radical cholecystectomy, 20, 23f
  Roux-en-Y choledochojejunostomy, 55
Major papilla cannulation, for ERCP, 32–33, 32f
Microwave ablation (MWA), of hepatic neoplasms, 133–134, 134f–135f, 136
Middle hepatic vein (MHV), 116f, 117
  intraoperative ultrasound (IOUS) of, 125, 125f
  in left hepatic trisegmentectomy, 225–226, 225f
  in right hepatic trisegmentectomy, 215, 215f
Minimally invasive choledochojejunostomy
  complications, 66
  differential diagnosis, 61
  imaging and diagnostic studies, 61
  laparoscopic choledochojejunostomy, 63–64, 64f–65f
  outcomes, 66
  patient history and physical findings, 61
  pearls and pitfalls, 66
  positioning, 62
  postoperative care, 66
  preoperative planning, 61–62
  robotic choledochojejunostomy, 65–66, 65f
Minimally invasive distal pancreatectomy
  complications, 330
  computed tomography (CT), 319, 320f
  diagnostic laparoscopy
    intraoperative ultrasound, 321–322, 322f
    peritoneum and viscera examination, 321
    port placement, 321, 321f
  differential diagnosis, 319
  endoscopic retrograde cholangiopancreatography (ERCP), 319, 320f
  endoscopic ultrasound (EUS), 319, 320f
  laparoscopic distal pancreatectomy and splenectomy, 322–328, 322f–327f
  magnetic resonance imaging (MRI), 319, 320f
  outcomes, 330
  patient history and physical findings, 319
  pearls and pitfalls, 330
  postoperative care, 330
  robotic distal pancreatectomy, 329
  spleen-preserving laparoscopic distal pancreatectomy, 328, 329f
  surgical management
    positioning, 320
    preoperative planning, 319–320
Minimally invasive left hepatic lobectomy, 187, 187f
  closure for, 192, 193f
  complications with, 194
  conversion in, 193
  cut surface evaluation in, 192, 192f
  drain placement in, 192, 193f
  exploration and lesion evaluation in, 189
  imaging and diagnostic studies for, 187, 187f
  liver exposure and mobilization in, 189, 189f
  outcomes with, 194
  parenchymal transection in, 191–192, 191f, 192f
  patient history and physical findings for, 187
  pearls and pitfalls of, 193
  port placement for, 188, 188f
  positioning for, 188
  postoperative care for, 194
  preoperative planning for, 188
  robot docking in, 189, 190f
  specimen retrieval in, 192
  vascular control in, 189, 190f–192f, 191–192
Minimally invasive pancreaticoduodenectomy, 257
  colon and duodenum mobilization in, 259–260, 259f–260f
  complications with, 265
  duodenum or stomach division in, 258–259, 258f–259f
  imaging and diagnostic studies for, 257
  indications for, 257
  jejunum transection in, 261, 261f
  outcomes with, 265, 265t
  pancreatic neck division in, 261, 261f
  patient history and physical findings for, 257, 257t
  pearls and pitfalls of, 264
  porta hepatis dissection in, 260–261, 260f
  positioning for, 258
  postoperative care for, 265
  preoperative planning for, 258
  PV identification in, 258–259, 258f–259f
  RPD, 264, 264f
  SMV identification in, 259–260, 259f–260f
  trocar placement for, 258, 258f
  uncinate process dissection from SMA in, 262–263, 262f, 263f
Minimally invasive right hepatectomy, 170
  complications with, 177
  hand-assisted laparoscopic, 171–174, 171f–174f
  imaging and diagnostic studies for, 170, 170f
  outcomes with, 177
  patient history and physical findings for, 170
  pearls and pitfalls of, 177
  postoperative care for, 177
  pure laparoscopic, 175, 175f
  robotic right hepatectomy, 175–177, 176f
  surgical management and operative technique for, 171
Minimally invasive segmental hepatectomy
  approach, 153
  definition, 153
  patient history and physical findings for, 153
  pearls and pitfalls, 159
  positioning for, 154
  preoperative imaging, 153, 153f
  preoperative planning for, 153
  rationale, 153
  robotic-assisted bisegmentectomy, 154–156, 154f–156f
  robotic-assisted right posterior sectorectomy, 156–159, 157f, 158f
Minimally invasive splenectomy
  laparoscopic splenectomy, 403–404, 404f
  robotic splenectomy, 404–405, 405f
Mitomycin-C, chemoembolization using, 140, 141f
MRI. See Magnetic resonance imaging (MRI)

N

Neuroendocrine tumors (NETs), 122, 122f

O

Obesity, 61–62
Octreotide, 138
Oily chemoembolization, 140, 141f
Omni-Trak retractor, open distal pancreatectomy, 312
Open cholecystectomy
  abdominal wall opening for, 14
  closure for, 17
  complications with, 18
  cystic duct and artery ligation in, 15–16, 16f
  gallbladder dissection in, 15
  imaging and diagnostic studies for, 12–13
  incision for, 14, 14f
  indications for, 13
  outcomes with, 18
  patient history and physical findings for, 12
  pearls and pitfalls of, 17
  peritoneum incision for, 15, 15f
  positioning for, 13
  postoperative care for, 17
  preoperative planning for, 13
  retractor placement for, 14, 14f
Open distal pancreatectomy
  closure, 316
  complications, 318
  computed tomography (CT), 311, 311f
  endoscopic ultrasound (EUS), 311
  incision, 312
  indications, 312, 312t
  Omni-Trak retractor, 312
  outcomes, 317–318
  pancreas exposure, 313, 313f
  pancreatic dissection
    spleen-preserving distal pancreatectomy, 314–315, 315f
    splenectomy, lateral to medial, 313–314, 314f
    splenectomy, medial to lateral, 314, 315f
  pancreatic transection, 315, 316f
  patient history and physical findings, 311
  patient positioning, 312
  pearls and pitfalls, 316–317
  postoperative care, 317
  preoperative planning, 312
  splenic flexure, 313
  surgical management, 312
Open splenectomy
  closure, 402
  incision, 400, 401f
  mobilization, 400–401, 401f–402f
  vessels and excision ligation, 402, 403f, 403t

P

Pancreas
  complications, 397
  diagnosis, 394
  EUS of, for pancreaticoduodenectomy, 246, 266
  exposure, open distal pancreatectomy, 313, 313f
  imaging and diagnostic studies, 394–395
  indications, 394, 394t
  patient history, 394
  pearls and pitfalls, 397
  physical findings, 394
  postoperative care, 397
  steps, 395–396, 395f–396f
  surgical management, 395

Pancreatic dissection, open distal pancreatectomy
　spleen-preserving distal pancreatectomy, 314–315, 315f
　splenectomy
　　lateral to medial, 313–314, 313f
　　medial to lateral, 314, 315f
Pancreatic duct, in ERCP
　cannulation of, 32–33, 32f
　sphincterotomy, 33, 33f
　stricture dilation, 34
　tissue acquisition, 36
Pancreatic necrosectomy
　complications, 380, 380t
　imaging and diagnostic studies, 372, 373f
　open necrosectomy
　　abdominal closure, 376
　　cholecystectomy, 375, 375f
　　debridement, 375, 375f
　　drains, 375, 376f
　　enteral access, 375, 375f
　　exposure, 374–375, 374f
　outcomes, 379
　patient history, 372
　pearls and pitfalls, 378
　physical findings, 372
　postoperative care, 379, 379f
　splenectomy, 378
　transgastric necrosectomy, 376–377, 377f–378f
Pancreatic neuroendocrine tumors (PNETs)
　abdominal exploration, 342
　closure and drain placement, 343, 343f
　complications, 344
　differential diagnosis, 340
　imaging and diagnostic studies, 340–341, 341f
　incision placement, 342, 342f
　mass dissecting, 342–343
　outcomes, 343–344
　pancreatic dissection, 342
　patient history, 340
　pearls and pitfalls, 343
　physical findings, 340
　positioning, 341
　postoperative care, 343
　preoperative planning, 341
　surgical management, 341
Pancreaticobiliary limb, clamping of, 53
Pancreaticobiliary obstruction, 29, 29t
Pancreaticoduodenectomy (PD), 245
　bile duct division in, 252, 253f
　Cattell-Braasch maneuver in, 247–248, 248f
　complications with, 256
　diagnostic laparoscopy in, 247
　dissection off superior mesenteric-portal vein confluence in, 254, 254f
　duodenum division in, 252, 252f
　imaging and diagnostic studies for, 245–247, 246f
　incision for, 247
　indications for, 245
　Kocher maneuver in, 247–248, 248f
　LT takedown in, 252
　outcomes with, 256
　pancreas division in, 253, 253f
　patient history and physical findings for, 245
　pearls and pitfalls of, 256
　porta hepatis dissection in, 250, 250f
　positioning for, 247
　postoperative care for, 256
　preoperative planning for, 247
　resectability assessment in, 247
　retroperitoneal and SMA dissection in, 255, 255f
　SMV exposure in, 248–249, 248f, 249f
　specimen labeling in, 255
　tunnel creation between neck and PV in, 251, 251f
Pancreaticogastrostomy (PG)
　complications, 288
　differential diagnosis, 284
　duct to mucosa, 287, 287f
　outcomes, 288
　patient history and physical findings, 284
　pearls and pitfalls, 288
　postoperative care, 288
　preoperative planning, 284
　surgical management, 284
　telescopic invagination, 284–286, 285f–286f
Pancreaticojejunostomy (PJ), 273, 284
　complications, 297, 361, 361t
　differential diagnosis, 355
　enterotomy preparation in, 277, 277f
　feeding jejunostomy, placement of, 360
　final steps in, 282
　imaging and diagnostic studies, 355, 355f–356f
　inner layer back row in, 280, 280f, 281f
　inner layer front row in, 275–276, 275f, 276f, 281–282, 281f
　laparoscopy, 289
　　end-to-end intussuscepting anastomosis, 291–293, 292f–294f
　　end-to-side, duct-to-mucosa (Blumgart) anastomosis, 295–296, 295f–296f
　　surgical management, 289, 289f
　　trocar placement, 290, 290f
　longitudinal pancreatic ductotomy, 359, 359f
　outcomes, 283, 297, 361
　outer layer back row in, 278, 278f, 279f
　outer layer front row in, 282, 282f
　pancreas exposure, 356
　pancreatic head resection, 357, 358f
　pancreatic transection for, 273–274, 273f
　patient history and physical findings, 273, 289, 355
　pearls and pitfalls, 283, 297, 360
　physical findings, 355
　positioning, 356
　postoperative care, 283, 297, 360–361
　preoperative planning, 356, 356t
　remnant pancreas, 291, 291f
　robotic surgery, 289
　　end-to-side, duct-to-mucosa (modified Blumgart) anastomosis, 296
　　surgical management, 289, 290f
　　trocar placement, 290f, 291
　Roux-en-Y pancreaticojejunostomy, 359, 360f
　setup for, 274, 274f, 275f
　surgical management, 356, 356t
　technical considerations for, 275
Pancreatic pseudocysts, enteric drainage
　acute necrotic collection (ANC), 363, 363f
　acute peripancreatic fluid collections (APFCs), 362–364, 362f–363f
　complications, 371
　differential diagnosis, 364
　extragastric cyst gastrostomy, 368
　imaging and diagnostic studies, 364–365
　laparoendoscopic intragastric cyst gastrostomy, 368–369, 368f–369f
　patient history, 364
　pearls and pitfalls, 371
　physical findings, 364
　positioning, 365
　postoperative care, 371
　preoperative preparation, 365
　procedures description, 366
　Roux-en-Y cyst jejunostomy, 369–370
　surgical management, 365
　transgastric cyst gastrostomy, 366–367, 366f–367f
　treatment, 365
　walled-off necrosis (WON), 363, 363f
Pancreatic transection, open distal pancreatectomy, 315, 316f
Pancreatic tumors excision, 350
Pancreatoduodenectomy, with portomesenteric venous resection, 298
Pancreatoscopy, 36
Papilloma, 73
Paraaortic node, assessment of, in HC resection, 76–78
Partial splenectomy (PS), 415–416
Patch closure, portal vein (PV) resection and reconstruction, 305, 306f
Pedicle tracking method, of liver intraoperative ultrasound (IOUS), 125
Percutaneous endoscopic necrosectomy, 391
Percutaneous transhepatic biliary imaging and intervention
　percutaneous transhepatic cholangiography. See Percutaneous transhepatic cholangiography (PTC)
　percutaneous transhepatic drainage (PTHD). See Percutaneous transhepatic drainage (PTHD)
Percutaneous transhepatic cholangiography (PTC)
　balloon dilation, 47–48, 47f–48f
　brushings/biopsy, 49, 49f
　cholangiogram, 46, 46f
　for choledochoduodenostomy (CDD), 67
　complications, 50
　duct cannulation, 45–46, 46f
　immediate preprocedure, 45, 46f
　intrahepatic biliary-enteric anastomosis, 81
　minimally invasive choledochojejunostomy, 61
　outcomes, 50
　patient history and physical findings, 44
　pearls and pitfalls, 50
　positioning, 45
　postoperative care, 50
　preprocedure planning, 45
　stent placement, 48–49, 48f–49f
　stone and debris removal with, 49
Percutaneous transhepatic drainage (PTHD)
　complications, 50
　digital subtraction angiography, 47, 47f
　internal/external biliary drainage catheters, 46, 47f
　outcomes, 50
　patient history and physical findings, 44
　pearls and pitfalls, 50
　positioning, 45
　postoperative care, 50
　preprocedure planning, 45
Perihepatic packing, for hepatic trauma, 238, 238f
Peritoneal cavity, entry into, for laparoscopic cholecystectomy, 3–4, 4f
Peritoneum incision of, for open cholecystectomy, 15, 15f
Peritonitis, after laparoscopic cholecystectomy, 10
PG. See Pancreaticogastrostomy (PG)
PJ. See Pancreaticojejunostomy (PJ)
Porta hepatis
　dissection of, in pancreaticoduodenectomy, 250, 250f, 260–261, 260f, 269, 269f
　palpation of, for right hepatic trisegmentectomy, 217, 217f

Portal dissection
  in biliary atresia management, 107–108, 107f
  in right hepatectomy, 172, 172f, 173f
Portal lymphadenectomy, in radical cholecystectomy, 25–26, 26f
Portal veins (PV)
  for choledochal cysts, 96
  for hilar cholangiocarcinoma (HC) resection, 78–79, 79f
  in hilar hepaticojejunostomy, 84, 84f
  intraoperative ultrasound (IOUS) of, 125–126, 125f–126f
  in left hepatic trisegmentectomy, 223–224
  in left lateral sectionectomy, 150, 150f
  in pancreaticoduodenectomy, 245–247, 246f, 251, 251f, 254, 254f, 258–259, 258f–259f
  resection and reconstruction
    complications, 309
    computed tomography (CT), 298, 298f
    dissection, 301–303, 302f–303f
    femoral/saphenous vein, 303
    incision and exposure, 301
    interposition graft, 307, 308f–309f
    jugular vein, 303
    left renal vein, 303
    outcomes, 309
    patch closure, 305, 306f
    patient history and physical findings, 298
    pearls and pitfalls, 309
    positioning, 300, 301f
    postoperative care, 309
    preoperative planning, 299–300, 299f–300f
    primary end-to-end anastomosis, 305, 307, 307f
    primary longitudinal closure, 305, 306f
    primary transverse closure, 304–305, 305f
    vascular control, 303–304, 304f
  in right hepatectomy, 164, 164f, 172, 172f, 173f
  in right posterior sectionectomy, 148
  in segment 3 hepaticojejunostomy, 88, 89f
  surgical anatomy of, 115–116, 116f
Portoenterostomy, in biliary atresia management, 108, 109f
Positron emission tomography (PET), 74
Posterior superior pancreaticoduodenal artery (PSPD), 77
Postoperative pancreatic fistula (POPF), 284
Prednisolone, in biliary atresia management, 109, 110t
Pregnancy, in open cholecystectomy, 13
Pringle maneuver, for hepatic trauma, 241, 241f
Pylorus-preserving pancreaticoduodenectomy (PPPD), 245, 252

R
Radical cholecystectomy, 19, 19f
  complications, 27
  extrahepatic biliary tree resection in, 25–26, 26f
  imaging and other diagnostic studies, 20–22
  incision and exposure, 24, 24f
  intraoperative ultrasound, 24, 24f
  outcomes, 27
  patient history and physical findings, 19–20
  pearls and pitfalls, 26
  portal lymphadenectomy in, 25–26, 26f
  positioning, 23, 23f
  postoperative care, 27
  preoperative planning, 22–23
  segment IVb/V resection in, 24–25, 25f
Radioembolization, for hepatic neoplasms, 138, 141–143, 142f
Radiofrequency ablation (RFA), of hepatic neoplasms, 133, 133f–134f, 136
Replaced left hepatic artery, 115, 115f
Replaced right hepatic artery, 115, 115f, 139, 139f
Retrogastric retrocolic debridement (transperitoneal), 382–384, 382f–384f
Retroperitoneal dissection, in pancreaticoduodenectomy, 255, 255f
Right hepatectomy, 160, 160f, 197–198, 197f–200f
  complications with, 168
  hilar dissection and vascular control in, 164–165, 165f
  imaging and diagnostic studies for, 160, 160f
  incision and exposure for, 162–163
  indications for, 160, 161t
  mobilization for, 163–164, 163f, 164f
  outcomes with, 168
  parenchymal transection in, 165–167, 166f
  patient history and physical findings for, 160
  pearls and pitfalls of, 167–168
  positioning for, 162
  postoperative care for, 168
  preoperative planning for, 161–162, 161f
  RHV dissection in, 164
Right hepatic artery (RHA)
  in choledochal cyst management, 96, 96f
  replaced, 115, 115f, 139, 139f
  in right hepatic trisegmentectomy, 217, 217f
  in right posterior sectionectomy, 147–148, 148f
  surgical anatomy of, 114–115, 115f
Right hepatic duct (RHD)
  in hilar hepaticojejunostomy, 86, 86f
  in right hepatectomy, 165, 173, 173f
  surgical anatomy of, 117, 118f
Right hepatic trisegmentectomy, 214, 214f
  closure for, 220
  complications with, 220
  exposure for, 216
  hepatic veins dissection in, 219, 219f
  hilar dissection in, 217–218, 217f, 218f
  hilar palpation for, 216–217, 217f
  imaging and diagnostic studies for, 214–215, 214f, 215f
  incision for, 216, 216f
  indications for, 214
  liver mobilization for, 217, 217f
  liver transection in, 219, 219f
  outcomes with, 220
  patient history and physical findings for, 214
  pearls and pitfalls of, 220
  positioning for, 216
  postoperative care for, 220
  preoperative planning for, 215–216
Right hepatic vein (RHV), 116, 117f
  in right hepatectomy, 165
  in right hepatic trisegmentectomy, 219, 219f
  robotic-assisted right posterior sectorectomy, 157–159, 158f
Right portal vein (RPV), 115
  intraoperative ultrasound (IOUS) of, 126, 126f
  in left hepatic trisegmentectomy, 224
  in right hepatectomy, 164, 165f
  in right hepatic trisegmentectomy, 217, 217f
  in right posterior sectionectomy, 148
Right posterior sectionectomy, 147–148, 148f
  robotic-assisted, 201–202, 202f
Robotic-assisted bisegmentectomy, 154–156, 154f–156f
Robotic-assisted pancreaticoduodenectomy, 266
  colon and duodenum mobilization in, 268, 268f
  complications with, 271
  imaging and diagnostic studies for, 266, 266f
  outcomes with, 271
  pancreas mobilization and division in, 270, 270f, 271f
  patient history and physical findings for, 266
  pearls and pitfalls of, 271
  porta hepatis dissection in, 269, 269f
  port placement for, 267, 268f
  positioning and room setup for, 267, 267f
  postoperative care for, 271
  preoperative planning for, 267
  stomach division and mobilization in, 269, 269f
Robotic-assisted right posterior sectorectomy, 156–159, 157f, 158f
Robotic choledochojejunostomy, 65–66, 65f
Robotic distal pancreatectomy, 329
Robotic liver resection
  complications with, 203
  differential diagnosis, 196, 196t
  imaging and diagnostic studies for, 196–197
  left hepatectomy, 201, 201f
  left lateral sectionectomy, 201, 201f
  outcomes with, 202–203, 203t
  patient history and physical findings for, 196
  pearls and pitfalls of, 202
  positioning, 197, 197f
  postoperative care for, 202
  right hepatectomy, 197–198, 197f–200f
  right posterior sector resections, 201–202, 202f
Robotic right hepatectomy, 175–177, 176f
Robotic splenectomy, 404–405, 405f
Round ligament approach. See Segment 3 hepaticojejunostomy
Roux-en-Y anatomy, 286, 287f
Roux-en-Y choledochojejunostomy, 55, 55f
  choledochojejunostomy anastomosis, 58, 59f
  closure, 60
  complications, 60
  differential diagnosis, 55
  imaging and diagnostic studies, 55–56, 56f
  incision and operative exposure, 56, 57f
  jejunojejunal anastomosis, 59
  outcomes, 60
  patient history and physical findings, 55
  pearls and pitfalls, 60
  positioning, 56, 57f
  postoperative care, 60
  preoperative planning, 56
  Roux limb creation, 58
Roux-en-Y cyst jejunostomy, 369–370
Roux-en-Y hepaticojejunostomy
  in biliary atresia management, 108, 108f
  for choledochal cyst, 98, 98f
Roux-en-Y pancreaticojejunostomy, 359, 360f
Roux limb
  creation of
    in hilar hepaticojejunostomy, 86, 86f
    laparoscopic choledochojejunostomy, 63–64, 64f–65f
    in Roux-en-Y choledochojejunostomy, 58
    in surgically assisted endoscopic retrograde cholangiopancreatography (ERCP), 52

INDEX   I-9

S
Sectionectomy
  left lateral, 149–150, 150f
    robotic-assisted, 201, 201f
  right posterior, 147–148, 148f
    robotic-assisted, 201–202, 202f
Sectorectomy, right posterior, robotic-assisted, 156–159, 157f, 158f
Segmental hepatectomy, 146, 146f
  caudate lobe resection, 150–151, 151f
  complications with, 152
  imaging and diagnostic studies for, 146
  indications for, 146, 147t
  left lateral sectionectomy, 149–150, 150f
  outcomes with, 152
  patient history and physical findings for, 146
  pearls and pitfalls of, 152
  positioning for, 147
  postoperative care for, 152
  preoperative planning for, 146–147
  right posterior sectionectomy, 147–148, 148f
Segment 3 hepaticojejunostomy, in intrahepatic biliary-enteric anastomosis, 88–90, 89f–90f
Segment IVb/V resection, in radical cholecystectomy, 24–25, 25f
Side-to-side choledochoduodenostomy
  choledochoduodenal anastomosis for, 69–70, 70f–71f
  incision and exposure, 68–69, 68f–69f
Sir-Spheres, 416
Specimen
  from minimally invasive left hepatic lobectomy, 192
  from pancreaticoduodenectomy, 255
Sphincter of Oddi dysfunction (SOD), 36, 37f
Sphincterotomy, 33, 33f
  endoscopic retrograde cholangiopancreatography (ERCP), 33, 33f
Spleen-preserving distal pancreatectomy, 314–315, 315f
Spleen-preserving laparoscopic distal pancreatectomy, 328, 329f
Splenectomy, 419–420
  complications, 406
  differential diagnosis, 398
  drains placement, 328
  laparoscopic, 399t
  lesser sack and short gastric vessels, 322, 322f–323f
  linear stapler, 326, 327f
  lymphadenectomy, 327–328
  minimally invasive splenectomy
    laparoscopic splenectomy, 403–404, 404f
    robotic splenectomy, 404–405, 405f
  open distal pancreatectomy
    lateral to medial, 313–314, 313f
    medial to lateral, 314, 315f
  open splenectomy
    closure, 402
    incision, 400, 401f
    mobilization, 400–401, 401f–402f
    vessels and excision ligation, 402, 403f, 403t
  outcomes, 406
  pancreatic body and tail mobilization, 323–324, 324f
  patient history, 398–399
  pearls and pitfalls, 405
  physical findings, 398–399
  port site closure, 328
  postoperative care, 406
  retroperitoneum, 327
  specimen extraction, 328
  spleen-preserving, 328, 329f
  splenic artery isolation, 324–325, 325f–326f
  splenic flexure, 322–323, 323f
  splenic vein division, 327, 327f
  splenic vein isolation, 324, 324f–325f
  surgical management, 399–400, 399f, 400t
  vascular stapler, 326, 327f
Splenic injury
  complications, 421
  differential diagnosis, 417
  exploration, 419
  imaging and diagnostic studies, 417, 418f, 418t
  patient history, 417
  pearls and pitfalls, 421
  physical findings, 417
  positioning, 418
  postoperative care, 421
  preoperative planning, 418
  skin incision, 419
  splenectomy. See Splenectomy
  splenic mobilization, 419, 419f
  splenorrhaphy. See Splenorrhaphy
  surgical management, 418
Splenic vessel preservation (Kimura) technique, 328, 328f–329f
Splenorrhaphy, 420, 420f–421f
  complications, 416
  differential diagnosis, 407, 407t
  high-grade splenic injuries, 410–412, 411f
  imaging and diagnostic studies, 407–408
  incision, 410
  low-grade splenic injuries, 410
  mobilization, 410
  outcomes, 415–416
  partial splenectomy, 412–413, 413f–414f
  patient history, 407, 407t, 408f
  pearls and pitfalls, 415
  physical findings, 407, 407t, 408f
  positioning, 409
  postoperative care, 415
  preoperative planning, 408–409
  surgical management, 408–409
Stand-off scanning, of liver, 124
Stenting
  of biliary duct, 35–36, 35f, 48–49, 48f–49f
  of pancreatic duct, 35–36, 35f
Steroids, in biliary atresia management, 109, 110t
Stomach
  division and mobilization of, in pancreaticoduodenectomy, 269, 269f
  division of, in minimally invasive PD, 258–259, 258f–259f
Subtotal cholecystectomy, 16–17, 17f
Sump syndrome, choledochoduodenostomy (CDD), 72
Superior mesenteric arteriogram, for TACE, 139, 139f
Superior mesenteric artery (SMA), 245–246, 246f, 254, 254f, 262–263, 262f–263f, 266, 266f
Superior mesenteric vein (SMV), 298. See also Portal vein (PV) resection and reconstruction
  in pancreaticoduodenectomy, 245–246, 246f, 248–249, 249f, 266, 266f
  in pancreatoduodenectomy, 259–260, 259f–260f
Surgically assisted endoscopic retrograde cholangiopancreatography (ERCP), 51
  complications with, 54
  differential diagnosis, 51
  draping and ERCP performance in, 53
  gastric pexy in, 52
  gastrostomy closure or tube placement in, 53, 53f
  indications for, 51
  outcomes with, 54
  pancreaticobiliary limb clamping in, 53
  patient history and physical findings, 51
  pearls and pitfalls of, 54
  positioning for, 51–52, 51f
  postoperative care for, 54
  preoperative planning for, 51
  transgastric trocar placement in, 52
  trocar placement in, 52, 52f

T
Technetium-99m macroaggregated albumin (Tc-99m MMA), lobar injection of, 142, 142f
TheraSphere, 141
Transabdominal ultrasound, hilar cholangiocarcinoma (HC), 73
Transarterial chemoembolization (TACE), for hepatic neoplasms, 138–141, 140f–141f
Transarterial embolization (TAE), for hepatic neoplasms, 141
Transcholedochal exploration, 41, 41t
Transcystic exploration, 40, 40f
Transgastric cyst gastrostomy, 366–367, 366f–367f
Tumor thrombus (TT), IVC, 206, 206f
  resection with, 209–211, 210f, 211f
  resection without, 207–209, 207f–209f

U
Ultrasound (US)
  for cholecystectomy
    laparoscopic, 1
    open, 12, 12f
  choledochal cyst, 93
  intrahepatic biliary ductal dilation, 44, 44f
  minimally invasive choledochojejunostomy, 61
  radical cholecystectomy, 20
  Roux-en-Y choledochojejunostomy, 55
Uncinate process, dissection of, in minimally invasive PD, 262–263, 262f, 263f

V
Vascular control
  in left lateral sectionectomy, 150, 150f
  in minimally invasive left hepatic lobectomy, 189, 190f–192f, 191–192
  and resection, 303–304, 304f
  in right hepatectomy, 164–165, 165f
  in right posterior sectionectomy, 148, 148f
Venovenous bypass (VVB), for IVC resection, 205, 206f
Video-assisted retroperitoneal debridement, 384, 384f

W
Walled-off necrosis (WON), 363, 363f, 386
Warshaw technique, 328

Y
Yttrium 90 (90Y), radioembolization with, 138, 142, 142f